HANDBOOK OF LEPROSY

Dr. Anand Anerao

ALLIED HEALTH PRESS

Handbook of Leprosy

Author: **Dr. Anand Anerao**

Allied Health Press
4164 Lakeshore Road
Burlington ON L7L 1A4
Canada
www.alliedhealthpress.com
Email: orders@arclereducation.com

ISBN: 978-1-77956-794-9

ABOUT THE AUTHOR

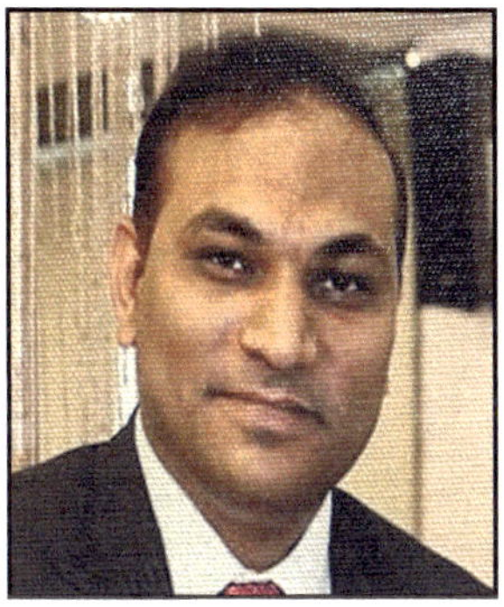

Dr. Anand Anerao is currently an Associate Professor at Parbhani Medical College. After completing his MBBS in 2001 from Indira Gandhi Medical College, Nagpur, he pursued his master's degree in Orthopedic Surgery from Shivaji University in 2007. Following his MS, he completed a fellowship in Arthroscopy from Kamineni Hospital, Hyderabad in 2009. He served as a Medical Officer at Sub-District Hospital, Gangakhed, for three years (2009-2012). Additionally, he has been in private practice for the past 18 years.

Brief Table of Contents

Detailed Table of Contents

CHAPTER 15

Ethical and Legal Considerations of Leprosy Care 359

Index 383

LIST OF FIGURES

LIST OF ABBREVIATIONS

AFB	Acid-Fast Bacilli
AI	Artificial Intelligence
ALERT	Addis Ababa Leprosy Research and Treatment Center
BB	Borderline Borderline
BCG	Bacillus Calmette–Guérin
BL	Borderline Lepromatous
BT	Borderline Tuberculoid
CBR	Community Based Rehabilitation
CD-RISC	Connor-Davidson Resilience Scale
CIDP	Chronic Inflammatory Demyelinating Polyneuropathy
CPD	Chronic Periodontal Disease
DALYs	Disability-Adjusted Life Years
DLQI	Dermatology Life Quality Index
DNA	Deoxyribonucleic Acid
DOT	Directly Observed Therapy
DTH	Delayed-Type Hypersensitivity
ELISA	Enzyme-Linked Immunosorbent Assay
ENL	Erythema Nodosum Leprosum
ENN	Erythema Nodosum Leprosum Necroticans
EQA	External Quality Checks
ERAT	Endoscopic Retrograde Appendicitis Therapy
GPZL	Global Partnership for Zero Leprosy
HD	Hansen's Disease
HLA	Human Leukocyte Antigens
ICA	Immunochromatography Assay
IFN-γ	Interferon-Gamma
ILEP	International Federation of Anti-Leprosy Associations

KTiOx	Potassium-Incorporated Titanium Oxide
LFA	Lateral Flow Assay
LILRA2	Leukocyte Immunoglobulin-like Receptor Subfamily a Member 2
LL	Lepromatous Leprosy
MAC	Membrane Attack Complex
MB	Multibacillary
MDT	Multidrug Therapy
mROM	Monthly Cocktail of Rifampicin, Ofloxacin, and Minocycline
MTT	Metatarsal
N-CAM	Neural Cell Adhesion Molecules
NCD	New Case Detection
NFI	Nerve Function Impairment
NGF	Nerve Growth Factor
NRG1	Neuregulin 1
NTD	Neglected Tropical Disease
P0	Protein Zero
PB	Paucibacillary
PBL	Paucibacillary Leprosy
PBMC	Peripheral Blood Mononuclear Cells
PCR	Polymerase Chain Reaction
PGL-1	Phenolic Glycolipid-1
PMP22	Peripheral Myelin Protein 22
PNL	Pure Neural Leprosy
POCUS	Point-of-Care Ultrasound
qPCR	Quantitative Polymerase Chain Reaction
SDI	Socio-Demographic Index
SHG	Second-Harmonic Generation
T1R	Type 1 Reactions
T2LR	Type 2 Leprosy Reaction
T2W	T2-Weighted
TLR	Toll-Like Receptor
TLR9	Toll-Like Receptor 9
TMT	Tarsometatarsal
TNF	Tumor Necrosis Factor
TT	Tuberculoid
WHO	World Health Organizations

PREFACE

Leprosy is one of the oldest known human diseases, with historical evidence of the disease in ancient Egypt and India. It is most commonly caused by the bacterium Mycobacterium leprae, with Mycobacterium lepromatosis playing a lesser role, presenting challenging problems for clinicians, scientists, and public health workers. Although the incidence has decreased markedly throughout the world since the introduction of multidrug therapy in the 1980s, new cases occur regularly in the endemic areas of Asia, Africa, and Latin America. The chronic course of leprosy and the complex clinical presentations—indeterminate and tuberculoid, borderline, and lepromatous forms—require an intimate understanding of microbiological and immunological factors. This range of host response is the reason for the widespread extent of tissue involvement and neurological damage of the disease, and the need for early diagnosis and prompt treatment to prevent irreversible nerve damage and resulting disability.

In addition to its biological complexity, leprosy also has severe social and economic consequences. Previously, patients were stigmatized, discriminated against, and deprived of livelihoods. While treatment regimens today can make patients non-infectious in a matter of weeks and frequently restore skin and nerve function, stigma remains. Disability caused by untreated or late disease, ranging from sensory deficit and deformity to blindness, has long-term consequences for quality of life.

The Handbook of Leprosy is a professionals' guide to the condition, whether in clinical practice, public health policy, laboratory work, or community work. It summarizes expert opinion from across a broad spectrum of professionals such as dermatologists, neurologists, immunologists, epidemiologists, rehabilitation workers, and sociologists, each of whom brings their expertise in a concise and detailed format. It is evidence-based and based on the best current practice, using a combination of tried-and-tested guidelines and groundbreaking new ideas. Case studies also bring to light real-world problems and solutions, highlighting the interface between medical treatment and patient-centered care.

Chapter 1, "Introduction to Leprosy," introduces the historical evolution of our understanding of the disease, covering initial misperceptions to modern-day classification systems, and outlining its current epidemiological patterns.

Chapter 2, "Pathophysiology and Immunology of Leprosy," addresses host–pathogen interactions responsible for clinical heterogeneity, such as the role of cell-mediated and humoral immune responses, formation of granulomas, and mechanisms of nerve damage.

Chapter 3, "Classification of Leprosy," outlines Ridley–Jopling classification in concorinteraction with the World Health Organization's operational criteria and explains how disease type determines prognosis and treatment regimen.

Chapter 4, "Clinical Features of Leprosy," offers a step-by-step process for diagnosing dermal lesions, peripheral nerve disease, and systemic symptoms through the range of the disease.

Chapter 5, "Diagnostic Methods of Leprosy," evaluates traditional methods like slit-skin smears and histopathologic examination, as well as modern methods that include polymerase chain reaction assays and immunological tests. The chapter provides practical recommendations on specimen collection, laboratory processing, and result interpretation to maximize diagnostic sensitivity, particularly in low-resource settings.

Treatment—past and present—is the focus of Chapter 6, "Treatment Options for Leprosy," which discusses multidrug therapy regimens, drug resistance management, and antileprosy agent pharmacology.

Chapter 7, "Complications of Leprosy," addresses prevention and management of impaired nerve function, secondary infections, and trophic ulcers, with guidelines for monitoring long-term outcomes.

Chapter 8, "Reactions to Leprosy and Their Treatment," discusses Type 1 (reversal) and Type 2 (erythema nodosum leprosum) reactions, such as pathogenesis, clinical presentation, corticosteroid treatment regimens, and adjunctive treatments such as thalidomide and immunosuppressants.

Chapter 9, entitled "Public Health Aspects of Leprosy," covers the public health aspects by considering a variety of surveillance approaches, contact tracing interventions, the incorporation of leprosy services within primary health care systems, and political and economic support strategies.

Chapter 10, entitled "Updates and Advances in Leprosy Research," emphasizes leading-edge vaccine promise, host genetics studies, advanced diagnostic tools, and mobile health interventions. Chapter 10 emphasizes the pivotal role of translational research in linking lab discoveries with clinical practice and programmatic uses.

Chapters 11 and 12 address special populations. "Pediatric Leprosy" (Chapter 11) addresses the presentation of the disease, disability risks, and treatment dosing and duration issues in children.

Chapter 12, "Leprosy in Pregnancy," discusses maternal and fetal outcomes, safety profiles of antileprosy drugs, and recommendations for perinatal care to reduce risks for mother and child. These chapters emphasize the need for individualized treatment in high-risk groups.

Chapter 13, "Leprosy-Related Disabilities and Rehabilitation," offers a model for evaluating impairment, planning programs of occupational and physiotherapy, and adapting protective equipment to avoid further damage.

Chapter 14, entitled "Psychosocial Aspects and Quality of Life," by the authors discusses the psychological impact of diagnosis, measures to minimize stigma, and community integration to enhance mental health and quality of life.

Lastly, Chapter 15, "Ethical and Legal Aspects of Leprosy Care," discusses patient rights, confidentiality, informed consent, and national and international legislation regulating discrimination and access to care.

This book is intended to meet the needs of a broad spectrum of readers. Clinicians, dermatologists, neurologists, infectious disease specialists, and primary care physicians, will welcome its clear advice on diagnosis, treatment, and management of related complications. Public health officials and program planners will learn to use it as a guide for planning and evaluating Leprosy control programs. Laboratory scientists and researchers will find concise summaries of current knowledge plus recommendations for research questions to pursue. Rehabilitation therapists, social workers, and mental health professionals will become familiar with the full spectrum of patient needs. Students of medicine, nursing, and allied health will find a cohesive, authoritative source that integrates the biomedical, social, and ethical dimensions of leprosy care.

This Handbook of Leprosy must not only be a handy reference for quick access to clinical and programmatic questions but also a foundation for continued effort toward fulfillment of the world's aspiration to end transmission of leprosy. By synthesizing data from all disciplines, we aim to make possible an integrated effort addressing both the health and the human rights aspects of this disease of centuries.

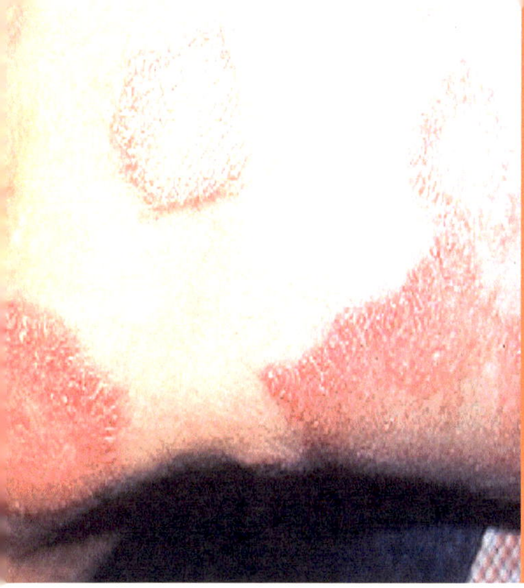

Chapter 1

INTRODUCTION TO LEPROSY

Contents

Introduction

Infectious diseases have long stimulated societies to shift their medical practices and public policies. Leprosy, for instance, is not just another infection—it carries a persisting nature and a heavy social stigma that sets it apart. Caused by *Mycobacterium leprae*, the disease usually messes with the skin, nearby nerves, parts of the respiratory system, and occasionally even the eyes. Its gradual onset and unpredictable symptoms have, in most cases, made early detection a real challenge; when unattended, this slow-moving illness often ends up causing deformities and disabilities over time. Understanding leprosy, which behaves quite differently from many fast-acting infections, generally calls for a special kind of intervention, as the chronic symptoms and intricate immune responses push for more comprehensive, sometimes even repeated, study. When it comes to its spread, the details remain under active investigation. Generally speaking, prolonged close contact with someone untreated seems to be key, yet, surprisingly, leprosy is not as contagious as acute infections. Many people exposed do not show signs, thanks in part to natural immunity. Characteristic warnings include skin patches that are either lighter or have a reddish hue along with reduced sensation from nerve damage—a pretty clear signal of the disease. And with nerve issues sometimes causing muscle weakness, delayed diagnosis can eventually lead to noticeable deformities. Its incubation period, ranging from a few months to several years, really complicates the issue when trying to trace infection sources, which only underscores the need for early, well-informed interventions and outreach to at-risk groups. Modern treatments have generally turned the tide for leprosy patients, largely thanks to multidrug therapy (MDT) protocols. This regimen combined antibiotics like dapsone, rifampicin, and clofazimine has reworked leprosy from a debilitating condition into one that is often curable, if treatment is followed steadily over 6–12 months. Even though knocking out the bacterium is the main aim, doctors still must tackle nerve damage and work hard to forestall disabilities. Despite these impressive medical advances, persisting social stigma sometimes stops patients from getting help as early as they would need to. Observations from other chronic diseases affecting marginalized groups suggest that combining community outreach with patient education is pretty crucial. To summarize, an effective approach to leprosy is not just about the medication—it is also about caring for the psychological and social fallout along the way (Elendu et al., 2023; Panahi et al., 2023) (Figure 1.1).

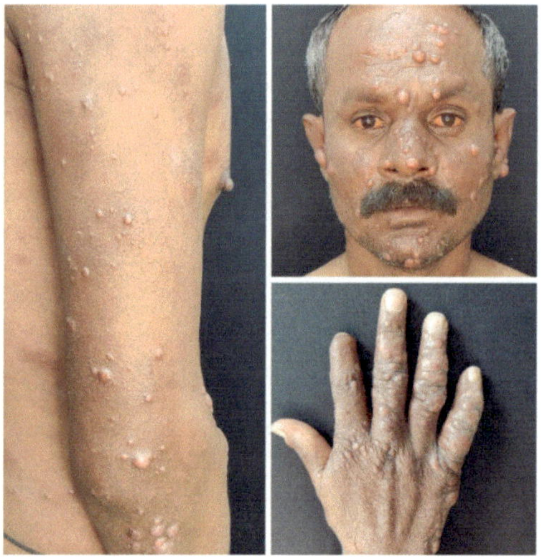

Figure 1.1. Leprosy.

Source: Lepra. (2023). *Leprosy image. Leprosy Review.*

Definition and Historical Context

Over the centuries, our grasp of diseases and ways to treat them kept changing in unexpected ways. Cultural trends, philosophical ideas, and scientific breakthroughs all stimulated our understanding along. Leprosy, for example, has long been wrapped in fear and error, which not only shaped medical views but also led to enduring social stigma. Back in medieval times, there was a curious shift when Ayurvedic practices started; this odd, hands-on trial combined everyday experimentation with fresh theories and even reshaped how illnesses like leprosy were seen (Wujastyk et al., 2019). In most cases, these early experiments hint at how vibrant and unpredictable medical progress can be. Looking at the history of leprosy, it is impossible to ignore the heavy social backdrop that always accompanies it. Being diagnosed was not just about health, it often meant being cast aside. Generally speaking, those with leprosy found themselves isolated and judged harshly, a response driven by deep-seated fear and moral assumptions. This social layer colored not only community interactions but also local health policies. In several instances, leprosy served as a symbol for broader anxieties about purity, contamination, and even moral decay. Similar patterns of exclusion show up with other marginalized groups throughout history (Beloso et al., 2017).

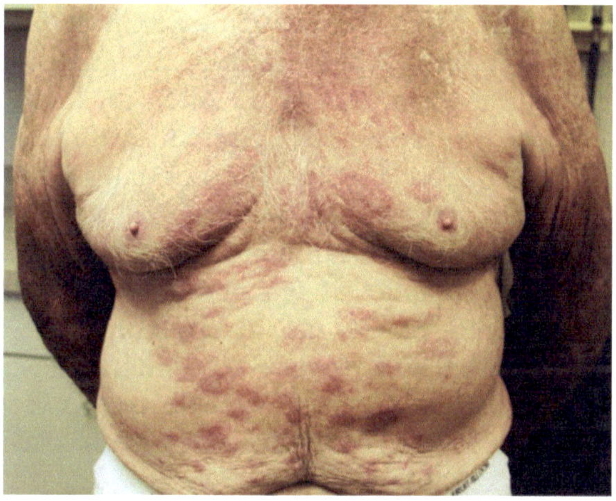

Figure 1.2. The definition of leprosy.

Source: By Luis A. Marcos, Stephen Conerly, and Sue Walker - https://www.ncbi.nlm.nih.gov/pmc/articles/PMC4125238/, CC BY 4.0, https://commons.wikimedia.org/w/index.php?curid=80168963

When you peel back the layers, you see that leprosy isn't merely a disease; it's a chapter in our social story. The way we label and understand leprosy has also twisted over time as both medical knowledge and societal views evolved. Early on, doctors recognized it by obvious physical signs and clung to misconceptions about how it spread, often combining in ideas of the religious or supernatural. Then, thanks to breakthroughs in microscopic and microbial science, experts came to see leprosy as an infection caused by *Mycobacterium leprae*—a realization that reshaped diagnostic criteria and treatment approaches. This progress, however, wasn't smooth; traditional beliefs often clashed with new therapeutic practices, induceing a kind of medical revolution that combined old ideas with new methods. One can spot echoes of these developments in ancient medicinal texts that dared to harness the power of diverse substances (Wujastyk et al., 2019). To summarize, the shifting definition of leprosy reflects a long and winding journey that mirrors broader changes in both science and society (Figure 1.2).

Overview of the Disease's Prevalence

Medical breakthroughs have come a long way, yet leprosy still persists as a stubborn issue globally. Many regions, especially those with scarce medical support and tougher economic conditions, continue to bear its weight. Roughly 200,000 new cases emerge every year , a sign that, even with improved control strategies, the disease keeps moving forward. Countries with low Socio-Demographic Index (SDI) often clock much higher age-adjusted rates, and this gap isn't solely about the microbes; it also shows how social factors affect its spread. In most cases, understanding these patterns helps set up the right interventions and direct resources, paving the way for a future where leprosy might finally be eliminated (Zhang et al., 2025). A closer look at demographics reveals some unique characterestics with respect to age and gender trends with leprosy. For example, new infections tend to peak for individuals aged between 25 and 35, while the overall numbers usually hit their highest in those around 35–40. This spread suggests long exposure periods and a lag before symptoms emerge, really underscoring the disease's chronic nature. Males, for reasons that might include job-related exposures, differing access to healthcare, and even a bit of social stigma, often register higher rates of infection and rack up more disability-adjusted life years than females. Such nuances, generally speaking, are key when it comes to fine-tuning public health strategies and boosting early detection efforts (Zhang et al., 2025). Looking back, the toll of leprosy was even heavier, with deep-rooted social stigma making life tougher for those affected. Also known as Hansen's disease, it arises primarily from the bacteria *Mycobacterium leprae* and *Mycobacterium lepromatosis*, and it mainly targets the skin and peripheral nerves. The early 1980s brought a big change with the advent of MDT, which really turned the tide in high-burden places like India. By 2005, India had impressively cut its leprosy numbers to below one case per 10,000 people—a clear win for public health. Still, some pockets of the disease hang around, meaning we must stay vigilant and keep pushing educational efforts to bust old myths and lessen the stigma that, at times, hampers treatment and stalls full eradication.

1.1. Historical Perspectives on Leprosy

Leprosy has been misunderstood and shrouded in stigma for centuries. People often saw it as a kind of divine retribution or a sign of personal failing, and that view led to real exclusion, both physically and in terms of honor and identity. Individuals weren't just isolated from society; families lost face too. Research on the cultural side, in most cases, shows these deep-seated fears connected to karma and shame still influence attitudes today (Visser et al., 2025). It's a complex history where old ideas held back public health efforts while intensifying isolation. Back when medical minds first began to untangle the mystery, the disease was mostly explained in supernatural or moral terms. Then, scientists identified the bacterial cause, inducing a shift toward more scientific treatment. Still, issues persisted. For instance, qualitative studies point out that reconstructive surgery can be a game changer for patients, even as economic hurdles and unreliable healthcare access hold many backs. Treatment delays often arise from not just infrastructural problems but also the persisting fear wrapped up in old beliefs about leprosy (Shrivastava et al., 2024). In most cases, efforts now have to juggle both clinical care and a slow, sometimes complex, psychosocial recovery. Looking at the past really matters when we shape today's public health plans. The long-held connection between leprosy and social disgrace means that fighting it isn't just about curing the body, it's about mending broken reputations, too. When families, communities, and healthcare providers all pitch in, there's a chance for someone affected by leprosy to restore their dignity. It's not only about smoothing out physical deformities; it's also about rebuilding social identity. The historical record, as complex as it sometimes appears, continues to remind us that deeply rooted perceptions affect how people experience illness and care, so comprehensive, culturally aware interventions are key (Shrivastava et al., 2024; Visser et al., 2025) (Figure 1.3).

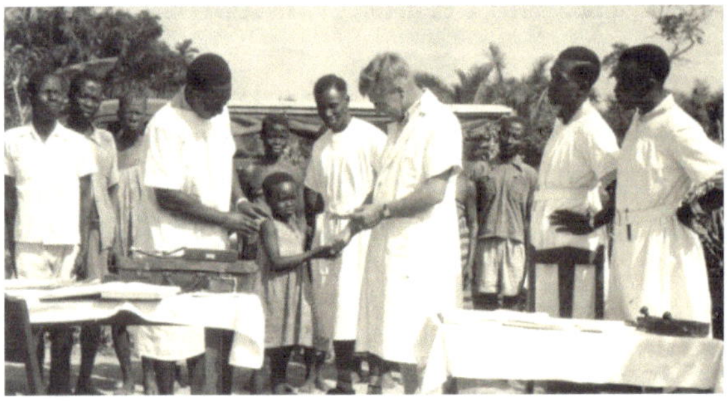

Figure 1.3. The history of leprosy.

Source: The Leprosy Mission International. (n.d.). *An Outdoor Clinic.*

1.1.1. Ancient References and Cultural Perceptions

Diseases like leprosy in ancient times were

deeply wrapped up in the myths and stories of the day. Old writings and religious texts often treated leprosy as if it were a punishment from the gods or a sign of a spiritual flaw. In many instances, these accounts reveal that people then thought of the illness as more than just physical, a marker of ethical or social failings too. Leprosy, as depicted in these narratives, stirred up fear and drove people to push the afflicted aside, combining ideas of purity with notions of contamination. In a very human way, these cultural snapshots show that leprosy was not only a medical problem but also a social label, steeped in tradition and the collective mindset of the time. Looking at how ancient societies made sense of leprosy, one finds that cross-cultural encounters and myth-filled traditions played key roles.

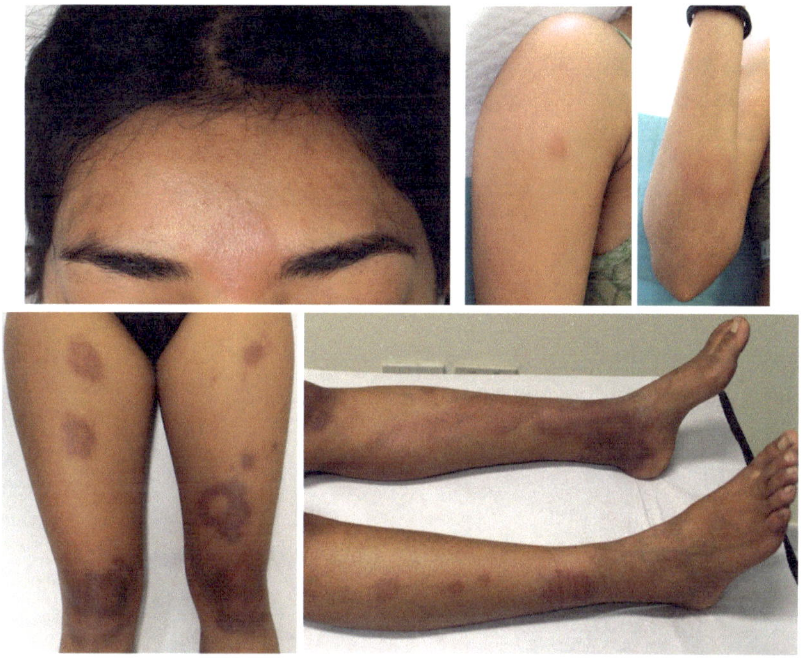

Figure 1.4. The back of a patient with leprosy.

Source: Beltrame A, Fargnoli MC, Avanzi C, Sollima L, Pomari E, Mori A, Longoni SS, Moro L, Orza P, Jackson M, et al. Leprosy in an Adopted Woman Diagnosed by Molecular Tools: A Case Report from a Non-Endemic Area. *Pathogens*. 2023; 12(2):165. https://doi.org/10.3390/pathogens12020165

Myth and moral thought often intermingled, framing leprosy as part of a grand cosmic design and a reminder of human vulnerability. Generally speaking, this pattern mirrors what happens when diverse cultural legends and ideas combine to rewrite the story of disease and its impacts. For example, comparing Eastern and European myths shows that symbols connected to illness and recovery reappear in different settings, subtly reshaping the overall narrative about leprosy. These cultural references weren't fixed, they evolved over time, adapting to answer both spiritual and ethical concerns (Yan, 2024). Beyond the realm of literature and philosophy, the real-life experience of dealing with leprosy in ancient communities carried its own deep cultural weight. Archaeological findings and various texts suggest that social responses to the disease were mixed—sometimes marked by strict rituals of exclusion and, in other cases, by acts of care. Local belief systems, with all their characterestics, often dictated ideas about contagion, cleanliness, and social stability. Even analyses of later visitor accounts, although a bit more modern, offer signals into how regional traditions might have shaped attitudes toward diseases in historically significant places (Zhu & Wang, 2024). In many ways, understanding these layers of ancient cultural thought sheds light on why stigma has persisted and how whole communities struggled with the inclusion or isolation of those suffering from leprosy (Figure 1.4).

1.1.2. The Impact of Leprosy on Societies

Leprosy's impact isn't just skin deep, it changes lives and shifts how communities come together. People living with leprosy often get sidelined and treated unfairly, and that kind of rejection can spiral into a persistent cycle of stigma that makes bouncing back even harder. Sometimes cultural mix-ups and rampant misinformation only worsen the stigma, which is exactly why using tools altered for local contexts is so key.

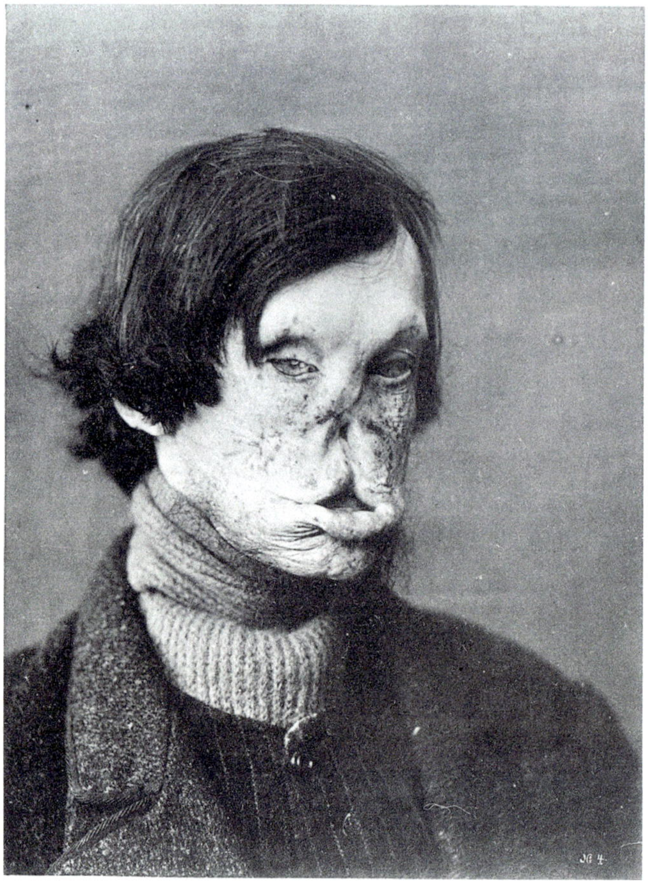

Figure 1.5. The impact of leprosy on societies.

Source: By https://wellcomeimages.org/indexplus/obf_images/a3/77/2b528f9e5c003ff89939b087573d.jpgGallery: https://wellcomeimages.org/indexplus/image/L0032810.htmlWellcome Collection gallery (2018-04-06): https://wellcomecollection.org/works/n9sqqkra CC-BY-4.0, CC BY 4.0, https://commons.wikimedia.org/w/index.php?curid=36056619

For example, adapting and testing The SARI (Stigma Assessment and Reduction of Impact) Stigma Scale in the Ambonese-Malay language has really made a difference in one endemic area, laying the groundwork for interventions that feel right for that community. That tool shows us that stigma isn't one uniform thing; it pops up in various ways, affecting a patient's mind and their role in society. All of this underscores that culturally sensitive strategies are critical in easing social isolation and boosting acceptance for those with leprosy (Rahayu et al., 2025). Beyond stigma, leprosy stokes a whole range of psychosocial challenges that interefere with everyday life and community bonds. In places like Mozambique, research has shown that people with leprosy, and even those battling similar neglected illnesses, , often face serious psychological pressure, find themselves increasingly isolated, and run into roadblocks when trying to join in on everyday activities. In many cases, nearly 70% of those affected experience significant mental distress, which really speaks to the emotional toll of the disease. When stigma combines with physical limitations, it tends to shut people out of essential social and economic opportunities, keeping poverty and marginalization alive. The harsher the physical effects, the more intense the emotional and social fallout, proving how intertwined physical health and social life are. Some community projects focusing on group self-care and local engagement have shown promising results, suggesting that a well-rounded support system can make a big difference (Robin van Wijk et al., 2024). When you add up the effects of stigma, mental health strains, and social exclusion, you end up facing a major roadblock to truly understanding leprosy's impact on society. It's clear that fighting the disease isn't only about medicine; it's equally about tearing down prejudiced views and promoting real inclusion. Stigma not only degrades a person's self-esteem but also undermines public health efforts by keeping individuals from seeking help when they need it. To make matters worse, the financial stress that comes with being socially discriminated against only deepens existing inequalities over time. That's why we need strategies that mix medical care with psychological and social support. Approaches using well-tested tools like the SARI Stigma Scalethat lean on community education to clear up misinformation, which can help build an environment where those affected by leprosy regain their dignity and join society fully (Rahayu et al., 2025; Robin van Wijk et al., 2024) (Figure 1.5).

1.1.3. Changes in Treatment and Understanding Over Time

Looking back, leprosy's history is a real mix of shifting medical ideas and changing social views. People used to think the disease was some sort of curse or punishment—almost like a contagious mark that demanded isolation. Early remedies were basic at best, relying more on individuallore than on solid science, and they didn't really help much. It wasn't until the late 1800s, when microbiology made some serious strides, that researchers finally pinpointed *Mycobacterium leprae* as the culprit. That discovery flipped the script from mystical explanations to a bacterial cause, which in most cases paved the way for better-targeted treatments and a fresh look at social responses. It kind of shows how mixcombining past insights with modern research can make all the difference (Bhattacharya, 2003). By the mid-1900s, multidrug therapy (MDT) really turned the tables on leprosy treatment. Before these advances, options like chaulmoogra oil did little more than offer dubious relief while bringing along a host of side effects. Then came antibiotics such as dapsone, rifampicin, and clofazimine—drugs that not only revolutionized medical care but also began to undermine the stubborn fears about leprosy being an incurable and highly contagious curse. Thanks to these new treatments, patients gradually found their way back into society; visible signs faded, and the risk of spreading the infection dropped. Of course, as with many infections (especially those prone to resistant strains), constant vigilance remains necessary to keep drug resistance at bay (Gillen et al., 2009). This ongoing need for caution really highlights how our understanding of infectious diseases is always evolving. Today, tackling leprosy means detecting it early, offering a combination of thorough treatment and social support, and not forgetting the mental and social side of recovery. Modern programs, like community awareness campaigns and integrating leprosy care into standard health services—are breaking down old stigmas and championing human rights, a far cry from past isolationist methods. At the same time, studies in genetics and immunology, believe it or not, continue to unveil why some people might be more vulnerable and how the disease progresses, opening up new avenues for therapy and prevention. When you consider how far we've come, , from fear-based segregation to evidence-driven, compassionate care, it underscores the point that our approach to leprosy is tightly linked to how we view the disease and those who suffer from it. Ultimately, this shift mirrors a broader trend in medical history where scientific breakthroughs meet a drive for social justice (Bhattacharya, 2003).

1.2. Causes and Transmission

Mycobacterium leprae, the microbe behind leprosy, has a unique trait, it tends to settle in the cooler parts of the body like the skin and peripheral nerves. It usually sneaks in through the nasal passages or minor skin lesions. Close, ongoing contact with untreated cases increases the risk, so catching the infection early matters. Cultural ideas and deep-rooted stigma often delay people from seeking help, which in turn lets the disease spread further (Prakoeswa et al., 2025).

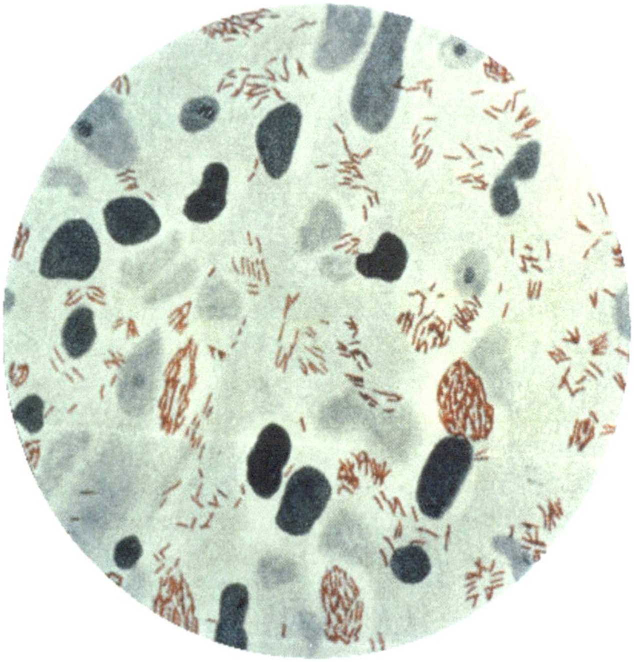

Figure 1.6. Leprosy causes.

Source: Public Domain, https://commons.wikimedia.org/w/index.php?curid=1783282*Mycobacterium leprae*

To summarize, the organism's natural characterestics mixed with these social hurdles set the stage for leprosy's persistence. The spread of leprosy gets even messier when you factor in age, lifestyle, and living conditions. Research generally shows that many cases emerge among men in their prime, likely connected to everyday work and social habits. At the same time, household interactions, genetic susceptibilities, and overcrowded homes all seem to raise the odds of catching the infection. Even though pinpointing each risk factor remains a bit elusive, evidence suggests that long-term exposure and delays in treatment are major causes. Early detection is especially crucial since patients with a heavy bacterial load tend to pass on the infection more readily. Clinical findings even hint that the longer someone struggles with the illness, the higher their risk of disability, pointing to the need for sharper surveillance and preventive measures (Jap et al., 2024). It isn't just the biology or the environment at fault; deep-seated social stigma also complicates the issue when it comes to controlling leprosy. Misunderstandings and fear about the disease have bred discrimination, leaving patients isolated and sometimes too embarrassed to talk about their symptoms. These social pressures, in many cases, slow down the move to get treated, which then fuels further transmission in communities. Limited education and low awareness in affected areas keep old myths alive about leprosy being permanently contagious. Tackling this effectively means embracing culturally sensitive education, boosting community engagement, and backing supportive policies. When these social dynamics mix with clinical realities, it becomes clear that only a well-rounded approach, addressing biology, behavior, and belief, will finally rein in leprosy (Prakoeswa et al., 2025) (Figure 1.6).

1.2.1. The Bacterium Mycobacterium leprae

In many parts of the world, infections just seem to hang around, reminding us that the links between microbes, the surroundings, and human bodies can be surprisingly complex. Take *Mycobacterium leprae*, for instance, the microbe behind leprosy, which keeps health officials on their toes with its unpredictable ways of spreading. Recent work using techniques like quantitative polymerase chain reaction has shown that the DNA of this microbe pops up not only in patients already diagnosed with leprosy but also in people who don't show clear symptoms, such as healthcare staff and local residents. It even appears that the bacterium might be persisting in the environment and could settle in spots like the tear film, hinting that we might have underestimated how it travels around (Sabage et al., 2025). In most cases, this makes us wonder if our usual ideas about contagion need a second look. Understanding how *M. leprae* causes trouble means we have to dig into both what the microbe does and how our bodies react. Generally speaking, its harmful effects aren't just about its own characteristics; our immune system plays a huge part too. Researchers have seen that when the bacterium invades, it often hits the peripheral nerves, leading to neuropathy, a classic sign of leprosy, and the degree of nerve damage seems to shift with how the immune system sets in. Studies even point out that our normal antigen presentation suffers, with reduced expression of major histocompatibility complex molecules in response to the microbe's phenolic glycolipid-1 (PGL-1), which in turn weakens adaptive immunity. This mix-up in the immune response lets the bacterium stick around longer and trigger further nerve injury, showing just how intertwined *M. leprae*'s survival can be with our body's defenses (Jess Mé Abrahão Silva et al., 2024). It's no small wonder that this clever microbe manages to dodge our immune system so well, making treatment and control extra challenging. Early responders like pattern recognition receptors do their best to spot *M. leprae* and start off inflammation, but what happens next—whether adaptive immune cells ramp up or pull back—affects the course of the disease. In most cases, patients can present very different immune profiles; some lean toward a tuberculoid form with robust cell-mediated responses, while others show a lepromatous form that's more about weak cellular reactions and heightened humoral responses. With regulatory T cells and unusual shifts in B cell behavior adding to the complexity, the picture becomes even messier. This mix of responses affects not only individual outcomes but also the way the disease spreads across communities, pushing experts to rethink early detection and control methods (Jess Mé Abrahão Silva et al., 2024; Sabage et al., 2025).

1.2.2. Modes of Transmission Among Humans

In many cases, the way infections spread isn't just about the microbes—it's also about how people live and the conditions they're in. Leprosy, for instance, comes from *Mycobacterium leprae* and is thought to pass mainly through long-term, close contact with untreated individuals, even though exactly how that happens still isn't totally clear.

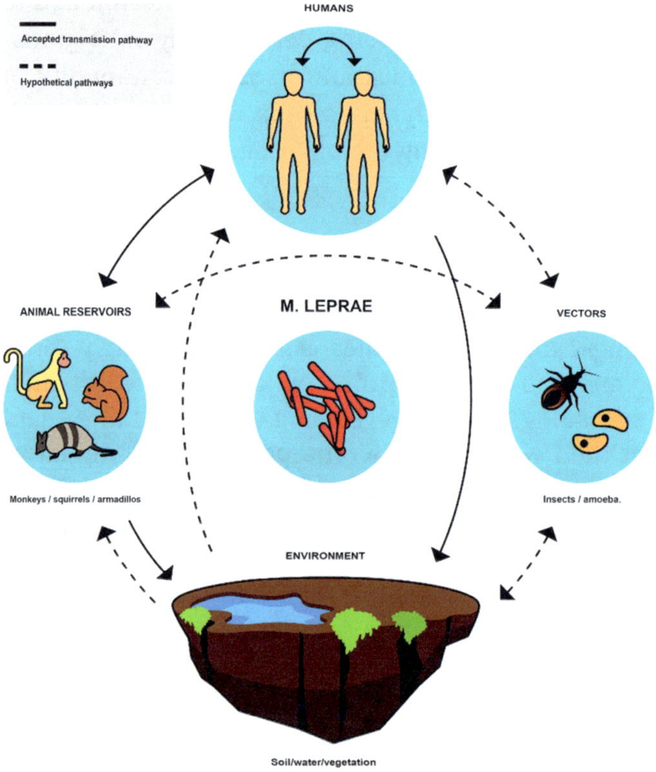

Figure 1.7. Transmission of *M. leprae* involves several factors and pathways.

Source: Truman, R. W., et al. (2020). *Transmission Pathways of M. leprae.* PLOS Neglected Tropical Diseases.

People might get infected when tiny droplets from a cough or sneeze float through the air; however, leprosy tends to need repeated, extended exposure because its infectivity is relatively low. Genetic factors, immune status, and even the local environment all mix into the chance of getting infected. It matters here that asymptomatic carriers or undiagnosed patients can end up quietly spreading the disease, which only makes controlling it complex. Looking at other diseases also shows us a complicated picture. Think of HIV and hepatitis B. With HIV, for example, the mother-to-child route plays a big role—this vertical transmission is heavily shaped by how much a mother knows about her own health, where she lives, and her access to prenatal care (Akinrefon et al., 2025). Just like leprosy, many of these infections are influenced not only by the microbe itself but also by socioeconomic and behavioral factors. Hepatitis B, on the other hand, can travel along perinatal, sexual, or even parenteral lines—a reflection of both local healthcare practices and the prevalence of the virus in a given area (Agboeze et al., 2023). All of these examples generally remind us that the spread of disease is complex, often woven from threads of human behavior, healthcare systems, and the natural characterestics of the pathogens. When you look closely at leprosy, its transmission isn't only about the microbe—it's deeply connected to everyday interactions and how people access care, especially in regions where it's common. Regular, prolonged contact, , like what you might see among family or close friends, is seen as the keyway the bacterium spreads, which stands in contrast to diseases that jump quickly through brief, casual encounters. It's also worth noting that the long incubation period of leprosy can hide the spread for several years, which complicates early detection and treatment. Much like other infections where early, even antenatal, care can make a difference (Agboeze et al., 2023; Akinrefon et al., 2025), catching and treating leprosy early is essential to breaking its cycle. In short, public health approaches need to mix proper medical treatment with social and economic strategies, because, more often than not, both are essential to effectively reducing the spread (Figure 1.7).

1.2.3. Risk Factors Associated with Leprosy

Risk factors for leprosy don't come from a single source – they mix environmental characterestics with individual habits. Crowded homes, for example, put people in prolonged close contact, which can let *Mycobacterium leprae* spread more easily. It turns out that the nature of our living spaces, think poor ventilation, high humidity or even dim lighting, can decide whether the bacteria stick around or not. In many cases, simply not keeping up with personal hygiene can wear down the skin's natural defenses, opening up more chances for the microbe to get in. Overall, where we live and how we look after ourselves are tightly combined together in affecting leprosy risk, so ensuring better living conditions and a bit more attention to cleanliness is pretty important to lower infection chances within communities (Pertiwi et al., 2024). Immune responses and basic demographics add another twist to the issue. The disease can show up in different ways depending on how an individual's immune system tackles it; generally speaking, some people end up with a more aggressive version or odd immunological reactions. Studies have even pointed out that being male is often linked to a higher risk for these reactions, possibly due to subtle biological factors or varied exposure levels. Patients carrying larger amounts of the bacteria—as flagged by a positive bacillary index—tend to face more severe outcomes, and when treatments for multibacillary forms aren't followed closely, complications can quickly pile up. In most cases, early detection, tailored therapy, and sticking with the treatment plan are keys to keeping the disease in check (Rakotoarisaona et al., 2023). Another layer is added when you consider vaccination and a person's immunological history. The Bacille Calmette-Guérin (BCG) vaccine, originally made for tuberculosis, seems to offer some protection against leprosy too, generally boosting a person's overall defense. Whether someone has received BCG can noticeably decide their chances of infection, which makes it a handy preventive factor on a larger scale. Oddly enough, even elements like the type of building materials used in a house or the local ambient temperature can affect how long *Mycobacterium leprae* survives around us. Put all these factors together, environment, hygiene, and immune history, and you get a pretty detailed picture of how biology, behavior, and surroundings intersect. Recognizing this complex mix is crucial for rolling out effective public health measures to lower the global burden of leprosy (Pertiwi et al., 2024).

1.3. Symptoms and Diagnosis

Leprosy doesn't usually announce itself loudly. It creeps in quietly, with patients noticing small skin patches, often lighter or sometimes reddish—that feel strangely numb or less reactive to heat, cold, or pain because the nerves aren't working right. Over time, the nerves in the arms and legs can get thicker, and that numbness might usher in muscle weakness or even disabilities if nothing is done. Sometimes the eyes get dry, and, in some cases, this can even lead to blindness, which complicates the overall picture.

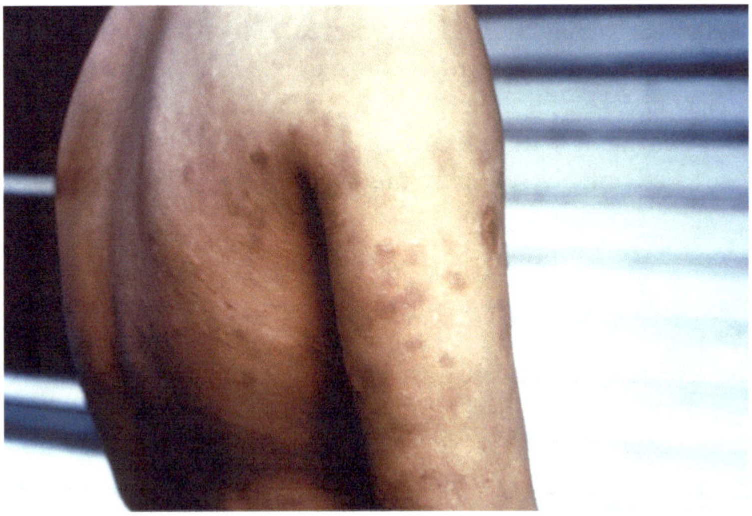

Figure 1.8. The symptoms and diagnosis of leprosy.

Source: Centers for Disease Control and Prevention (CDC). (2024). *HD Lesions on Back and Arms.*

All these symptoms come straight from the infection slowly attacking the skin, nerves, and mucosal tissues—a clear sign that the disease touches multiple areas. Detecting these signs early on is important to ward off permanent damage and disability, so doctors make sure to do complete examinations and take detailed patient histories (Ahmed et al., 2021). When it comes to figuring out if someone has leprosy, doctors mix hands-on clinical checks with lab tests to nail down the presence of *Mycobacterium leprae* and see how bad the infection is. Typically, they're on the lookout for those characteristic skin spots, altered sensations, and thick nerves, all of which they check during a neurological exam. They also use skin smears and sometimes biopsies; looking under a microscope, they can spot acid-fast bacteria, which gives them direct proof of infection. Further, examining the tissue samples further helps in sorting out which type of leprosy is present, which then shapes the treatment plan. Still, in many areas with fewer resources, the diagnosis leans heavily on clinical judgment despite these tests. This mix of clinical insight and lab support stands as a cornerstone in managing leprosy, ensuring that the diagnosis stays on target and reducing the risk of mistakes (Newport & Myrvang, 2009). Because leprosy is so multifaceted, its diagnosis demands extra vigilance, its signs can easily be confused with other skin or nerve conditions. Fungal infections, vitiligo, or even various peripheral neuropathies can show up with similar-looking skin changes or issues with sensation, making things even more complicated. That's why health authorities have set firm guidelines: typically, a combination of pale or reddish lesions with clear loss of sensation, thickened nerves, and positive lab findings like skin smears or biopsies form the diagnostic triad. Early, spot-on diagnosis is key to kicking off multidrug therapy before the disease can progress further and spread. Although leprosy is treatable, the persisting stigma and the hurdles in diagnosis mean that continued medical education and better testing methods are still very much needed, especially in regions where resources are scarce and cases are more common (Newport & Myrvang, 2009; Ahmed et al., 2021) (Figure 1.8).

1.3.1. Common Symptoms of Leprosy

Leprosy shows up in several ways that can mix up how we spot it early on. The skin might have uneven patches—sometimes lighter, sometimes with a reddish tint, and these spots can lose that normal feel, which is mostly due to nerve issues underneath. Often, nerves near the skin get thicker and even a bit sore, and when that happens, muscles can start to weaken, and the usual sense of touch goes out the window. Without that natural warning from their bodies, people can easily end up with injuries or infections they never saw coming. The skin changes are usually the clear indicators, but the slow creep of the disease means it sometimes persists long enough to be unknowingly passed along before anyone gets treated. Catching these early signs is generally key to stepping in before more serious damage sets in. Beyond just what you see on the skin, eye problems emerge too, although they're talked about less often. In severe cases, especially in the lepromatous form—loss of eyebrows or eyelid issues can lead to situations like not fully closing the eyes or experiencing constant irritation on the surface. You might also get ongoing inflammation inside the eye, which can be connected to a combination of factors: direct bacterial effects, some hiccups in nerve function, and even overactive immune responses.

These shifts can sometimes pave the way for complications like glaucoma or cataracts, adding another layer to the trouble. In most cases, this eye involvement shows that the microbes causing leprosy reach way beyond just the skin and major nerves, so it's important to check the eyes early, as part of a full examination (Blagojevic et al., 1990). Leprosy continues to be a stubborn public health challenge, especially in places like India where it's still pretty common. Sure, visible skin marks and nerve issues are the go-to signs of the disease, but it can emerge in different forms, from milder types to more severe cases with widespread lesions. The tougher, multibacillary variant not only brings along more extensive skin damage and a higher chance of disability but also carries a greater load of acid-fast bacteria in the tissues. Even with all the progress in treatment methods these days, the steady number of new cases hints that many individuals with early symptoms slip through the diagnostic cracks or aren't treated soon enough. That's why health strategies need to focus on recognizing these signs early and making care accessible to help cut down on transmission and prevent long-term issues from a delayed diagnosis (Beauclair et al., 2015) (Figure 1.9).

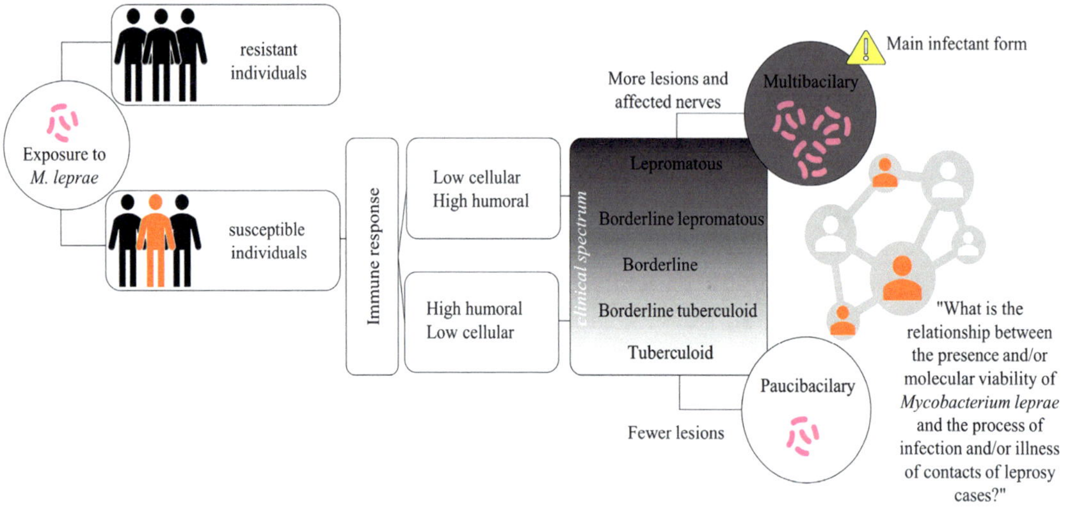

Figure 1.9. Symptoms of leprosy.

Source: Vidal SL, Batista LCF, Lages DdS, Bortolomai BE, Bueno IdC, Niitsuma ENA, Oliveira NGd, Baptista IMFD, Lana FCF. Molecular Detection of *Mycobacterium leprae* and the Process of Infection and Illness in Contacts of Leprosy Patients: A Systematic Review. *Tropical Medicine and Infectious Disease*. 2025; 10(2):32. https://doi.org/10.3390/tropicalmed10020032

1.3.2. Diagnostic Methods Used by Healthcare Professionals

Getting the diagnosis right for leprosy stays at the heart of controlling this age-old disease and lessening its impact on public health. Clinicians mix careful check-ups with lab tests to spot *Mycobacterium leprae* infections, often, patients turn up with pale or reddish patches along with some sensory loss, which leads to more detailed nerve and skin exams. In many cases, skin smears and biopsies offer a glimpse of acid-fast bacilli under a microscope, although how well they work can shift along the disease's spectrum. In regions with fewer resources, where fancy laboratory setups are hard to come by, skilled clinical judgment sometimes has to fill in the gaps. So, tailoring a combination of diagnostic techniques to local conditions becomes pretty much a must for catching the disease early and curbing its spread (Perez et al., 2024). New diagnostic approaches are cropping up to work alongside traditional methods by offering quicker, more sensitive ways to detect *M. leprae*. Techniques like polymerase chain reaction (PCR) have changed the game by directly detecting bacterial DNA in patient samples – something that is especially valuable in those paucibacillary cases where the bacterial load is low and microscope checks might miss a thing. Still, putting PCR and similar advances into practice is often slowed down by cost, infrastructure limitations, and shortages in technical know-how. It's also worth mentioning that immunological assays, which gauge a host's response to leprosy-specific antigens, are currently under investigation as potential point-of-care tools. In most cases, filling these diagnostic holes is crucial because delays or oversights can let the disease progress and keep community transmission going (Perez et al., 2024). Using these tests effectively is deeply intertwined with health system factors that influence leprosy control efforts. Research generally shows that delays in diagnosis can stem both from patient-related issues, like stigma and inadequate awareness, and from broader system hiccups, for instance, logistical problems in healthcare delivery. Some hands-on case-finding initiatives, when mixed with community engagement, seem to help individuals come forward sooner for testing. Moreover, offering better training for health workers in detecting and confirming leprosy is key to boosting both diagnosis accuracy and treatment adherence. Strengthening overall oversight, communication tools, and service frameworks can all add up to a wider diagnostic reach and better outcomes in affected areas, stimulating us closer to the goal of leprosy elimination (Gusmao et al., 2022) (Figure 1.10).

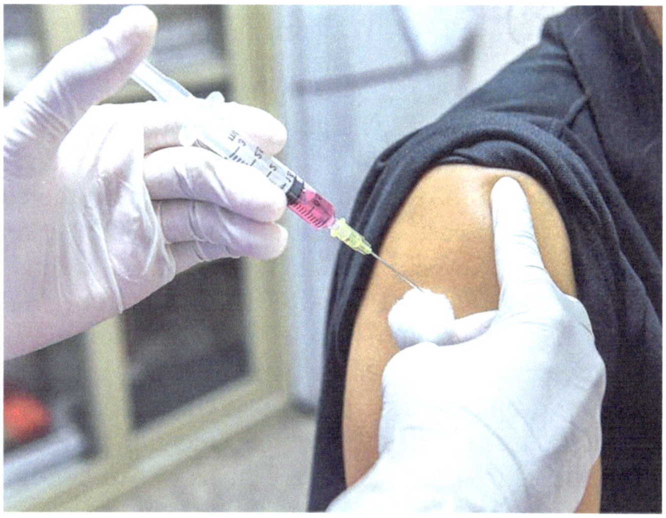

Figure 1.10. The diagnostic methods used by healthcare professionals.

Source: RVO Health. (2020). *Female receiving shot.* https://media.post.rvohealth.io/wp-content/uploads/2020/09/6357-female_recieving_shot-732x549-thumbnail-732x549.jpg.

1.3.3. Challenges in Diagnosing Leprosy

Leprosy can be complex to diagnose, in most cases because its signs creep in so slowly that they often go unnoticed. It may take years before symptoms become noticeable, and when they do, they're sometimes so mild they get mixed up with other skin conditions. The disease isn't uniform either, skin spots, nerve issues, and a broad range of lesions emerge depending on how the body reacts. In areas where this illness is common, getting a good diagnosis is even harder because specialized tests aren't always available; Further, the weight of social stigma can keep people from seeking help early on, which only makes things worse (Chandiok, 2024). Confirming leprosy in the lab adds another layer of challenge. *Mycobacterium leprae*, the microbe behind the disease, simply won't grow in a standard lab setup, which means doctors have to depend on skin smears and detailed tissue checks, procedures that require a certain level of expertise that isn't always at hand. Immunological tests sometimes lend a hand, but they often miss cases where only a few bacteria are present. Sure, PCR and other molecular tools offer better accuracy, yet in many resource-poor areas, these tests are just not an option. To complicate things further, leprosy can mimic other mycobacterial or skin conditions, so clinicians have to lean on both their judgment and available tests to reach a solid diagnosis (Bhavika, 2024). Diagnosing the disease in kids brings its own set of hurdles. Since children can show only faint or unusual symptoms, leprosy in young patients is frequently mistaken for common childhood skin issues. This overlap means early signs can easily fly under the radar, making it tough to get a timely diagnosis. Pediatric cases are especially important for mapping how the disease spreads, but they don't get enough attention, partly because factors like migration change the game entirely. To summarize, enhancing access to diagnostic tools and boosting awareness among health professionals are key steps to catching the illness early and helping to lower its global impact (Bhavika, 2024).

1.4. Treatment and Management

Early detection is absolutely key when dealing with leprosy because catching it early can help keep any lasting problems from taking hold. The go-to treatment here is multidrug therapy, often known as MDT, which throws together drugs like dapsone, rifampicin, and clofazimine to fight off *Mycobacterium leprae*. In most cases, this combo not only speeds up the clearance of the harmful bacteria but also cuts down on the chance of spreading and stops drug resistance from creeping in. It's important to jump on treatment early since nerve damage—the major source of long-term issues—can sneak up quietly before you even notice anything wrong. Keeping an eye on nerve function and stepping in at the right moment is crucial to prevent serious, disabling complications. On top of that, newer approaches are experimenting with neuroprotective and immunomodulatory agents to try to guard against or even reverse nerve injury, which shows how our grasp of leprosy's nerve damage and immune responses is steadily evolving (Rashidi et al., 2025). Overall, combining pharmacological, neurological, and rehab-focused care turns out to be a must for a well-rounded approach to managing leprosy.

It isn't just the bacteria that need attention – leprosy brings its own set of complications. Many patients suffer from nerve issues that require extra help such as wound care, physiotherapy, and sometimes even reconstructive surgery to regain function and avoid deformities. Because nerve problems can flare up suddenly, leading to sharp inflammation and faster damage, doctors often rely on quick corticosteroid use or other immunosuppressive treatments to put a lid on the swelling. Then there's the social side of things; the stigma and psychological toll can be heavy, prompting the need for mental health support and community engagement programs that encourage patients to stick with their treatment. In some cases, trouble compounds when infections like tuberculosis emerge, making it necessary to dig deep into a differential diagnosis and use treatments like anti-Koch's therapy as needed (Patel et al., 2024). So truly, care goes beyond just clearing bacteria, it calls for a comprehensive, often complex approach that touches on medical, mental, and social realms. Long-term success in battling leprosy depends on keeping up with follow-ups and making sure patients are well-informed about their own care. Regular check-ins help catch any sudden changes or reactional states early so that nerve problems don't turn into permanent damage. Patients who stick with the full MDT course tend to have a much better outlook , not only does it help them individually, but it also keeps the greater community healthier. It's equally vital to teach patients how to protect areas that have lost sensation because those parts are at risk for injuries and secondary infections that often lead to deformities. New diagnostic tools, from molecular tests to advanced neuroimaging—are slowly reshaping how we keep track of the disease, enabling doctors to step in faster and with more precision (Rashidi et al., 2025). MixCombining these fresh techniques with strong public health measures is generally speaking key to easing the overall impact of leprosy and boosting life quality for people around the globe (Figure 1.11).

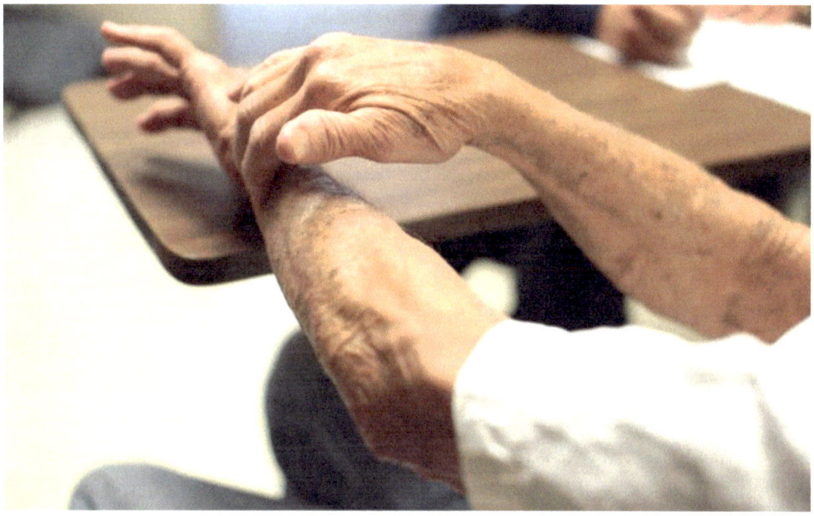

Figure 1.11. Early detection method for subclinical leprosy.

Source: Universitas Airlangga. (2020). *Ilustrasi oleh FK UNAIR 1.* https://unair.ac.id/wp-content/uploads/2020/10/Ilustrasi-oleh-FK-UNAIR-1.jpeg.

1.4.1. Current Treatment Options Available

Managing leprosy has come a long way over the past several decades. MDT still stands as the main treatment, mixcombining rifampicin, dapsone, and clofazimine to tackle *Mycobacterium leprae* and cut down on its spread. It's generally effective at curing people, slowing the disease's course, and keeping drug resistance at bay—but new cases still emerge, showing that antibiotics alone aren't a catch-all solution. That's why researchers are now eyeing extra treatments that boost a person's own defenses, acknowledging the complex interaction between the microbe and our immune system, and pressing for plans that go beyond just antimicrobials (Kimberly et al., 2024). Alongside the traditional approach, drugs that stimulate the immune system in one direction or another have started to attract attention. These immunomodulatory agents can either ramp up or quiet down immune responses, helping clear the bacteria more quickly or easing the harmful inflammation that sometimes builds up. In many cases, treatments like levamisole, thalidomide, a combination of vitamins (A, D, E, and C), zinc, and selenium have been tried out in clinical settings. Their role? To shift the body's internal balance towards fighting off the invasion and mending tissue damage caused by long-term infection. Still, exactly how these agents work together and which combinations hit the sweet spot remains a matter of active research—using them might just lower risks like nerve damage and disability in the long run (Kimberly et al., 2024). Treating leprosy where resources are tight has its own set of curves to navigate. The challenges here aren't so different from what we see with other deep-seated infections like tuberculosis or leishmaniasis, where both biology and economic factors get in the way. Limited healthcare infrastructure, complex early diagnoses, and socio-economic hurdles make it hard to roll out both MDT and its add-ons smoothly. This mix of obstacles has spurred efforts like the VALIDATE Network, which pushes for strategies that bridge different infections. By leaning into these broader, interconnected approaches, drug development can better reflect what happens in hard-hit regions—potentially opening the door to easier access to effective treatments and easing the overall disease burden.

1.4.2. The Role of Multidrug Therapy (MDT)

Decades ago, treating leprosy felt like a steep climb until MDT burst onto the scene and flipped the script. Before this approach came around, options were few and often ran headlong into problems like drug resistance and the incomplete clearing of *Mycobacterium leprae*. A combination usually made up of dapsone, rifampicin, and clofazimine turned out to be a sort of multi-angled attack on the bacilli, hitting it from several sides at once. This way of fighting not only bumped up cure rates but also slashed treatment times, generally cutting down the chances for resistance to emerge. Around the globe, MDT's rollout is linked with a noticeable drop in both disease spread and prevalence. Still, its true power depends heavily on patients staying the course and starting treatment early, a task that, in many endemic areas, is easier said than done. MDT's benefits stretch beyond just zapping the bacteria; they seem to influence the broader impacts of the disease, too. Studies show that people who never get treated tend to suffer more oral and dental troubles, think decayed or missing teeth, and even lesions like abrasion and abfraction. In contrast, those on MDT often enjoy better oral hygiene, with lower readings on measures like the Plaque Index and Papillary Bleeding Index, which hints that the drugs help ward off extra complications (Choudhari & Bajaj, 2023). Interestingly, however, some findings note that treated patients sometimes experience more clinical attachment loss, perhaps pointing to the long-term effects of the therapy or persisting issues from leprosy itself. It all paints a picture of a complex interplay between treatment and the disease's many faces, hinting that a well-rounded care plan is needed to tackle both the bacteria and its other consequences. Even with all its wins, multidrug therapy isn't without its bumps in the road. A big concern is the rise of antimicrobial resistance and the constant need to fine-tune treatment protocols. New research has even explored alternatives, like lymecycline—as either add-ons or replacements to the standard WHO-MDT. Comparative analyses generally agree that while WHO-MDT still takes center stage, weaving in newer drugs might boost outcomes, especially when patients show resistance or can't tolerate the regular regimen (Catrisse et al., 2023). The stubbornness of drug resistance keeps pushing us to keep a close watch and alter guidelines as needed. Moreover, factors such as local economies and how easily people can access healthcare play a huge role. For all these reasons, continually refining MDT—coupled with improved diagnostic, preventive, and rehabilitative efforts—remains key to keeping leprosy numbers down and lessening its overall global impact (Figure 1.12).

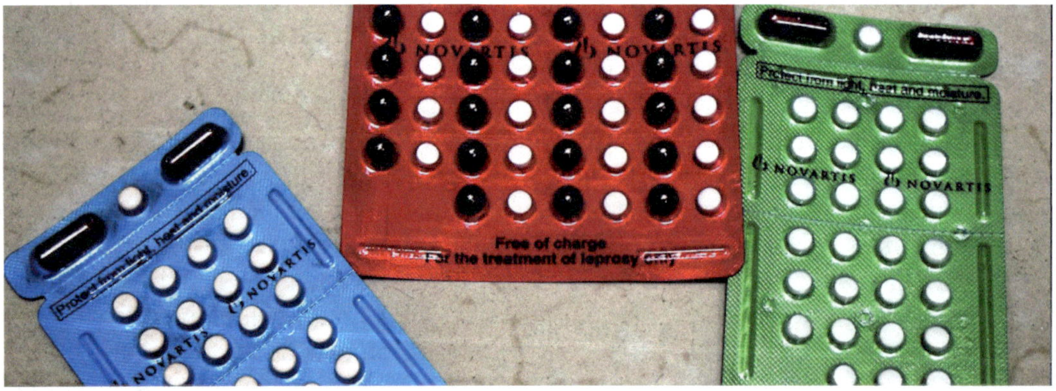

Figure 1.12. The role of multidrug therapy (MDT).

Source: The Leprosy Mission Trust India. (n.d.). *Multidrug Therapy (MDT) for Leprosy Disease.*

1.4.3. Importance of Early Intervention and Follow-Up Care

Early detection makes a big difference in managing leprosy. Often, the signs of the disease show up gradually, so diagnosis can get pushed back—this delay increases nerve damage and disability. Acting fast helps stop the disease from spreading in a community and can cut down on the physical issues later on. Starting treatment early usually means better outcomes and fewer long-term problems. People also get a chance to learn about the disease and why sticking with multidrug therapy matters, which can help keep functioning intact and life a bit more normal. Without that prompt care, the risk of lasting deformities goes up, showing just how crucial early clinical detecting and treatment is for controlling leprosy. Keeping in touch through follow-up care matters just as much. Chronic conditions like leprosy need regular check-ups so that reactions, relapses, or secondary infections don't sneak up on someone after therapy. Routine follow-up opens the door for doctors to spot even the faintest sign of nerve trouble before it turns into something worse. It also gives patients a little extra support with the social and emotional baggage that often comes with the disease, stigma and isolation can be real issues here. When health systems stick with consistent clinical and rehab care, they can adjust treatments to fit what the patient needs, which helps maintain both function and a sense of belonging. In a lot of cases, this ongoing care echoes what's done in managing other chronic illnesses, reminding us that good care goes well beyond the first round of treatment. Tailored follow-up approaches hit the mark across different healthcare settings. Research in neurodevelopmental practice shows that when follow-up services line up with what families prefer, it tends to boost both engagement and adherence, which improves overall health outcomes (Sharma et al., 2024). Tools like ultrasound, used a lot in managing vascular access, demonstrate that precise monitoring and timely alters to treatment can extend benefits significantly (Veneziano et al., 2025). MixCombining these insights from various fields allows leprosy care programs to fine-tune their follow-up routines, making them more accessible, cutting down barriers, and addressing not just medical but also educational and emotional needs. With a follow-up strategy that respects cultural and individual differences, the early wins from rapid treatment get bolstered by a comprehensive, ongoing care plan that lowers the chance of relapse and builds stronger community health (Figure 1.13).

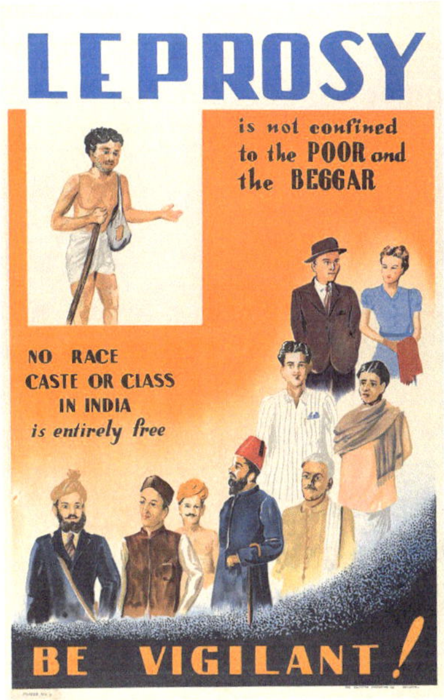

Figure 1.13. The importance of early intervention and follow-up care.

Source: By https://wellcomeimages.org/indexplus/obf_images/38/f5/9cca7b895752fe0dce6baa90f9c3.jpgGallery: https://wellcomeimages.org/indexplus/image/L0077162.htmlWellcome Collection gallery (2018-03-30): https://wellcomecollection.org/works/ephaug8v CC-BY-4.0, CC BY 4.0, https://commons.wikimedia.org/w/index.php?curid=37709067medication

A CLOSER LOOK

PHYLOGEOGRAPHY OF LEPROSY

In the past decade, it has become increasingly apparent that one can retrace the evolutionary history of peoples and their migrations by studying the genotypes of the pathogens they carry. In this regard, disease-causing bacteria such as Helicobacter pylori, Yersinia pathogenis, and *M. leprae* have served as valuable tools. Conversely, understanding the structure of human populations and their immunogenetics can also provide insight into the evolution of pathogens.

Phylogenetic studies of *M. leprae* have allowed us to infer relationships between different strains and to attempt to retrace their history. There is a fairly strict correlation between the geographical origin of the leprosy patient and the SNP profile: types 1A–D occur predominantly in Asia, the Pacific region, and East Africa; types 3I–M in Europe, North Africa, and the Americas; and types 4 N–P in West Africa, the Caribbean region, and South America. *M. leprae* belonging to SNP types 2E–H appears to be the rarest, although this may be due to under-sampling, and has only been detected in Ethiopia, Malawi, Nepal/North India, and New Caledonia (Figure 1.14).

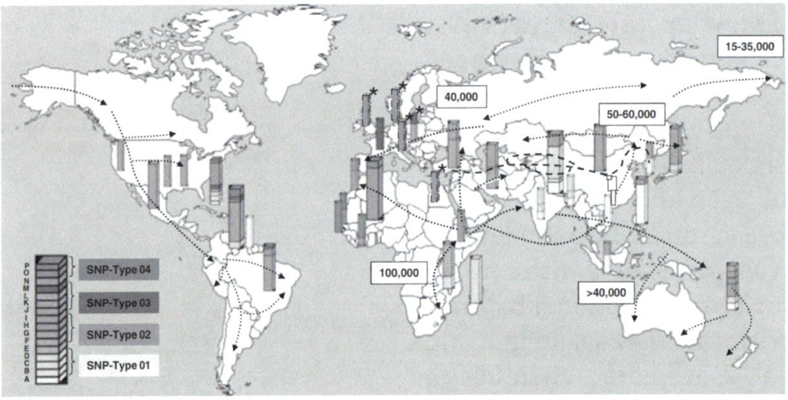

Figure 1.14. Global dissemination of *M. leprae* from SNP typing. Pillars are located on the country of origin of the *M. leprae* sample and color coded according to the scheme for the 16 SNP subtypes.

Source: Nunzi, E., & Massone, C. (2012). Leprosy: A Practical Guide. Springer Italia.

Applying the principles of maximum parsimony, two plausible evolutionary schemes arise. In the first scheme, which we consider more probable, *M. leprae* of SNP type 2, present in the region of East Africa/Near East, preceded SNP type 1, which migrated eastward, and SNP type 3, which disseminated westward in human populations, before SNP type 3 gave rise to type 4. In the second scenario, type 1 was the progenitor of type 2, with SNP types 3 and 4 following in numerical order. Comparison of what is known of human migrations with the phylogeny of *M. leprae* is highly informationrmative and reveals general agreement with the historical record and several contradictions.

The proposition that leprosy originated in the Indian subcontinent and was introduced into Europe by Greek soldiers returning from the Indian campaign of Alexander the Great is not compatible with the phylogeny of *M. leprae* since SNP type 1 predominates in India, whereas SNP type 3 afflicted European populations. From India, leprosy is thought to have moved to China, in about 500 BC, and then to Japan, reaching Pacific islands such as New Caledonia as recently as the 19th century. Once again, this is partly contradicted by the results of *M. leprae* genotyping, as leprosy appears to have been introduced into Asia by two different routes. The first of these, which is historically consistent, is the southern one associated with the SNP type 1 strains present in the Indian subcontinent, Indonesia, and the Philippines. The second is a more northerly route beginning in the eastern Mediterranean region and extending via Türkiye and Iran to China, and hence to Korea and Japan. The strains encountered along this route are mainly of SNP subtype 3K, and the Silk Road appears to have been a likely means of transport and disease transmission. The Plague or Black Death, caused by *Yersinia pathogenis*, is thought to have reached Europe in the 14th century from China via the Silk Road, being carried by humans and their fleas. Concerning leprosy, the opposite route of transmission may have been traveled, with the disease originating in Europe or the Near/Middle East and then spreading to the Far East.

Nothing is known of the history of leprosy in sub-Saharan Africa except that the disease was present before the colonial era. The phylogeny of *M. leprae* suggests that the disease was most likely introduced into West Africa by infected explorers, traders, or colonialists of European or north African descent, rather than by migrants from East Africa, as *M. leprae* of SNP type 4 is endemic in West Africa and much closer to type 3 than to type 2. West and southern Africa are believed to have been settled by migrants from the eastern part of the continent before the arrival of humans in the Eurasian regions. It seems unlikely that early humans brought leprosy into West Africa unless clonal replacement has since occurred. From West Africa, leprosy was then introduced by the slave trade from the 17th century onward into the Caribbean region, Venezuela, Brazil, and other parts of South America, as isolates of *M. leprae* with the same SNP type, 4N or O, are found there as in West Africa, which is consistent with the history of slavery. Strains of SNP subtype 4P are restricted to South America or the Caribbean, and they must have branched off during the last 400 years, since the introduction of the ancestral strain from West Africa, which was likely of SNP type 4 N or O. It appears improbable that leprosy was introduced into the Americas by early humans via the Bering Strait; instead, it seems more likely that immigrants from Europe brought the disease, as most of the *M. leprae* strains found in North, Central, and South America have the 3I genotype associated with European leprosy cases. In the 18th and 19th centuries, when the Mid-Western states of the USA were settled by Scandinavian immigrants, many cases of leprosy were recorded at a time when a major epidemic was underway in Norway. Further support for the "European origin" hypothesis is provided by the finding that wild armadillos from Louisiana, USA, which are naturally infected with *M. leprae*, also harbor the SNP type 3 strain, indicating that they were contaminated from human sources of European origin. Immigrants from France and Spain primarily were the main settlers in the state of Louisiana. It is also noteworthy that, on islands such as the French West Indies and New Caledonia, there is much greater SNP variety of *M. leprae*, reflecting the passage of, and settlement by, successive human populations. It is known that migrations by sea rather than over land or via coastal routes lead to more diversity in humans through intercombining, and a greater range of diversity is also apparent among their pathogens.

SUMMARY

Looking back at leprosy research and treatment, key breakthroughs have shifted how we handle this enduring infection. The BCG vaccine, which started out for tuberculosis, now surprisingly shows benefits when used against leprosy. Studies generally speaking reveal that BCG induces the immune system and may even lower how severe the disease gets. It's clear these kinds of interventions still matter—even with the heavy stigma and complications that leprosy brings along. Meanwhile, researchers keep noticing extra immune-boosting effects from BCG, hinting at fresh ways for better prevention and patient outcomes (Locht et al., 2020). Taking on leprosy in a full, real-world way also means keeping in mind the broader backdrop in which long-lasting diseases persist, especially among aging individuals. The challenges of chronic infection mix with the natural hurdles of getting older, physical limitations, memory slips, and even social roadblocks that pile on the difficulties. Recent work usually stresses that early diagnoses, steady support, and combined treatments can mitigate these age-related issues and help preserve independence. In most cases, the idea is that our health systems need to keep evolving so that care truly fits individual circumstances (Mare Pšová et al., 2019). In the end, pushing forward with leprosy care and control comes down to ongoing research, bolstered healthcare resources, and raising public awareness to impact old stigmas. The ups and downs learned from vaccine work and managing other chronic conditions tell us that a diverse mix of approaches is key. Continued investments in new treatments – paired with community-level support – aim to tackle not just the medical aspects, but also the social and economic hurdles. And, by encouraging global cooperation and fair treatment access, there's a real shot at reaching the people who need it most. The road toward leprosy elimination might be bumpy sometimes, but mixcombining insights from immunology, public health, and care for older populations shows that this goal is within reach in our time (Mare Pšová et al., 2019; Locht et al., 2020).

Viewing leprosy through the lens of different social and cultural experiences shows just how complex the challenges can be when it comes to helping communities recover. Sometimes, the usual top-down fixes leave people feeling more helpless than empowered, making them depend on outside help instead of figuring things out for themselves. On the other hand, when locals get involved in choosing and running their own programs, there's a induce of hope and ownership that can change the game. You might even see that some modern, industrial-style management methods fit in snugly here, helping to build a framework for lasting progress in post-leprosy villages. It seems clear that using approaches that respect cultural nuances and put community voices first could break the cycle of disenfranchisement and lead to stronger, more resilient development (Redington et al., 2019). Medical care remains a big deal in fighting leprosy, with antibiotic treatments working hard to cure the infection and slow its spread. Still, models like Directly Observed Therapy and case management, although common nationwide, often miss the mark when it comes to matching the real cultural and social needs of communities, especially Indigenous ones. Some experts, drawing on decolonial ideas, argue that these standard models can lack the kind of warm, personalized care that truly fits people's lives. Insights coming from patients, families, and local health workers keep reminding us that trust, clear communication, and shared decision-making are key to sticking with treatment plans. In short, when treatment strategies weave in community stories and cultural identity, they tend to work better and feel more acceptable to those who need them most (Oliver, 2022). Combining a community's historical backdrop with its cultural diversity and today's healthcare challenges is essential when rethinking how to beat leprosy. Even though medical science has moved forward, the disease still persists in the most overlooked corners, a sign that there are deep-seated issues within our health systems. Family support, cultural connections, and a sense of belonging are all huge parts of how well people cope with their illness. Not to mention, the long shadow of colonization still affects modern healthcare practices, often breeding distrust and keeping disparities alive. Rethinking our treatment plans with a mix of local know-how and a respectful nod to history might just smooth the path to better health outcomes. In the end, combining community engagement with a healthy dose of historical awareness offers a more rounded way to tackle both the medical and social hurdles of leprosy (Redington et al., 2019; Oliver, 2022).

KEY TERMS FROM THIS CHAPTER

- Antibiotics
- Chronic diseases
- Hansen's disease
- Leprosy
- Microbial science
- Mycobacterium leprae,
- Ayurvedic practices
- Clofazimine
- Infectious diseases
- Medical history
- Multidrug therapy
- Mycobacterium lepromatosis

References

1. Abdul, S., Adeghe, E., Adegoke, B. O., Adegoke, A. A., & Udedeh, E. H. (2024). Promoting health and educational equity: Cross-disciplinary strategies for enhancing public health and educational outcomes. *World Journal of Biology Pharmacy and Health Sciences, 2024, 18(02), 416–433.*
2. *Article DOI: 10.30574/wjbphs.2024.18.2.0298*(accessed on 10th May 2025).
3. Agboeze, J., Igwe, N., & Ukaegbe, C. (2023). Hepatitis B virus seroprevalence and potential perinatal transmission among pregnant women in Abakaliki, Nigeria. *Nigerian Medical Journal: Journal of the Nigeria Medical Association*, *64*, 582–590. https://www.semanticscholar.org/paper/aae045dd79de9357d0b96b246b0658f158999828 (accessed on 10th May 2025).
4. Akinrefon, A.A.; Adeniyi, O.I.; Afolabi, B.N.; Olatoregun, O.J. Impact of Maternal Factors on Vertical HIV Transmission in Jigawa State, Nigeria: A Multilevel Analysis of Antenatal Care and Knowledge of HIV Status. Int. J. Dev. Math. (IJDM) 2025, 2, 244–250, https://doi.org/10.62054/ijdm/0201.19.(accessed on 10th May 2025).
5. Deribe, K., Meribo, K., Gebre, T., Hailu, A., Ali, A., Aseffa, A., & Davey, G. (2012). The burden of neglected tropical diseases in Ethiopia, and opportunities for integrated control and elimination. *Parasites & vectors*, *5*, 240. https://doi.org/10.1186/1756-3305-5-240(accessed on 10th May 2025).
6. Alhumaid, N. K., Alajmi, A. M., Alosaimi, N. F., Alotaibi, M., Almangour, T. A., Nassar, M. S., Memish, Z. A., et al. (2023). *Reported Bacterial Infectious Diseases in Saudi Arabia: Overview and Recent Advances.* Research Square. https://doi.org/10.21203/rs.3.rs-3351846/v1 (accessed on 10th May 2025).
7. Allen, I., Lockwood, D. N., & Hay, R. (2024). The centenary of the Leprosy Relief Association (Lepra)—A moment for celebration and reflection. *Transactions of the Royal Society of Tropical Medicine and Hygiene*, *118*, 299–303. https://www.semanticscholar.org/paper/e8c69dc6284fc20d955f8e0660a75015b7267fbd (accessed on 10th May 2025).
8. Anbessie, M., Belete, Y., Ayele, B. A., Valcour, V., Kavanagh, N., Prioleau, C., & Yohannis, K. (2023). Media for advocacy of mental health in the Ethiopian context: Current practice, gaps, and future directions. *Frontiers in Psychiatry*, *14*. https://www.semanticscholar.org/paper/068c3470b67b412870dbcd60bd5795549224973f (accessed on 10th May 2025).
9. HABIBALLA AHMED, M. M., ANURADHA, and P. WADHWA. "A REVIEW ON AGENTS FOR THE TREATMENT OF LEPROSY INFECTION". *Asian Journal of Pharmaceutical and Clinical Research*, vol. 14, no. 3, Mar. 2021, pp. 25-29, doi:10.22159/ajpcr.2021.v14i3.40373. (accessed on 10th May 2025).
10. Auliyah, A. N., Pertiwi, M., & Syahrul, F. (2024). Risk factors for leprosy: A systematic review. *The Indonesian Journal of Public Health*. https://www.semanticscholar.org/paper/71bb510198ab18cff0e877d9e4e421d9471a46fd (accessed on 10th May 2025).
11. Beauclair, R., Brook, C. E., Galvani, A. P., Lietman, R., et al. (2015). *Spatial Heterogeneity in Projected Leprosy Trends in India.* https://core.ac.uk/download/74708493.pdf (accessed on 10th May 2025).
12. Beloso, B. M. (2017). *Queer Theory, Sex Work, and Foucault's Unreason*. https://core.ac.uk/download/129032536.pdf (accessed on 10th May 2025).

13. Blagojevic, M., Bonnici, M. R., Depasquale, G., Schiro, A., et al. (1990). *Ocular Manifestations in Lepromatous and Tuberculoid Leprosy.* https://core.ac.uk/download/46601751.pdf (accessed on 10th May 2025).

14. Chandiok, T. (2024). Leprosy: A comprehensive review of epidemiology, diagnosis, and public health challenges. *International Journal of Science and Research (IJSR).* https://www.semanticscholar.org/paper/4a533d61ce8530edeacb7d1374b3ac660f7d1eaa (accessed on 10th May 2025).

15. Perez, R. L., Chase, J., & Tanner, R. (2024). Shared challenges to the control of complex intracellular neglected pathogens. *Frontiers in public health, 12,* 1423420. https://doi.org/10.3389/fpubh.2024.1423420(accessed on 10th May 2025).

16. Choudhari, M., & Bajaj, P. (2023). Evaluation of dental and periodontal health status in leprosy patients during three different stages of drug regimen: A cross-sectional study. *Journal of Clinical and Diagnostic Research.* DOI: https://doi.org/10.7860/JCDR/2023/64907.18760 (accessed on 10th May 2025).

17. Diaz, J. C. D., Abad-Venida, M. L., Espinoza-Thaebtharm, A., Cathryn Salonga, M. E., & Abad-Casintahan, M. F. (2023). Comparison between lymecycline with multidrug therapy and standard multidrug regimen (WHO-MDT) in the treatment of multibacillary leprosy patients: a retrospective cohort study. *International journal of dermatology, 62*(9), 1186–1192. https://doi.org/10.1111/ijd.16767(accessed on 10th May 2025).

18. Franklin, H., Tora, A., Deribe, K., Reda, A. A., & Davey, G. (2013). Development of a scale to measure stigma related to podoconiosis in Southern Ethiopia. *BMC public health, 13,* 298. https://doi.org/10.1186/1471-2458-13-298 (accessed on 10th May 2025).

19. Elendu, C., Amaechi, D. C., Alakwe-Ojimba, C. E., Elendu, T. C., Elendu, R. C., Ayabazu, C. P., Aina, T. O., et al. (2023). Understanding sickle cell disease: Causes, symptoms, and treatment options. *Medicine, 102.* https://www.semanticscholar.org/paper/29cd6291d9b14c8e8129c07af8733241e6b8c1c6 (accessed on 10th May 2025).

20. Kimberly, Kesya; Ferina, Siti Aisha Nabila; and Esti, Prima Kartika (2024) "Immunomodulators in leprosy: A narrative review," *Journal of General - Procedural Dermatology & Venereology Indonesia*: Vol. 8: Iss. 1, Article 10. DOI: 10.7454/jdvi.v8i1.1123 Esti, P. K., Ferina, S. A. N., & Kimberly, K. (2024). *Immunomodulators in Leprosy: A Narrative Review.* https://core.ac.uk/download/639387425.pdf (accessed on 10th May 2025).

21. Fadilla, U. S., & Choiriyah, I. U. (2024). Enhancing Maternal Engagement for Effective Lowering Prevention Strategies. *Indonesian Journal of Cultural and Community Development, 15*(3), 10.21070/ijccd.v15i3.1102. https://doi.org/10.21070/ijccd.v15i3.1102 lower (accessed on 10th May 2025).

22. Fastenau, A., Willis, M., Vettel, C., Stuetzle, S. C. W., Penna, S., Chahal, P., Schlumberger, F., et al. (2024). Integrating community engagement in zero leprosy efforts: A pathway to sustainable early detection, control and elimination. *Tropical Medicine and Infectious Disease, 9.* https://www.semanticscholar.org/paper/b1dcb54f7b36622ddb4d15e783c65203af2fa65a (accessed on 10th May 2025).

23. Filipek, K. L., Gowland, R. L., Roberts, C., Tucker, K., et al. (2021). Alloparenting adolescents: Evaluating the social and biological impacts of leprosy on young people in Saxo-Norman

England (9th to 12th centuries AD) through cross-disciplinary models of care. *The Family in Past Perspective.* Routledge; eBook ISBN9780429355912 https://core.ac.uk/download/578137914.pdf (accessed on 10th May 2025).

24. Gillen, A.A. 2009. The Genesis of Methicillin-Resistant *Staphylococcus aureus*: A Modern Day "Leprosy" and Hospital Menace. *Answers in Depth*, July 1, 2009. Web. (accessed on 10th May 2025).

25. Pinheiro, M. G. C., Lins, S. L. D. F., Gomes, B. R. D. S., Simpson, C. A., Mendes, F. R. P., & Miranda, F. A. N. (2019). Contextual analysis of health care at discharge in leprosy: an integrative review. Análise contextual da atenção à saúde na alta em hanseníase: uma revisão integrativa. *Revista gaucha de enfermagem, 40*, e20180258. https://doi.org/10.1590/1983-1447.2019.20180258 (accessed on 10th May 2025).

26. Gusmao, C., Soares, D., Da Costa, F., Sarmento, J. C. J., Afliana, L., Afliana, L., Martins, N., et al. (2022). *Contributing Factors to the Resurgence of Leprosy Cases in Timor-Leste.* https://core.ac.uk/download/539601846.pdf (accessed on 10th May 2025).

27. Jaiswal B, Rajpurohit P, Munot Y, et al. International journal of therapeutic innovation. Medic Scientific. 2024; 2 (4) : 192-202. (accessed on 10th May 2025).

28. Ayleen Nathalie Jap , Hawari I. Community Medicine and Education Journal. Hanif Medisiana Publisher. 2024; 5 (2) : 517-524.(accessed on 10th May 2025).

29. Lima, R. B., Vivian, G. F., Alba, L. M. R., de Gois, K. S. N., Tomaz, V. A., Pinto, M. C., Ramos-Silva, F. F., et al. (2023). Bacilloscopy for leprosy in Brazil's public health system between 2013 and 2022. *Revista Ciências em Saúde, 13*, 38–45. https://doi.org/10.21876/rcshci.v13i4.1458 (accessed on 10th May 2025).

30. Locht, C., & Lerm, M. (2020). Good old BCG – What a century-old vaccine can contribute to modern medicine. *Journal of Internal Medicine, 288*, 611–613. https://doi.org/10.1111/joim.13195 (accessed on 10th May 2025).

31. Maresova, P., Javanmardi, E., Barakovic, S., Barakovic Husic, J., Tomsone, S., Krejcar, O., & Kuca, K. (2019). Consequences of chronic diseases and other limitations associated with old age - a scoping review. *BMC public health, 19*(1), 1431. https://doi.org/10.1186/s12889-019-7762-5(accessed on 10th May 2025).

32. Mariyani, Istiarsyah, Ardiansyah, Maisura, Zikrullah, & Mena Sari. (2024). HIV/AIDS AND DRUG PREVENTION STRATEGIES FOR THE HIGHER EDUCATION CONTEXT. *Jurnal Pengabdian Bangsa, 4*(1), 17-25. https://doi.org/10.61992/jpb.v4i1.200(accessed on 10th May 2025).

33. Newport, M. J., & Myrvang, B. (2009). Proceedings of a joint meeting between the Norwegian Society of Infectious Diseases and the Royal Society of Tropical Medicine and Hygiene, Oslo, 20 June 2008. *Transactions of the Royal Society of Tropical Medicine and Hygiene, 103*(4), 321–324. https://doi.org/10.1016/j.trstmh.2008.11.010 (accessed on 10th May 2025).

34. Bhattacharya, S. (Ed.) (2003). Public health in Calcutta. *Wellcome History, 22*, 1-24. http://www.wellcome.ac.uk/stellent/groups/corporatesite/@msh_publishing_group/documents/web_document/wtd006093.pdf (accessed on 10th May 2025).

35. Niu, Y. (2024). The polygenetic nature of K.D. Balmont's poetics and cultural traditions of ancient China. *Solov'evskie Issledovaniya*. https://www.semanticscholar.org/paper/ffa9596912c4ed58af432bd12fdc1179c8976939 (accessed on 10th May 2025).

36. Nogueira, A. S., Garcia, M. A. C., Silva, M. B. D., Costa, P. F. D., Frade, M. A. C., Salgado, C. G., & Barreto, J. G. (2024). Clofazimine-induced cutaneous hyperpigmentation as a source of stigma in the treatment of leprosy: A cross-sectional study. *Tropical medicine & international health : TM & IH, 29*(4), 327–333. https://doi.org/10.1111/tmi.13977(accessed on 10th May 2025).

37. Oliver, S. J. (2022). From Isolation to Inclusion: Embracing Local Perspectives in Examining the Treatment Model of Care for Aboriginal Persons Affected by Tuberculosis or Leprosy in the Kimberley Region, North Western Australia [Doctor of Philosophy (College of Medicine)]. The University of Notre Dame Australia. https://researchonline.nd.edu.au/theses/386(accessed on 10th May 2025).

38. Panahi, Y., Gorabi, A. M., Talaei, S., Beiraghdar, F., Akbarzadeh, A., Tarhriz, V., & Mellatyar, H. (2023). An overview on the treatments and prevention against COVID-19. *Virology journal, 20*(1), 23. https://doi.org/10.1186/s12985-023-01973-9 (accessed on 10th May 2025).

39. Patel, H., Pundkar, A., Shrivastava, S., Goyal, S., & Chandanwale, R. (2024). Navigating Foot Tuberculosis in a Leprosy Survivor: A Case Managed Solely With Medical Strategies. *Cureus, 16*(2), e53991. https://doi.org/10.7759/cureus.53991(accessed on 10th May 2025).

40. Prakoeswa, F., Maharani, F., Sari, W. A., & Risanti, E. D. (2025). Overcoming negative stigma towards leprosy patients. *Berkala Ilmu Kesehatan Kulit dan Kelamin*. https://www.semanticscholar.org/paper/92f2a909871ac23e96914ed1104049a1a2647367 (accessed on 10th May 2025).

41. Rahayu, T., Friska, D., Sopamena, Y., Menaldi, S. L., Gibran, K., Dadun, Ruwaida, I., & Irawati, Y. (2025). Validity and reliability of local endemic language version of the SARI Sigma Scale questionnaire for assessing stigma in leprosy patients. *Frontiers in public health, 12*, 1474745. https://doi.org/10.3389/fpubh.2024.1474745(accessed on 10th May 2025).

42. Mendrika Fifaliana Rakotoarisaona, Malalaniaina Andrianarison, Onivola Raharolahy, Fandresena Arilala Sendrasoa, Volatantely Ratovonjanahary, et al. (2023). Epidemiological and Clinical Features of Leprosy Reactions and Associated Risk Factors in Malagasy People from 2012 to 2021. International Journal of Clinical Dermatology, 6(1), 1-9. https://doi.org/10.11648/j.ijcd.20230601.11(accessed on 10th May 2025).

43. Rashidi, M., Pitton Rissardo, J., Byroju, V. V., Fornari Caprara, A. L., Rashidi, F., Prathiraja, O., Moharam, H., Elendu, C. C., Bahar, M., & Jayasinghe, M. (2025). Exploring the Neurological Manifestations of Leprosy: Clinical Insights and Implications. *Cureus, 17*(1), e77799. https://doi.org/10.7759/cureus.77799 (accessed on 10th May 2025).

44. Redington, W. (2019). The story of a village: A case study in strategic planning at Enyinndakurom, Ankaful, Central Region, Ghana. *Project Management Research and Practice*, 5 https://core.ac.uk/download/213631192.pdf (accessed on 10th May 2025).

45. Senyurek, G., Kavas, M., & Ulman, Y. (2021). Stigmatization, discrimination, violation of autonomy, and compromised confidentiality: A descriptive qualitative analysis of the lived experiences of people living with HIV in healthcare settings in Turkey. https://doi.org/10.21203/rs.3.rs-33490/v2(accessed on 10th May 2025).

46. Sharma, P., Kularatna, S., Abell, B., McPhail, S. M., & Senanayake, S. (2024). Preferences for Neurodevelopmental Follow-Up Care for Children: A Discrete Choice Experiment. *The patient, 17*(6), 645–662. https://doi.org/10.1007/s40271-024-00717-3 (accessed on 10th May 2025).

47. Shrivastava, K., Ray, S., Rathod, H., Wahegaonkar, A. L., Jadhav, S. L., Mahajan, A., S, J., Verma, P., Palal, D., & Sengupta, S. (2024). Transforming Lives: A Qualitative Study Seeking Insights Into Reconstructive Surgery for Leprosy Patients in Western Maharashtra. *Cureus*, *16*(9), e68416. https://doi.org/10.7759/cureus.68416(accessed on 10th May 2025).

48. Silva, M. J. A., Silva, C. S., Brasil, T. P., Alves, A. K., Dos Santos, E. C., Frota, C. C., Lima, K. V. B., & Lima, L. N. G. C. (2024). An update on leprosy immunopathogenesis: systematic review. *Frontiers in immunology*, *15*, 1416177. https://doi.org/10.3389/fimmu.2024.1416177(accessed on 10th May 2025).

49. Sleet, D. (2024). Injury prevention and public health. *Italian Journal of Public Health*. https://www.semanticscholar.org/paper/99212b4818c1fe105ba761163e24242326719a81 (accessed on 10th May 2025).

50. Srivastav, Y., Prajapati, A., Jaiswal, A., Yadav, S., Prajapati, A., & Madhaw, K. (2023). Overview of leprosy, including the diagnosis and current available treatments. *Journal of Innovations in Applied Pharmaceutical Science (JIAPS)*, *8*(3), 24-33. https://doi.org/10.37022/jiaps.v8i3.495(accessed on 10th May 2025).

51. Shafee Ullah, Ulhaq, F., Basit, A., Imtiaz, F., Noreen, A., Elahi, A., & Attiq-Ur-Rehman. (2024). HIV/AIDS Stigma and Discrimination in Pakistan: A Qualitative Study. *Indus Journal of Bioscience Research*, *2*(02), 531–540. https://doi.org/10.70749/ijbr.v2i02.219(accessed on 10th May 2025).

52. van Wijk, R., Raimundo, L., Nicala, D., Stakteas, Y., Cumbane, A., Muquingue, H., Cliff, J., van Brakel, W., & Muloliwa, A. M. (2024). Leprosy and lymphatic filariasis-related disability and psychosocial burden in northern Mozambique. *PLoS neglected tropical diseases*, *18*(8), e0012342. https://doi.org/10.1371/journal.pntd.0012342(accessed on 10th May 2025).

53. Veneziano, A., Franchin, M., Cervarolo, M. C., Monteleone, S., Ros, L., & Tozzi, M. (2025). Optimizing the life of vascular access during follow-up. *The Journal of cardiovascular surgery*, *66*(1), 26–29. https://doi.org/10.23736/S0021-9509.24.13263-6(accessed on 10th May 2025).

54. Visser MJ, KC EA, Sopamena Y, et al. Cultural Mechanisms of Leprosy-Related Stigma: A Gendered Analysis Using the What Matters Most Framework in Far-Western Nepal. *Qualitative Health Research*. 2025;0(0). doi:10.1177/10497323251318604(accessed on 10th May 2025).

55. Wujastyk, D. (2019). Iron Tonics: Tracing the Development from Classical to Iatrochemical Formulations in Ayurveda. (2019). *HIMALAYA: The Journal of the Association for Nepal and Himalayan Studies*, *39*(1), 74-90. https://doi.org/10.2218/himalaya.2019.7878 (accessed on 10th May 2025).

56. Zhang, K., Zhang, W., & Lu, H. (2025). Global Trends in the Incidence, Prevalence and Disability-Adjusted Life Years of Leprosy from 1990 to 2019: An Age-Period-Cohort Analysis Using the Global Burden of Disease Study 2019. *Clinical, cosmetic and investigational dermatology*, *18*, 883–898. https://doi.org/10.2147/CCID.S508600(accessed on 10th May 2025).

57. Zhu, F., & Wang, W. (2024). The Study of Tourist Experience in Historical and Cultural Towns Based on Online Texts: A Case Study of Gongtan Ancient Town. *Frontiers in Business, Economics and Management*, *15*(2), 309-314. https://doi.org/10.54097/0m81b407(accessed on 10th May 2025).

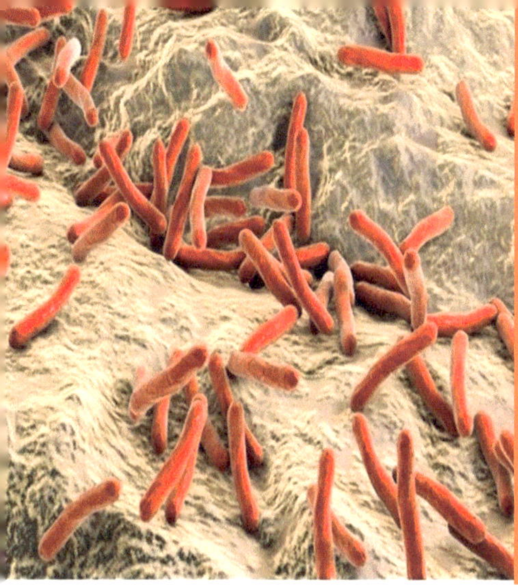

Chapter 2

PATHOPHYSIOLOGY AND IMMUNOLOGY OF LEPROSY

Contents

Introduction

Hansen's disease, or leprosy, is a long-lasting infection that mainly attacks the skin, the nerves on the edges, and even the lining of the upper airways. In many cases, even though we've seen progress with medicines and public health fixes, the disease still persists globally, especially in areas where healthcare is hard to come by. Its hidden beginning and slow, drawn-out progression mean that it's difficult to catch in its early stages, which in turn tends to lead to severe issues. To grasp what leprosy does, you do have to examine how *Mycobacterium leprae*, the microbe responsible for the whole thing—makes contact with our immune system. This give-and-take not only alters the way the symptoms present themselves but also affects how the disease progresses, reminding us just how critical our immune defenses play in keeping both infection and tissue destruction at bay. A brief survey of these host-pathogen dynamics lays the groundwork for further exploration into the complicated world of leprosy's underlying biology. To summarize, the course of leprosy is largely determined by how effectively our body resists *M. leprae*. On the positive side, there's the tuberculoid type, in which an effective cell-mediated immunity suppresses the bacteria and induces granuloma formation. On the negative side, there's the multibacillary—or lepromatous—type, in which an ineffective cell-mediated response allows the bacteria to grow, producing more severe skin eruptions. This division appears to boil down to variations in T-helper cell cues; generally, Th1-type responses dominate in the tuberculoid patients and Th2 cytokines such as IL-4, IL-5, and IL-10 in the lepromatous patients (Anggraeni et al., 2018). These adjustments to the immune system not only appear to determine the coarseness of the disease but contribute to the pattern of spread of the infection, as individuals with the multibacillary form are typically the principal reservoirs for the pathogen. In addition to the battle within the immune system, leprosy also disrupts body tissues in a manner that results in a combination of symptoms and complications. For instance, when the bacteria infect the nerves, it can lead to numbness and even deformities, seriously disrupting a person's everyday life. The entire scenario, the immediate bacterial attack combined with the body's occasional overaggressive defense maneuvers, conveys the unexpected character of the disease, in which the microbe and our own reactions determine the outcome. Current research into treatments that stimulate the immune system (such as applying agents to increase interferon-gamma production) holds the potential shiftto shift the balance in favor of clearing the infection in those more challenging multibacillary cases (Anggraeni et al., 2018). Excavating into such processes is important not only for creating improved therapies but also for coping with the types of complications that usually accompany leprosy and demonstrating how complex its biology is with our immune responses (Figure 2.1).

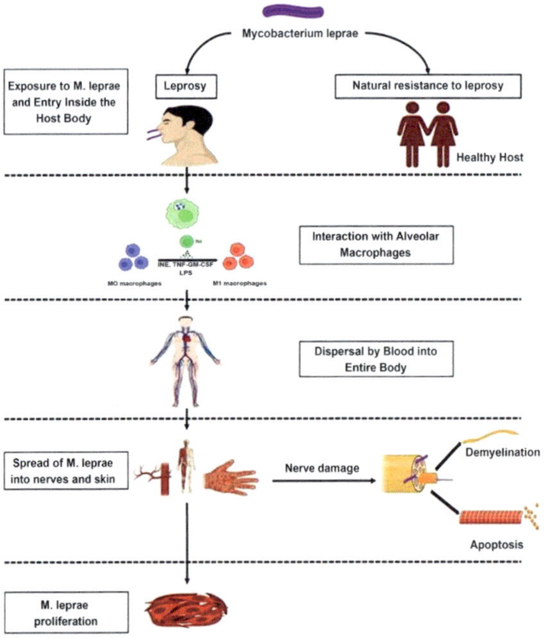

Figure 2.1. Schematic representation depicting the interaction between the host and *M. leprae*. (Biorender).

Source: Frontiers in Pharmacology. (2024). *Interaction Between Host and M. leprae.*

Definition of Leprosy

Leprosy, also known as Hansen's disease from the history books, is a chronic infection caused by the bacterium *Mycobacterium leprae*. It primarily affects the skin, peripheral nerves, regions of the respiratory tract, and even the eyes. Based on the way an individual's immune system responds, the symptoms can go haywire—sometimes appearing in the form of less severe, localized tuberculoid cases and at other times evolving into the extensive lepromatous type. Its slow, near-hidden onset and extended incubation period have a way of throwing early detection off, tending to allow the damage to accumulate before anyone intervenes. Essentially, gaining control of leprosy is about examining both the microbe itself and our body's response to it and determining that this is more than just an infection but a complex immunological puzzle in and of itself with its own array of complications. At the center of the progression of the disease, the immune response of the host takes center stage. Tuberculoid leprosy patients tend to have a robust cell-mediated response against *M. leprae*, which leads to more localized lesions and fewer bacteria. On the other hand, the people afflicted with what has been popularly known as multibacillary or lepromatous leprosy experience a poor cellular defense that permits the bacteria to advance far and wide, bringing about more sensational symptoms. Overall, this disruption of immune function is correlated with increased levels of Th2 cytokines such as IL-4, IL-5, and IL-10, a combination that has the effect of suppressing effective cell defense, while important Th1 cytokines, including interferon-gamma (IFN-γ), remain abnormally low. This cytokine signal imbalance underlies the entire complex picture of leprosy and the reason why certain individuals end up carrying high bacterial loads, nearly qualifying as natural reservoirs for the infection (Anggraeni et al., 2018). Identifying these immunological patterns, in the majority of instances, is the key to unlocking both the mechanics of the disease and its optimal treatment pathways. Leprosy is not merely a simple infection—after all, it's tightly married to the complex ballet between a pathogen and the immune response of the host. The clinical course depends on how the body detects and responds to *M. leprae* antigens; if the cell-mediated response is deficient, the bacteria are free to multiply, leading to skin lesions and nerve damage. Current research is even experimenting with additional therapies, like immune-stimulating supplements designed to increase IFN-γ levels among multibacillary patients, which may assist in maintaining control of the infection (Anggraeni et al., 2018). Recent scholarly endeavors, driven by both new findings and grant money explain leprosy's intricate pathophysiology, but there remains a well-documented need for more integrated approaches to diagnosis, treatment, and immune modification. Overall, this wider picture illustrates that controlling leprosy is more than fighting off an infection; it's more about managing a complex interplay of microbial stimuli and immune reactions.

2.1. Overview of Leprosy

Leprosy is known as a scary disease around the world, thanks in large part to its long history and societal impact—but if you want to know what's going on, you have to look at the microbe behind it and how it shows up in patients. This infection is caused by a slow-growing microbe called *Mycobacterium leprae* that tends to damage the skin, peripheral nerves, the lining inside the nose and throat, and even the eyes. Its long incubation period, often lasting several years, makes detecting it early tough. You can see leprosy in different ways: sometimes it appears as a milder version where the body's response is strong and only a few bacteria are present, and other times it comes as a more severe, widespread form where the immune system barely fights back. That range, with varied nerve damage and disabilities, reflects the many ways our immune systems react to the infection, and getting a grip on these trends is key to understanding both how the disease advances and how treatments can work overtime. At the cellular level, *M. leprae* sets off a complex interaction with our immune system that shapes the illness in surprising ways. The bacterium tends to zero in on Schwann cells—the cells that help insulate our nerves, and by disrupting them, it triggers demyelination and the nerve damage we typically see. There's an interesting split here too: on one hand, strong Th1 responses help corral the pathogen through active macrophages, while on the other, weaker Th2 responses just can't keep the bacteria in check. Along with that, our body's innate sensors, like pattern recognition receptors, play their part by altering inflammatory pathways and stimulating the adaptive immune response. Further, the fact that *M. leprae* can survive inside cells for such long periods—by dodging and even altering our own defenses—points to a clever, if frustrating, host-pathogen back-and-forth that makes the ultimate eradication of the disease a real challenge (Cedzy Mński et al., 2019). Recent work in immunology is starting to reveal fresh insights about leprosy that might line up with discoveries in other infections, hinting at new ways to treat it. Generally speaking, toll-like receptors (TLRs) have come up as key players in noticing and fighting off microbes in chronic infections; some evidence even hints that altering TLRs could change inflammatory cascades and help keep the bacteria under control, much like ideas seen in studies of other diseases where the body's immune response goes awry (Gillina et al., 2021). Small adjustments in these innate immune pathways could open up promising paths for treatment and possibly cut down on tissue damage. In the end, mixcombining what we learn from molecular immunology with what health professionals observe in the clinic seems essential in developing both new biomarkers and treatments that take care of the infection and manage its inflammatory side effects (Figure 2.2).

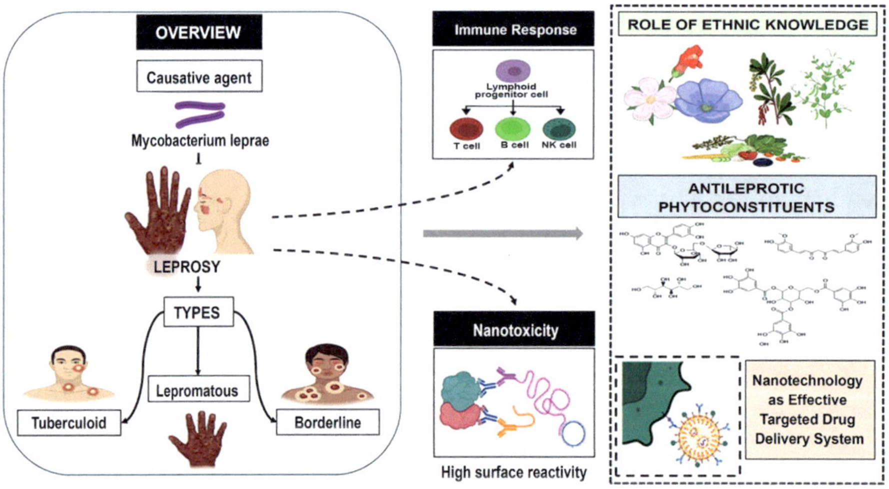

Figure 2.2. Overview of leprosy.

Source: Kimta N, Majdalawieh AF, Nasrallah GK, Puri S, Nepovimova E, Jomova K and Kuča K (2024) Leprosy: Comprehensive insights into pathology, immunology, and cutting-edge treatment strategies, integrating nanoparticles and ethnomedicinal plants. Front. Pharmacol. 15:1361641. doi: 10.3389/fphar.2024.1361641

2.1.1. Causative Agent: Mycobacterium leprae

Leprosy shows its complex clinical picture mostly because of its culprit, *Mycobacterium leprae*. This microbe isn't like other pathogens—it tends, in most cases, to settle into macrophages and Schwann cells, the very cells that help defend the body and keep nerves working properly. By sticking with these targets, it ends up causing the classic nerve damage and skin lesions we expect. Its tendency for persisting inside these cells, frankly, makes diagnosis complex and delays detecting the disease early. Traditional tests such as skin biopsies and bacilloscopy often miss early signs since they can be invasive and lack the needed sensitivity. Lately, though, mass spectrometry, which detects lipid markers directly from skin imprints, has shown promise as a rapid, noninvasive alternative—sometimes flagging infected individuals even before the typical symptoms appear (Lima et al., 2018). In short, *M. leprae* not only dodges immune defenses but also alters the lipid makeup of host cells in ways that stand out. Looking at its cell wall and metabolism, *M. leprae* plays with fire when it comes to interacting with our immune system.

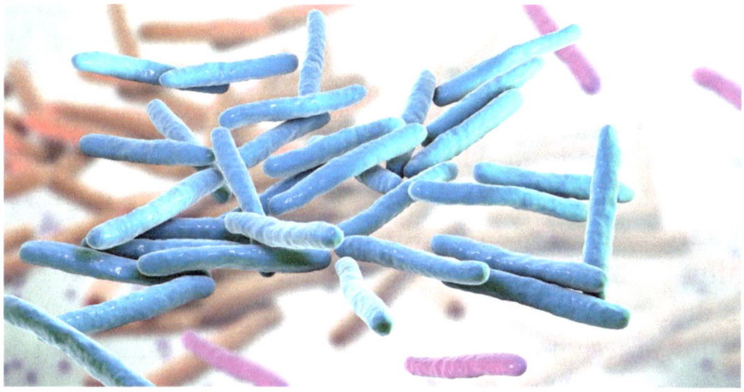

Figure 2.3. *Mycobacterium leprae* bacteria, the causative agent of Hansen's disease, also known as leprosy.

Source: University of Florida Epidemiology. (2023). *Mycobacterium leprae.*

The bacterium sports a complex, lipid-rich envelope—packed with unusual fatty acids like mycolic acids—that makes it acid-fast and tough when facing host attacks. Quite interestingly, these same lipids might mix with immune cells and decide cytokine production, subtly shifting immune responses. High-resolution lipidomic analyses have even found markers such as phthiocerol and other lipid signals in infected tissues; these act as hints of the disease's presence. By upsetting both the structural integrity and signal pathways in macrophages and Schwann cells, the bacterium ensures its survival and spread in unpredictable ways. This complex interplay accounts for the wide range of clinical forms seen in leprosy, from the milder paucibacillary to the more aggressive multibacillary cases—all corresponding to different immune reactions (Lima et al., 2018). It turns out that grasping these biochemical characterestics is key to developing therapies that hit the mark. On the immune side, *M. leprae* sets off a complicated interaction between bacterial trickery and our body's defenses. Generally speaking, the pathogen is pretty adept at interfering with cell-mediated immunity—a factor that, in many cases, largely determines the outcome of the disease. In multibacillary leprosy, for instance, the body shifts toward a Th2-type response, with higher levels of IL-4, IL-5, and IL-10, which then usually come at the expense of protective Th1 cytokines like IFN-γ. This kind of immunosuppressive environment lets the bacterium multiply more freely, leading to a high bacterial load and plenty of skin lesions that further spread the infection. Interestingly, recent clinical trials using adjunct therapies, like a bit of black seed extract supplementation, have hinted at the possibility of boosting IFN-γ production in these patients, perhaps reviving the Th1 response needed to clear the bacteria. To summarize, these findings remind us that *M. leprae* not only induces immune dysregulation but also becomes a potential target for smart immunomodulatory strategies in leprosy treatment (Figure 2.3).

2.1.2. Modes of Transmission

Understanding how microbes attack and move around communities begins with observing how they enter and go about. The case of leprosy is a good example—its transmission largely occurs due to people having close contact for extended periods, particularly when untreated individuals discharge droplets teeming with *Mycobacterium leprae*. This process is consistent with the microbe's preference for inhabiting the body's cooler regions and its consciously slow movement. The microbe can lie dormant within cells, evading the immune system long enough to persist; actually, that complicates things. There are also genetic variations between individuals that enter into the picture, influencing not only individual cases but general trends in local outbreaks. The combination of how virulent the microbe is and individual characteristics results in varying levels of spread, with close living quarters posing additional risk (Nadel, 2002). Not all leprosy transmission relies on direct, face-to-face contact. Some findings hint that the microbe might persist in soil or water, causing incidental exposure, even if we're still figuring out how important these routes are. In certain regions, armadillos have been mentioned as a potential link in the chain, stimulating us to think about leprosy's entire ecological picture. The persistence of the microbe is in part due to its peculiar biochemical loweractivities that allow it to remain viable outside the human body in certain circumstances (Cox, 1983). Such peculiarities complicate control efforts since disrupting the cycle of environmental or animal transmission isn't as simple as stopping direct transmission. For most situations, a mixed strategy that encompasses all these avenues is required, particularly in high-risk settings where close-contact matters converge with exposure to the environment or animals. Aside from the biological parts, how our immune systems respond is a big part of the picture—affecting both the dose of microbes required for infection and the likelihood of the disease continuing to spread. In general, individuals with robust cell-based immunity can keep *M. leprae* in check or eliminate it rapidly, decreasing the likelihood of future transmission. Conversely, individuals who have poorer defenses tend to be more likely to become latent carriers. Genetic differences that affect cytokine release and overall immune control account for why levels of transmission differ even among individuals with comparable exposure (Nadel, 2002). And let's not overlook, the fact that the incubation period is so long means some people may unknowingly pass along the microbe, which contaminates tracing cases. The virus's ability to evade detection and its slow replication only make it harder to catch it early. Overall, figuring out the immune terrain is important to de-mystifying how leprosy spreads and to informing public health efforts that target the right areas.

2.1.3. Global Prevalence and Demographics

Leprosy is an age-old illness that still damages public health in many parts of the world. Over 200,000 new cases emerge every year , and places like India, Brazil, and Indonesia shoulder much of that burden. Scarce healthcare, stubborn poverty, and delayed diagnosis fueled by social stigma all mix into a complex situation. Sometimes cultural practices and local geography blur the lines further. Overall, knowing where the cases occur matters, since the level of exposure and immune response can differ a lot from one population to another. Looking closer at who gets leprosy reveals some interesting twists. Kids under 15 in regions where the disease is common account for a sizable share of new cases, which generally points to ongoing transmission. Males appear more often in the statistics – but this might partly be due to unequal access to healthcare rather than any deep biological differences. In many cases, the varied data by age and gender shows a complex interaction between our natural defenses and what our surroundings throw at us. Studying these patterns, even with a bit of repetition, helps pinpoint the most at-risk groups and guides how we interpret the immune response that affects disease severity.

Everyday living conditions and socioeconomic factors also play a huge role in how leprosy takes hold and how our bodies fight back. Crowded homes, poor sanitation and even malnutrition all weaken our immune systems, making it easier for *Mycobacterium leprae* to tip the balance from a hidden infection to an active disease. Recent advances have been aiming at detecting early markers—biomarkers that might indicate infection before clear symptoms appear, which, in most cases, could transform early diagnosis and treatment. Some studies, for example, have tested parts of the bacterium (antigens, to be specific) to detect subclinical cases among close contacts (Rivoire et al., 2012). Adapting sensitive immuno-assays to local realities may very well boost efforts to monitor and control the spread, cut transmission, and reduce disabilities. To summarize, mixcombining social and economic insights with immunological research is key to tackling leprosy effectively (Figure 2.4).

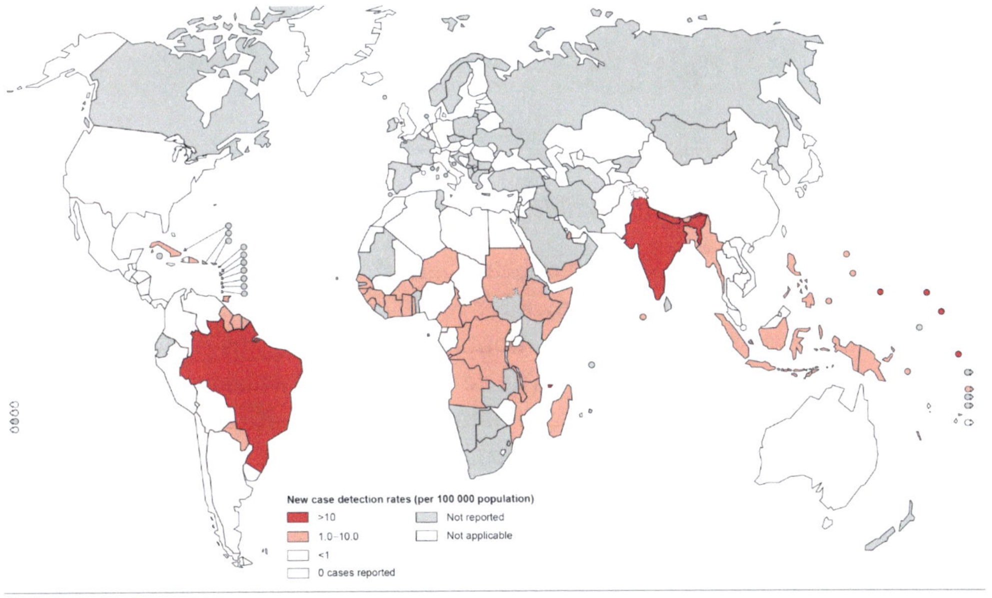

Figure 2.4. Global prevalence of leprosy.

Source: By World Health Organization - World Health Organization, CC BY-SA 3.0 igo, https://commons.wikimedia.org/w/index.php?curid=85056456

2.2. Pathophysiology of Leprosy

Leprosy shows itself in many ways. It starts out as a peculiar tug-of-war between the microbe, *Mycobacterium leprae*, and the body's own immune efforts. When the bacteria sneak into skin and nerves, they get busy multiplying, which in many cases stokes up everything from a pretty active cell-based defense to a rather weak immune reaction. In short, how the body reacts ends up shaping how severe the disease becomes. In more spread-out forms of the condition—what we often call multibacillary leprosy—the immune system just can't seem to get its act together. Generally speaking, the body misses generating a sharp, cellular response. This seems to happen because the cytokine balance tips in favor of a Th2-dominant pattern, with unusually high levels of IL-4, IL-5 and IL-10; these molecules end up putting the brakes on the protective Th1 response that's normally essential to keep the microbe in check. As a result, a high bacterial count builds up, turning patients into inadvertent reservoirs, which complicates the whole host-pathogen conversation and promotes a more chronic, persisting condition (Anggraeni et al., 2018).

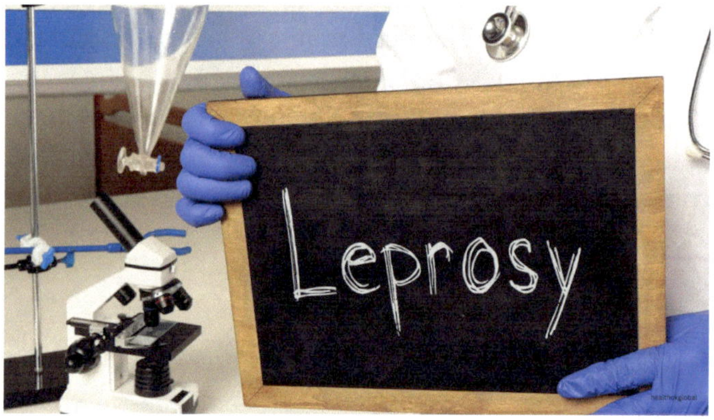

Figure 2.5. Pathophysiology of leprosy.

Source: Health OK Global. (n.d.). *Pathophysiology of Leprosy.*

Looking closer at the immune side of things, one finds that T-helper cell responses tell a big part of the story. The Th1 side, for instance, is known for releasing IFN-γ—a key that helps macrophages chase down and clear out *M. leprae*. Yet, in patients with lepromatous or multibacillary forms of leprosy, this Th1 activity tends to be blunted. The consequence? A weakened cellular defense gives the bacteria free rein to multiply, which in turn damages the formation of granulomas that would normally help encapsulate the infection. In most cases, research hints that stimulating the immune system to boost IFN-γ levels could help re-establish that missing defense. There's even some early evidence that supplements like black seed extracts, , with immunomodulatory properties, might boost IFN-γ production, thereby hopefully sharpening the cell-mediated response and leading to better outcomes for severe cases (Anggraeni et al., 2018). Beyond skin and nerves, the reach of leprosy can sometimes extend to internal organs, throwing in further complexity. For example, kidney involvement shows just how far immune dysfunction can go. Leprosy, which is grouped with other neglected tropical illnesses, may trigger kidney injury through processes like immune complex deposition and ongoing low-level inflammation. This, in turn, can cause significant damage to the organs. Understanding these complex, interwoven mechanisms is pretty crucial for catching complications early and managing them effectively. New work on biomarkers for detecting kidney injury in infectious diseases has, in many cases, opened up fresh avenues for detecting organ damage sooner highlighting that leprosy is a disease with both local and systemic consequences (Figure 2.5).

2.2.1. Mechanism of Infection

M. leprae initiates its attack in a rather subdued, near-hidden manner. When it infiltrates the body, it targets Schwann cells in peripheral nerves and skin macrophages. Its ruse is easy but effective—it grows slowly and resides within cells, evading those initial immune warning signs. In most instances, the bacterium sets up shop in cooler areas such as the skin and the nerves close to the body's surface. This clandestine lifestyle slowly erodes nerve tissues, which is why individuals eventually feel numbness and nerve damage; in general, this slow, behind-the-scenes process makes early detection and intervention a true challenge. One interesting twist in the infection process is the way *M. leprae* toys with the immune system. In more intense, multibacillary infections, the microbe prods the body into a kind of Th2 mode—this involves increased amounts of IL-4, IL-5, and IL-10, while vital factors as interferon-gamma (IFN-γ), which assist in clearing the bacteria, remain in short supply. Patients in such cases have high loads of bacteria and feature numerous skin lesions, and they usually turn them into unsuspecting reservoirs for transmitting the disease. Conversely, when the body is going full-on Th1, the disease remains more limited with fewer bacteria present. This complex game of immune responses quite literally illustrates how changing immune responses have a bearing on how leprosy appears and develops (da Lino et al., 2018). More recent research even suggests that *M. leprae*'s antics are not restricted to the skin and nerves. Under chronic immune activation, the infection could extend its influence on organs such as kidneys—occasionally causing renal issues, similar to that of other tropical conditions as well. It appears that the continuous immune reaction has the potential to cause damage within both glomerular and tubular parts of the kidney. In most instances, the knowledge of these additional effects would help to shed some light on the global influence of leprosy. There's also promising research into treatments that boost IFN-γ production—a move that may help restore effective immune control against the bacterium. To summarize, tying together these infection mechanisms with immune modulation strategies might pave the way for better treatment approaches in the future (Anggraeni et al., 2018; da Lino et al., 2018).

2.2.2. Clinical Manifestations and Symptoms

Leprosy often starts sneaking up on you with hardly noticeable changes. At first, a person might see patches on the skin that are either lighter or have a bit of redness, and these spots usually don't feel normal because the bacteria tend to interefere with the peripheral nerves. You'd notice the affected areas don't register touch, which is a sign that nerve damage is quietly setting in. In many cases, the nerves themselves get thicker—a clear sign that things are off, and this thickening can later bring on muscle weakness or, in bad situations, even muscle wasting. Generally speaking, how the disease shows up depends a lot on the body's immune response. One form, known as the localized tuberculoid type, usually shows strong cellular immunity that keeps the spread in check, while the lepromatous form sports more widespread skin lesions with lots of bacilli because the immune system isn't able to fight it as effectively. Sometimes, subtle systemic symptoms join the picture, hinting at a complex interplay between the microbe and the body's defenses. Beyond those skin and nerve changes, there are other complications that tend to emerge from inflammation and secondary infections. As nerve damage steadily worsens, the loss of protective feeling makes it easier for someone to accidentally hurt themselves, which can lead to trauma or even small ulcerations, especially on the hands and feet.

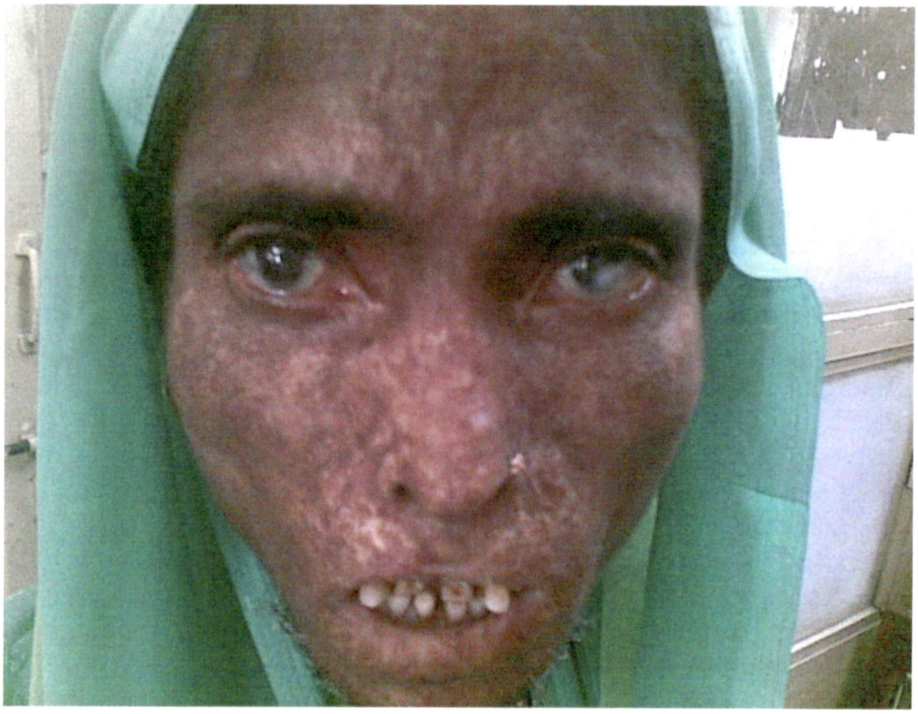

Figure 2.6. Chronic insensate patch due to leprosy infection.

Source: By Varsha.zadokar - I took this picture during my undergraduate programme at medical school., CC BY-SA 3.0, https://commons.wikimedia.org/w/index.php?curid=26822964Medication

Over time, those minor issues can turn into chronic wounds and even deformities that further impact quality of life. Then there are the so-called leprosy reactions. For example, Type 1 (reversal) or Type 2 (erythema nodosum leprosum) episodes can flare up unexpectedly, not only worsening nerve damage but also induceing systemic symptoms like fever, malaise and swollen lymph nodes. In most cases, these episodes might spill over into multiple organs—kidney problems have been mentioned in some studies, adding a layer of complexity to an already complex condition (da Lino et al., 2018). Being aware of these issues is important so treatment can keep up with the disease before irreversible harm sets in. Sometimes the fallout from leprosy isn't confined to the skin and nerves; it can also twist itself into broader immune problems, occasionally paving the way for things like amyloidosis or other secondary conditions. Although the bulk of leprosy's damage shows up on the skin and nerves, the constant inflammation and buildup of immune complexes can harm other parts of the body, including the gastrointestinal tract, which mirrors reports of similar issues in other infectious diseases (Chyntia et al., 2008). In most cases, noticing non-skin symptoms, like unexpected weight loss, tummy damages, or that persistent overall malaise—is key in advanced cases. To summarize, the way leprosy affects multiple systems underscores a pretty intricate bond between a persisting infection and an overactive or misdirected immune response, making management a real challenge. This complex overlap between ongoing infection, immune dysregulation and tissue damage calls for a treatment plan that brings together expertise from several fields, allowing a more rounded approach to care (Figure 2.6).

2.2.3. Stages of Disease Progression

Leprosy sets its silent stage with a long incubation period when the minuscule pathogen *Mycobacterium leprae* enters the host nearly undetected. It establishes a comfortable niche in the skin cells and peripheral nerves, all the while without any overt symptoms. This is the quiet period that can last for several years, which in most instances makes the initial diagnosis difficult. While, slowly, the immune defenses of the body begin to rouse and attempt to keep things under control, the initial response is capricious—now it keeps the bacteria relatively contained, and then it allows the infection to wander into other areas. That early, symptom-free period lays the groundwork, frequently deciding if the disease ends up as a lesser or a more serious variant later on. After that low-key start, the symptoms at last come through and the picture is transformed pretty dramatically. Individuals may experience bumpy patches on the skin, numbness, or even nerves that appear to enlarge without warning—obvious indicators of what is happening to Schwann cells and along peripheral nerve pathways. The vigor of the body's cell-mediated immune drive tends to influence what emerges: a robust response will tend towards a tuberculoid variety with only a few lesions, while a weak response may produce the more scattered, lepromatous form with issues widely distributed. More often than not, this disparity isn't merely a matter of how the disease appears, it also affects the danger of complications such as nerve damage and even longer-term disablement. In reality, keeping a close eye on these developments yields important information for designing treatment protocols that softly stimulate the immune system. When leprosy descends into its chronic phase under untreated conditions, it gets a lot worse. Bacterial growth goes on unchecked and recurrent inflammation ultimately leads to nerve degeneration that is frequently irreversible, resulting in loss of sensation, muscle weakness, and even deformity. By this stage, the immune system occasionally can become a bit unstable, precipitating abrupt type 1 or type 2 lepra reactions that merely worsen the damage to the nerve. Additional infections can also be added to the mix, imposing further health impediments. Each of these exacerbates the all-important need for early diagnosis and prompt immune modulation to prevent ongoing damage. Learning these phases in tandem provides us with a better idea of how the complex interaction between the pathogen and our body determines the long-term prognosis (Buckley et al., 2020).

2.3. Immune Response to Leprosy

The immune system's complex interplay is key in how leprosy shows up and progresses. When someone encounters *Mycobacterium leprae*, things can go one of two ways, basically, the immune reaction branches out unexpectedly. One branch leans on cell-driven defense while the other banks on antibodies. In cases where the body mounts a robust cell-based response, tuberculoid leprosy tends to appear, with Th1 cytokines like IFN-γ stepping in to keep the bacilli under control. On the other hand, if that cell response lags, the disease turns multibacillary or lepromatous; here, Th2 cytokines (including IL-4, IL-5, and IL-10) come to dominate, spurring a high bacillary load and widespread impact. Generally speaking, this imbalance helps explain why untreated multibacillary cases continue to spread the bacteria, underscoring the complex interaction between host and pathogen (Anggraeni et al., 2018). Scientists have recently been tinkering with ways to boost this lagging cellular response in multibacillary leprosy. One intriguing approach involves the use of black seed extract—yes, that natural remedy seems to help stimulate the immune system toward a Th1-focused reaction.

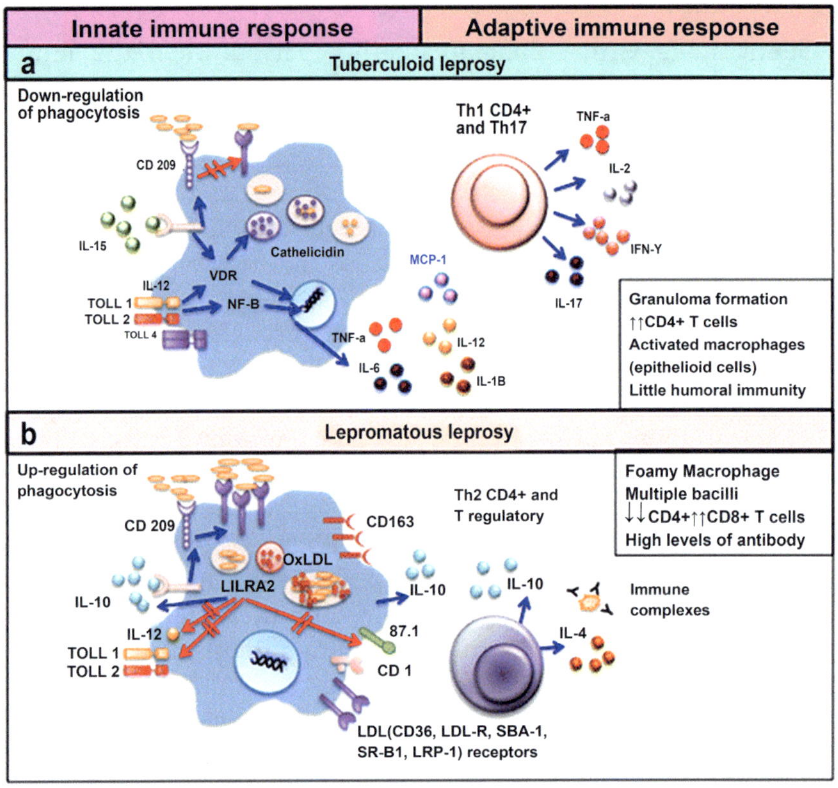

Figure 2.7. Immune response in the polar clinical forms of leprosy. (a) In tuberculoid leprosy (TT) patients, the innate immune response is activated by *M. leprae* through toll-like receptors 2/1 (TLR2/1). IL-15 stimulates the vitamin D-dependent antimicrobial program in macrophages and inhibits phagocytosis of mycobacteria. (b) In lepromatous leprosy (LL) patients, IL-4, IL-10, leukocyte immunoglobulin-like receptor subfamily A member 2 (LILRA2), and oxidized phospholipids inhibit TLR2/1-induced cytokine responses but preserve IL-10 release.

Source: Silva, C. A., et al. (2016). Immune Response in Leprosy. *Infectious Diseases of Poverty*, *5*(1), 1–12.

In one randomized controlled trial, patients treated with the extract alongside standard multidrug therapy saw a noticeable bump in IFN-γ levels. Since IFN-γ is pretty important for activating macrophages and cleaning up bacteria, these results point to a promising path where targeting immune pathways might improve outcomes. In most cases, mixcombining antimicrobial drugs with strategies tuning the immune response could open up a more integrative way to counter the lepromatous form of the disease (Anggraeni et al., 2018). Beyond these immune-driven paths, leprosy's effects go further afield in the body. Even organs like the kidneys get dragged into the damage. This happens because immune complex deposits and ongoing inflammation, induced by persisting bacillary antigens, start to wear down renal function. Recognizing these mechanisms is crucial; it lets clinicians spot the early signs of kidney involvement and step in sooner. There's also a buzz around biomarker research, which might lead to catching kidney damage earlier, thus helping prevent long-term complications. Tying together what we know about leprosy's systemic reach with its immune characterestics underscores the need for a whole-body approach in caring for affected individuals (Figure 2.7).

2.3.1. Innate Immune Response

When *Mycobacterium leprae* first meets a human, it induces off a swirl of immediate defense reactions that seem to set the stage for what leprosy might become. Once the bacillus slips into the skin and edges of peripheral nerves, pattern sensors, like those Toll-like receptors on macrophages and dendritic cells—spot its familiar molecular signature and promptly start gobbling it up while sending off inflammatory signals.

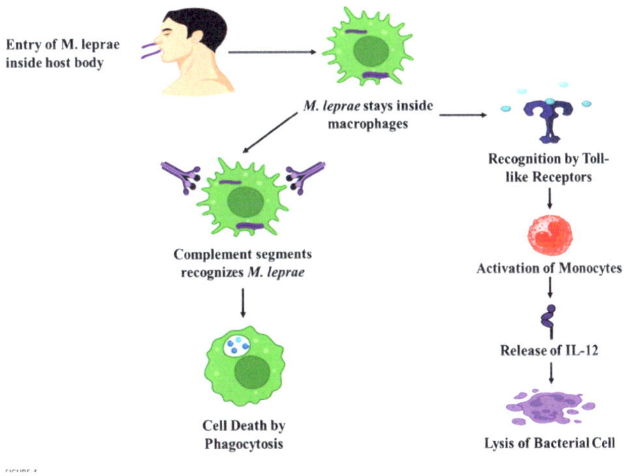

Figure 2.8. Diagrammatic representation of innate immune response against *M. leprae* (Biorender).

Source: Kimta N, Majdalawieh AF, Nasrallah GK, Puri S, Nepovimova E, Jomova K and Kuča K (2024) Leprosy: Comprehensive insights into pathology, immunology, and cutting-edge treatment strategies, integrating nanoparticles and ethnomedicinal plants. Front. Pharmacol. 15:1361641. doi: 10.3389/fphar.2024.1361641

This rapid-fire response is meant to block the spread of the bacteria by firing up antimicrobial processes and calling in extra immune cells, yet *M. leprae* has learned a few tricks to slip past these early safeguards. In most cases, whether the bacteria stay contained or pushes ahead into a more serious infection comes down to just how effective that initial immune scramble is, underlining the vital role of our innate defenses in the whole leprosy picture. Macrophages and natural killer cells take center stage as frontline fighters against the invader. When activated, macrophages churn out reactive nitrogen intermediates and release pro-inflammatory signals, tumor necrosis factor-alpha and interleukin-12, that try both to neutralize the pathogen and set up later, more refined immune responses. Natural killer cells join the fray too, their production of interferon-gamma giving macrophages an extra boost in microbe-killing power. Interestingly, recent studies have hinted those interventions, such as adding black seed extracts, might crank up that interferon-gamma release further, potentially enhancing the innate cellular burst seen in multibacillary leprosy patients (Anggraeni et al., 2018). This mix of innate immune activity and possible therapeutic alters paints a picture of how early internal responses might be modulated to manage the infection better. Diving a bit deeper, our own genetic makeup seems to weigh in on the battle, too. Variations in immune response genes—think those coding for human leukocyte antigens or killer-cell immunoglobulin-like receptors—can shift how well our innate system fends off *M. leprae*, ultimately affecting who might be more prone to severe forms of leprosy (Alves et al., 2018). These genetic differences influence how effectively antigens are presented and how natural killer cells operate, meaning that even tiny alters in our DNA can shape how quickly and robustly our body reacts to the invasion. Generally speaking, understanding these genetic nuances not only clarifies the wide array of leprosy symptoms seen in different patients, but also reinforces the idea that our early immune responses play a key role in the disease's unfolding drama (Figure 2.8).

2.3.2. Adaptive Immune Response

Leprosy shows us that the way our immune system works can change what happens during the disease. After *Mycobacterium leprae* gets into the body, the response sets in almost immediately. T-helper cells step in, but they don't all act the same—some become Th1 and others Th2. Generally speaking, a strong Th1 response, which releases cytokines like IFN-γ, sets off cell-based defenses that keep the bacteria in check; on the other hand, a more dominant Th2 reaction—marked by interleukins such as IL-4, IL-5, and IL-10—tends to hold back these cell responses, leaning instead toward antibody-based (humoral) action. This weaker cellular push may let the bacteria multiply, leading eventually to what we call the multibacillary or lepromatous form of the disease (Anggraeni et al., 2018).

It's important to note that figuring out how these two reaction routes balance out can be the difference between clearing the bacteria and letting them stick around. Our genes also have their say in this whole process, and it turns out that individual genetic differences can decide the immune response against *M. leprae*. Variations in genes, such as those for human leukocyte antigens (HLA), killer immunoglobulin-like receptors (KIR), and MHC class I chain-related proteins, alter how antigens are recognized and how signals bounce around in the immune system. In many cases, these alters decide whether someone mounts a more effective cell-based fight or develops a bias toward humoral responses, setting the stage for anything between the tuberculoid and lepromatous spectrums. Sometimes, these genetic characterestics also seem to intersect with immune reactions later on, like type 1 and type 2 complications that can make the disease even complex. Overall, digging into these genetic factors not only unpacks the immune misadventures of leprosy but might also light the way toward more personalized treatments (Alves et al., 2018). Some treatments are starting to look at this balance as a way to help patients, especially those with multibacillary leprosy, get better outcomes. For example, adding immunomodulatory agents to the mix seems to give a boost to IFN-γ production, in turn strengthening the Th1 response that's key for battling the bacteria. Experimental work shows that when patients get this kind of supplementation along with the usual multidrug therapy, they often end up with noticeably higher IFN-γ levels than those on a placebo. In many cases, this indicates that the extra support helps their cell-based immunity better handle the heavy bacterial load typical of multibacillary cases. These observations suggest that altering or even enhancing the body's natural adaptive immunity could play an important part in how we manage and treat leprosy (Anggraeni et al., 2018) (Figure 2.9).

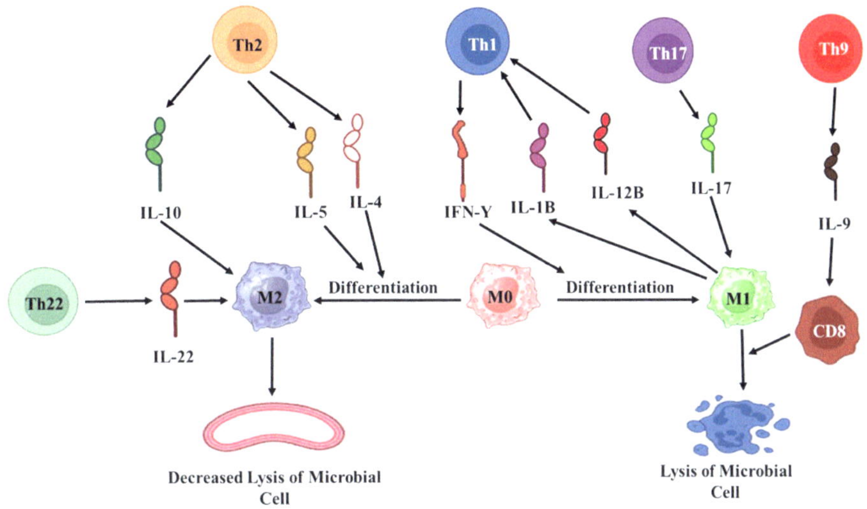

Figure 2.9. Diagrammatic representation of acquired immune response against *M. leprae* (Biorender).

Source: Kimta N, Majdalawieh AF, Nasrallah GK, Puri S, Nepovimova E, Jomova K and Kuča K (2024) Leprosy: Comprehensive insights into pathology, immunology, and cutting-edge treatment strategies, integrating nanoparticles and ethnomedicinal plants. Front. Pharmacol. 15:1361641. doi: 10.3389/fphar.2024.1361641

2.3.3. Role of Cytokines and Immune Mediators

Immune mediators mix together in ways that change how leprosy appears. In multibacillary cases, having an extra condition like chronic periodontal disease (CPD) seems to further increase both local and systemic cytokine levels, which in most cases impacts how the disease moves along and what reactions show up. For example, patients with both CPD and leprosy reactions usually have much lower serum IL-4 and IL-6, with a peculiar rise in IFN-γ. This pattern points to a lean toward the Th1 type response—a shift that may just make inflammation and tissue damage worse. You can also notice that reduced IL-4 matching with increased TNF-α gene expression, along with a positive link between IL-6 and IFN-γ, creates a complex cytokine network that seems to run immune regulation in the skin's microenvironment during these flare-ups (Cortela et al., 2018). Dendritic cells come into play as the conductors of the immune orchestra in leprosy, setting off both innate and adaptive responses by presenting antigens and sending out cytokine signals. Their activity isn't uniform though; in tuberculoid leprosy, a robust DC presence goes hand in hand with strong cellular immunity and good bacterial control, while in the lepromatous form, weaker DC activation is often linked to a diluted immune response and more widespread disease. Interestingly, new work with nano-formulations, like those potassium-incorporated titanium oxide (KTiOx) nanostructures—offers a fresh take on tuning DC function. These tiny constructs seem to boost phagocytic activity and stimulate the balance of inflammatory signals by increasing the activation of interferon-regulating factors, which are key for antiviral and antibacterial tasks; at the same time, they help moderate cytokine secretion in a rather dual-edged way, gearing the system up to fight off hidden intracellular bacteria such as *Mycobacterium leprae* (Barragan et al., 2023). Looking at the whole picture, shifting cytokines and other immune mediators is critical not just for defending the host but also for shaping how leprosy unfolds. The push-and-pull between pro-inflammatory and anti-inflammatory signals, like IFN-γ, TNF-α, IL-4, and IL-6—seems to govern granuloma formation, nerve injury, and overall tissue pathology. When patients face overlapping inflammatory conditions, these altered cytokine patterns show that our systemic immune control can affect local responses, underscoring the need for integrated treatment approaches. Further, the idea of using nanotechnologies to alter dendritic cells offers a promising avenue for immunotherapy, particularly in lepromatous leprosy where the usual immune kick-start just isn't enough. Taken together, these insights hint that cytokine networks and other immune messengers can serve as both markers and targets for therapy within leprosy's complicated immune landscape (Barragan et al., 2023; Cortela et al., 2018) (Figure 2.10).

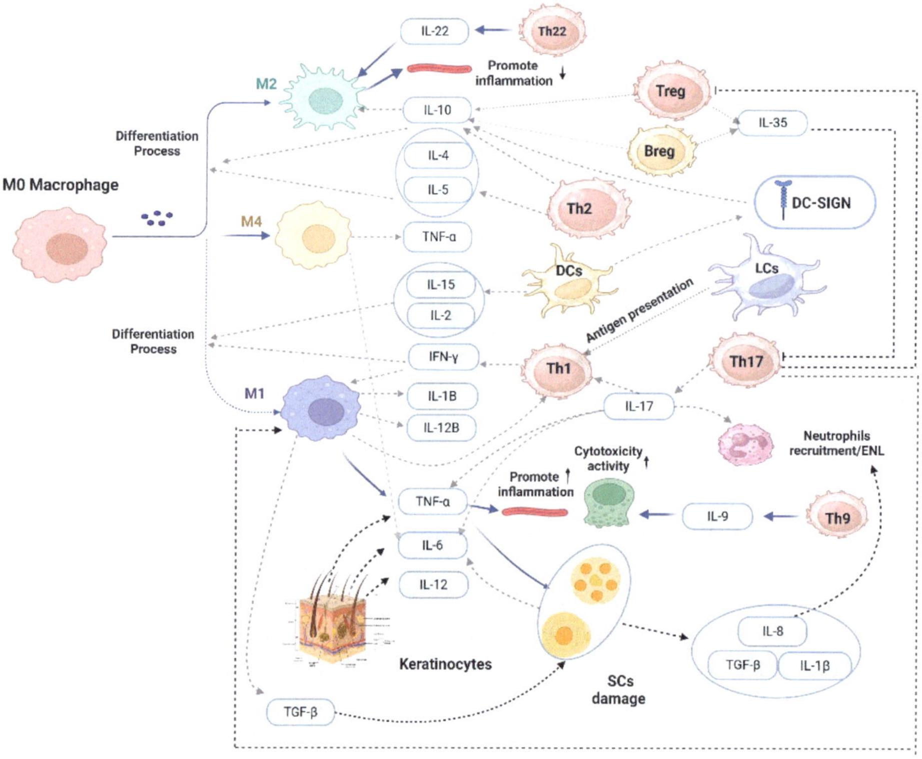

Figure 2.10. The secretion of cytokines during the immune response of leprosy infection.

Source: Kimta N, Majdalawieh AF, Nasrallah GK, Puri S, Nepovimova E, Jomova K and Kuča K (2024) Leprosy: Comprehensive insights into pathology, immunology, and cutting-edge treatment strategies, integrating nanoparticles and ethnomedicinal plants. Front. Pharmacol. 15:1361641. doi: 10.3389/fphar.2024.1361641

2.4. Challenges in Leprosy Management

Understanding leprosy has come a long way, yet handling it remains a complex business for clinicians. Early signs can be so subtle and varied that many patients slip through undetected—

approximately 30% might not show the usual light skin patches or lose sensation, making a timely diagnosis tough. The go-to tests—skin biopsies and bacilloscopy—are invasive and simply not sensitive enough, especially when the disease isn't heavy on bacteria. What's needed is a gentler, more accurate test that catches the illness early, cuts down its spread, and lets treatment start right away. Recent studies, like those checking for lipid markers with skin imprint mass spectrometry, seem to be pointing in a promising direction (Buckley et al., 2020). The immune system's role only complicates the issue further. Leprosy can look wildly different from one person to the next, ranging from a tuberculoid form, where a strong cell-driven response keeps the infection in check, to the lepromatous type, which shows a feeble immune reaction and lets bacteria run rampant. This flip-flop in immune behavior not only complicates treatment plans but also affects how well patients do overall. In many cases, immune reactions, like a Type 1 (reversal) or a Type 2 (erythema nodosum leprosum) response, induce sudden bouts of inflammation that, if left unchecked, can hurt nerves and lead to disability. These episodes point, generally speaking, to the need for close monitoring and more personalized immune treatments. MixCombining these immune insights into everyday practice still stands as one of the bigger hurdles in raising leprosy care. On top of that, social and healthcare system pitfalls deepen the challenge. Leprosy often strikes in poor, resource-limited areas where healthcare isn't readily available. The social stigma and discrimination connected up with the disease tend to keep people from seeking help when they need it, which in turns fuels its spread. Further, many healthcare facilities just don't have enough trained staff or the proper resources to consistently roll out multi-drug treatment—the backbone of leprosy therapy. Ultimately, addressing these socioeconomic factors and ensuring fair access to the latest diagnostic and treatment tools are vital steps. Merging biomedical innovation with smart public health strategies seems to be the most promising path for reducing the disease's overall burden and its social impact (Lima et al., 2018; Buckley et al., 2020).

2.4.1. Stigma and Social Implications

Leprosy still persists in many underprivileged groups, making daily life that much tougher. Advances in medicine might be impressive, but *Mycobacterium leprae* nestles inside cells so quietly that diagnosis often gets pushed back, leaving old, stubborn misconceptions in its wake. Outdated ideas—rooted in history and prejudice, often lead people to see nerve damage or skin changes not just as clinical issues but as signals of personal failing or risk of contagion. This warped view boosts social isolation, shrinks job prospects, and messes with mental well-being, all of which throw a wrench into public health work. Generally speaking, when you look at leprosy, you can't separate its biological side from the social environment in which it spreads and gets treated (Perez et al., 2024). People's fear of being shunned because of obvious signs, or just because of baseless fears about contagion, , often stops them from getting help or sticking to treatments. In many cases, this reluctance leads to later diagnoses and enables the disease to persist longer in communities, especially where resources are thin. Standard diagnostic tests can be pretty invasive and with early screening being scarce, the obstacles only multiply. Some newer ideas, like non-invasive tests that use lipid markers, might not only ease the clinical load but also help ease some of the heavy social fallout by getting treatment started sooner (Lima et al., 2018). The effects of leprosy ripple out far beyond the individual. Families and whole communities often bear the economic and emotional brunt of it all—social shunning can mean losing touch with friends and job opportunities, which in turn deepens cycles of poverty and generally lowers quality of life. When stigma creeps in, community unity suffers and effective health measures become harder to pull off. Tackling this issue means combining on-the-ground education, mental support, and active community engagement with modern medical advances. Only by combining our understanding of body processes with everyday social realities can we hope to break the cycle of transmission and improve care. This kind of broad, if sometimes a bit unefficient, approach is crucial for stopping neglected diseases in their tracks (Perez et al., 2024) (Figure 2.11).

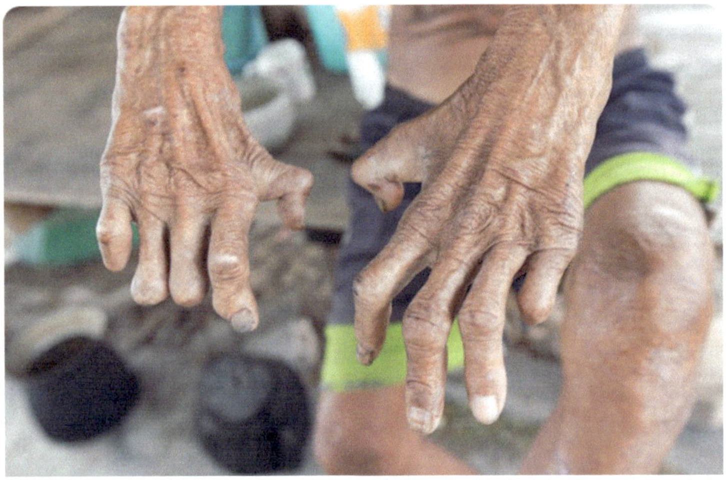

Figure 2.11. The stigma and social implications.

Source: Kon, K. (2017). *Hand Injuries from Leprosy*. News-Medical.net.

2.4.2. Drug Resistance Issues

Mycobacterium leprae's interactions with its host's immune responses shape how leprosy shows up in patients and make treatment a bit of a maze. The bacterium, for instance, tends to persist in host cells, which isn't something we see with many infections, and this shady behavior can throw a wrench in our efforts to deal with drug resistance. Patients with the multibacillary form, who generally end up with high bacterial counts, might unwittingly offer a refuge for resistant strains. The way Th1 and Th2 responses sort of swing back and forth influences how well the bacteria get cleared Further, an immunosuppressive setting in some individuals might even let those pathogenic resistant bacilli thrive. In most cases, mutations in *M. leprae* that interefere with rifampicin, dapsone, and clofazimine performance have turned into a pretty big hurdle for our standard multi-drug treatments, meaning ongoing monitoring and new drug ideas remain a must (Fr LARóes et al., 2022). Drug resistance in leprosy is, frankly, a complex issue. There aren't many reliable markers available for catching resistance early, and the bacterium's slow replication—coupled with the fact that we don't have a solid *in vitro* culture system—makes quick testing almost impossible. This delay, along with a limited grasp of how immunological processes kick off resistance, means treatment alters come too late sometimes. It appears that host-related factors might even alter drug metabolism or alter bacterial sensitivity, further complicating the issue. When resistance mutations hit the genes connected to antibiotic targets, treatment efficacy takes a nosedive, resulting in persisting infections and higher relapse risks, which not only complicate individual care but also keep transmission chains alive. Clearly, mixcombining immunological insights with molecular diagnostics is a critical move if we're going to outsmart drug-resistant leprosy and push for better outcomes (Fr LARóes et al.,

2022). Looking at other infectious diseases like COVID-19, one can see some interesting, albeit not entirely straightforward, immunological parallels that might light the way for leprosy drug resistance strategies. For example, toll-like receptor 9 (TLR9) has been linked to shaping immune responses and controlling inflammation in various conditions. Generally speaking, steering TLR9 activity could serve a double purpose: it might enhance the host's defense while at the same time cutting down on harmful inflammation that can lower treatment effectiveness. Given that immunomodulatory agents impacting TLR9 have shown promise as adjunct treatments in other infections, it's worth exploring if similar approaches could back up antibiotic regimens in leprosy. Such strategies could help maintain drug sensitivity and reduce relapse chances, even if the approach still feels a bit emergent. In most cases, this integrated immune-antibiotic approach could offer a new angle on overcoming the present challenges with drug-resistant leprosy (Fr LARóes et al., 2022).

2.4.3. Access to Healthcare and Resources

Barriers to getting proper healthcare play a big role in how leprosy shows up and spreads, especially in areas where poverty is widespread. Leprosy, which tends to hide inside cells, needs to be detected fast and treated continuously to keep nasty complications at bay. In most low-resource settings, however, vital diagnostic tools and tailored treatments are in short supply, which ends up hampering care. At the same time, basic healthcare systems, often lacking enough skilled staff and solid lab facilities—make it harder to spot cases early on, and that, in turn, lets the disease keep spreading. On top of that, stigma and social isolation almost always discourage people from seeking help as soon as they should, further complicating control efforts. All this shows how closely biological challenges and social hurdles mix together to affect individual care and broader public health outcomes (Perez et al., 2024). In areas hit hard by neglected tropical diseases, the mix of poverty, poor sanitation, and shaky healthcare access makes handling leprosy even complex. People in these tough-to-reach communities often face hurdles like long distances from health centers and steep transportation costs, which means they rarely take advantage of available services. Sometimes, there isn't enough clear public health education, so symptoms end up being misunderstood or noticed too late, delaying early treatment. It seems that all these challenges call for a more joined-up approach—one that boosts local infrastructure, raises community awareness, and sharpens the health system's response. Recognizing that these constraints are layered and complex is pretty key to crafting strategies that work in settings with few resources (Rodriguez-Morales, 2019).

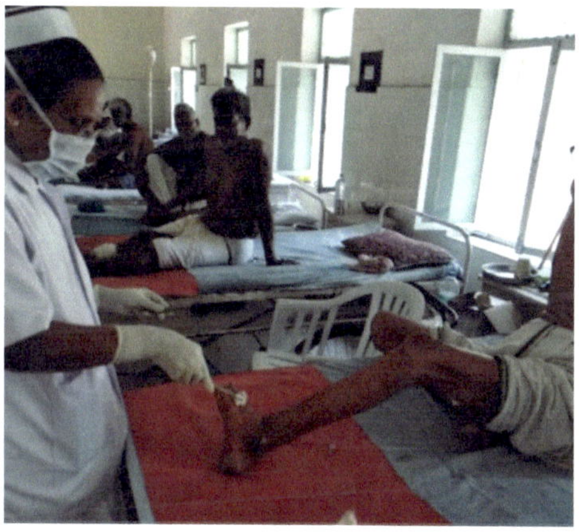

Figure 2.12. The access to healthcare and resources.

Source: The Leprosy Mission Trust India. (2023). *Access to Healthcare for People with Leprosy.*

On a wider scale, global efforts to fight leprosy stress the need to upgrade healthcare systems and spread resources in a fair way. Training health workers, so they can spot both the immune and pathological signals of the disease, helps catch it sooner and cuts down on misdiagnoses with other skin problems.

Prioritizing access to multidrug therapy paired with supportive care is crucial to stop the disease from progressing and to reduce the disabilities it can cause. Additionally, throwing in some psychosocial , —albeit in modest doses, can ease the stigma that sometimes keeps patients from sticking with treatment. Merging solid biomedical actions with an understanding of social issues, then, lays the groundwork for sustainable leprosy control, making it clear that better healthcare access is vital for breaking transmission and lessening the overall disease burden (Perez et al., 2024; Rodriguez-Morales, 2019) (Figure 2.12).

A CLOSER LOOK

GENETICS OF LEPROSY

Leprosy, like other infectious diseases, was widely accepted as hereditary in the pre-microbiological era. The revolutionary finding of a microorganism—originally named Bacillus leprae—in lesions of leprosy-affected individuals led Gerhard H. Armauer Hansen to fiercely refute the belief that leprosy was inherited. Today, scientists have clearly shown that exposure to *M. leprae* is necessary but not sufficient to explain leprosy occurrence, and several genes and genomic regions have been implicated in the complex genetic mechanism controlling host susceptibility to leprosy at different stages of the disease (Figure 2.13).

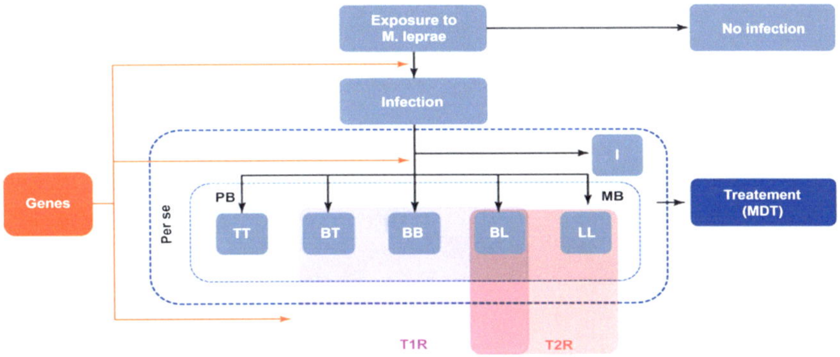

Figure 2.13. Schematic representation of the clinical classification spectrum of leprosy.

Source: Springer Nature. (n.d.). *Clinical Classification Spectrum of Leprosy.*

The complete sequence of the *M. leprae* genome was first published in the early 2000s. Compared to *M. tuberculosis*, the *M. leprae* genome shows strong reductive evolution as the bacteria specialized as an obligatory intracellular parasite in humans. Since then, whole genome analysis has provided insights about several aspects of leprosy, including the history of the disease. For example, in 2018, genome sequences of 10 *M. leprae* DNA samples obtained from the remains of medieval Europeans produced a snapshot of the last 1500 years of leprosy history in the European continent. *M. leprae* from four distinct phylogenetic branches were found among the 10 samples, some matching modern strains from different locations around the world. This study highlights the diversity of *M. leprae* strains in medieval Europe, and the authors proposed new models for leprosy dissemination: (i) the introduction of strains from different parts of the world into Europe, which may have happened before the medieval era; or (ii) the onset of leprosy occurred in Western Eurasia or in Europe, and not in western Africa, as previously proposed.

Regarding leprosy pathogenesis, bacterial genomics also identified a novel mycobacterial species named *M. lepromatosis*, a rare mycobacterium that apparently causes a distinct form of leprosy and is mainly found in Central America.

Comparative analysis of *M. leprae* isolates from different parts of the world confirmed the conserved nature of its genome. The low variability of the *M. leprae* genome suggests that the wide variety of responses observed upon exposure to the pathogen is largely controlled by host genetic factors. The hypothesis has been reinforced by observations such as familial aggregation of cases, a higher concorinteraction rate of leprosy phenotypes in monozygotic as compared to dizygotic twin pairs, and the presence of a strong major gene effect controlling leprosy, as demonstrated by complex segregation analysis. Although powerful to detect the existence of a genetic component controlling a specific trait, these observational studies do not provide any information about the identity of the genes or the nature of the genetic variants underlying the identified effect; for that, molecular studies are necessary

SUMMARY

Mycobacterium leprae's interaction with the host immune system molds the way leprosy shows up. In many cases, a slip in our immune defenses lets the microbe hang around and multiply, which often ends up causing the heavy, multibacillary version with widespread skin spots and nerve damages. When our Th1 defense sets in stronger, though, the infection tends to be more on the milder side—a paucibacillary form that stays more contained. There are even emerging ideas, like using black seed extracts to boost IFN-γ production—that hint at extra ways to shore up our natural barriers (Anggraeni et al., 2018). This fresh perspective gently stimulates us to mix these immune-targeting alters into our old multidrug routines, aiming to fix the deeper issues behind the disease. Detecting leprosy fast is key for good management and to curtail its spread. Traditional tests, which lean heavily on invasive skin biopsies and bacilloscopy, sometimes miss early or unusual cases because of limited sensitivity. Lately, though, researchers have been exploring a new trick: noninvasive skin imprinting to pick up lipidomic biomarkers combined with high-resolution mass spectrometry. This approach often catches the infection quickly—even in individuals who don't show classic signs, paving the way for prompt treatment (Lima et al., 2018). In most cases, these diagnostic advances could help bridge the gap by reducing delays and enabling a smoother fight against the disease. To wrap it all up, the way leprosy unfolds depends a lot on how strong our immune responses are. Digging into its immunology and embracing new diagnostic tricks not only broadens our understanding but also shifts us from focusing solely on killing bacteria to restoring immune balance. Testing out immunomodulatory adjuncts, like those black seed derivatives, along with cutting-edge lipidomic methods, might boost both patient care and public health outcomes. This kind of whole-picture approach promises not only to ease the heavy toll for patients but also to slow down transmission—pushing global efforts closer to effective leprosy control and, eventually, eradication (Anggraeni et al., 2018; Lima et al., 2018).

When looking into infectious diseases, you quickly notice that you have to study both the microbe itself and how our bodies react. Take leprosy, for example—*Mycobacterium leprae* tends to attack nerves and skin, resulting in a range of clinical pictures that depend on how the immune system answers the call. The microbe's tendency for invading Schwann cells disrupts normal nerve signals and induces a kind of persisting inflammation. Generally speaking, whether the disease turns out mild or severe hinges on the immune response: a strong Th1 response usually holds the infection in check, leading to tuberculoid leprosy, while a shift toward a Th2 response often shows up as a more spread-out, lepromatous form. In most cases, this shift in immunity underlines leprosy's double-sided nature—it's as much about the infection as it is about how the body fights it. Early in *M. leprae* infection, our innate defenses jump into action, with macrophages eating up the bacteria and setting off inflammation. Recent findings suggest that these cells aren't simply sitting back; they instead adjust themselves into a more aggressive, proinflammatory state that's key to stopping the bacteria from multiplying. This adaptability—a kind of macrophage plasticity—is central in both clearing the microbe and, unfortunately, in sometimes causing tissue damage. For instance, the way tumor necrosis factor (TNF) signaling stimulates macrophages to undergo apoptosis highlights how pivotal early, innate responses are in managing disease progression and keeping our tissues intact. These insights fit into wider models of immunotherapy, showing that innate cells often directly help clear pathogens without waiting for the adaptive system to catch up (Mart et al., 2024). Looking at leprosy as a whole, it's also important to factor in environmental and animal aspects that twist contagion dynamics. Even though *M. leprae* mainly bothers humans, animal reservoirs, like armadillos and other organisms, add an extra layer of challenge for eradication efforts. Further, other skin infections caused by similar bacteria reveal the ever-changing hurdles in managing these cutaneous diseases and understanding their immune interactions (Chase et al, 2023). All this puts the spotlight on leprosy's multifaceted nature, where aspects like bacterial invasion, shifting immune responses, and broader ecological factors together demand a thorough approach when it comes to diagnosis, treatment, and public health measures.

KEY TERMS FROM THIS CHAPTER

Bacterial loads
Chronic infections
Host-pathogen
Immune reactions
Immunological patterns
Malnutrition
Cell-mediated response
Healthcare
Immune modification
Immune response
Interferon-gamma
Mass spectrometry

References

1. Chyntia Olivia MJ*, Tito Ardi*, Evy Yunihastuti**, Ari Fahrial Syam***, Murdani Abdullah*** (2008). *Intractable Diarrhea Due to Secondary Gastrointestinal Amyloidosis in a Patient with History of Leprosy.* The Indonesian Journal of Gastroenterology, Hepatology, and Digestive Endoscopy; Volume 9, Number 1, April 2008. https://media.neliti.com/media/publications/66279-EN-intractable-diarrhea-due-to-secondary-ga.pdf (accessed on 10th May 2025).
2. Vicentin Alves H, Tiaki Tiyo B, Maria Sell A, Eliete Laguila Visentainer J. Immunogenetics of MHC and KIR in the Leprosy [Internet]. Hansen's Disease - The Forgotten and Neglected Disease. IntechOpen; 2019. Available from: http://dx.doi.org/10.5772/intechopen.75253f (accessed on 10th May 2025).
3. Anggraeni, P., Himbawani, M., Susanto, R. S. D., Widayati, S., et al. (2018). *Effects of Black Seeds Extracts Supplementation on IFN-γ Level of Multibacillary Leprosy Patients Receiving WHO-MDT.* https://core.ac.uk/download/234033649.pdf (accessed on 10th May 2025).
4. Barragan, J., Cervantes, J., Kositangool, P., Warren, J., et al. (2023). *Potassium-Incorporated Titanium Oxide Nanoparticles Modulate Human Dendritic Cell Immune Response to Mycobacterium leprae.* https://core.ac.uk/download/598023287.pdf (accessed on 10th May 2025).
5. Bezemer, G. F. G., & Garssen, J. (2021). TLR9 and COVID-19: A Multidisciplinary Theory of a Multifaceted Therapeutic Target. *Frontiers in pharmacology*, *11*, 601685. https://doi.org/10.3389/fphar.2020.601685 (accessed on 10th May 2025).
6. WITEK, Aleksandra, PARYS, Jakub, MIKOSIŃSKA, Agnieszka, KAŹMIERCZAK, Martyna, MOSSAKOWSKI, Maciej, KAŁUZIAK, Patrycja, JAJCZAK, Marta, LITWIN, Mateusz, JESIONEK, Stanisław and WITEK, RAfał. Vitiligo Review: etiopathogenesis, diagnosis and treatment. *Quality in Sport*. Online. 13 January 2025. Vol. 37, p. 57367. DOI 10.12775/QS.2025.37.57367. (accessed on 10th May 2025).
7. Buckley, H. R., Domett, K., Higham, C., Higham, T., et al. (2020). Two probable cases of infection with *Treponema pallidum* during the Neolithic period in Northern Vietnam (~2000–1500 B.C.). *Bioarchaeology International, 4*(1), 15–36. https://core.ac.uk/download/351177968.pdf (accessed on 10th May 2025).
8. Cedzyński, M., Thielens, N. M., Mollnes, T. E., & Vorup-Jensen, T. (2019). Editorial: The role of complement in health and disease. *Frontiers in Immunology*, *10*. https://doi.org/10.3389/fimmu.2019.01869 (accessed on 10th May 2025).
9. Perez, R. L., Chase, J., & Tanner, R. (2024). Shared challenges to the control of complex intracellular neglected pathogens. *Frontiers in public health*, *12*, 1423420. https://doi.org/10.3389/fpubh.2024.1423420(accessed on 10th May 2025).
10. Cortela, D. C. B., Ignotti, E., Nogueira, M. R. S., Pereira, M. C., et al. (2018). *Inflammatory Cytokines in Leprosy Reactions and Periodontal Diseases.* https://core.ac.uk/download/268295011.pdf (accessed on 10th May 2025).
11. Cox, F. (1983). Handbook of medical parasitology. V. Zaman and Loh Ah Keong. 218 pages. ISBN 0 86792 000 9. ADIS Health Science Press, New York, 1982. £17.00. *Parasitology*, *87*, 536–537. https://www.semanticscholar.org/paper/8efdeb2a75fc8348e82209571989217488b6268a (accessed on 10th May 2025).

12. Bezerra da Silva Junior G, Amélia Reis Jereissati A, Karoline Medina Neri A, Oliveira da Costa Lino D, Gomes Ramalho de Oliveira J, De Francesco Daher E. Neglected Tropical Diseases with an Impact on Kidney Function [Internet]. Current Topics in Tropical Emerging Diseases and Travel Medicine. IntechOpen; 2018. Available from: http://dx.doi.org/10.5772/intechopen.78981 (accessed on 10th May 2025).
13. Fróes, L. A. R., Sotto, M. N., & Trindade, M. Â. B. (2022). Leprosy: Clinical and immunopathological characteristics. *Anais Brasileiros de Dermatologia*, *97*, 338–347. https://doi.org/10.1016/j.abd.2021.08.006 (accessed on 10th May 2025).
14. Lima, E. de O. (2018). *Innovation in Leprosy Diagnosis: Potential Non-Invasive Method Associated to High Resolution Mass Spectrometry. https://core.ac.uk/download/296880362.pdf* (accessed on 10th May 2025).
15. Martínez-López, M. F., de Almeida, C. R., Fontes, M., Mendes, R. V., Kaufmann, S. H. E., & Fior, R. (2024). Macrophages drive the earliest anti-tumoral response to BCG therapy by directly killing bladder cancer through TNF signaling. *bioRxiv (Cold Spring Harbor Laboratory)*. https://doi.org/10.1101/2024.01.05.574391 (accessed on 10th May 2025).
16. J. Rodriguez-Morales, A. (Ed.). (2019). Current Topics in Neglected Tropical Diseases. IntechOpen. doi: 10.5772/intechopen.73918 (accessed on 10th May 2025).
17. Nadel S. (2002). Helping to understand studies examining genetic susceptibility to sepsis. *Clinical and experimental immunology*, *127*(2), 191–192. https://doi.org/10.1046/j.1365-2249.2002.01781.x (accessed on 10th May 2025).
18. Rivoire, B. L. (2012). *Development and Evaluation of New Leprosy Skin Test Antigens as Diagnostic Tools*. https://core.ac.uk/download/354378292.pdf (accessed on 10th May 2025).

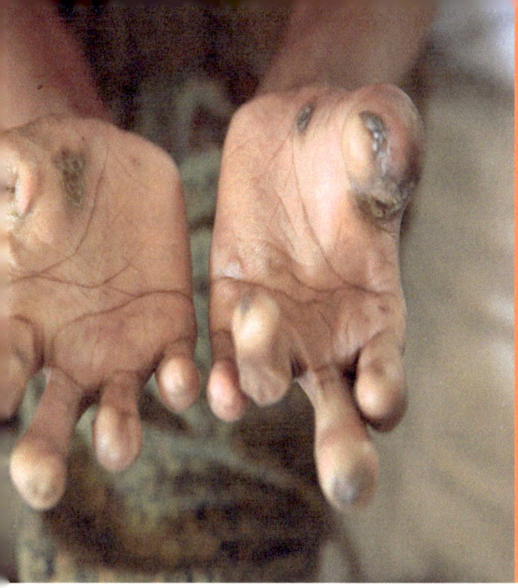

Chapter 3

CLASSIFICATION OF LEPROSY

Contents

Introduction

Leprosy remains a stubborn health problem in many parts of the world. Caused by *Mycobacterium leprae*, it stubbornly challenges public health despite modern tests and treatments. The disease can show up as anything from a minor skin blemish to severe nerve damage, a reflection of the complex interplay between the microbe and the body's immune response. This complex mix pushed experts to create different systems for sorting leprosy to diagnose and treat it more effectively. Accurate classification isn't just key for treating patients—it also helps in tracking the disease across communities. Misdiagnosis still pops up in regions where the disease is common, influenced by factors like gender, age, and the way symptoms present themselves, which clearly signals the need for better frameworks (Ignotti et al., 2020). Understanding how leprosy spreads and how it behaves overall is pretty crucial when coming up with control strategies. Research looking at pediatric cases, for instance, reveals that kids generally show milder symptoms, with nerve involvement being relatively rare, which suggests that close, long-term contact might be required for transmission. In many cases, the fact that youngsters often fall into the less severe, paucibacillary category over the multibacillary type points to differences in immune response. These small yet important differences mean that any system used to classify the disease needs to be adaptable enough to account for varying levels of severity and the body's response (Kattan et al., 2006). The shifting scene of leprosy classification proves that we need methods that can handle diagnostic challenges and fit different global resource settings. The Ridley-Jopling system, for example, takes a deep dive into the disease by using clinical, histopathological, and immunological signals, ranging from tuberculoid to lepromatous forms, so doctors can better gauge disease progression and tailor treatments. However, the WHO's operational approach pares things down into two groups, paucibacillary and multibacillary, for practical multidrug therapy decisions. In most cases, these frameworks try to balance in-depth clinical insight with real-world practicality, all aimed at reducing misdiagnosis and bettering patient outcomes around the globe (Ignotti et al., 2020) (Figure 3.1).

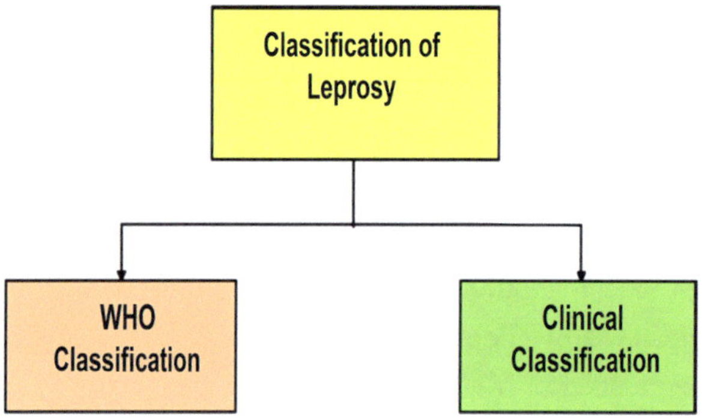

Figure 3.1. Classification of leprosy.

Source: Studocu. (n.d.). *Document thumbnail image.* https://website-assets.studocu.com/img/document_thumbnails/198452f4c77011f86b51c042e3455594/thumb_1200_927.png.

3.1. Ridley-Jopling Classification: An Overview

Leprosy is pretty complex, and trying to figure it out meant we needed a more layered way to sort its many faces. The Ridley-Jopling method jumps in by looking closely at immune responses—it breaks the disease into five parts: tuberculoid (TT), borderline tuberculoid (BT), borderline borderline (BB), borderline lepromatous (BL), and lepromatous (LL). Instead of neat, separate boxes, this system sees leprosy as falling along a spectrum, where the body's reaction to *Mycobacterium leprae* steers what you end up seeing. Generally speaking, when someone's cell-based immunity is strong, they often show milder forms like TT; if the immune response is weak, the disease tends to shift toward the more severe multibacillary LL type. This gradual shift even gives doctors useful hints about how the bacterial load connects with overall immune health, making the whole approach key for understanding the disease's pathogenesis and for shaping treatment plans based on each patient's profile (Hambridge, 2024). At the heart of this approach is the fusion of visible symptoms with what the immune system is doing. Skin biopsies, for instance, remain the top method—revealing granulomas and bacterial clusters that line up with what we'd expect from each category. Still, the real-life picture isn't always crystal clear; sometimes features overlap enough that extra tests become necessary. In most cases, recent advances have offered less invasive options, like checking alpha PGL-I IgM antibody levels via a quick fingerstick, which often corresponds nicely with what's seen in the biopsy. These blood tests help flag patients with the multibacillary form who might have a higher risk of transmitting the disease. In effect, these new techniques link up with classic tissue analysis in a natural, sometimes surprising way, paving the road for earlier diagnosis and more targeted intervention aligned with Ridley-Jopling's ideas (Braet et al., 2021). Even though the World Health Organization tends to simplify things by dividing leprosy into just two groups—paucibacillary and multibacillary—for treatment purposes, the detailed picture provided by the Ridley-Jopling system remains indispensable. Its nuanced scale gives clinicians signs about how the disease might progress, recur, or lead to disabilities. It also shines a light on the interplay between the host and the pathogen, revealing variations in how the disease shows up in different populations. In most cases, research has shown that delays in diagnosis can worsen disability rates and keep the spread going, highlighting just how important accurate categorization is (Hambridge, 2024). Combining the classic Ridley-Jopling framework with newer diagnostic techniques creates a solid foundation that supports both individual patient care and broader public health strategies in the ongoing battle to control leprosy (Figure 3.2).

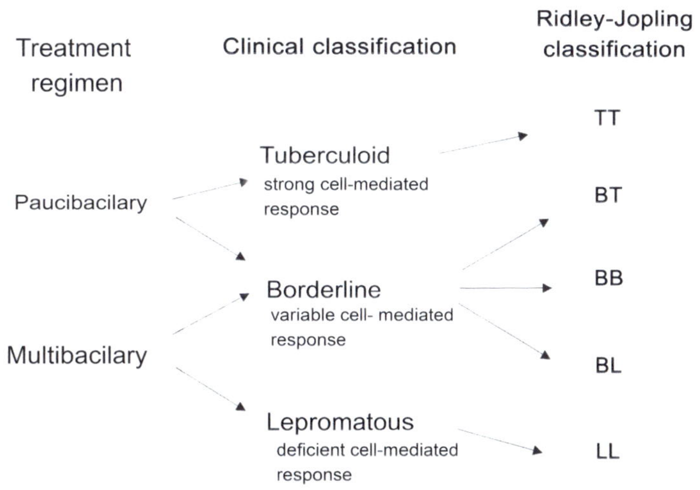

Figure 3.2. The Ridley-Jopling classification of leprosy.

Source: Chaves LL, Patriota Y, Soares-Sobrinho JL, Vieira ACC, Lima SAC, Reis S. Drug Delivery Systems on Leprosy Therapy: Moving Towards Eradication? *Pharmaceutics*. 2020; 12(12):1202. https://doi.org/10.3390/pharmaceutics12121202

3.1.1. Development and Purpose of the Ridley-Jopling Classification

Leprosy classification hasn't stayed the same over the years—it's shifted as doctors ran into all kinds of disease presentations. Early ideas were pretty simple and just didn't cover the wide range of immune responses seen in patients. Then came the Ridley-Jopling method, which, generally speaking, treats leprosy as a fluid condition along a continuous immune spectrum. This approach sorts cases along a line from tuberculoid to lepromatous, with borderline forms scattered in between, using markers from tissue samples, immune signals, and clinical signs. It offers a more layered view that helps us get a better feel for how the disease evolves and what it might mean for those affected. Further, it reminds us that the body's own attack, not to mention its varying strength, plays a big role in how the disease symptoms, which is key for treatment choices and for grasping how the infection spreads (Hambridge, 2024). Ridley and Jopling, in their own way, jointly collected lots of detailed pathology and immune information to capture the full range of leprosy's behavior. Unlike older, clumsier models, their system zeroes in on how a person's cell-based immune response , which can differ a lot from one patient to the next when dealing with *Mycobacterium leprae* – shapes what the disease does. Put simply, individuals with a strong immune system tend to develop limited tuberculoid spots, whereas a softer immune response leads to the more spread-out lepromatous picture. This range of reactions, in most cases, explains why patients can end up with very different outcomes and why doctors needed a model that linked what they observe with lab results. This combining of immune insights and clinical details marked a turning point in leprosy diagnosis and care, opening up more personalized treatment and fresh research into better control measures (Hambridge, 2024). More than just a way to slot patients into neat groups, the Ridley-Jopling framework acts as a backbone for making treatment calls and keeping tabs on disease trends. Breaking down leprosy according to immune strength and bacterial load, it not only hints at prognosis and risks for complications but also steers clinicians toward the right therapeutic routes. It builds a kind of common language for practitioners and researchers all over the world—even if sometimes the punctuation and phrasing wander a bit, which helps keep diagnoses and treatment reviews consistent. Notably, flagging those borderline cases shows why it's important to watch for shifts in immune response that might trigger sudden changes. With newer diagnostic tools like skin test antigens and immunoassays popping up (as recent studies have pointed out), this classification still holds up well for interpreting complex clinical pictures and steering effective case detection efforts aimed at reducing both disability and spread (Hambridge, 2024).

3.1.2. Categories Within the Ridley-Jopling Classification

Leprosy shows up in lots of unexpected ways—much of which comes from the complex immune reaction that *Mycobacterium leprae* induces in different people. Generally speaking, many clinicians use the Ridley-Jopling approach to slot the disease into a handful of groups. This method isn't just a neat checklist; it paints a picture of a continuous range that stretches from the tuberculoid end, with a strong, cell-based immune push, a few clear skin spots, and very little bacterial presence—to the lepromatous end, where the body's response is much weaker, leading to more lesions and a bigger bacterial load. In between, there are several intermixed states that, in most cases, show a combination of immune activity and varying disease severity—a gradation that helps in fine-tuning diagnoses and treatments. Right in the middle, one finds the so-called borderline variants—a trio of forms sometimes labeled BT, BB, and BL—each one fluctuating in its immune stance. Often, the borderline tuberculoid cases capture some features of the tuberculoid type, yet with a few extra lesions and a slightly increased bacterial count. The borderline group, by contrast, can flip between a more tuberculoid or a more lepromatous picture, depending on the strength of the host's immune response, which isn't always consistent. Meanwhile, borderline lepromatous cases lean toward the lepromatous side (but not completely), marked by multiple skin spots and some nerve involvement. To summarize, these varied shapes of the disease underline its dynamic nature and remind us that a patient's immune status plays a crucial role in how things progress

(Ignotti et al., 2020). In children, the spread of these Ridley-Jopling categories tends to be a bit different than in adults—a factor that's pretty important for understanding both how the disease spreads and how best to handle it in younger patients. Typically, the forms with lower bacterial counts, like the tuberculoid and borderline tuberculoid types, occur more often among kids, likely reflecting their mostly intact immune defenses that keep the bacteria in check. On the other hand, the multibacillary types, including borderline lepromatous and full-blown lepromatous leprosy, show up less frequently, yet they can be especially complex—think more nerve problems and odd hypersensitivity reactions, even though nerve damage overall seems less common in these younger individuals. This might be due, in most cases, to a shorter period during which the disease makes its mark coupled with different immune system dynamics (Kattan et al., 2006). Recognizing these nuances gives doctors a better handle on diagnosis, what to expect down the road, and how to choose therapies that best fit each age group (Figure 3.3).

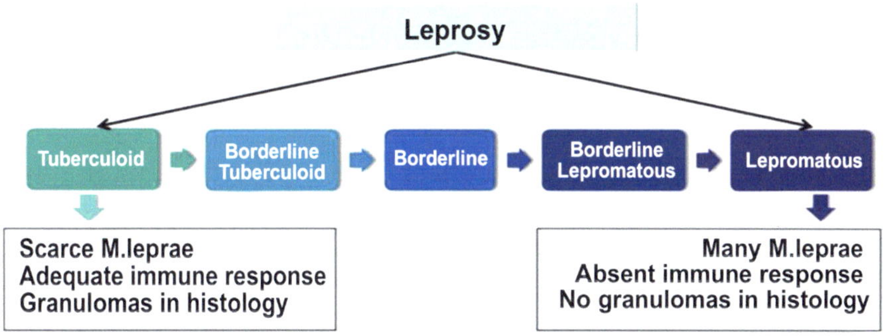

Figure 3.3. Forms of leprosy.

Source: Springer Nature. (n.d.). *Forms of Leprosy.*

3.1.3. Significance of the Classification in Clinical Practice

Treating leprosy effectively comes down to detecting its different forms and correctly sorting patients. The Ridley-Jopling approach, which leans on signals from immune responses and tissue details, gives doctors an insightful look at how the body handles *Mycobacterium leprae*. It breaks the disease into forms, from the tuberculoid end to the lepromatous end, with each type showing its own signs and bacterial counts. In everyday clinical work, noticing these differences early is key to stopping treatments that might miss the mark and even induce drug resistance. Proper classification also helps in predicting outcomes and jumping in early to avoid issues like nerve damage or disability. To summarize, using this scheme to guide multidrug therapy is critical both for improving individual patient outcomes and for shaping broader public health strategies aimed at controlling leprosy. But classification isn't just for fine-tuning treatment—it also plays a big role in keeping tabs on the disease at the community level. The WHO took the detailed Ridley-Jopling method and simplified it into two main categories, commonly known as paucibacillary and multibacillary, focusing squarely on bacterial load to set treatment length and tailor public health actions. This kind of quick, no-fuss approach is especially important in resource-poor settings, where speedy decisions are needed without a lot of laboratory back-up. By matching the intensity of treatment to how infectious a person might be, this method helps break the cycle of transmission in areas where leprosy still persists. It also supports on-the-ground things like contact tracing and early checks, all of which work together to curb the spread and even lower the stigma that often sticks with the disease (Hambridge, 2024). New diagnostic advances have teamed up with these classification systems to catch leprosy earlier and with greater accuracy. Work on skin test antigens and immune assays is aimed at catching hints of the disease before full-blown symptoms show up (Rivoire et al., 2012. Detecting early immune signals can refine how both the Ridley-Jopling and WHO classifications get applied, ensuring that treatment starts on time and helps prevent further disability. When modern diagnostic tools combined with tried-and-true classification strategies, doctors are better equipped to match treatments with how severe or what type of leprosy a patient has. This combination ultimately leads to improved patient outcomes and backs global efforts aimed at treating leprosy. In reality, these classification systems aren't just tools for individual care; they're a backbone for the larger fight to reduce leprosy's overall burden.

3.2. Types of Leprosy in Ridley-Jopling Classification

Leprosy shows up in a range of forms that reflect how a person's immune system deals with *Mycobacterium leprae*. Generally speaking, the Ridley-Jopling system splits it into five main types – starting with TT and ending with LL, with the borderline types (BT, BB, BL) mixed in between. Tuberculoid leprosy, for example, comes with a strong cell-based response that limits the number of well-outlined skin spots and some nerve complications.

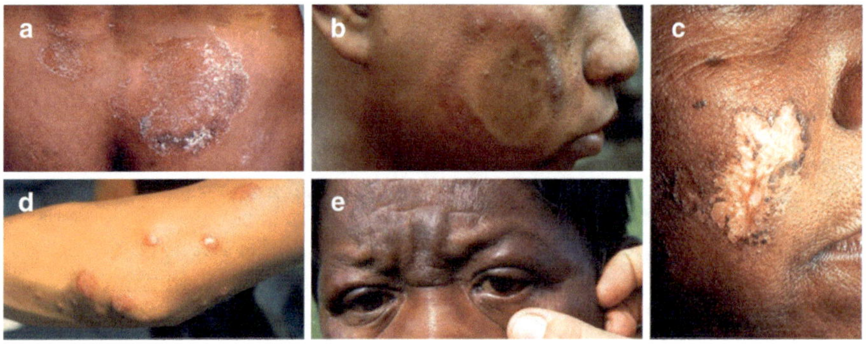

Figure 3.4. Types of leprosy in Ridley-Jopling classification: (a) Tuberculoid (TT) leprosy; (b) borderline tuberculoid (BT) leprosy; (c) borderline borderline (BB); (d) borderline lepromatous (BL) leprosy; and (e) lepromatous (LL) leprosy.

Source: ResearchGate. (n.d.). *Ridley-Jopling classification of leprosy. https://www.researchgate.net/publication/261443499/figure/tbl1/AS:601751736565773@1520480202581/Ridley-Jopling-classification-of-leprosy.png.*

On the other hand, lepromatous cases tend to muster a weak reaction, letting the bacteria spread and causing multiple, usually symmetric, lesions. You could say the borderline forms are a bit all over the map in terms of immune status, which makes them show up in diverse ways both clinically and under the microscope. In most cases, this kind of detailed breakdown helps steer treatment decisions by mapping out the disease's behavior over time. In everyday clinical practice, those borderline forms tend to keep doctors on their toes. BT looks much like the tuberculoid form but shows up with extra lesions and a touch of bacteriological positivity. Then there's the so-called BB type – smack in the middle with traits and bacterial loads that sort of balance between the strong and weak ends, and which sometimes flips into reactional states. Meanwhile, BL generally shifts closer to the lepromatous end with heftier bacillary loads and most often, a lot more lesions. These types, sort of fluid and dynamic in how the immune system handles them, can even change over time, and getting an accurate read on them is key because missteps might lead to the wrong treatment choices and worse outcomes (Ignotti et al., 2020). Another interesting piece of the puzzle is the indeterminate form – a sort of early or even abortive version of leprosy that doesn't fit efficiently into the other categories. It typically shows up as vague, lightly pigmented spots and hardly any nerve issues, which usually makes early diagnosis pretty complex. This form might clear up on its own or, depending on how the immune system plays along, evolve into one of the more clearly defined Ridley-Jopling types. Kids, in particular, often present with this indeterminate style, and that gives us valuable hints about how the disease spreads among younger individuals who, by the way, tend to have milder symptoms and fewer nerve problems (Kattan et al., 2006). To summarize, catching these early signs early on is super important to nip transmission and progression in the bud (Figure 3.4).

3.2.1. Tuberculoid Leprosy

Tuberculoid leprosy is one of the extreme forms you see in leprosy—it shows a strong cell-based defense against *Mycobacterium leprae*. Usually, people get just a few distinct, light-colored patches on their skin that come with a marked loss of feeling because nerves are involved. The immune system fights off the bacteria so well that hardly any manage to stick around, which generally makes this type less contagious than others. Under the microscope, you spot clusters of epithelioid cells and those big Langhans giant cells, which hint at a Th1-style immune kick. In the classic Ridley-Jopling layout, tuberculoid leprosy sits on the opposite end from lepromatous leprosy (Alrehaili, 2023). This difference is pretty key when doctors decide on treatment plans and even figure out the likely course of the disease according to WHO's multidrug therapy guidelines. Looking more into the Ridley-Jopling system, you find that tuberculoid leprosy shows off strong immunity that limits bacterial growth. Fewer microbes mean the condition sticks to a paucibacillary profile with only minimal spread of skin lesions. Typically, positive lepromin skin tests reveal a strong delayed-type hypersensitivity reaction, which stands in stark contrast to the multibacillary varieties that spread widely. Because of these differences, the WHO's classification helps in assigning the most suitable therapy. In most cases, the recommended treatment is a shorter stint of multidrug therapy since the bacterial load is lower, leading to fewer complications and generally better outcomes (Alrehaili, 2023). Both systems together give a fairly complete picture for diagnosis and management. Recent improvements in diagnostic tools, especially rapid point-of-care tests—have shed new light on detecting tuberculoid leprosy despite its low bacterial count. Although these tests were mainly honed for multibacillary situations, their sensitivity can vary when the bacteria are scarce in tuberculoid cases. Early identification is important if we want to avoid the nerve damage that can happen with delayed treatment. Some systematic reviews have indicated that while serological assays and immunohistochemical methods hold promise, they sometimes fall short because the immune response in tuberculoid leprosy is so aggressive. This means that clinicians still lean on good old clinical exams and histopathology, as outlined by both Ridley-Jopling and WHO standards, to make the right call on starting multidrug therapy (Figure 3.5).

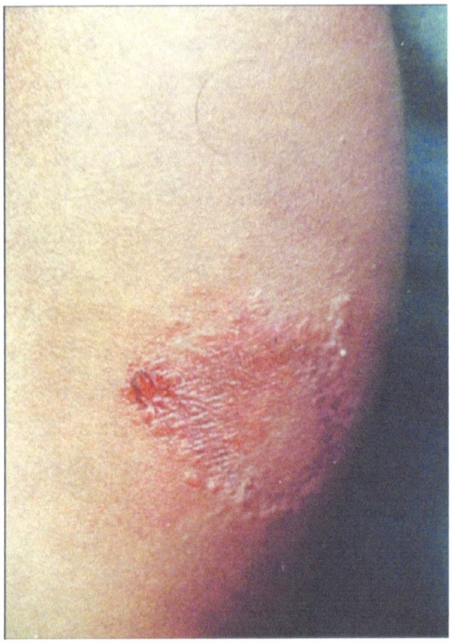

Figure 3.5. Tuberculoid leprosy.

Source: ResearchGate. (n.d.). *Tuberculoid Leprosy.*

3.2.2. Lepromatous Leprosy

Lepromatous leprosy sits at the multibacillary end of the spectrum set by Ridley-Jopling. It carries a high bacterial load and a generally weak cell-mediated response. People with this type tend to show many symmetric, loosely defined skin patches – nodules, plaques, and areas of diffuse infiltration emerge in various spots. The abundance of *Mycobacterium leprae* in these lesions, a telltale sign, sets it apart from the tuberculoid form and often leads to widespread nerve damage and disability. Some labs have even tried using anti-phenolic glycolipid-I serology to support the classification (though, truth be told, diagnosis still leans mostly on clinical grounds). This sort of categorization directs the choice of long-term, multi-drug therapy. The WHO, on the other hand, operates a simpler classification by eyeing the bacterial load and the clinical picture, lumping cases into either paucibacillary or multibacillary groups. Generally speaking, lepromatous leprosy drops into the multibacillary bucket because of its heavy bacterial burden and widespread lesions – factors that demand a longer, more aggressive treatment plan.

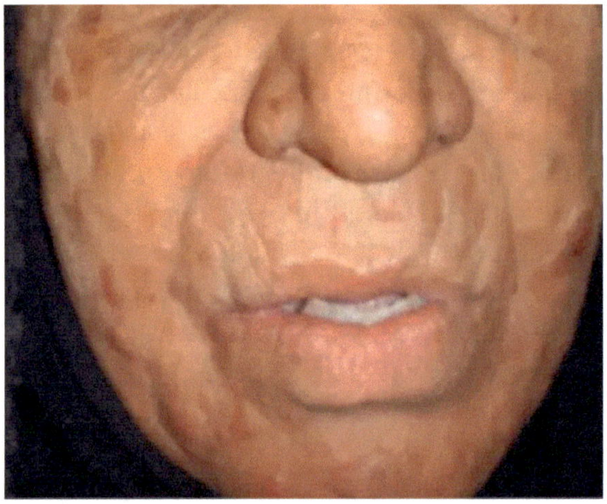

Figure 3.6. Lepromatous leprosy.

Source: WebPathology. (n.d.). *Lepromatous Leprosy.*

This framework, built more for public health management than for fussing over immunological nuances, sometimes ends up blurring the finer differences that the Ridley-Jopling system so clearly highlights. Even so, it remains essential for rolling out multidrug therapy in places where lab tests are scares. In most cases, understanding how these systems overlap helps clinicians balance accurate diagnosis with effective treatment. Studies on leprosy in children reveal an interesting twist: severe forms like lepromatous are quite rare among younger individuals. Often, children present with the more limited, paucibacillary form; severe nerve involvement or the hypersensitivity reactions seen in lepromatous cases hardly emerge. This pattern suggests that age-related immune factors play a big role in how the disease unfolds. Besides, the frequent occurrence of infections within families points to the importance—sometimes even the necessity—of close, prolonged contact in catching such multibacillary infections. To summarize, these insights underline why both classification systems remain valuable for refining public health strategies and tailoring patient care (Figure 3.6).

3.2.3. Borderline Leprosy

Borderline leprosy boils down to the host's immune fight against *Mycobacterium leprae*, which in turn shapes the entire look of the disease both on the skin and under the microscope. You see, this form isn't fixed—it kind of hangs in the balance between tuberculoid and lepromatous leprosy, showing up with a combination of cellular and antibody-driven responses. Often, patients sport uneven skin spots and nerve damages, a sign of the immune system reacting in more ways than one. This jumble definitely makes figuring out the right diagnosis and treatment complex. In most cases, doctors lean on systems like the Ridley-Jopling classification, which splits borderline leprosy into borderline tuberculoid and borderline lepromatous types—to guide treatment and forecast the outlook (Alrehaili, 2023).

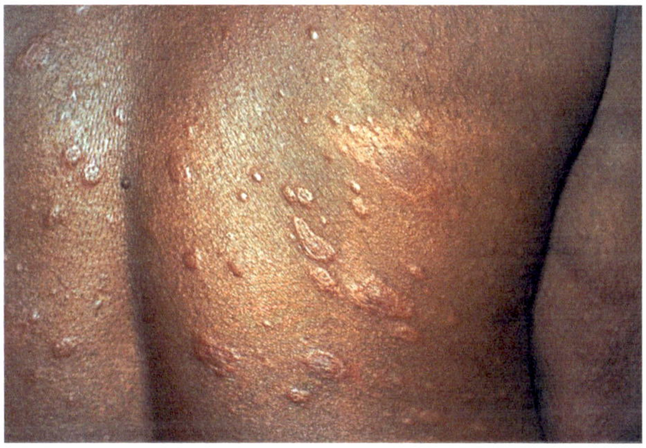

Figure 3.7. Borderline lepromatous (BL) leprosy.

Source: Wellcome Collection. (n.d.). *Borderline Lepromatous Leprosy.*

In essence, the way the body and microbe interact here explains a lot of the disease's ups and downs. Clinically, the unpredictable traits of borderline leprosy throw quite a wrench into the work of health providers, especially in areas where the disease is common. Unlike the pretty clear-cut polar types, borderline cases tend to show a middling immune response that leaves skin lesions and nerve issues all over the place. This uncertainty shapes medical decisions for multidrug therapy because the chance for immune overreactions (say, reversal reactions or erythema nodosum leprosum) goes up—something that, if not handled quickly, might edge up nerve damage and disability. The WHO uses a simpler split into paucibacillary and multibacillary forms, usually grouping borderline cases as multibacillary due to a heftier bacterial load, even though that method sometimes misses the finer details compared to Ridley-Jopling (Alrehaili, 2023). Meanwhile, as efforts ramp up to control leprosy, detecting borderline cases early remains crucial. Generally speaking, the mid-range nature of the immune response in these cases offers a prime chance to step in before the disease takes a turn for the worse. Tools like contact tracing and more advanced tests—including molecular assays such as 16S rRNA qPCR—have proven quite useful in catching early or even hidden infections, particularly among household contacts who might not show clear symptoms yet seem more at risk. All these improvements, when woven into existing classification tricks, boost both the sensitivity and accuracy of a diagnosis, which can lead to better outcomes for patients. Also, keeping an eye on factors like a patient's age and specific immune characteristics can help fine-tune treatment plans. Altogether, this combination of classic clinical classification with modern molecular diagnostics plays a big role in the global push Toward Zero Leprosy, striving to cut down transmission and ease the disease burden via solid, evidence-based steps (Alrehaili, 2023) (Figure 3.7).

3.3. World Health Organization (WHO) Operational Classification: An Overview

Leprosy care, in most cases, needs an approach that's simple and easy to roll out across various health settings, especially in places where the disease is common. The WHO method jumps right in by counting skin spots on patients, which naturally leads to quicker treatment plans. Instead of relying on those complicated lab tests or tissue studies, it simply splits cases into just two groups, paucibacillary and multibacillary that help steer the use of multidrug regimens without too much fuss. Sure, some clinical fine points get lost in translation, but overall, this strategy cuts down on diagnosis hurdles and increases treatment access in resource-tight areas. To summarize, its practical, straightforward nature vibes well with the need to balance clinical precision with real-world feasibility in global leprosy control programs (Bouceiro-Mendes et al., 2019). A big plus of the WHO system is its sheer ease of use; pretty much anyone in healthcare, even if they aren't skin specialists, can apply it. Since it zeroes in mainly on the number of lesions, making that first diagnosis becomes a lot simpler—a real win considering leprosy's often odd and unpredictable presentations.

That being said, this streamlined method can sometimes miss the broader picture; it might not capture every twist in the immune response or nerve involvement (sometimes even spelling it out a bit challengingly). While the Ridley-Jopling classification dives deeper into those nuances, its complexity doesn't lend itself too well to wide use in regions hit hardest by the disease. Consequently, although the WHO approach prioritizes a sort of one-size-fits-all treatment, it might overlook some of the finer details needed for tailoring care to each individual (Aftab et al., 2016). Even with these trade-offs, the WHO classification remains a trusty tool in battling leprosy, especially with the disease's long hidden period and its many clinical faces. It's pretty effective at speeding up diagnosis, getting treatment started without delay, and setting up standard care routines that help curb disability and block further spread. This method also helps bridge the gap between primary care providers and specialized centers by offering a sort of common ground for making both diagnosis and treatment choices. Combining in insights from other systems, like the Ridley-Jopling method—can boost overall clinical understanding while keeping things operationally sound. So, overall, the WHO system serves as a clever compromise, putting practical public health action first even if it means some clinical intricacies slip through the cracks (Aftab et al., 2016; Bouceiro-Mendes et al., 2019) (Figure 3.8).

Clinical classification	SLPB	PB	MB
Number of skin lesions	Only 1 lesion	2 to 5 lesions	6 or more lesions
	AND	AND	OR
Skin smears	Negative at all sites	Negative at all sites	Positive at any site
Distribution	-	Asymmetrical distribution	More symmetrical distribution
Sensation loss	Definite loss of sensation	Definite loss of sensation	Extensive sensation loss
Nerve damage (loss of sensation or muscle weakness)	No nerve trunk involvement	Only 1 nerve trunk	Many nerve trunks
Ridley-Jopling correlation	I, TT, some BT	TT, most BT	Some BT, BB, BL, LL

Figure 3.8. World Health Organization (WHO) classification of leprosy.

Source: ResearchGate. (n.d.). *WHO Classification of Leprosy.*

3.3.1. Development and Purpose of the World Health Organization (WHO) Operational Classification

Leprosy shows up in many unpredictable ways, and its immune response can leave health workers in a spin worldwide. Because of this, individuals began looking for a simpler way to diagnose and treat it. The older Ridley-Jopling system just didn't cut it, especially in places without plenty of resources, so the WHO came up with an operational classification. Basically, this new system splits cases into two groups: paucibacillary (PB) and multibacillary (MB). It mainly looks at how many skin lesions are present and whether bacilli show up on a skin smear, which cuts down on the fuss when deciding on treatment. This practical approach, which combined what you see in the clinic with real-world needs (particularly in regions that lack high-tech labs), makes it easier to manage leprosy on a global scale. Generally speaking, the whole point of adopting this WHO system was to meet the hands-on challenges in endemic areas, where health workers sometimes have only basic training and little access to advanced diagnosis. By cutting away the more complicated aspects of categorizing leprosy, the system made it simpler to roll out multidrug therapy (MDT) – a change that's improved outcomes and lowered transmission rates. It zeroes in on counts and transmission risks rather than getting too detected up in subtle immune details, encouraging quick treatment interventions. This is key for stopping the disease early and avoiding the disabilities that come from delayed diagnosis—a concern that especially hits vulnerable groups, like children. Studies even suggest that kids often show the PB form, so catching these cases early via a simpler system helps improve health overall and breaks the cycle of household spread (Kattan et al., 2006). To summarize, this method has become a crucial tool in broad leprosy control efforts. On top of that, the WHO operational classification helps with international comparisons and in tracking leprosy control efforts as part of global health planning. Its clear, straightforward criteria let different countries report cases in a consistent way, which in turn sharpens the picture of leprosy prevalence and how well MDT works. In regions where cases are rare or mostly imported—Scandinavian countries, for instance, the system nicely complements clinical judgment and even histopathologic analysis by offering an easy-to-use framework for front-line providers dealing with a combination of patients (Aftab et al., 2016). This flexibility shows that its use isn't limited to high-incidence areas; it also aids clinicians in detecting leprosy amid its varied clinical presentations and complex immune reactions. In the end, the WHO's classification not only smooths out treatment protocols but also plays a major role in uniting global efforts to eliminate leprosy.

3.3.2. Categories Within the World Health Organizations (WHO) Operational Classification

Leprosy control in many regions has long demanded a simpler way to diagnose and treat patients, especially where resources are stretched thin. The reality on the ground pushed experts to adopt a system that groups cases into just two types—PB and MB. Instead of getting complex in the elaborate details found in older classifications like the Ridley-Jopling system, this approach uses basic clinical signs and bacteriological checks to decide how to treat individuals.

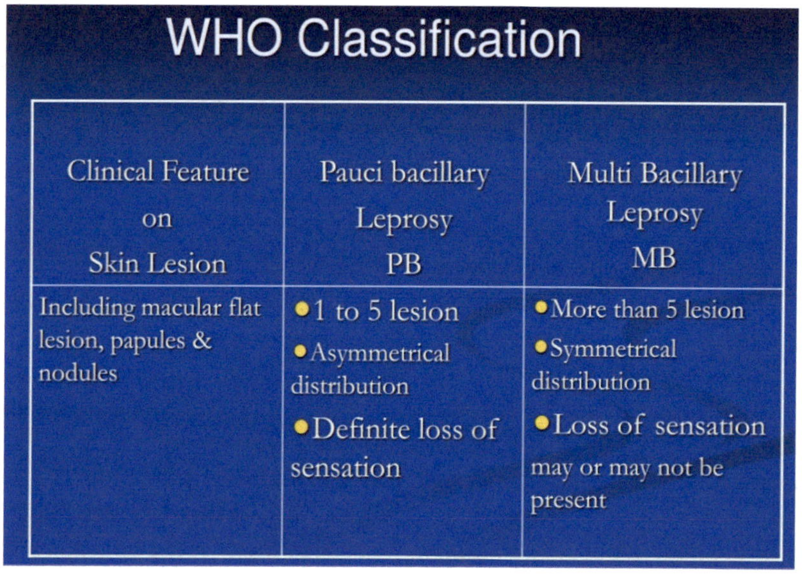

Figure 3.9. World Health Organizations (WHO) classification.

Source: SlideServe. (n.d.). *WHO Classification.*

It basically boils down to checking how many skin lesions there are and whether bacilli show up on a slit-skin smear. Such distinctions are not arbitrary; they tie directly to the bacterial load and infection risk, playing a crucial role in tailoring both treatment length and follow-up care. In many endemic areas, however, the picture isn't always crystal clear. Misdiagnoses still emerge quite a bit, primarily because the body's signals can vary widely and access to confirmatory tests isn't always at hand. Some studies – generally speaking – have shown that certain groups, such as females, children, or those with nerve issues but no obvious skin lesions, are more prone to falling into the wrong category (Ignotti et al., 2020). This means that while the two-tier WHO system is handy for standardizing therapy, it often relies on a doctor's careful judgment and additional checks to make sure every case is handled correctly, even if there's sometimes a bit of overlap in symptoms. On top of that, the WHO setup takes into account shifting trends in who gets affected and how the disease spreads, especially among vulnerable populations like children. Research shows that kids usually show up with the PB form, indicating a lower bacterial presence and, possibly, a smaller chance of severe progression (Kattan et al., 2006). This trend supports the focus on PB and MB categories, ensuring that treatment can be initiated quickly to slow down transmission, particularly among family members who live closely together. It's worth noting that, although nerve involvement and reaction states are critically important for managing the disease clinically, they don't fit efficiently into this system. So, while the WHO method cuts through some of the complexity for global health efforts, it still works best when used alongside the more detailed Ridley-Jopling approach, offering a practical yet somewhat approximate tool for leprosy control (Figure 3.9).

3.3.3. Role of the World Health Organizations (WHO) Classification in Global Health Initiatives

Global health efforts rest a lot on keeping diagnostic and treatment guidelines consistent, especially when fighting infections. Take leprosy as an example—the WHO's approach groups patients using simple checks like counting skin bumps and gauging bacterial loads. This method works hand-in-hand with the more detailed Ridley-Jopling system, letting healthcare workers in areas with limited resources spot cases fast and start a multidrug plan. That straightforward design makes it a go-to for large-scale monitoring and control, keeping reporting and treatment on track across different regions. Its ease of use means it can slip right into national health plans, which is essential for tackling leprosy in places where it still runs rampant (Costa et al., 2024). The system's impact goes beyond just treating patients; it also has a broader role in global plans to wipe out the disease. By keeping case definitions consistent, it backs epidemiological comparisons and helps track trends over time and between populations.

In most cases, that standardization is key when checking the effects of public health efforts and shaping big policy decisions internationally. It even stimulates early case detection, a step that's important for avoiding disability and the stigma that comes with late diagnosis. You'll also find new digital aids and AI-driven tools coming into play here, all designed to boost accuracy and access in areas that struggle with resources. All of this fits in with the WHO's push to speed up leprosy elimination by making sure treatment gets to individuals when they need it (Barbieri et al., 2022). It's also worth noting that the role of the WHO system in worldwide health shows why we need practices that are both sturdy and flexible tools that work across the board but still cut it for local challenges. Since leprosy tends to hit marginalized communities harder, this classification system is crucial for steering resources and fine-tuning interventions for vulnerable groups. It even builds bridges among healthcare providers, researchers, and policymakers by giving everyone a common way to talk about issues like underreporting and social stigma. Bolstered by a solid base of epidemiological data, the WHO method stands behind educational campaigns and community-building efforts in places where the disease is common. Basically, it isn't just another diagnostic approach but a core piece of a broader strategy to reduce leprosy's biopsychosocial impact and bring a greater sense of fairness in health outcomes worldwide (Barbieri et al., 2022; Costa et al., 2024).

3.4. Types of Leprosy in World Health Organizations (WHO) Operational Classification

Leprosy is an infection caused by *Mycobacterium leprae* that sticks around for a long time, and it can be pretty complex to diagnose since it shows up in so many different ways. To deal with that, the World Health Organization came up with a classification system meant to simplify figuring out treatment, especially in places with limited resources. Instead of laying everything out in neat boxes, they kind of lump the disease into two main types - one called PB and the other MB. PB usually means you have five or fewer skin spots, and when doctors run a skin smear, they often find little or even no bacteria, suggesting only a low number of bacilli are present. On the other hand, MB involves more than five lesions and is often paired with skin smears that light up with bacteria, hinting at a heavier load. This simple, two-pronged method helps individuals on the ground make quick decisions about diagnosis and treatment, although it isn't as detailed as the Ridley-Jopling approach, which dives into immune responses and examines tissues under a microscope. Interestingly, even though the straightforwardness of the WHO system has boosted case detection in many instances, misdiagnoses still emerge (especially with PB cases) since the signs can overlap with other skin problems (Ignotti et al., 2020). Looking closer at how leprosy spreads and what it means for patients, you notice some real differences between the PB and MB forms. Generally speaking, PB cases tend to cause fewer complications and have a lower chance of nerve damage, whereas MB cases often show a wider spread of bacteria and trigger more aggressive immune reactions that lead to nerve issues. This isn't just a minor detail, it changes how treatment is approached and even shapes public health strategies to keep the disease in check. For example, children often lean toward the PB type, showing milder symptoms and rarely progressing to the multibacillary form, which suggests that their immune systems might work a bit differently. These small but important differences underline why it's so crucial to assign patients the right classification under the WHO guidelines, ensuring treatment plans hit the mark and disabilities are kept at bay. Further, the fact that leprosy tends to spread through close, prolonged contact, especially among family members, shows why targeted contact tracing and preventive treatments are so necessary in areas where the disease is common (Kattan et al., 2006). Still, even with all its practical perks, the WHO system isn't perfect and does have some limitations when it comes to accuracy and thoroughness. Since it mainly depends on counting lesions and checking smear results, it might miss early or unusual cases that don't fit the normal picture, which can lead to diagnostic errors. Research has pointed out that misdiagnoses emerge more often among groups like women, kids, or patients whose symptoms are mostly nerve-related rather than the typical skin lesions—indicating a need for better training and additional diagnostic tools. It's also interesting that there isn't a clear link between misdiagnosis rates and how common leprosy is in a region, which suggests that individual and disease-specific factors play a major role. So, while the WHO system stays a cornerstone in managing leprosy worldwide, mixcombining it with more detailed clinical checks and follow-up measures is pretty much crucial for sharpening diagnostic precision and improving patient outcomes (Ignotti et al., 2020).

3.4.1. Multibacillary Leprosy

Leprosy is a complex disease, and its overall complexity means doctors need clear, more or less practical, ways to break it down so treatment and expected outcomes become manageable. In many cases, one of the toughest forms, multibacillary leprosy, shows up with a heavy bacterial load and a wide range of symptoms. This type fits in quite snugly with what's called the borderline lepromatous and the classic lepromatous categories in the Ridley-Jopling framework, with patients often having several skin lesions, broad skin infiltrations, and notable nerve issues. WHO's method, for instance, divides these cases by noting if there are more than five skin lesions or a positive bacilloscopy index, a sign that the case is more infectious and needs a longer multidrug treatment plan. In most cases, these multibacillary situations end up being harder to diagnose and manage because they lead to serious nerve damage and other immune complications that demand quick, hands-on intervention. Lab tests have been brought in to support what you see in the clinic when trying to pick apart multibacillary leprosy. Tests that look for anti-phenolic glycolipid-I (PGL-I) antibodies have proved pretty useful in telling patients apart. For example, the ML Flow and the ML immunochromatography assay (ICA) tests give point-of-care options, though their performance can vary by region—this might be because of differences in patients' immune responses and the actual bacterial load. These tools naturally back up the Ridley-Jopling and WHO classification methods, especially when it comes to fine-tuning treatment plans and keeping a check on progress. Even if these blood tests can't completely take the place of in-person clinical and bacteriological examinations, combining them into the overall classification routine does boost sensitivity in identifying multibacillary cases, ultimately helping optimize treatments and maybe even easing transmission. The range of symptoms seen in multibacillary leprosy shows that one single approach just won't do, especially in regions where the disease is common. Cases left untreated for a long time tend to show off some unusual features like erythema nodosum leprosum and pronounced lymphatic involvement, which highlights how varied this condition can be. Such uneven presentations not only make diagnosis complex but also stress the need for experts to get together and for institutions to team up for the sake of accurate diagnosis, classification, and management. By taking the time to understand the little immune characterestics and the clinical diversity in these cases, teams can keep altering the classification systems, ensuring that, generally speaking, care stays both accessible and effective for patients worldwide (Bouceiro-Mendes et al., 2019) (Figure 3.10).

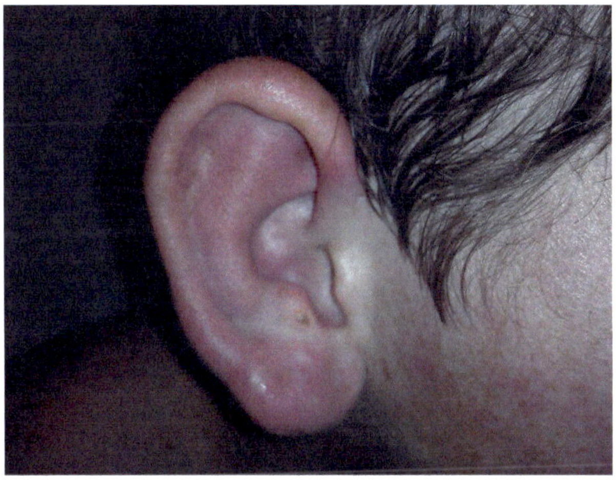

Figure 3.10. Multibacillary leprosy.

Source: Wikimedia Commons. (2019). *Multibacillary Leprosy.*

3.4.2. Paucibacillary Leprosy

Leprosy shows a complex interaction between how the body fights off invaders and the *Mycobacterium leprae* microbe. Out of its many faces, the paucibacillary type stands out for having a vigorous, cell-based defense that usually keeps the bacteria in check—even though, in many cases, you barely spot them in the lesions. If you observe the Ridley-Jopling system, you'll notice that forms like tuberculoid leprosy tend to have few, if any, bacilli, only a handful of skin patches, and nerve issues that stick closely around those spots. This kind of strong immune reaction sits in stark contrast to the multibacillary presentation, where higher bacterial counts are common; genes like HLA and KIR, for instance, seem to wiggle how our bodies recognize and combat the bacteria (Alves et al., 2018). Generally speaking, understanding these genetic alters is key to fine-tuning leprosy classification and improving predictions about its outcomes. When it comes to making treatment decisions in areas hit hard by leprosy, the World Health Organization usually opts for a simpler, more hands-on approach. Essentially, they break the disease into two groups—paucibacillary and multibacillary, based largely on how many skin lesions a patient has and the results from slit-skin smears. In most cases, if someone shows up with five or fewer lesions and no detectable bacilli, the diagnosis lands as paucibacillary. While this clear-cut system works well on the ground, it doesn't quite capture the full range of immune-related details that the detailed Ridley-Jopling scheme offers. Still, because these guidelines help steer standard multidrug therapy regimens (which, incidentally, are shorter for paucibacillary cases) and keep public health efforts on track, they're crucial for lowering the risks of disability and the stigma that often follows (Hambridge, 2024). Looking closer at the nuances reveals some real challenges in detecting and managing paucibacillary leprosy early enough to avoid nerve problems. Even though the bacterial load is usually low, waiting too long for a diagnosis can lead to worsening nerve damage and, eventually, a higher chance of disability. Researchers are busy exploring how genetic factors alter the immune response—not only to shed light on how the disease develops, but also to find early markers that might lead to quicker case detecting and even more tailored treatments (Alves et al., 2018). Some epidemiological models also hint that ramping up our detection methods for these cases might do a lot to cut down both transmission and long-term disability (Hambridge, 2024). To summarize, combining insights from both the Ridley-Jopling system and WHO's classification seems pretty central to sharpening treatment plans, boosting surveillance, and stimulating us closer to the goal of wiping out leprosy (Figure 3.11).

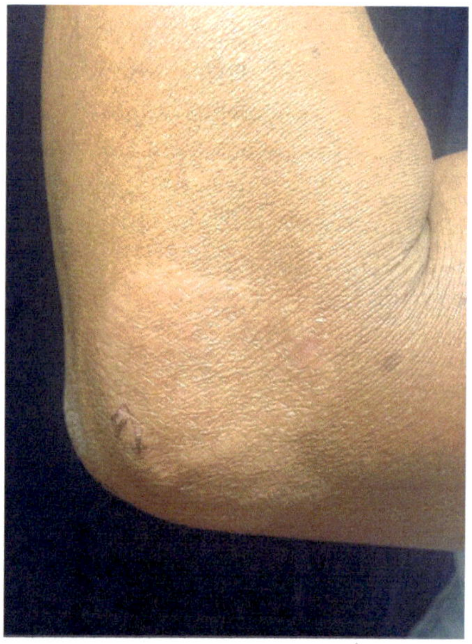

Figure 3.11. Paucibacillary leprosy (PB).

Source: Wikimedia Commons. (2019). *Paucibacillary Leprosy (PB).*

3.4.3. Implications for Treatment Based on Classification

Leprosy shows up in so many ways that the treatment has to match the way the patient's body fights the infection—this isn't just a neat textbook rule but a practical guide. The Ridley-Jopling system, which sorts patients based on their immune response, helps decide how long and intense the MDT should be. Take tuberculoid leprosy, for example; when the immune response is strong, treatment tends to be shorter because there aren't many bacteria around. In contrast, lepromatous leprosy, with its high bacterial count and weak host response, almost always needs a longer, tougher MDT course. Detecting signs like numb patches on the skin and nerve involvement can steer doctors toward early treatment, helping to prevent irreversible nerve damage and disability. To summarize, a thorough clinical check—mixcombining what you see with lab results—keeps treatment on track and improves outcomes in both high- and low-prevalence areas (Aftab et al., 2016). The immune system's own reactions add another twist during treatment. Patients sometimes face Type 2 lepra reactions (think erythema nodosum leprosum [ENL]) that tend to emerge in borderline lepromatous and lepromatous cases, and these reactions can complicate matters. The frequency, strength, and duration of these ENL episodes can even throw off MDT adherence, often pushing doctors to add medications like corticosteroids or thalidomide into the mix. In most cases, keeping an eye on risk factors such as bacterial load, and even something like the patient's age—helps clinicians prepare for flare-ups. Breaking down ENL into its forms—acute, multiple acute, and chronic—is key for tailoring a plan that tackles both the infection and the immune fallout, thereby boosting long-term prognosis (Pocaterra et al., 2006). On another note, the World Health Organization's classification smooths out treatment decisions by splitting patients into two groups—paucibacillary and multibacillary. This method works especially well in places with limited resources because it leans on visible signs rather than relying on detailed immune testing. For multibacillary cases, a longer treatment plan is used to wipe out the heavier bacterial burden and manage immune complications, while the paucibacillary approach keeps drug exposure low yet still effective. Still, mixcombining the WHO's system with the Ridley-Jopling method can fine-tune the strategy, especially for borderline cases where immune responses can be unpredictable. Such a combined approach underlines how getting the classification right helps balance potent treatment with side effects and resource needs (Pocaterra et al., 2006; Aftab et al., 2016).

A CLOSER LOOK

PURE NEURAL LEPROSY

Pure neural leprosy (PNL), often called neural leprosy, is an exceedingly rare variant of leprosy, primarily affecting one or more peripheral nerves. According to consensus, individuals presenting one or two enlarged nerves are classified as having paucibacillary leprosy (PBL). In contrast, those with more than two affected nerves are categorized as having MB leprosy. The indications of nerve damage in PNL encompass sensory loss, muscle weakness, diminished sweating ability, and swollen or painful nerves. Other indications of PNL include motor impairment by developing weakness, muscle wasting (atrophy), and paralysis in the affected limbs due to damage to the motor nerves. Furthermore, enlargement of peripheral nerves, known as nerve hypertrophy or neuritis is also an indication of PNL. This enlargement is caused by inflammation and infiltration of the nerves by immune cells in response to the infection. Identifying whether a nerve is swollen is not always straightforward. For patients with challenging-to-diagnose PNL cases, procedures like biopsy, involving fine needle aspiration and PCR or electroneuromyography, can be particularly valuable whenever feasible. Recent studies indicate that asymptomatic leprosy cases with nerve swelling, with or without pain, can be identified and treated early through the use of high-resolution ultrasound. Specifically, individuals who fall outside the normal range for nerve thickness in the principal nerves affected by leprosy can be diagnosed and treated early. By identifying abnormal nerve thickness in these individuals, even in the absence of symptoms, healthcare professionals can diagnose silent peripheral neuropathy associated with leprosy and initiate early treatment (Figure 3.12).

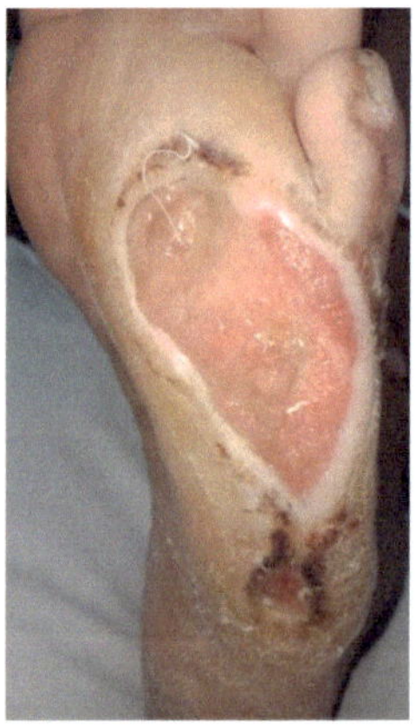

Figure 3.12. Pure neural leprosy (PNL).

Source: Authorea. (n.d.). Pure Neuritic Leprosy Presenting with Type 1 Reaction: A Rare Case Report.

SUMMARY

Leprosy classification methods like the Ridley-Jopling system and the WHO approach help untangle the many faces of the disease. They cover a wide range of immune responses, from tuberculoid to lepromatous, and in most cases, influence both the outlook and how treatment gets combined to patient needs. Even though we've made real progress, catching the disease early remains complex because its symptoms show up all over the place. When nerve issues take center stage, timely detection becomes even more complicated. Combining these systems into routine practice can boost case detection and help lessen disabilities. With leprosy still a heavy global burden despite elimination efforts, there's a clear call for better diagnostic methods. A broad grasp of these schemes not only lets clinicians tailor therapies but also supports ongoing monitoring necessary to push toward zero leprosy worldwide (Alrehaili, 2023). Looking closer, the WHO's simplified method shines in busy field settings, especially where resources are tight—it basically sorts cases into paucibacillary and multibacillary groups for treatment. However, the Ridley-Jopling model dives deeper into the immune pathways, offering signals about disease progression and possible pitfalls. Still, both systems definitely have their limitations, signaling that altering them based on real data and patient symptoms might be needed. Recent studies analyzing symptom patterns point out that nerve-specific signs, which often slip by and delay diagnosis, can raise the risk of disability. This insight generally pushes us toward more awareness campaigns and targeted clinical training, particularly in neurology—to catch the disease earlier and reduce both complications and spread (Chen et al., 2021). In the end, while the Ridley-Jopling and WHO Operational classifications remain the bedrock for managing leprosy from both a clinical and public health angle, their real strength lies in being part of a broader plan that includes sharper diagnostic vigilance and active patient education. The ongoing occurrence of new cases and related disabilities shows that simply classifying isn't enough; proactive case-finding and stronger health systems are just as crucial. Future efforts should zero in on boosting symptom recognition, especially for those nerve-related hints that often go unnoticed, and on widening training for multidisciplinary teams. Marrying these classification methods with wider strategies will better position global health initiatives to hit the ambitious mark of "Towards Zero Leprosy," aiming for a more holistic eradication, beyond just neat categories (Alrehaili, 2023; Chen et al., 2021).

Leprosy classification plays a key role in both diagnosing and managing this long-lasting infection. The Ridley-Jopling system dives into immune details by breaking the disease into five types—based on what doctors see, what lab tissues reveal, and how many bacteria each case carries. On one end, tuberculoid leprosy shows a strong cell response; on the other, lepromatous leprosy is marked by a much weaker defense and broader spread. Further, the WHO method groups cases into just two categories, paucibacillary and multibacillary, to streamline treatment decisions. These differing approaches remind us that leprosy's symptoms can be pretty complex and that tailored treatment is necessary to lessen disability and cut transmission. Early detection, in most cases, is crucial since delays only worsen outcomes and fuel the spread (Hambridge, 2024). Speeding up early diagnosis still tops the agenda given the huge public health stakes. New tools, like skin test antigens and interferon-gamma assays, are now being used to pinpoint an infection even before clear symptoms appear. These methods seem pretty promising at catching tuberculoid leprosy with good specificity, though they occasionally stumble with sensitivity. Ongoing tests and clinical trials hint at a future where catching the disease pre-symptomatically could ease the burden of stigma and help prevent nerve damage from becoming permanent. The mix of serological markers together with immune tests might just boost overall accuracy, efficiently supplementing established classification methods and improving patient outcomes (Rivoire et al., 2012). To summarize, combining the detailed insights of the Ridley-Jopling approach with the straightforward WHO categories gives us a broader view of leprosy, from its varied immune responses to practical treatment steps. The Ridley-Jopling system unpacks the disease's immune characteristics, while the WHO method keeps treatment accessible and simple. New diagnostic tests that align with these frameworks could increase early detection and enhance overall disease control. Studies show that diagnostic delays still pose a serious challenge by increasing both transmission and long-term disability. Clearly, ongoing research, and the smart integration of new techniques with older methods—is vital if we're to reduce leprosy's impact and move closer to eliminating it on a global scale (Hambridge,Rivoire et al., 2012; Hambridge, 2024).

KEY TERMS FROM THIS CHAPTER

- Bacteria
- Borderline lepromatous
- Epithelioid cells
- Hypersensitivity reactions
- Immune assays
- Light-colored patches
- Borderline borderline
- Borderline tuberculoid
- Full-blown lepromatous leprosy
- Immune activity
- Lepromatous
- Positive lepromin skin tests

References

1. Aftab, H., Nielsen, S.D. & Bygbjerg, I.C. Leprosy in Denmark 1980–2010: a review of 15 cases. *BMC Res Notes* **9**, 10 (2016). https://doi.org/10.1186/s13104-015-1768-6 (accessed on 10th May 2025).
2. Alrehaili J. (2023). Leprosy Classification, Clinical Features, Epidemiology, and Host Immunological Responses: Failure of Eradication in 2023. *Cureus*, *15*(9), e44767. https://doi.org/10.7759/cureus.44767(accessed on 10th May 2025).
3. Vicentin Alves H, Tiaki Tiyo B, Maria Sell A, Eliete Laguila Visentainer J. Immunogenetics of MHC and KIR in the Leprosy [Internet]. Hansen's Disease - The Forgotten and Neglected Disease. IntechOpen; 2019. Available from: http://dx.doi.org/10.5772/intechopen.75253 (accessed on 10th May 2025).
4. Braet SM, van Hooij A, Hasker E, Fransen E, Wirdane A, Baco A, et al. (2021) Minimally invasive sampling to identify leprosy patients with a high bacterial burden in the Union of the Comoros. PLoS Negl Trop Dis 15(11): e0009924. https://doi.org/10.1371/journal.pntd.0009924 (accessed on 10th May 2025).
5. Barbieri, R. R., Xu, Y., Setian, L., de Souza-Santos, P. T., Trivedi, A., Cristofono, J., Bhering, R., et al. (2022). Reimagining leprosy elimination with AI analysis of a combination of skin lesion images with demographic and clinical data. *The Lancet Regional Health – Americas*, *9*, 100192–100192. https://doi.org/10.1016/j.lana.2022.100192 (accessed on 10th May 2025).
6. Bouceiro-Mendes, R., Ferreira, J., Filipe, P., Freitas, C., et al. (2019). *Um Caso Clínico de lepra Multibacilar com Vários Surtos de Eritema Nodoso Leproso*. Revista SPDV 77(1) 2019; Lepra multibacilar com surtos de eritema nodoso leproso; https://core.ac.uk/download/322632732.pdf (accessed on 10th May 2025).
7. Chen, X., Zha, S., & Shui, T. (2021). Presenting symptoms of leprosy at diagnosis: Clinical evidence from a cross-sectional, population-based study. *PLoS Neglected Tropical Diseases*, *15*, e0009913–e0009913. https://doi.org/10.1371/journal.pntd.0009913 (accessed on 10th May 2025).
8. Costa, A. K. M., Souza e Silva, D. C., da Rocha Rosa, P. H., Vaz Gonçalves, R. B., Santos, V. O., Guimarães, Y. P., & Carneiro, V. S. M. (2024). *Leprosy in Brazil: From the Social Developments to the Diagnosis-Therapeutic Evolution of the Disease*. Seven Editora eBooks. https://doi.org/10.56238/sevened2024.001-058 (accessed on 10th May 2025).
9. Hambridge, T. (2024). *Shortening Leprosy Case Detection Delay: Narrowing the Window of Transmission and Disease Progression*. Hambridge T. Department of Public Health. Erasmus University Rotterdam. 2024;(accessed on 10th May 2025).
10. Neves, K. V. R. N., Nobre, M. L., Machado, L. M. G., Steinmann, P., & Ignotti, E. (2021). Misdiagnosis of leprosy in Brazil in the period 2003 - 2017: spatial pattern and associated factors. *Acta tropica*, *215*, 105791. https://doi.org/10.1016/j.actatropica.2020.105791 (accessed on 10th May 2025).
11. Kattan, Jessica Anne, "The Epidemiology and Clinical Presentation of Leprosy in the Pediatric Population of Paraguay" (2006). Yale Medicine Thesis Digital Library. 251. http://elischolar.library.yale.edu/ymtdl/251 (accessed on 10th May 2025).

12. Manta, F. S. N., Barbieri, R. R., Moreira, S. J. M., Santos, P. T. S., Nery, J. A. C., Düppre, N. C., Sales, A. M., et al. (2019). Quantitative PCR for leprosy diagnosis and monitoring in household contacts: A follow-up study, 2011–2018. *Scientific Reports, 9.* https://doi.org/10.1038/s41598-019-52640-5 (accessed on 10th May 2025).

13. Mawardi P. Leprosy: The Ancient and Stubborn Disease [Internet]. Current Topics in Tropical Emerging Diseases and Travel Medicine. IntechOpen; 2018. Available from: http://dx.doi.org/10.5772/intechopen.79984 (accessed on 10th May 2025).

14. Pocaterra, L., Jain, S., Reddy, R., Muzaffarullah, S., Torres, O., Suneetha, S., & Lockwood, D. N. (2006). Clinical course of erythema nodosum leprosum: an 11-year cohort study in Hyderabad, India. *The American journal of tropical medicine and hygiene, 74*(5), 868–879. (accessed on 10th May 2025).

15. Rivoire, B. L. (2012). *Development and Evaluation of New Leprosy Skin Test Antigens as Diagnostic Tools.* Thesis & Dissertations. Colorado State University; http://hdl.handle.net/10217/88338(accessed on 10th May 2025).

16. Romero, C. P., Castro, R., do Brasil, P. E. A., Pereira, D. R., Pinheiro, R. O., Toscano, C. M., & de Oliveira, M. R. F. (2022). Accuracy of rapid point-of-care serological tests for leprosy diagnosis: a systematic review and meta-analysis. *Memorias do Instituto Oswaldo Cruz, 117*, e220317. https://doi.org/10.1590/0074-02760220317 (accessed on 10th May 2025).

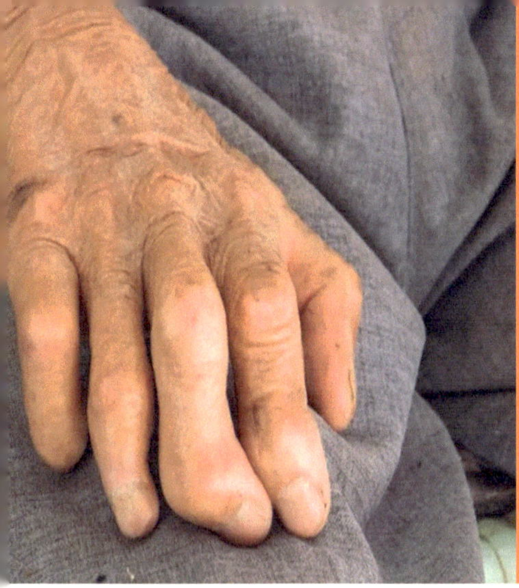

Chapter 4

CLINICAL FEATURES OF LEPROSY

Contents

Introduction

Hansen's disease, or leprosy as most call it, is still a heavy burden on health in many parts of the globe, especially in areas where poverty mixes with limited healthcare. Caused by Mycobacterium leprae, this infection shows up on the skin, nerves at the body's edges, the lining of the upper airways, and even the eyes. We've known about leprosy for what feels like forever, yet its signs can shift unexpectedly from just a few light spots on the skin to more severe nerve damages that might cause deformities. Recognizing these varied signs early on is important, since catching it sooner can help avoid irreversible problems and cut down the stigma. In tropical and subtropical areas, where neglected tropical diseases (NTDs) are more common, leprosy continues to demand fresh research and careful attention (Bélard et al., 2016). Honestly, leprosy's clinical picture isn't clear-cut at all. Our immune system reacts in many different ways when faced with Mycobacterium leprae, which means that, generally speaking, the disease can show up in more than one form. You have the tuberculoid kind, which usually brings well-outlined, lighter patches on the skin along with a loss of feeling, and then there's the lepromatous form, full of widespread nodules, plaques, and a kind of overall complex infiltration. Nerve damage stands as a key, if harsh, feature that often leads to numbness and disability. And then there's the additional twist of leprosy reactions—whether it's type 1 (often called reversal reaction) or type 2 (known as erythema nodosum leprosum)—that can further worsen nerve damage. Such nuances in presentation help clinicians, in most cases, adjust treatment plans to reduce long-term harm (Rodriguez-Morales, 2019). In most tropical and subtropical regions, diagnosing and managing leprosy is a tough battle because diagnostic tools and quality care are hard to come by. Quite like other NTDs, where fancy imaging equipment is a rarity, many doctors rely on good old clinical judgment and basic lab tests to pin down the diagnosis. There's some promise in using point-of-care technologies, however, their role in tackling leprosy is still pretty underexplored (Bélard et al., 2016). Added to this are factors like poverty, unsanitary conditions, and the close contact people have with untreated cases, all of which help the illness spread. Looking at leprosy against this backdrop not only deepens our overall understanding of the disease but also underscores just how urgently sustainable, community-based health solutions are needed (Rodriguez-Morales, 2019) (Figure 4.1).

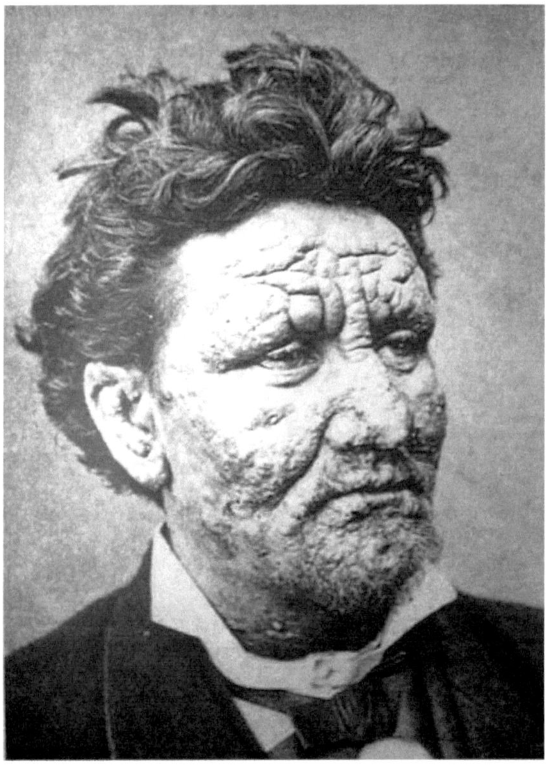

Figure 4.1. Clinical manifestations of leprosy caused by Mycobacterium leprae.

Source: By Pierre Arents - Pierre Arents printed the photographs for Leloir's monograph on leprosy titled, Traité pratique et théorique de la lèpre, published in 1886. This image is Plate VIII from that atlas. Vide: http://www.artandmedicine.com/biblio/authors/french/Leloir.html, Public Domain, https://commons.wikimedia.org/w/index.php?curid=325260

4.1. Incubation Period

Leprosy tends to appear in a manner that may surprise you, at least in part because the interval between exposure to infection and being ill may be quite lengthy, and it varies from person to person. The so-called incubation period, just the interval between initial infection and the onset of symptoms, may be several years in duration, with some indicators suggesting at least a minimum of two years. This lag in time may put both doctors and patients in a squeeze; there may be a carrier without any apparent symptoms. Often, this lag translates into the disease not being found until much later, and it tends to spread where individuals persist together nearby, consider family members who spend large amounts of time together. For instance, if you observe children with leprosy, you realize that the older ones look more likely to contract it, perhaps because they have been exposed for a longer period. Overall, these facts reveal just how hidden Mycobacterium leprae can be and how there needs to be careful observation of groups that could be at risk (Kattan et al., 2006).

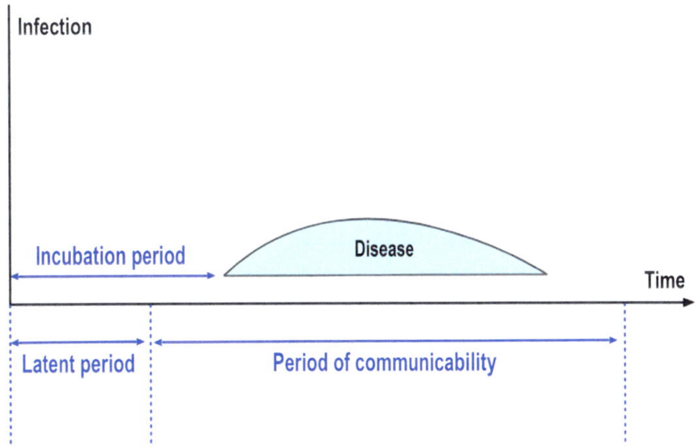

Figure 4.2. In some diseases, as depicted in this diagram, the latency period is shorter than the incubation period. After the latency period (but before clinical infection) the infected person can transmit the disease without signs of any symptoms. Such infection is called subclinical infection.

Source: Wikimedia Commons. (n.d.). Concept of Incubation Period.

The identification of symptoms becomes difficultas it significantly differ from individual to individual. Because the incubation period is so extended, it's not unusual for individuals to relocate or even travel before ever realizing something's amiss, so it's difficult to track where the disease may have initiated. In areas where leprosy is not commonly encountered, physicians usually only become familiar with it after the condition is quite far along—usually when patients present with symptoms like numb spots on the skin or obviously inflamed nerves. Since early symptoms can be fairly evasive and inconstant, hearing the complete history, particularly information regarding travel, exposure risk—is important. Generally speaking, clinicians focus on where someone has lived and what risks they might have been under. It's also noteworthy that immune responses, observed in up to 40% of cases in some populations, can further complicate by obscuring the clinical picture; these responses typically engage after the onset of symptoms, suggesting the prolonged incubation doesn't merely postpone signs but could also modify the behavior of the disease (Aftab et al., 2016). Understanding the effect of this extended incubation period is important for both public health measures and improved patient management. The extended duration of the condition in most instances requires monitoring for a lengthy period and close follow-up with individuals who have had contact with patients, eventually leading to the detection of the condition before permanent nerve destruction occurs. The variations in how long this duration is also tell us something about the struggle between the host and the disease—implying that an individual's immune system can influence how soon symptoms of leprosy appear and how severe they are. Surprisingly, kids tend to have less severe symptoms and fewer overactive immune reactions, perhaps because they've only been exposed to the bacteria for a shorter period of time or because their immune systems respond differently during the initial stages. Connecting what we have learned regarding the incubation period with the signs of illness not only increases the chances of a proper diagnosis but also assists in making treatment decisions, which is at the heart of controlling and containing the transmission of leprosy (Kattan et al., 2006; Aftab et al., 2016) (Figure 4.2).

4.1.1. Duration of Incubation

Leprosy often shows up so subtly that it's hard to identify early on, mainly because the pathogen tends to persist for a long time before symptoms visible. The disease can take anywhere from several months to, in most cases, up to three to five years to get going, and sometimes even longer in younger kids. Because the signs build up so gradually, doctors might not catch it until the symptoms are more obvious. In kids under five, for example, there often isn't enough time for all the typical features to appear, which is why leprosy seems less common in that age group. This delay can also jumble the link between when someone was exposed and when problems start showing up, making it complex to trace the infection through communities; in short, the slow onset not only clouds early detection but also complicates timely treatment and broader public health management (Mehta et al., 2022). Consider, too, how the incubation time plays into patterns of relapse and treatment effectiveness.

Research generally suggests that relapses emerge several years after the main therapy wraps up, on average, about six years later. It turns out that the type and length of the multidrug treatment matter a lot; briefer regimens might even bring on a quicker relapse, hinting that cutting treatment short can let the bacteria hang on and later reawaken. To summarize, the combination of different incubation lengths across disease forms and treatment courses points to the need for personalized monitoring and extended post-treatment follow-up so as to lessen relapse risks and improve outcomes (Shetty et al., 2011). The unpredictable incubation period also complicates efforts to rein in the spread of leprosy. Since the infection can be silent for years, detecting new cases relies heavily on watchful screening, especially among high-risk individuals and close contacts of those already diagnosed. In fact, catching leprosy in kids often signals that fresh infections are happening in the community, underlining ongoing transmission and hidden reservoirs of the disease. This scenario highlights why a broad public health approach—including early diagnosis, preventive immunization, and careful contact tracing—is so crucial. All things considered, taking on the challenges posed by this long, hidden incubation period with extra caution and swift action remains key to reducing both the clinical impact and the spread of the disease (Mehta et al., 2022).

4.1.2. Factors Influencing Incubation

Leprosy's progression depends on a combination of factors that don't always fall into neat categories. In most cases, the time between first coming into contact with Mycobacterium leprae and noticing any symptoms—what we commonly call the incubation period—can be as short as a few months or extend well past a decade. Generally speaking, the body's own defenses play a major role: a strong cell-mediated response might lead to milder forms of the disease or delay symptoms, while a weaker immune system could speed things up and cause more severe signs. Genetics and even nutrition come into play, subtly affecting how the immune system handles the bacteria. This interplay, with a sort of repeated reminder of how key immune health is, makes early diagnosis complex, and delays in treatment only add to the risk of spreading the infection and increasing disability. Everyday living conditions are also part of the picture.

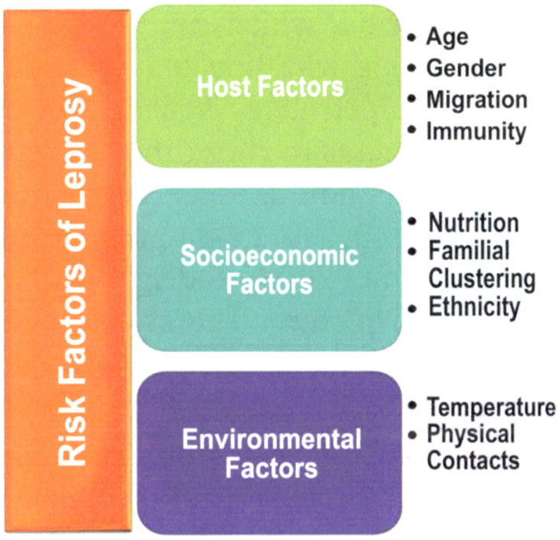

Figure 4.3. Various risk factors of leprosy.

Source: Cureus. (2023). Various Risk Factors of Leprosy.

People who live in crowded or unsanitary spaces tend to have more constant exposure to the bacterium, which can sometimes shorten that waiting period before symptoms appear because the body faces a heavier bacterial load. Climate factors and socioeconomic challenges often blur the lines even further; for instance, areas with poor healthcare access may not only extend the period before symptoms turn obvious but also hinder early recognition and treatment. In various settings, underlying conditions or other infections can also interfere with how the body manages the bacteria, further influencing how quickly the disease takes hold. Essentially, a complex interaction of environmental and personal factors means that public health measures aimed at better living conditions, improved nutrition, and increased clinical awareness are crucial to curbing the spread and impact of leprosy. Looking deeper, insights from pharmacology and immunology help us understand just how complex leprosy's behavior can be. Treatment plans often try to temper the immune response just enough to avoid worsening symptoms or triggering drug resistance—a strategy not too different from those used in other immune-related issues (Neunert et al., 2019). Although these methods were originally laid out for autoimmune disorders, they seem to fit well when we consider that a person's immune state is central to how the disease unfolds. At the molecular level, some studies suggest that changes in immune regulation, like shifts in transcription activity—might affect the way the bacterium interacts with its host, a pattern also observed in other illnesses where factors like transcription factor degradation come into play (Katherine et al., 2018). Ultimately, these molecular details help explain why some individuals experience a delayed onset while others do not, and they hint at the possibility of targeted treatments that could help shorten or stabilize the incubation period, thereby improving outcomes (Figure 4.3).

4.1.3. Implications for Disease Spread

Leprosy's spread depends on a combination of who gets it and where they live. It usually spreads through long periods of close contact, often among family members when Mycobacterium leprae is passed along in respiratory droplets. Sometimes you see skin spots or nerve issues that can, in many cases, delay recognizing the disease; this lets undetected cases persist longer in the community. Then there's the incubation period, which can vary wildly, from several months to over a decade—making it complex to untangle who infected whom. Individuals living in poverty with limited access to good healthcare, cramped living spaces, and unsanitary surroundings are especially at risk, which means the infection tends to stick around in these regions. Animal sources, like armadillos, though a less common route, add another twist by hinting at the possibility of zoonotic spread. All of these factors together suggest that a broad, careful watch is needed to keep leprosy's transmission in check (Gardner et al., 2008; Rodriguez-Morales, 2019). Socio-economic factors also mix in heavily with the clinical picture. The stigma and social isolation that come with leprosy often deter people from seeking help early, thereby stretching out the time they might, even inadvertently, spread the disease. Movement of populations, from rural areas where the disease is endemic to bustling urban centers—can shuffle the pathogen into new pockets of susceptible people. There's also an indirect nod to climate; shifts in weather that influence how people and insects interact might change transmission risk a bit (even though, to be clear, leprosy is not spread by insects). Generally speaking, these social and environmental issues are just as important as the clinical signs in shaping the epidemic's path (Rodriguez-Morales, 2019). Beyond the typical human-to-human spread, there are wider ripples that call for fresh approaches in research and intervention. Studies with nonhuman primates have, in most cases, opened up new insights about how hosts and microbes interact ; insights that help explain why leprosy tends to persist. Research using macaque models has revealed some of the long, quiet phases and chronic infection mechanisms that mirror the slow course of the disease. These findings, arguably, could steer the development of vaccines or treatments designed to break the chain of spread. Moreover, tackling neglected tropical diseases like leprosy calls for tougher health infrastructure and more community education to catch cases early and trim the stigma. To summarize, bridging clinical signals, environmental factors, and lab research in a multidisciplinary way looks promising for curbing leprosy's global impact (Gardner et al., 2008; Rodriguez-Morales, 2019).

4.2. Skin Manifestations

Leprosy shows up in many unpredictable ways, mostly depending on how each person's body fights off Mycobacterium leprae. You might notice a few lights, pale spots or red patches on the skin—sometimes even raised lumps that seem to pop out unexpectedly. Often these marks go hand in hand with changes in feeling, since the microbes tend to focus on the nerves right in the skin;

this loss of sensation is a big clue for most clinicians. In many cases the range of these skin signs (from the mild tuberculoid type to the more spread-out lepromatous forms) mirrors just how robust—or not—the body's immune defenses are. Further, these skin damages don't just show an infection is present; they also help the disease move along if it isn't detected early.

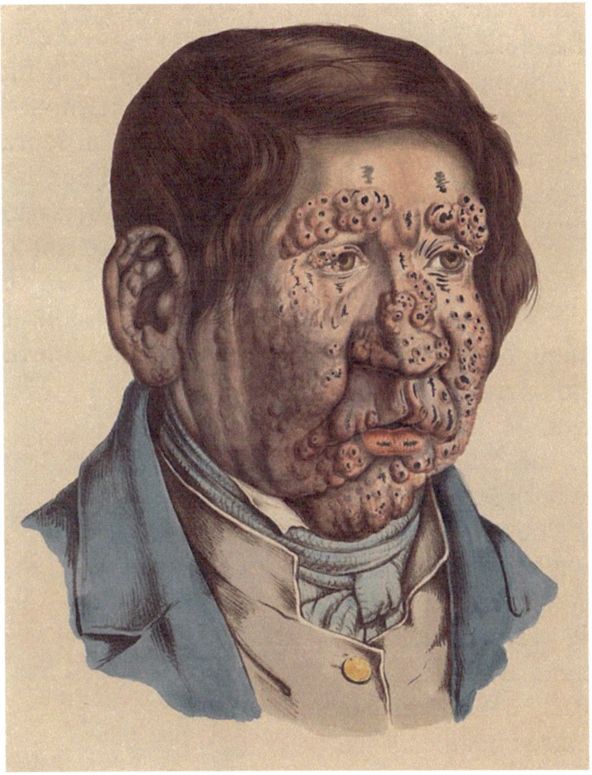

Figure 4.4. Skin manifestations.

Source: By https://wellcomeimages.org/indexplus/obf_images/6c/06/31c42b21852bf000b0523b6b7e61.jpgGallery: https://wellcomeimages.org/indexplus/image/L0074842.htmlWellcome Collection gallery (2018-03-21): https://wellcomecollection.org/works/xkekcuxr CC-BY-4.0, CC BY 4.0, https://commons.wikimedia.org/w/index.php?curid=36302224

Sometimes, leprosy even sneaks up in odd spots like the ear. It can affect the external ear, including the lobules, completely pain-free—a bit surprising when you compare it to conditions like relapsing polychondritis, where individuals usually feel pain and the lobules remain untouched. This subtle symptom, especially when mixed with joint aches and unusual skin patches, easily throws off the diagnosis. In many cases, only a close look through histopathology can clear up whether it's leprosy or maybe an autoimmune mix-up, preventing the mistake of using immunosuppressive drugs when they shouldn't be used (Pruthi et al., 2016). On a practical level, these complex presentations remind doctors to keep leprosy in mind, even in cases that don't fit the classic textbook picture. Leprosy isn't just about what you see on the surface; sometimes it reaches the genitals or other mucous areas, which makes figuring things out that much harder. These lesions might look just like common sexually transmitted infections, with ulcerations, bumpy, wart-like growths, or even deeper tissue damages that confuse the issue. And in cases of lepromatous leprosy, issues like hypogonadism can sneak in, adding yet another twist to an already complicated picture. Even though these genital signs don't always get the spotlight, they do add to the social stigma and overall health burden carried by patients. Being aware of these mixed-cut presentations is key for catching the disease early and handling not just the physical, but also the sensitive social side of things (Richens, 2004) (Figure 4.4).

4.2.1. Types of Skin Lesions

People with leprosy can show a whole range of skin changes that seem to mirror the body's varied immune responses to Mycobacterium leprae. In many cases, early marks, often rather vague, appear as pale spots with softly blurred edges and reduced feeling. These spots might be so understated they could be confused with other skin conditions, which can make detecting the disease in its early stages pretty complex. As things progress, the lesions tend to become more obvious—sometimes as clearly defined pale or reddish patches, or even as raised nodules. Their shape and spread usually reflect the person's immune status; for instance, tuberculoid leprosy generally shows a few sharply outlined plaques along with notable nerve problems, whereas lepromatous leprosy typically brings about many symmetrical nodules or a more diffused skin involvement. This varied clinical picture of skin lesions helps guide both classification and treatment, usually relying on careful physical exams paired with tissue studies (Rajshri et al., 2021). A look under the microscope often gives the final word on the different skin marks seen in leprosy. The Ridley-Jopling scheme, which connects what you see clinically with what appears in the tissue, generally splits the condition into five types: indeterminate, tuberculoid, borderline tuberculoid, borderline lepromatous, and lepromatous. For example, tuberculoid lesions usually feature nicely formed granulomas with only a few bacteria, a sign of a strong cell-mediated response. However, lepromatous lesions reveal a rather diffuse mix of macrophages loaded with bacilli, hinting at a weaker immune reaction. The borderline forms show a combination of these features, with the amount of granulomatous activity and bacillary counts varying a bit. Special stains, like the Fite-Faraco method—are often key for detecting Mycobacterium leprae in these lesions, which then helps clinch both the diagnosis and the proper categorization. All these microscopic signals tend to line up with the varied clinical appearances seen in patients (Rajshri et al., 2021). Skin lesions due to leprosy sometimes get mixed up with those from other infectious diseases.

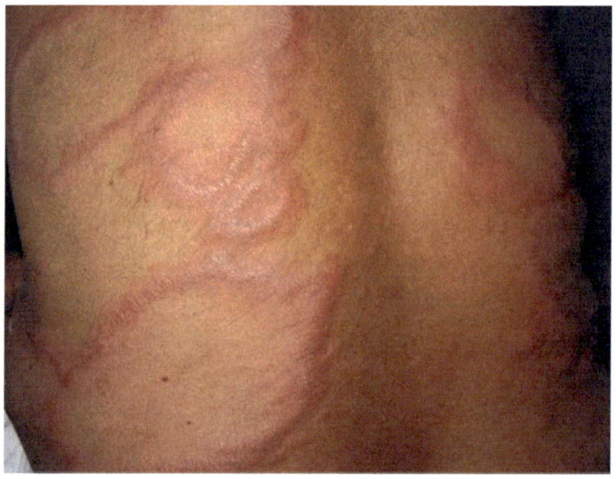

Figure 4.5. Skin lesions.

Source: Dermacosm. (n.d.). Leprosy Skin Lesions.

Take leishmaniasis, for instance: though it too can produce lesions ranging anywhere from ulcers to nodules, its cause lies in an intracellular parasite transmitted by sand flies, a clear difference from the bacterial origin found in leprosy. Especially in areas where several infectious skin issues overlap, knowing exactly what a leprosy lesion looks like is pretty critical. Recognizing these lesions through both clinical checks and tissue analysis can lead to quicker treatment, which in turn helps cut down on long-term disability, and yes, even the stigma that often tags along. In most cases, sorting out these nuanced lesion types not only guides more focused therapy but also backs up public health efforts aimed at controlling the spread and complications of the disease (Rajshri et al., 2021) (Figure 4.5).

4.2.2. Distribution of Lesions on the Body

Leprosy diagnosis often hinges on where its signature skin spots appear. Lesions tend to show up in the cooler parts of the body—on the face, ears, hands, feet, and even along the outer areas of the limbs. Generally speaking, these patches vary in color, texture, and even hair growth. The uneven distribution is a striking marker, hinting at nerve problems that disturb normal feeling and skin maintenance. Since these regions are also more likely to experience minor injuries, the resulting damage can worsen the condition, so doctors must weigh both environmental influences and body structure when considering leprosy. Environmental exposure also plays a role in shaping the pattern of these lesions, adding another layer to our understanding of the disease. For example, in other mycobacterial infections such as Buruli ulcer, lesions often cluster around joints like the elbows and ankles—a pattern that hints at the impact of mechanical stress and blood flow. However, leprosy does not efficiently follow patterns seen with common insect bites or superficial injuries; its lesion spread instead points to unique pathogen-specific processes. In most cases, this differentiation underscores the need to closely examine both the bacteria and how its lesions are spread as a key part of the clinical evaluation (Bolz et al., 2013). Nerve damage is a major factor in how leprosy lesions evolve. When the trigeminal nerve gets involved, for instance, the resulting sensory loss can lead to trophic ulcers on the face after repeated minor traumas. Although trigeminal trophic syndrome is rare, instances such as bilateral facial ulcerations following surgical nerve damage clearly demonstrate how disrupted nerve signals can alter lesion patterns and their persistence (Di Luca et al., 2017). Overall, it becomes essential to assess both the skin changes and underlying nerve issues, since sensory deficits heavily influence where lesions form and how long they last.

4.2.3. Changes in Skin Pigmentation

Skin color changes often give doctors early hints about various skin issues; leprosy, for instance, shows some pretty unique pigment shifts. You might see patches that come off as lighter or even a bit red, and that usually means there's some deeper inflammation at work along with nerve involvement. Basically, these changes happen because Mycobacterium leprae messes with the pigment cells, so they don't work like they should. Often the affected areas feel numb, which helps set leprosy apart from other skin conditions. There's also a tendency for these spots to show extra little signs like hair loss or dryness. Recognizing these shifts early is quite important, especially in places where leprosy is a common misdiagnosis can delay treatment and even worsen the outlook (Patel et al., 2017). How leprosy changes skin color varies a lot, depending on the type of the disease and how the body reacts. In cases like tuberculoid leprosy, you generally get well-defined lighter patches with a notable loss of feeling—a reflection of a strong immune response that keeps the bacteria in check. On the other hand, the lepromatous form tends to bring about more diffusely spread red patches or even nodules that might darken, because here the bacteria have spread more widely in the skin. This kind of contrast shows why paying attention to the way skin color changes work along with other signs is key in figuring out the disease. You might also run into secondary changes, like areas getting darker or lighter after treatment, which can make things a bit more confusing. So, having a solid grasp of these pigment shifts can boost diagnostic accuracy and help guide treatment plans (Patel et al., 2017). Leprosy isn't like other skin problems that affect color—its changes also mirror nerve damage, which often makes things more complicated. Since the lighter patches usually lose feeling, patients can end up with repeated injuries or even minor infections that further alter how the skin looks. Interestingly, nerve issues sometimes show up before any obvious skin changes are visible, prompting doctors to use nerve tests or even small biopsies to catch what's called pure neurotic leprosy, a form that might not show clear skin lesions but can still have subtle pigment shifts (Jayaraman et al., 2012). Generally speaking, the interplay between the immune response, bacterial load, and skin color leads to a pretty complex picture. In most cases, combining careful clinical checks with nerve studies and lab tests is crucial to piece together the full story of these pigment alterations in the broader context of leprosy (Figure 4.6).

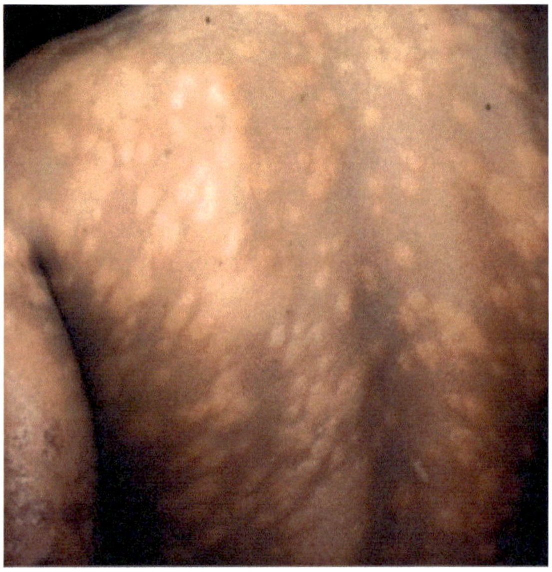

Figure 4.6. Changes in skin pigmentation.

Source: The Leprosy Mission International. (n.d.). Patch of Discolored Skin Due to Leprosy.

4.3. Neurological Symptoms

Leprosy hits the nerves in some pretty dramatic ways, often shaping how the disease unfolds and how treatments get planned. Patients often mention that they feel numb, experience tingling, or even lose the sense of pain , all signs pointing to damage with the peripheral nerves. This usually happens when Mycobacterium leprae sneaks into Schwann cells, inducing inflammation and causing the myelin to break down.

As things progress, patients might notice muscle weakness or even paralysis—a real blow to everyday life. You also see nerve pain and deformities cropping up from this damage, which makes the situation even messier. Catching these issues early on is key to keeping permanent damage at bay, and paying close attention to nerve function ends up being a central part of managing the disease. Nerve problems in leprosy aren't limited only to the peripheral nerves; they can create a real diagnostic puzzle, much like other infectious nerve conditions. In forms like borderline or lepromatous leprosy, the nerve damage tends to be more widespread, often linked with a stronger inflammatory reaction. Generally speaking, the body's own immune response can trigger sudden flare-ups, sometimes known as lepra reactions, which bring on extra issues such as neuritis and a loss of sensation.

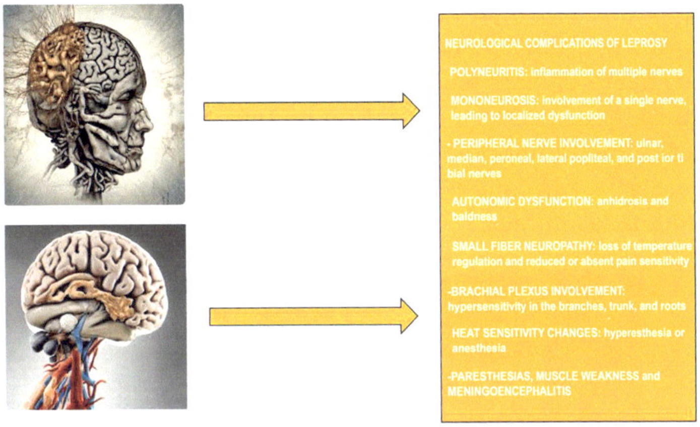

Figure 4.7. Neurological complications of leprosy.

Source: Neurology International. (2024). Neurological Complications of Leprosy.

New imaging techniques—though not perfect—help doctors get a clearer look at nerve inflammation and structural changes, making it easier to keep track and diagnose accurately. By combining what patients say they feel with lab results and even molecular signals, clinicians can better tell apart leprous neuropathy from other causes, which is pretty vital for timely treatment and for cutting down long-term nerve problems. Sometimes the struggle with nerve issues in leprosy isn't just the medical side of it, but also a tangle of social and economic challenges, especially in regions where the disease is common. In many cases, subtle signs like a slight numbness or early muscle weakness go unnoticed in resource-poor settings, often leading to higher disability rates. These delays mirror what we see with other infectious nerve disorders, where early, almost whispered symptoms prevent swift diagnosis (Ahmad et al., 2024). Financial and social pressures can limit access to good healthcare – including high-tech imaging or advanced molecular tests – which might otherwise pick up the problem sooner. As a result, these neurological complications can creep up unobserved until they're quite severe, sometimes showing as nerve swelling, deformities, or even secondary infections. Tackling these barriers, along with boosting early recognition of nerve issues, is crucial for lowering the overall impact of the disease on various populations (Ahmad et al., 2024) (Figure 4.7).

4.3.1. Peripheral Nerve Involvement

In leprosy, what happens to the peripheral nerves matters, it shapes not only how the disease shows up but also its long-term effects. Mycobacterium leprae creeps into these nerves, inducing a kind of chronic inflammation that makes them thicken over time, eventually leading to both loss of feeling and weak movement. Patients frequently mention feeling numb in spots that later match up with their skin patches, a sign that the sensory nerves have taken a hit. The ulnar nerve, for example, often gets noticeably thick (you can feel it during examination), which generally hints at the bacterium's odd fondness for cooler parts of the body. These changes tend to lower protective sensations, thereby upping the risk of injuries, ulcers, and even further infections. In most cases, the journey from early nerve damage to serious disability stresses the need for swift diagnosis and treatment to keep permanent deformities at bay (Rao, 2023). Generally speaking, the underlying process begins when the bacteria trigger a persistent granulomatous inflammation that slowly messes with the nerve's fiber structure. As the axons start breaking down, demyelination often tags along, so that nerve signals just don't get through as effectively as they once did. This disruption typically shows up as reduced sensation in a glove-and-stocking pattern—pretty much what you'd expect when thickened nerves stop doing their job properly. Weakness in the muscles, and sometimes even paralysis, can follow as the motor fibers give way, leading to physical issues like claw hand, foot drop, or even facial palsy.

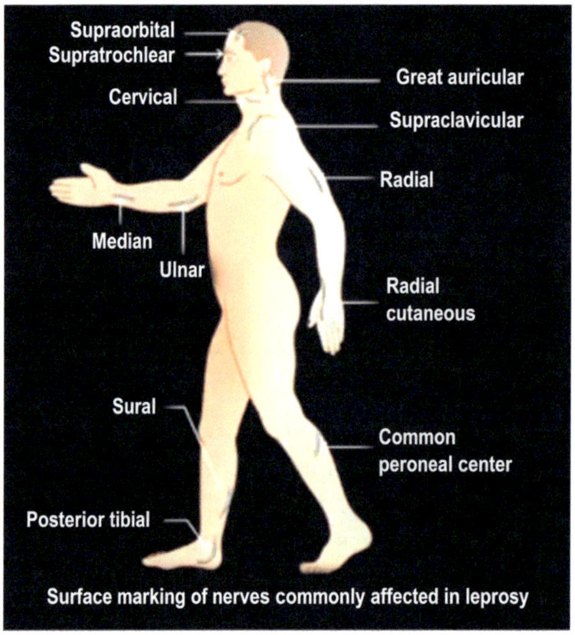

Figure 4.8. Nerve involvement in leprosy.

Source: Calderone A, Aloisi MC, Casella C, Fiannacca S, Cosenza B, Quartarone A, Calabrò RS. The Neurological Impact of Leprosy: Manifestations and Treatment Approaches. *Neurology International.* 2024; 16(6):1492-1508. https://doi.org/10.3390/neurolint16060111.

Often, the nerve damage keeps chugging along over time and may even worsen during treatment because of immune reactions, namely Type 1 and Type 2 lepra reactions, which makes ongoing neurological checks and treatment alters all the more important (Rao, 2023). When you compare other peripheral neuropathies, like those seen in neurosyphilis, a similar interplay between infections and nerve damage pops up. Although the microbes behind the conditions aren't the same, both illnesses show that peripheral nerves are surprisingly vulnerable to attacks—whether from an infectious trigger or an immune response, which then leads to that tell-tale sensorimotor loss. Overlapping signs such as diminished sensation and nerve thickening can complicate the issue diagnostically, so it usually takes a full workup—clinical checks, blood tests, and electrophysiological studies—to sort things out. Ultimately, effective management depends on identifying the exact cause and using a combination of tailored antimicrobial therapy and immune modulation to slow down, or even halt, further nerve damage. To summarize, this understanding supports the idea that tackling leprosy's nerve involvement calls for an integrated approach in both diagnosis and treatment (Figure 4.8).

4.3.2. Symptoms of Nerve Damage

Peripheral nerve damage plays a major role in how leprosy shows up. Sometimes it appears even before skin changes become obvious, and in other cases, it arrives hand in hand with them. Early on, when the nerve injury begins its slow, hidden march, doctors might miss it, especially if skin lesions are barely there. People can start to feel odd sensations like numbness, tingling, or burning in the affected spots. This happens because Mycobacterium leprae seems to zero in on Schwann cells, setting off a long-term inflammation and a kind of granulomatous breakdown of the nerve. In most cases, when the motor nerves get involved, muscle weakness and atrophy follow, often leading to deformities if nothing is done.

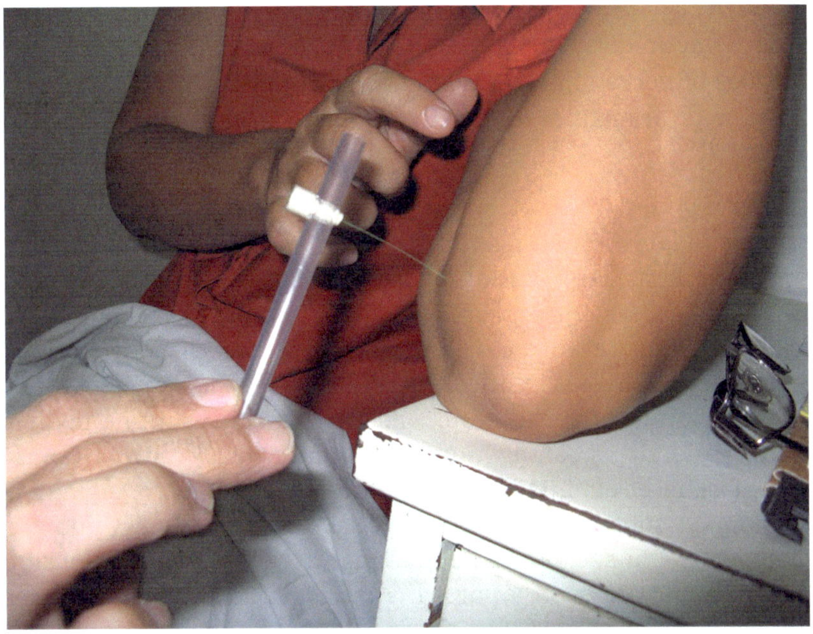

Figure 4.9. The symptoms of nerve damage.

Source: By Gadogado123 - Own work, CC BY-SA 4.0, https://commons.wikimedia.org/w/index.php?curid=84521471Medication.

That's why it's so important to check the nerves thoroughly. Tests such as nerve conduction studies might pick up changes even before someone notices symptoms, although these electrical signals aren't exclusively linked to leprosy, making a nerve biopsy the most reliable method for confirmation (Jayaraman et al., 2012). Looking at the bigger picture, enlarged nerves and loss of sensation are key warning signs that add to the overall burden of leprosy. Often, anesthetic skin lesions that come with noticeably thickened nerves point to peripheral nerve involvement, a pattern frequently seen in regions where the disease is common. The severity of nerve issues tends to shift depending on how the body's immune system reacts; for example, tuberculoid cases often show more confined damage, whereas lepromatous forms tend to cause far more widespread nerve compromise. Generally speaking, the immune responses seen in leprosy can even worsen nerve injury, triggering bouts of acute neuritis and painful tenderness. These changes can hit fast and hard, highlighting how unpredictable leprosy neuropathy can be. Physicians need to keep their guard up, especially with patients coming from or visiting endemic areas, to catch and treat the condition before any permanent damage occurs (Aftab et al., 2016). Over time, the ongoing nerve damage from leprosy can lead to serious functional impairments that deeply affect one's quality of life. As motor nerve problems gradually sap muscle strength, deformities like claw hand or foot drop are common stumbling blocks for many. Meanwhile, the loss of pain and temperature sensation often opens the door to repeated injuries and secondary infections, which only adds to the disability. It's clear that catching nerve changes early is important to avoid these later complications. Treatment isn't just about the antibiotics needed to clear the infection; it also involves immunomodulatory therapies to rein in the inflammation that harms nerves. Often, a team effort, bringing together rehabilitation, and sometimes even surgery, is required to manage the damage already done. In short, keeping a close, sometimes even obsessive, eye on neurological signs is crucial for lessening the lasting consequences of nerve injury, underscoring just how central these symptoms are to the overall course of leprosy Jayaraman et al., 2012; (Aftab et al., 2016) (Figure 4.9).

4.3.3. Consequences of Untreated Nerve Damage

Untreated nerve damage in leprosy often sets off a chain reaction of damages that goes far beyond the original infection. Numbness and a loss of sensation can show up early on but are too frequently missed or misread by primary care providers—so patients end up waiting for help way too long. This lapse is especially harmful because once one can't feel pain or temperature changes, injuries sneak in and may lead to lasting disabilities. In some cases, the nerves in the arms suffer too, causing muscles to waste and strength to drop, which in turn slices into daily function and overall quality of life. Research generally speaking hints that multibacillary leprosy tends to tangle up with several cranial nerves (Islam et al., 2016), making the neglect of early signs a major contributor to long-run socioeconomic issues. Besides physical harm, continued nerve damage in leprosy also takes a heavy psychological and social toll. People might end up with very visible changes , think clawed hands, a dropped foot, or even a partially paralyzed face , that often lead to stigma and isolation. When the peripheral nerves giving us, everyday functions are compromised, the impact is as much mental as it is bodily. When the body's reaction to Mycobacterium leprae isn't kept in check, nerve injury can spiral further (especially in patients whose immunity is already on the wane) (Mawardi et al., 2018). In most cases, these persisting effects make it hard to secure a job or stay involved with one's community, feeding into cycles of poverty and discrimination, which underlines the need for earlier, clearer diagnosis and management. Perhaps the most critical fallout from untreated nerve damage is the onset of lifelong disability—a burden on both the individual and health care systems. Damaged nerves tend to suffer from ongoing inflammation and even develop fibrosis, meaning their capacity to heal is severely stifled. As a result, patients face a cascade of problems like chronic ulcers, secondary bacterial infections, and even limb deformities. Studies have shown that many leprosy patients endure diagnostic delays extending beyond six months, during which irreversible nerve damage accumulates (Islam et al., 2016). Worse still, when cranial nerves get involved, conditions such as lagophthalmos and corneal ulceration can threaten eyesight. Hence, this cluster of complications not only deepens personal suffering but also places a heavy long-term strain on treatment and rehabilitation services, making early detection and prompt treatment absolutely essential (Figure 4.10).

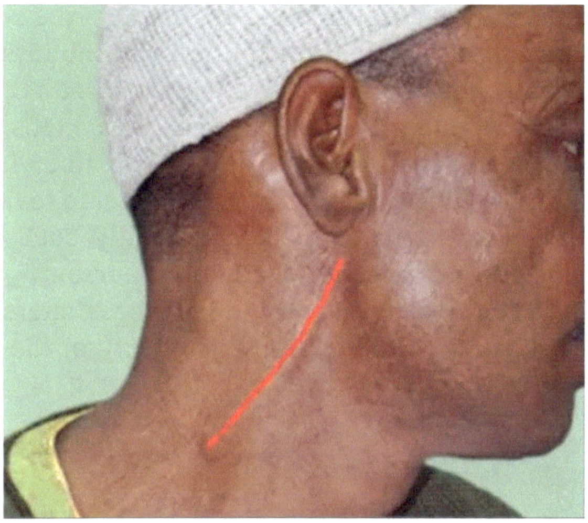

Figure 4.10. The consequences of untreated nerve damage.

Source: PrepLadder. (2023). Greater Auricular Nerve Damage in Leprosy.

4.4. Systemic Effects

Leprosy mostly shows up as skin spots and nerve issues, but it doesn't stop there. The infection can stir up a full-body reaction that leaves patients with symptoms like fever, a general sense of tiredness, and swollen lymph nodes, often cropping up during those Type 1 and Type 2 flare-ups. In many cases, these wider signs sneak in before or right when a major bout begins, pushing the immune system into overdrive and worsening nerve damage alongside other organ damages. Detecting these broader effects early is important, since catching them in time can help avoid long-lasting disabilities and keeps treatment on track. The damage to nerves is a well-known mark of leprosy, yet this very harm can trigger a cascade of other issues. For instance, nerve inflammation (neuritis) might bring on sharp pain, muscle weakness, and even disrupt functions like heart rhythm or digestion. Sometimes the body's own overactive immune response, an internal inflammatory storm, leads to joint pain, eye damages such as iridocyclitis, and recurrent fevers. Essentially, the infection goes far beyond just skin marks, reaching and affecting multiple systems in unpredictable ways. Given that these symptoms can flare up intermittently, keeping a close watch with a team of experts becomes vital to manage the disease effectively. All this means doctors have to think about more than just skin and nerve problems. Because leprosy's systemic impact can make patients more open to other infections when the immune system is low, it's a bit like what happens in other chronic mycobacterial diseases. Balancing antibiotic treatment with drugs that calm down the immune overreaction (Haworth et al., 2017) is a real juggling act. In most cases, noticing similarities with other intracellular infections shows just how key it is to grasp the ups and downs between the body's defenses and the microbe (Torres et al., 2017). Overall, mixcombining this broader understanding into treatment plans is crucial for fine-tuning care and boosting patient outcomes in the wider battle against infections.

4.4.1. Immune Response to Infection

Mycobacterium leprae's interaction with our immune system sets the stage for how leprosy shows itself. In some cases, like with the tuberculoid form, the body mounts a pretty vigorous cellular defense, macrophages get activated and even form granulomas that help corral the bacteria. These immune cells end up with a proinflammatory gene pattern, which tells us they're doing their part to keep the infection in check. Then again, however, the lepromatous form seems to have a much weaker cellular reaction, so the bacteria end up multiplying inside foamy macrophages that seem more tuned to anti-inflammatory or scavenging roles. Basically, such differences in macrophage behavior, often decideed by factors like infection load and a person's genes, play a central role in how the disease turns out. And, interestingly, the way the pathogen alters its own surroundings (e.g., by infecting Schwann cells) only adds to the overall complexity of the host–pathogen interaction (Leal-Calvo et al., 2021).

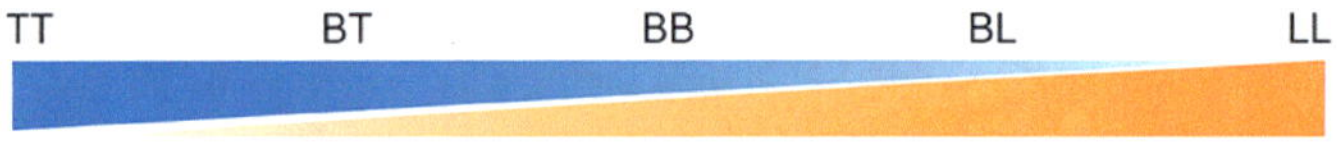

Cell types	T-lep immune responses	Leprosy associated genes	L-lep immune responses
Macrophage	M1 macrophage Microbicidal function	*VDR, OPA1, SLC7A2* *RAB32, SLC29A3, LRRK2* *IRGM, CTSB, DEFB1* *PARK2, PACRG, TNF*	M2 macrophage Phagocytosis
Dendritic Cell	Langerhans cells ↑ Plasmacytoid dendritic cells ↑ Dermal dendrocytes ↑	*TLR1, TLR2, NOD2* *HLA genes, MICA, MICB*	Langerhans cells ↓ Plasmacytoid dendritic cells ↓ Dermal dendrocytes ↓
Keratinocyte	HLA-DR + ICAM-1 ↑	*FLG*	HLA-DR - ICAM-1 ↓
T cell	Th1 ↑ Th17 ↑ Th9 ↑ IL-2, IL-18, IFN-γ ↑	*IL23R, IL12B, TNFSF15* *TYK2, SOCS1, IL18R1* *LTA*	Th2 ↑ Treg ↑ Th22 ↑ IL-4, IL-5 ↑

Figure 4.11. Genes and gene products involved in the immune response to M. leprae. Molecular and cellular interactions known or postulated to play a role in the immune response to M. leprae are depicted, as are genes with evidence of an association with susceptibility to leprosy and/or leprosy immune reactions through candidate gene studies, linkage analyses, or genome-wide association studies.

Source: Mi Z, Liu H and Zhang F (2020) Advances in the Immunology and Genetics of Leprosy. Front. Immunol. 11:567. doi: 10.3389/fimmu.2020.00567

Leprosy isn't just about the immediate, innate immune hit; it also pulls in adaptive strategies, where T-cell subsets and their cytokine outputs shape how the disease evolves. Generally speaking, patients with fewer bacteria (the paucibacillary type) tend to show a lively T-cell mix—both $CD4^{+}$ and $CD8^{+}$ cells releasing IFN-γ, IL-4, and IL-10, which suggests a balanced but strong push aimed at clearing the bacteria. On the other hand, the multibacillary cases mostly show a narrower cytokine profile, leaning mainly on IL-10 and IL-4, and this might help the bacteria slip past the immune defenses. Even among household contacts, there's evidence, like an extra boost in IFN-γ, that could be an early hint of either protective immunity or an unnoticed, subclinical infection. In most cases, these immune markers double as signals that might one day improve how we diagnose and predict disease progression (Marçal et al., 2020). Understanding our immune system's response to Mycobacterium leprae is key to interpreting why the disease appears in so many different ways and to coming up with better treatment strategies. In most instances, a strong Th1-type response is linked with a more confined and generally milder form of leprosy, while a shift toward Th2 or regulatory responses favors a more widespread infection packed with bacteria. It turns out that the state of macrophage activation, the mix of cytokines, and the delicate back-and-forth between pro- and anti-inflammatory signals together come into play when causing nerve damage and tissue changes. Advances in immunogenomics and biomarker research have been steadily peeling back the layers of these complex responses, thereby influencing ideas for early detection, treatment follow-up, and even monitoring those in close contact with patients. To summarize, the way our body fights back defines not only the clinical features of leprosy but also helps shape more personalized treatment and public health strategies (Marçal et al., 2020; Leal-Calvo et al., 2021) (Figure 4.11).

4.4.2. Impact on Overall Health

Leprosy isn't just a skin problem—it messes with a person's whole health and everyday living. The disease often hits the nerves—Mycobacterium leprae has a tendency for targeting peripheral nerves, so people end up with lost sensations and muscle weakness. When you can't feel things properly, you're more likely to suffer from additional injuries or get ulcers that, if ignored, might lead to serious disabilities or even deformities. These physical changes can get in the way of daily activities and, in most cases, add to social stigma and mental strains. Because leprosy sticks around for a long time, its effects usually persist, hitting not just health but also a person's social and economic well-being. The slow but steady nerve damage shows why finding the problem early and acting fast is so important – what looks like a simple clinical sign soon balloons into wider health issues needing both medical help and community support. It isn't only the nerve issues that are troublesome. Leprosy also brings along whole-body complications—secondary infections and a constant state of inflammation become key players in the disease's drama. People often get detected in cycles of painful flare-ups, known as lepra reactions, which cause swelling, extra pain, and even worsen the nerve damage. These bouts, in many cases, make tissue damage worse and slow down recovery, underlining just how complex the illness can be for the immune system. This persisting inflammation sometimes pushes patients into disabilities that require long-term care and increases pressure on healthcare services. Further, the mental toll, with bouts of anxiety or depression from both stigmatization and ongoing physical issues, means that treatment has to consider the whole person, not just the symptoms. And it gets even more complicated when you factor in that leprosy often coexists with other neglected tropical diseases among people in less advantaged communities. For example, podoconiosis, a condition marked by crippling leg swelling and ongoing inflammation (Molla et al., 2012), shares a similar pattern, where enduring morbidity limits mobility and the ability to work. Simple, cost-effective measures to control these infections can provide big public health wins by preventing disabilities and boosting community resilience (Fenwick et al., 2005). Programs that mix early detection, solid treatment, and rehabilitation might help lessen the long-term impacts of leprosy. Not only do these efforts cut down on the raw physical problems, but they also begin to tackle the deep-seated social and economic challenges that come hand-in-hand with the disease, making it clear that a broad, sustainable approach is needed to improve overall health outcomes in regions where the disease is common.

4.4.3. Co-Morbid Conditions Associated with Leprosy

Leprosy is a persistent infection from Mycobacterium leprae and, in many cases, lands patients in a complex situation with other health issues. This disease often shows up along with extra infections that complicate both diagnosis and treatment. Tuberculosis, for example, is another mycobacterial pathogen that sometimes tags along with leprosy, especially in places where resources are thin. When TB joins the mix, it doesn't just shift the immune response, it also makes drug schedules and side effects harder to handle. And then there's the fact that leprosy reactions can weaken the immune system, opening up room for other infections like HIV, which ups the ante on managing the illness. In most cases, grasping the complex interactions between these conditions is key to offering tailored and comprehensive care. People with leprosy don't just wrestle with infectious threats; they also battle the consequences of chronic nerve damage. Nerve impairment can lead to a range of issues such as sensory loss, deformities, and a predisposition to secondary infections; sometimes, these even result in ulcers or amputation. Chronic conditions like diabetes can make things even messier by intensifying neuropathic pain and stalling wound healing. Overall, the concurrence of metabolic issues with leprosy forces doctors to keep a watchful eye through careful, integrated management strategies. This overlap, in turn, piles on the physical burden, boosts healthcare costs, and increases the need for prolonged rehabilitation. Social and immune factors add further layers to the challenge. Immunosuppression—whether from HIV, malnutrition or other causes—can spell damage, leading to higher risks for severe infections like abdominal TB and other opportunistic diseases (Chalya et al., 2013; Olaye & Beke, 2018). Advanced age, delays in getting treatment, and having multiple illnesses often make patient care even complex, generally speaking. Early intervention and constant vigilance are crucial here while integrating public health initiatives helps lighten the overall load. Hence, a more relaxed approach to addressing these intertwined conditions could help reduce negative outcomes and improve the quality of life for those affected by leprosy, something every clinician strives for (Figure 4.12).

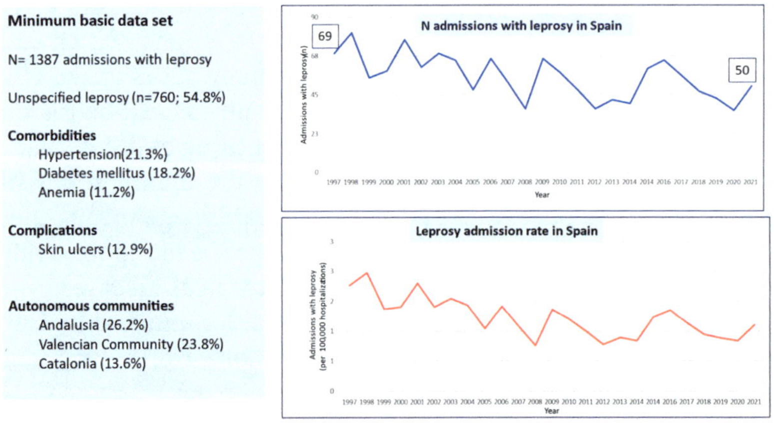

Figure 4.12. Comorbidities and complications in people admitted with leprosy in Spain, 1997–2021.

Source: Life. (2024). Comorbidities and Complications in People with Leprosy in Spain.

A CLOSER LOOK

INDETERMINATE LEPROSY (I)

An early, temporary form of the disease is indeterminate leprosy. The indeterminate form appears in subjects who have not developed CMI against *Mycobacterium leprae* (*M. leprae*) yet. It can be seen in children in endemic areas or in adults moving from countries without leprosy to endemic areas. The macule is the only skin lesion in indeterminate leprosy:

- A single macule or multiple macules (in which case there are no more than three lesions grouped together).
- No more than 3–4 cm wide.
- Red in light-skinned patients, or coppery in dark-skinned patients. They may also be hypopigmented with a homogeneous decrease in color.
- Permanent.
- Smooth surfaced, no scaling.
- With vague edges.
- Non-pruriginous.
- With normal sweating.
- With normal or slightly decreased thermal and/or tactile sensitivity.
- With normal body hairs.
- Resistant to topical therapies (Figure 4.13).

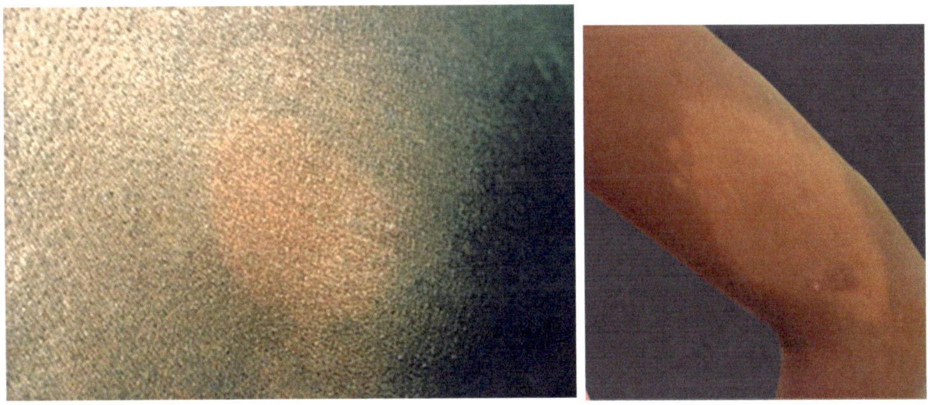

Figure 4.13. Indeterminate leprosy (I).

Source: CASE REPORT • An. bras. dermatol. 88 (6 Suppl 1) • Nov-Dec 2013 • https://doi.org/10.1590/abd1806-4841.20132050

Open-access Indeterminate leprosy and lepromatous index case: four cases in the same famil

In children, cutaneous manifestation is frequently localized on the face, buttocks, and upper or lower limbs. Peripheral nerves are not clinically affected. Acid-fast bacilli (AFB) are absent from skin smear.

Most patients affected by indeterminate leprosy heal spontaneously, while others evolve to a borderline form of the spectrum.

Careful clinical examination can identify changes in the indeterminate macule which can predict evolution onto the disease spectrum.

Moving from I to BT leprosy, the macule presents a series of differences, namely, anesthesia and prominent edges. There is also the presence of anhidrosis, which causes rough and dry surfaces.

The evolution from I to BL leprosy is characterized by central infiltration of the macule.

SUMMARY

Leprosy shows up in many different ways – sometimes with barely noticeable light patches on the skin, and other times with clear nerve damage that leads to real deformities. It's a long-term illness that often surprises doctors with its unpredictable course, including sudden reaction episodes like erythema nodosum leprosum (ENL), which further complicates treatment decisions. Catching these subtle signs early is key to avoiding lasting harm, even if the symptoms can feel all over the place. As we keep learning from new clinical findings, it becomes clear that tailoring treatments to each patient's specific situation isn't just helpful—it's essential. Getting to grips with the underlying biological factors gives clinicians a chance to predict and tackle problems before they get out of hand. New treatment ideas have been shaking up how we manage the complex immune reactions associated with leprosy, especially in cases with multiple bacteria, where ENL becomes a serious concern. Researchers, for example, have been exploring immunosuppressants like ciclosporin; these drugs seem to slow down flare-ups and cut down on the need for heavy corticosteroid use, although results for chronic ENL have been mixed (Bryceson et al., 2016). There's always that delicate balance: you want to ease the body's overactive immune response without inviting a host of unwanted side effects, particularly when patients end up on long courses of steroids. Ongoing trials and smaller pilot studies keep testing these newer methods, suggesting that treatment plans might need alters based on local factors and patient needs. Generally speaking, these efforts underline the vital need for flexible treatment guidelines and careful, ongoing patient check-ups. Besides finding better treatments, improving how we diagnose leprosy remains a core piece of the puzzle. New testing methods – sometimes borrowed from research in related infections like tuberculous lymphadenitis – offer a glimpse into faster, more accurate ways to spot the disease (Cruz et al., 2016). Doctors now combin the old-fashioned clinical exam with extra tools, such as molecular assays and cell-based evaluations, to catch the infection earlier and get treatment started without delay. By combining sharper diagnostic techniques with targeted therapies and a watchful approach to patient care, we might just cut down the overall impact of leprosy and prevent long-term disability that too often shadows the illness. To summarize, ongoing research and keeping a careful clinical eye on things remain key to battling this complex disease.

Leprosy shows up in a lot of different ways, and that comes down to how a person's immune system reacts. Sometimes the first signs are just light or red patches on the skin, with a bit of numbness hinting that nerves are getting involved. You might notice that some nerves seem thicker than usual or that feeling is off; these are the kinds of signals doctors watch out for. When the infection is heavy—what we often call the multibacillary form—you might see many scattered lesions, bumps, and noticeably thick nerves, whereas the paucibacillary type usually brings just a few spots with more focused nerve issues. If the disease isn't picked up and treated soon enough, it can eventually lead to permanent disabilities. In most cases, recent data still show a fair number of people arriving with grade 2 disabilities, meaning that there are visible deformities by the time diagnosis happens (Diabaté et al., 2025). Age and gender also seem to add a twist to how leprosy presents. While the illness can affect anyone, adult males are more commonly seen with the severe multibacillary type, where there's a higher bacterial load and tougher symptoms. At the same time, quite a few children end up with the disease, which hints at new and ongoing transmission. It's interesting, then, to see that multibacillary leprosy tends to emerge more in men, while women more often have the paucibacillary kind—a pattern that might be connected not only to differences in the immune response but also to various social factors that affect exposure and how quickly a diagnosis is made. When many patients arrive already showing disability, it underscores the issue of delayed detection and the continuing spread of the disease in these communities (Diabaté et al., 2025). Leprosy isn't just about skin spots and nerve damage, though; it often mingles with more systemic signs that can make diagnosis complex. Although it primarily deals with the skin and nerves, sometimes secondary infections or unusual immune reactions get in the mix, complicating the overall picture. In a way, this resembles other infections that affect several organs, reminding us that catching these conditions early can make a big difference. For instance, reactions like erythema nodosum leprosum and bouts of neuritis substantially add to the suffering, so keeping an eye on them is essential. To summarize, understanding the full range of leprosy's effects, even when it sometimes feels a bit complex or out of sync, is crucial for managing treatment, especially when other health issues might be persisting nearby.

KEY TERMS FROM THIS CHAPTER

- Armadillos
- Autoimmune disorders
- Bumpy
- Careful contact tracing
- Early diagnosis
- Histopathology
- Immunology
- Incubation period
- Lepromatous form
- Leprosy's clinical picture
- Neglected tropical diseases
- Personalized monitoring

References

1. Bélard, S., Tamarozzi, F., Bustinduy, A. L., Wallrauch, C., Grobusch, M. P., Kuhn, W., Brunetti, E., Joekes, E., & Heller, T. (2016). Point-of-Care Ultrasound Assessment of Tropical Infectious Diseases--A Review of Applications and Perspectives. *The American journal of tropical medicine and hygiene*, *94*(1), 8–21. https://doi.org/10.4269/ajtmh.15-0421 Bélard, S., Tamarozzi, F., Bustinduy, A. L., Wallrauch, C., Grobusch, M. P., Kuhn, W., Brunetti, E., Joekes, E., & Heller, T. (2016). Point-of-Care Ultrasound Assessment of Tropical Infectious Diseases--A Review of Applications and Perspectives. *The American journal of tropical medicine and hygiene*, *94*(1), 8–21. https://doi.org/10.4269/ajtmh.15-0421 (accessed on 10th May 2025).
2. Gardner, M. B., & Luciw, P. A. (2008). Macaque models of human infectious disease. *ILAR journal*, *49*(2), 220–255. https://doi.org/10.1093/ilar.49.2.220(accessed on 10th May 2025).
3. Aftab, H., Nielsen, S.D. & Bygbjerg, I.C. Leprosy in Denmark 1980–2010: a review of 15 cases. *BMC Res Notes* **9**, 10 (2016). https://doi.org/10.1186/s13104-015-1768-6 (accessed on 10th May 2025).
4. Khurshid Ahmad, Vypashi, and Iftikhar Ali (2024); CHILDHOOD TUBERCULAR MENINGITIS: INSIGHTS INTO CLINICAL PRESENTATION, RADIOLOGICAL FINDINGS, AND OUTCOME DETERMINANTS *Int. J. of Adv. Res.* (Jul). 1569-1573] (ISSN 2320-5407(accessed on 10th May 2025).
5. Pruthi, P., Munganda, H., Bangia, A., Rani, U., Budhiraja, R., & Brajpuriya, S. (2016). Leprosy with Atypical Skin Lesions Masquerading as Relapsing Polychondritis. *Case reports in infectious diseases*, *2016*, 7802423. https://doi.org/10.1155/2016/7802423 (accessed on 10th May 2025).
6. Olaleye A, Beke A. Determinants of Survival of Patients with Tuberculosis in Developing Countries [Internet]. Tuberculosis. InTech; 2018. Available from: http://dx.doi.org/10.5772/intechopen.75890 (accessed on 10th May 2025).
7. Bolz, M., Bratschi, M. W., Grize, L., Kerber, M., et al. (2013). Geographic distribution, age pattern and sites of lesions in a cohort of Buruli ulcer patients from the Mapé Basin of Cameroon. PLoS Negl. Trop. Dis., 7(6), e2252. https://core.ac.uk/download/18261771.pdf (accessed on 10th May 2025).
8. Bryceson, A., Moreira, A. L., Kumar, B., Voorend, C. G. N., Johnson, C., Faulds, D., Lockwood, D., et al. (2016). Comparison of efficacy and safety of ciclosporin to prednisolone in the treatment of erythema nodosum leprosum: Two randomized, double blind, controlled pilot studies in Ethiopia. PLoS Negl. Trop. Dis. https://core.ac.uk/download/42635363.pdf (accessed on 10th May 2025).
9. Cruz, A. T., Wright, C. A., Anunobi, C. C., Boehme, C. C., Murray, C. J. L., et al. (2016). Evaluation of Xpert® MTB/RIF and ustar easyNAT™ TB IAD for diagnosis of tuberculous lymphadenitis of children in Tanzania: A prospective descriptive study. BMC Infectious Diseases. https://core.ac.uk/download/46605185.pdf (accessed on 10th May 2025).
10. Damle, R. P., Vasaikar, M. S., & Bora, S. A. (2021). Clinico-pathological study of leprosy: A descriptive study. National Journal of Laboratory Medicine. National Journal of Laboratory Medicine. 2021 Jul, Vol-10(3): PO62-PO65 https://doi.org/10.7860/njlm/2021/47272.2516 (accessed on 10th May 2025).

11. di Luca, A., Ralli, M., Hemied, S., de Vincentiis, M., & di Luca, N. M. (2017). An atypical case of trigeminal trophic syndrome: A legal medicine perspective in medical responsibility. *SAGE open medical case reports, 5,* 2050313X17723548. https://doi.org/10.1177/2050313X17723548 (accessed on 10th May 2025).

12. Diabaté, A., Loumingou, L. A., Aba, Y. T., Gbandama, K. K. P., Sule, M. A., Kouakou, H. B., Bini, J. C., et al. (2025). Epidemiology and clinical features of new leprosy cases at the Raoul Follereau Institute of Cote D'Ivoire (Adzope) from 2013 to 2023. ARC Journal of Dermatology Volume 8, Issue 2, 2025, PP 31-35; ISSN No. (Online) 2456-0022; DOI: https://doi.org/10.20431/2456-0022.0802003(accessed on 10th May 2025).

13. Donovan, K. A., An, J., Nowak, R. P., Yuan, J. C., Fink, E. C., Berry, B. C., Ebert, B. L., & Fischer, E. S. (2018). Thalidomide promotes degradation of SALL4, a transcription factor implicated in Duane Radial Ray syndrome. *eLife, 7,* e38430. https://doi.org/10.7554/eLife.38430 (accessed on 10th May 2025).

14. Fenwick, A., Molyneux, D. H., & Hotez, P. J., (2005). "Rapid-impact interventions": How a policy of integrated control for Africa's neglected tropical diseases could benefit the poor. PLoS Med., 2(11), e336 https://core.ac.uk/download/pdf/3775709.pdf (accessed on 10th May 2025).

15. Haworth, C., Banks, J., Capstick, T., Fisher, A. J., Gorsuch, T., Laurenson, I. F., Leitch, A., et al. (2017). British Thoracic Society guidelines for the management of non-tuberculous mycobacterial pulmonary disease (NTM-PD). Thorax, 72, ii1–ii64. https://doi.org/10.1136/thoraxjnl-2017-210927 (accessed on 10th May 2025).

16. Hsieh C-L, Hsiao P-F. Diagnosis and Treatment of Leprosy in Taiwan during the COVID-19 Pandemic: A Retrospective Study in a Tertiaty Center. *Diagnostics.* 2023; 13(24):3655. https://doi.org/10.3390/diagnostics13243655 (accessed on 10th May 2025).

17. Islam, A. T., Sultana, S., Rahman, M., & Hoque, M. A. (2016). Neurological Manifestations in Leprosy: A Study in Tribal Community of Hill Tracts. *Journal of Enam Medical College, 6*(1), 10–14. https://doi.org/10.3329/jemc.v6i1.26373 (accessed on 10th May 2025).

18. Jayaraman, R. (2012). A Study on Diagnostic Significance of Nerve Conduction Studies in Early Detection of Pure Neuritic Hansen's Disease. https://core.ac.uk/download/287236524.pdf (accessed on 10th May 2025).

19. Kararizou, E., Anagnostou, E., Kapaki, E., & Davaki, P. (2015). Chronic inflammatory demyelinating polyneuropathy associated with neurosyphilis. The American Journal of the Medical Sciences, Volume 349, Issue 1, 90 – 91 https://www.semanticscholar.org/paper/32b5a0c5ece74a171c75e1527f6e81ead75755d1 (accessed on 10th May 2025).

20. Kattan, Jessica Anne, "The Epidemiology and Clinical Presentation of Leprosy in the Pediatric Population of Paraguay" (2006). Yale Medicine Thesis Digital Library. 251. http://elischolar.library.yale.edu/ymtdl/251 (accessed on 10th May 2025).

21. Leal-Calvo, T., Martins, B. L., Bertoluci, D. F., Rosa, P. S., de Camargo, R. M., Germano, G. V., Brito de Souza, V. N., Pereira Latini, A. C., & Moraes, M. O. (2021). Large-Scale Gene Expression Signatures Reveal a Microbicidal Pattern of Activation in *Mycobacterium leprae*-Infected Monocyte-Derived Macrophages With Low Multiplicity of Infection. *Frontiers in immunology, 12,* 647832. https://doi.org/10.3389/fimmu.2021.647832 Mycobacterium leprae(accessed on 10th May 2025).

22. Marçal, P. H. F., Gama, R. S., Pereira de Oliveira, L. B., Martins-Filho, O. A., Pinheiro, R. O., Sarno, E. N., Moraes, M. O., & de Oliveira Fraga, L. A. (2020). Functional biomarker signatures of circulating T-cells and its association with distinct clinical status of leprosy patients and their respective household contacts. *Infectious diseases of poverty*, *9*(1), 167. https://doi.org/10.1186/s40249-020-00763-7(accessed on 10th May 2025).

23. Mawardi P. Leprosy: The Ancient and Stubborn Disease [Internet]. Current Topics in Tropical Emerging Diseases and Travel Medicine. IntechOpen; 2018. Available from: http://dx.doi.org/10.5772/intechopen.79984 (accessed on 10th May 2025).

24. Mehta, H., Narang, T., Dogra, S., & Kumar, B. (2022). Pediatric leprosy: no child's play. *International journal of dermatology*, *61*(7), e244–e245. https://doi.org/10.1111/ijd.16152(accessed on 10th May 2025).

25. J. Rodriguez-Morales, A. (Ed.). (2019). Current Topics in Neglected Tropical Diseases. IntechOpen. doi: 10.5772/intechopen.73918 (accessed on 10th May 2025).

26. Neunert, C., Terrell, D. R., Arnold, D. M., Buchanan, G. R., Cines, D. B., Cooper, N., Cuker, A., et al. (2019). American Society of Hematology 2019 guidelines for immune thrombocytopenia. Blood Advances, 3, 3829–3866. https://doi.org/10.1182/bloodadvances.2019000966 (accessed on 10th May 2025).

27. Patel, K. B., Patel, R., & Sharma, N. (2017). Dermatological disorders during pregnancy: a study from tertiary care hospital. *International Journal of Reproduction, Contraception, Obstetrics and Gynecology*, *5*(5), 1354–1359. https://doi.org/10.18203/2320-1770.ijrcog20161287 (accessed on 10th May 2025).

28. Rao, N. N. (2023). Epidemiological and clinical pattern of leprosy in a tertiary care center in Bareilly, Uttar Pradesh, India: A retrospective study. Journal of Clinical and Diagnostic Research. JCDR Research and Publications. 2023; 7 (6) : 1-4. https://www.semanticscholar.org/paper/bf18391daf87adead2e4905b79421243a6c7e7e1 (accessed on 10th May 2025).

29. Richens J. (2004). Genital manifestations of tropical diseases. *Sexually transmitted infections*, *80*(1), 12–17. https://doi.org/10.1136/sti.2003.004093 (accessed on 10th May 2025).

30. Chalya, P.L., Mchembe, M.D., Mshana, S.E. *et al.* Clinicopathological profile and surgical treatment of abdominal tuberculosis: a single centre experience in northwestern Tanzania. *BMC Infect Dis* **13**, 270 (2013). https://doi.org/10.1186/1471-2334-13-270 (accessed on 10th May 2025).

31. Tian, Y., Hao, D., Du, J., Wang, H., & Wen, X. (2024). Summary of clinical features of 1800 cases of pyogenic liver abscess. European Journal of Gastroenterology & Hepatology, 37, 483–487. https://www.semanticscholar.org/paper/e9f124e08c1631141328c2a2936dd8d378305792 (accessed on 10th May 2025).

32. Molla, Y. B., Tomczyk, S., Amberbir, T., Tamiru, A., & Davey, G. (2012). Podoconiosis in East and West Gojam Zones, northern Ethiopia. *PLoS neglected tropical diseases*, *6*(7), e1744. https://doi.org/10.1371/journal.pntd.0001744 (accessed on 10th May 2025).

33. Torres-Guerrero, E., Quintanilla-Cedillo, M. R., Ruiz-Esmenjaud, J., & Arenas, R. (2017). Leishmaniasis: A review. F1000Research, 6, 750–750. https://doi.org/10.12688/f1000research.11120.1 (accessed on 10th May 2025).

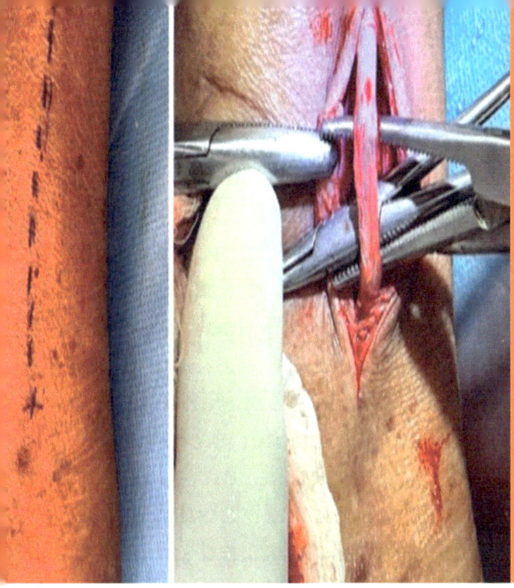

Chapter 5

DIAGNOSTIC TECHNIQUES OF LEPROSY

Contents

Introduction

Disease identification has always played a huge role in how medicine evolved. Leprosy, for example, throws a wrench in the works with its complex symptoms and long incubation period. This stubborn infection, caused by *Mycobacterium leprae*, reminds us just how vital it is to catch problems early with the right tests. There have been long-running debates, due to archaeological finds and old human remains—about how common leprosy was (Farro & Podgorny, 2015). Looking at these ancient signals adds layers to our understanding, even if the big picture remains a bit murky. All that history, as rough as it might have been, definitely sets the scene for why modern, quick detection and treatment are so important today. Today's testing methods are central to keeping leprosy from spreading, even though the disease still shows up in communities around the globe despite big medical strides. Doctors usually mix things up by doing straightforward physical checks, examining tissue samples under microscopes, and sometimes hunting down the bacteria's genetic code. New molecular tests, borrowing ideas from work done on other infections, have boosted both precision and reliability. For instance, testing frameworks originally designed for diseases like Buruli ulcer, focusing on local lab strength, regular quality checks, and smoother workflows have helped reframe how we approach diagnosing leprosy (Beissner et al., 2013). In most cases, combining solid lab practices with hands-on clinical skills means diagnoses come in faster, guiding public health policies and resource use more smartly. Leprosy diagnosis these days is a combination of classic clinical instincts and modern molecular techniques, each offering its own edge. Early on, detecting key skin and nerve signs is crucial, even though those signals can be subtle or sometimes look like other conditions, which makes things complex. The introduction of PCR-based tests has shifted the balance, letting doctors confirm the disease at a molecular level where regular microscopy might fail. Insisting on strong external quality checks and comprehensive training across labs—a lesson picked up from other mycobacterial studies (Beissner et al., 2013)—helps keep results consistent and reliable. All these methods together build a fuller picture that tackles the inherent complexities of leprosy detection, paving the way for better patient care and long-term disease control (Figure 5.1).

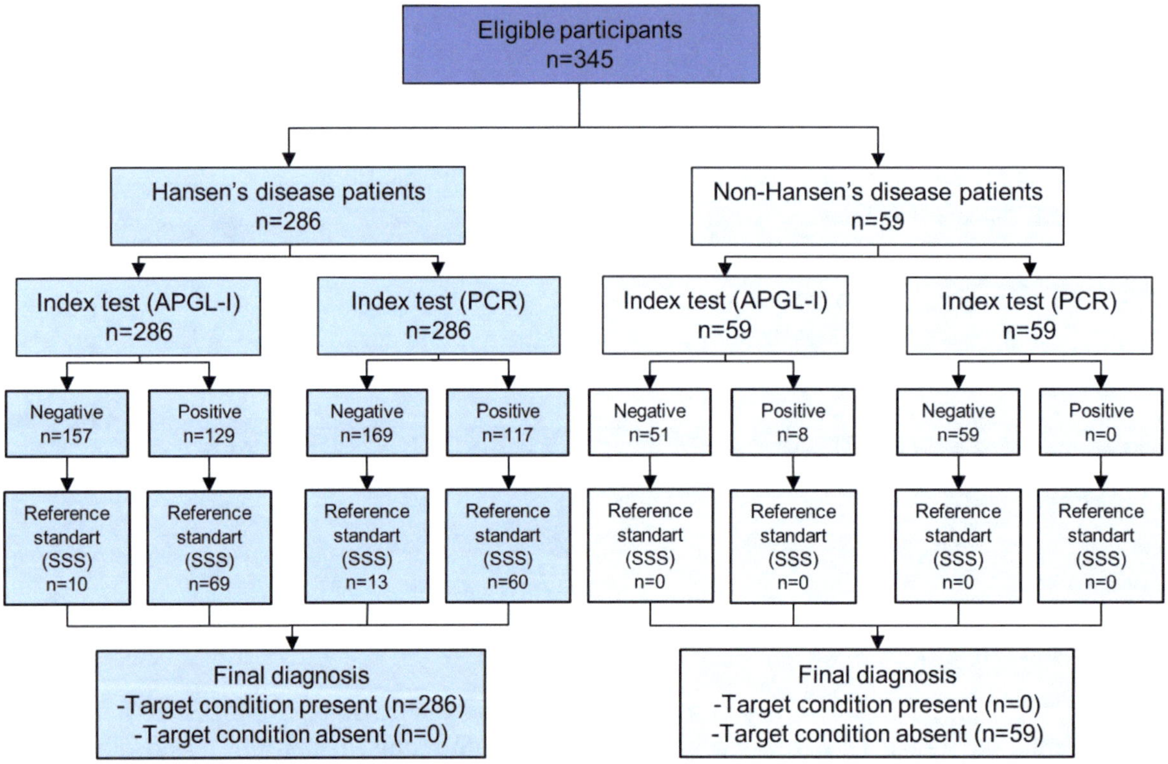

Figure 5.1. The diagnostic techniques of leprosy.

Source: Lima FR, de Paula NA, Simões MMR, Manso GMdC, Albertino GS, Felisbino GC, Antunes VMG, Perecin FAMC, Westin AT, Lugão HB and Frade MAC (2022) Bacilloscopy and polymerase chain reaction of slit-skin smears and anti-phenolic glycolipid-I serology for Hansen's disease diagnosis. Front. Med. 9:972244. doi: 10.3389/fmed.2022.972244

Importance of Accurate Diagnostic Techniques

Early detection of infections is key to getting proper treatment and keeping them under control, especially for individuals who are most at risk. Leprosy, for instance, is a chronic condition caused by *Mycobacterium leprae* that often shows only very subtle signs, so it can easily fly under the radar. A good and timely diagnosis isn't just about treatment; it also helps ease the stigma and social isolation that often come along with the disease. Diagnosing leprosy is complex because its clinical signs vary a lot and it sometimes looks a lot like other skin conditions, which means you need both reliable lab tests and a careful clinical look. In low-resource settings, where leprosy tends to occur more often, not having access to advanced technologies just makes these challenges even tougher, highlighting the need for methods that are both practical and dependable (Perez et al., 2024). The overall socioeconomic and epidemiological backdrop of leprosy further underscores how important accurate diagnostics are. Neglected tropical diseases like leprosy strike mostly at marginalized groups with limited healthcare, which increases the chance of underdiagnosis or even misdiagnosis. When mistakes in diagnosis happen, they mess up disease surveillance, slow down effective public health responses, and put extra pressure on already stretched-out healthcare systems. Climate shifts, migration, and urban growth add further complexity by making it even harder to separate leprosy from other infections in places where these diseases are common. In most cases, ensuring diagnostic accuracy is not just a clinical necessity—it's also a big part of the broader goal of health equity and reducing the overall socioeconomic impact (Rodriguez-Morales, 2019). Recent advances in molecular and immunological diagnostic techniques are changing the picture for leprosy detection. Methods like PCR and serological assays now offer much better sensitivity and specificity compared to traditional clinical checks and histopathological methods, which means even subclinical or early-stage infections can be spotted. Getting the diagnosis right sets the stage for choosing the proper treatment, helps limit the rise of drug resistance, and even supports contact tracing to keep further spread at bay. That said, putting these new techniques into practice isn't simple, especially in low-resource areas, where there are major logistical and financial hurdles. Generally speaking, overcoming these challenges calls for collaboration across different fields and tailoring strategies to local needs, aligning with global efforts against neglected tropical diseases. This approach not only improves outcomes for individual patients but also moves us closer to the ultimate goal of eliminating the disease (Perez et al., 2024).

5.1. Clinical Diagnosis

Precise diagnosis matters a lot when dealing with leprosy – the disease can show itself in so many complex ways that simply noting obvious symptoms just won't cut it. Traditional clinical exams, when combined to newer immunodiagnostic techniques, have helped pick out *Mycobacterium leprae* more accurately. In many cases, tools like the enzyme-linked immunosorbent assay (ELISA) jump to the forefront because they pinpoint infection markers and give doctors biochemical proof of what they suspect. Labs sometimes even use mimetic peptides as substitutes for protein antigens; these alternatives, which mimic natural markers in unexpected ways, sharpen diagnostic specificity. And then there are portable gadgets – lateral flow assays and biosensors – that let clinicians make rapid decisions out in the field, an essential step for early intervention. All these approaches, combined in a somewhat unpredictable fashion, ultimately boost diagnostic accuracy in regions where the disease is common (Lima et al., 2019). Even though modern lab techniques offer a lot of support, the art of diagnosing leprosy still leans heavily on a clinician's ability to spot the subtle signs and symptoms as the disease unfolds. Experience and on-the-job training become indispensable when it comes to telling leprosy apart from other skin or nerve conditions. In most cases, nabbing the diagnosis early helps cut down on severe complications and can even break the chain of transmission. Look at similar conditions like Buruli ulcer – enhanced quality assurance and local diagnostic capacity have often sped up early detection and reduced delays. Generally speaking, these improvements point to why continuous training, clear operating procedures, and rigorous yet sometimes inconsistently applied external quality checks (EQA) are so important to clinical practice (Beissner et al., 2013). Beyond the narrow focus of diagnosis, thinking about leprosy in the wider framework of public health is key. Early and correct identification paves the way for timely treatment, which helps stave off disabilities and eases the stigma around the disease. Combining sharp clinical judgment with molecular and immune-based assays creates a kind of diagnostic patchwork that covers more ground. This mixed approach also opens up possibilities for decentralized diagnosis, making it easier for healthcare workers in remote areas to take swift action. In essence, joining traditional clinical insights with modern diagnostic technologies is fundamental to advancing global efforts against leprosy – it balances patient care with the need for solid epidemiological tracking (Beissner et al., 2013; Lima et al., 2019) (Figure 5.2).

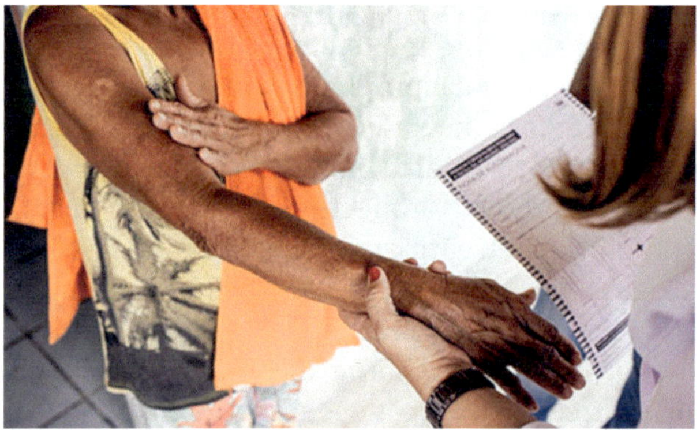

Figure 5.2. Clinical diagnosis.

Source: World Health Organization. (n.d.). *Leprosy Control.*

5.1.1. Patient History and Symptom Assessment

Taking a complete patient history is crucial when working with leprosy since it often lays out signals that might otherwise be missed. Doctors find that a patient's narrative, even when it starts with just a hint of numbness or a small patch of lighter skin, can point to potential exposure risks—details like past contact with known cases, where someone has lived or even worked can be unexpectedly revealing. In many cases, patients don't immediately connect these subtle changes with anything serious, so digging into previous treatments or even earlier misdiagnoses becomes key to understanding why proper care may have been delayed. This mix of background information and clinical insight steers medical professionals to choose further directed tests and helps sort leprosy apart from other skin or nerve issues, making a thorough history more than just a formality, it's an essential piece of the diagnostic puzzle. Evaluating symptoms of leprosy requires a careful, sometimes circuitous approach because the disease can appear in a variety of ways. Often, the loss of feeling in affected areas—where a person might not sense pain, heat, or even a light touch, stands out as a key indicator, and clinicians typically check by palpating peripheral nerves for any unexpected thickening or tenderness. A small patch of skin that seems less responsive might not sound like much at first, but once spotted, it can prompt earlier intervention and help slow down further transmission. Add to that the occasional presentation of broader signs like muscle weakness or even slight deformations and you see why a close look at each symptom, even the mild ones, is so important for guiding both diagnosis and overall management. Delayed diagnosis remains a stubborn problem in leprosy control—a challenge that has similarities to what happens in conditions like tuberculosis, where it's not uncommon for patients to show up only after symptoms have become a big deal (Cattamanchi et al., 2012; Hella et al., 2019). Often, early signs get overlooked by healthcare providers or are missed because patients aren't fully aware of what to look for; sometimes cultural or socioeconomic factors also mean that people hesitate to seek care right away. By combining a careful review of patient history with a mindful check for even the smallest early signs, doctors can help speed up referrals and confirmatory testing. When you factor in local trends, typical health-seeking behaviors, and even past interactions with healthcare, you get a richer diagnostic picture. To summarize, digging deep into a patient's story and keeping a keen eye on the symptoms isn't just about making a diagnosis, it's about cutting down on treatment delays, improving outcomes, and ultimately keeping the spread of leprosy in check (Figure 5.3).

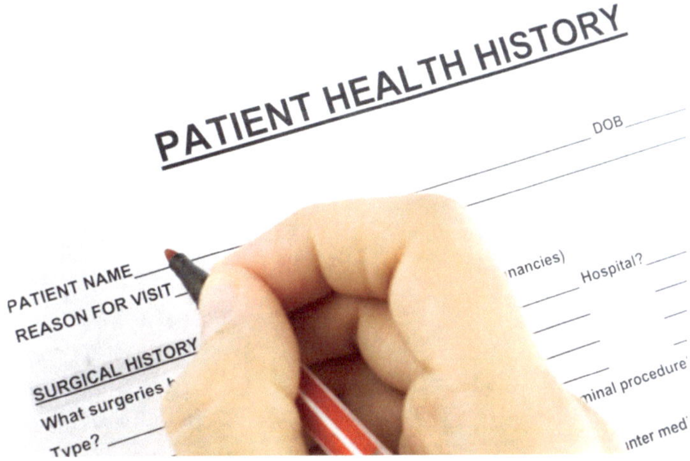

Figure 5.3. Patient health history.

Source: HealthChatPro. (2017). *Medical History.*

5.1.2. Physical Examination Findings

Patients suspected of leprosy can show lots of skin and nerve signals that help steer the diagnosis. Doctors sometimes notice light-colored or barely felt spots, plaques, or little nodules—details that might sneak past without a careful check of how the skin feels to temperature or touch. A quick press around common spots like the ulnar, median, and even the back of the ankle often finds nerves feeling thicker or softer than usual; these tactile hints, in most cases, lend weight to the idea that nerves are involved. In a way, these findings not only back up a leprosy diagnosis but also give a observe how the disease might behave, which naturally affects treatment choices.

Detecting these signs early, generally speaking, is key to staving off long-term disability. Further, when patients show muscle weakness or numbness along with skin spots, a careful look often beats lab tests in places with scarce resources, proving that a good physical check still holds plenty of value. Looking beyond just the skin and nerves, a broader body check can sometimes unearth signs of leprosy that mimic other infections. Sometimes, leprosy might even interefere with genital health, showing up as issues like hypogonadism or other related symptoms, which can make it complex to tell apart from sexually transmitted infections or nasal tropical microbes like filariasis or schistosomiasis (Richens, 2004). In most cases, clinicians need a high level of suspicion and a careful exam to separate these subtle signs from similar conditions. It's almost like the more systemic signals paint a bigger picture of how diverse and multi-layered leprosy can be. This wider glance—beyond just a skin check—not only deepens understanding but also helps tailor the diagnosis for both local cases and those linked to travel. Even though lab tests and molecular methods are advancing rapidly, a hands-on physical exam remains absolutely essential, especially where high-tech tools aren't easy to come by. For example, in areas with a high HIV rate (Cattamanchi et al., 2012), overlapping infections can complicate the issue, forcing clinicians to lean on cues like swollen nerves, specific numbness patterns, or distinct skin lesions to pick out leprosy from other mycobacterial issues. Detailed examinations, combined with a patient's history, often point the way well before confirmatory tests come back. This all-around, sometimes imperfect, yet effective approach allows early warning signs to be detected and tackled in time. So, despite all the new gadgets in diagnostics, the good, old-fashioned physical check-up still stands strong as a low-cost, reliable diagnostic tool (Figure 5.4).

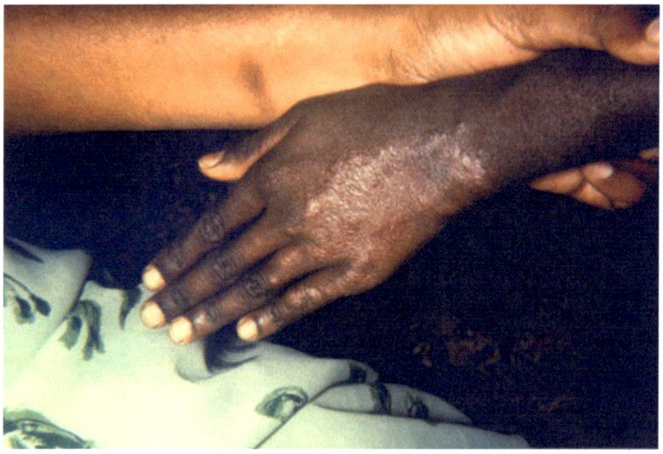

Figure 5.4. Leprosy physical examination.

Source: WikiDoc. (n.d.). *Leprosy Physical Signs.*

5.1.3. Differential Diagnosis Considerations

Diagnosing leprosy is pretty complex. It demands a careful look at many conditions that can mimic its symptoms, which, in most cases, makes the whole process feel a bit complicated. Nerve problems, for example, are a key sign of leprosy but they also emerge in other chronic neurological issues. CIDP (chronic inflammatory demyelinating polyneuropathy) often shows similar sensory and motor glitches, along with some noticeable nerve thickening—features that can easily be confused with leprosy. In most cases, doctors lean on electrodiagnostic tests and check how well patients respond to immunomodulatory treatments to tell CIDP apart since its treatment path is quite different from that for leprosy. Given the varied ways CIDP can appear, clinicians must weigh these signals in a bigger clinical picture to call the right diagnosis (Peter et al., 2021). This shows how a hands-on evaluation paired with targeted tests is essential for sorting out leprosy from its look-alike neuropathies. It doesn't end with neurological disorders, other granulomatous conditions also complicate the issue when trying to pinpoint leprosy. Diseases such as sarcoidosis or even cutaneous tuberculosis can mimic the skin and tissue changes seen in leprosy, pushing healthcare providers to go deeper with lab and histology workups. Biopsies come in handy here, often revealing the unique cellular clusters and granuloma patterns that set these diseases apart. Lately, molecular tests aimed at finding *Mycobacterium leprae* DNA have become a useful extra, especially when clinical signs are ambiguous. Generally speaking, ruling out these other possibilities is critical since each disorder carries its own treatment strategy and outcome expectations. In this way, adding extra lab and molecular evaluations helps boost the certainty of a leprosy diagnosis, ultimately reducing the risk of giving the wrong treatment (Peter et al., 2021). Beyond these challenges, there's also the issue of other neuropathies that share some common ground with leprosy. Diabetic neuropathy and various hereditary nerve conditions can both lead to sensory loss and muscle weakness, though their causes differ a lot. Diabetic neuropathy, for instance, stems from metabolic problems and usually shows up as a symmetrical condition—unlike leprosy, which often gives you asymmetrical nerve damage and accompanying skin lesions. Gathering a detailed patient history (including potential exposures) along with targeted neurophysiological tests usually paves the way for detecting these differences. By carefully ruling out these other causes, healthcare professionals can confidently apply the proper multidrug therapy meant for leprosy, thereby bettering patient outcomes and avoiding needless complications (Peter et al., 2021).

5.2. Laboratory Techniques

Getting an accurate diagnosis for infections almost entirely comes down to lab methods that, at their core, help clear up what a patient might be experiencing. In leprosy, for example, the lab tests have shifted over time to back up what doctors see in the clinic by using both traditional microscopy and more modern molecular tools. Microscopy remains a go-to strategy, labs stain skin smears with acid-fast dye to look for *Mycobacterium leprae*, but its sensitivity isn't always top-notch and it does lean on having well-trained technicians. Quality assurance measures and regular refresher training programs play a big role in keeping these tests reliable; in most cases, similar efforts in diseases like Buruli ulcer even reached inter-lab agreement rates of around 94% after strict external checks (Beissner et al., 2013). This drives home the point that having standardized lab practices is key for boosting leprosy diagnostics. Switching gears, molecular tests are increasingly in the spotlight because they generally offer sharper sensitivity and specificity when hunting for the bacteria's genetic material. For instance, PCR assays can pick up on *Mycobacterium leprae* DNA even in cases where the bacteria are scarce—something traditional microscopy might miss. Dry-reagent PCR methods and quantitative PCR help simplify the lab workflow and cut down on waiting times, which is especially important in resource-limited settings (Beissner et al., 2013). You might say that these PCR-based techniques are critical for early detection, as they pave the way for timely treatment, helping to reduce the spread and prevent disabilities. That said, these methods do require a solid lab infrastructure and experienced hands, and that can be a real challenge in some leprosy-endemic areas. On top of everything, sorting out leprosy from other mycobacterial infections adds another layer of complexity. Often, a more nuanced mix of tests is needed. Drawing on experience with tuberculosis in HIV-heavy regions, a combination of smear microscopy, cultures, and molecular techniques has been shown to boost diagnostic accuracy. In most cases, this hints at the promise of combining bacterial detection with clinical and even immunological assessments to nail down a leprosy diagnosis. Further, labs that keep up with continuous training and regular quality checks tend to have more consistent results—even if, occasionally, the process isn't perfectly streamlined. All of this plays a crucial role in ensuring that the diagnostic methods remain both sensitive and accessible, which is absolutely essential when managing leprosy as a public health challenge (Figure 5.5).

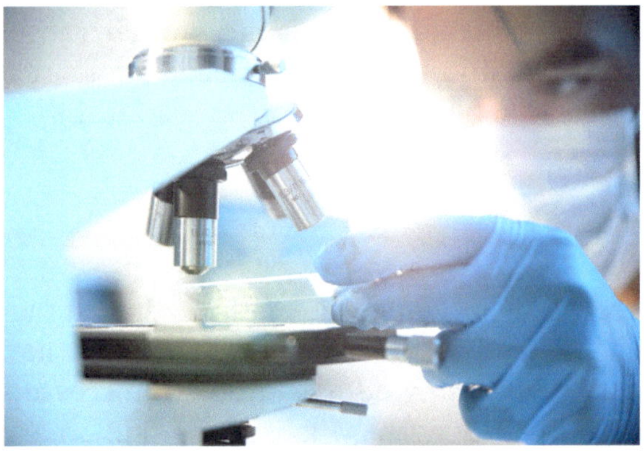

Figure 5.5. Laboratory techniques.

Source: Centers for Disease Control and Prevention. (2024). *Person at Microscope with PPE.*

5.2.1. Skin Smears and Histopathological Examination

Leprosy diagnosis depends on both what you see in the clinic and what lab tests confirm, rather than relying on one method alone. You might start with a skin smear, for instance, where superficial skin samples are taken to flag acid-fast bacilli (AFB) using stains like Ziehl-Neelsen; this simple test not only hints at the number of bacteria but also helps sort the disease along the Ridley-Jopling scale. At the same time, looking at a skin biopsy under the microscope often reveals changes, like granulomatous inflammation and nerve involvement—that, together with the bacilli spotted in samples, help solidify the diagnosis and track how the disease is evolving. Taken together, these tools usually boost the overall accuracy, laying a proper foundation for treatment, especially in common areas (Nandwani et al., 2017). Even though skin smears and histopathology are pretty handy, they aren't without their hiccups. For example, in cases like tuberculoid leprosy, the bacterial load tends to be low, so you might get a negative smear even when the disease is active—a fact that generally complicates early detection. And sure, while histopathological exams provide a clearer picture, they require invasive biopsies and someone with a keen eye to interpret them, which isn't always possible in resource-scarce settings. Still, combining skin smear analysis with a microscopic look at tissue (and sometimes advanced staining methods) tends to raise the diagnostic yield noticeably. This combined approach helps differentiate forms of leprosy, from the vague indeterminate type to the full-blown lepromatous form, which is crucial for both predicting how the disease might progress and picking the right treatment. Recent developments in techniques like fine needle aspiration cytology with acid-fast staining also offer quicker, less invasive alternatives that align well with traditional methods, boosting overall precision (Nandwani et al., 2017). Recent studies, generally speaking, have begun to underline how useful histopathological examinations can be when they work in tandem with molecular diagnostics for catching leprosy. While skin smear analysis is often the go-to frontline tool, the structural and pathological details revealed in histology prove indispensable when clinical features are ambiguous or when the initial smears come back negative. Moreover, pairing these methods with molecular tests, for example, PCR-based assays—helps in detecting subclinical or early-stage infections that might otherwise slip under the radar. In effect, a step-by-step diagnostic plan that weaves together clinical insights, tissue analysis, and molecular techniques can usually enhance detection accuracy and patient care. With continuous research lending more support to these combined strategies, it's becoming more important for health systems in affected regions to bolster histopathology services alongside traditional skin smear diagnostics, ultimately aiding efforts to reduce leprosy-related complications (Figure 5.6).

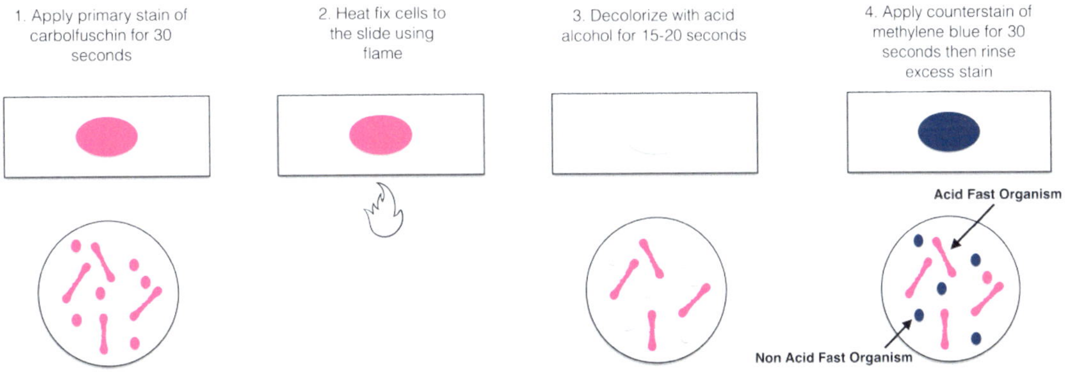

Figure 5.6. Staining kit used in modified Ziehl–Neelsen staining for demonstration of acid–fast bacilli (AFB).

Source: By Elizabeth Gray - File:Acid Fast Stain.pdf is a PDF version of this file.It should be used in place of this image when not inferior.File:Basic steps of acid fast staining procedure.svg → File:Acid Fast Stain.pdf. +/−, CC BY-SA 4.0, https://commons.wikimedia.org/w/index.php?curid=135137580

5.2.2. Serological Tests for Leprosy

Diagnostic improvements are front and center when it comes to detecting and tracking infectious diseases. Take leprosy, for example—serological tests have become a notable asset because they pick up antibodies aimed at specific *Mycobacterium leprae* targets. Antibodies like those reacting with phenolic glycolipid-I (PGL-I) and others such as LID-1 and NDO-LID often serve as key biochemical hints that help confirm a clinical suspicion. In contrast to traditional clinical diagnosis, which can be subjective and sometimes delay detection due to the disease's slow pace—these tests give a more direct, sensitive edge. In most cases, studies indicate that these assays not only help nail down a diagnosis but also flag neuritis, check how effective treatments are, and screen people in close-contact settings (Fabri et al., 2016). Overall, this approach reinforces the broader diagnostic framework by supporting both case confirmation and epidemiological oversight. New diagnostic approaches remain crucial in tackling diseases with long incubation periods like leprosy. Generally speaking, ELISAs have gained favor because they're sensitive and adapt well to various lab settings. These tests use antigens, or even mimetic peptides—, capture antibodies from a person's serum, indirectly hinting at an infection. Then there are lateral flow assays (LFAs) and portable biosensors, which, though a bit experimental at times, deliver rapid results with minimal sample fuss; these alternatives are particularly promising for remote or resource-thin regions. Their inclusion in public health plans underscores how serology can both verify an infection and prompt early intervention to break transmission cycles (Lima et al., 2019). In essence, such innovative tools help build a more flexible and accessible diagnostic landscape for leprosy. Even with all the progress, serological diagnostics aren't without their hitches. Variability in antibody responses across the leprosy spectrum—where multibacillary cases usually give off stronger signals compared to paucibacillary forms, which might show very low or undetectable antibody levels—means that relying on serology alone can be complex. However, when these tests are combined with clinical examinations and molecular methods, they notably improve diagnostic accuracy and patient monitoring. Also, serology does a solid job at screening larger populations, especially among high-risk contacts, by flagging potential cases even before obvious symptoms emerge (Fabri et al., 2016). Ongoing efforts to refine antigen targets and alter assay formats promise to raise both specificity and sensitivity, ultimately making serological assays a more integral part of combined leprosy diagnostic strategies (Figure 5.7).

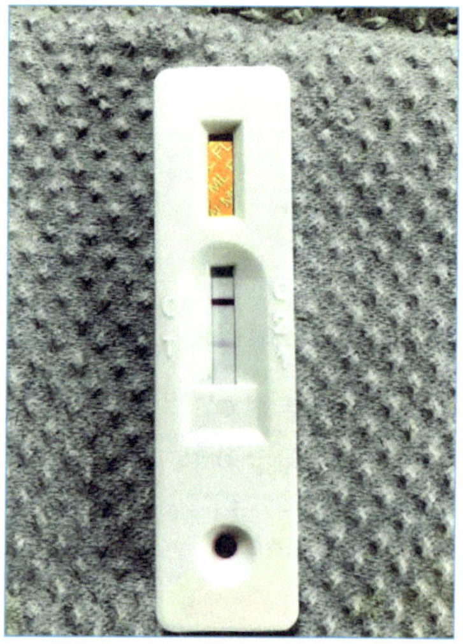

Figure 5.7. Positive result of ML flow serological test for leprosy.

Source: ResearchGate. (2024). *Positive Result of ML Flow Serological Test for Leprosy.*

5.2.3. Molecular Techniques: Polymerase Chain Reaction (PCR) and Deoxyribonucleic Acid (DNA) Analysis

The ability to pick up and gauge *Mycobacterium leprae* DNA with molecular methods has shifted leprosy diagnosis. Instead of relying solely on old techniques, like slit skin smears or histopathological exams, which often miss the mark in cases with very few bacteria—researchers now use PCR aimed at the Rlep gene to catch *M. leprae* DNA in several sample types (urine, blood, skin smears). Generally speaking, quantitative PCR (qPCR) even lets us measure bacterial load, a detail that tends to line up with how severe the disease is and what subtype it might be, a kind of precision older methods just couldn't match. In fact, some studies have noted the pathogen's DNA popping up in every single urine sample tested (Diana & Harish 2024), highlighting PCR's promise for non-invasive diagnosis and monitoring treatment response. Beyond just urine and blood, nasal swabs are getting a lot of attention as a less invasive way to nab *M. leprae* DNA. PCR assays focusing on targets such as the proline-rich antigen have detected the bacteria's genetic material in nasal samples taken from patients at different stages—whether they're just starting treatment, still actively undergoing it, or have finished therapy. This method not only backs up the diagnosis but also hints at how long bacterial DNA sticks around during and after treatment. Detection rates tend to be higher among multibacillary patients while dropping off in individuals who have completed treatment, making PCR a handy tool for disease monitoring. Further, gene sequencing of these PCR products shows there's a fair bit of genetic variation among *M. leprae* strains, an insight that's crucial for understanding how the pathogen behaves and spreads. Such molecular details, in most cases, are key to shaping better public health responses. We also have to remember that *M. leprae* simply won't grow in lab cultures, which used to be a huge hurdle for developing diagnostic tests. PCR and DNA analysis step in nicely by allowing for direct detection of the bacterium without needing live cultures. Since the PCR primers are finely tuned to *M. leprae*'s unique genes, they help avoid mix-ups with related mycobacteria. Advances in quantitative PCR further boost diagnosis by accurately tracking bacterial loads—an essential factor when judging treatment progress and disease development. When you combine these molecular techniques with traditional clinical data, early case detection becomes more practical and treatment management much more effective, especially in regions where early intervention is critical for lowering disability risks. To summarize, PCR and DNA analysis are, generally speaking, a major leap forward in the fight against leprosy (Diana & Harish 2024) (Figure 5.8).

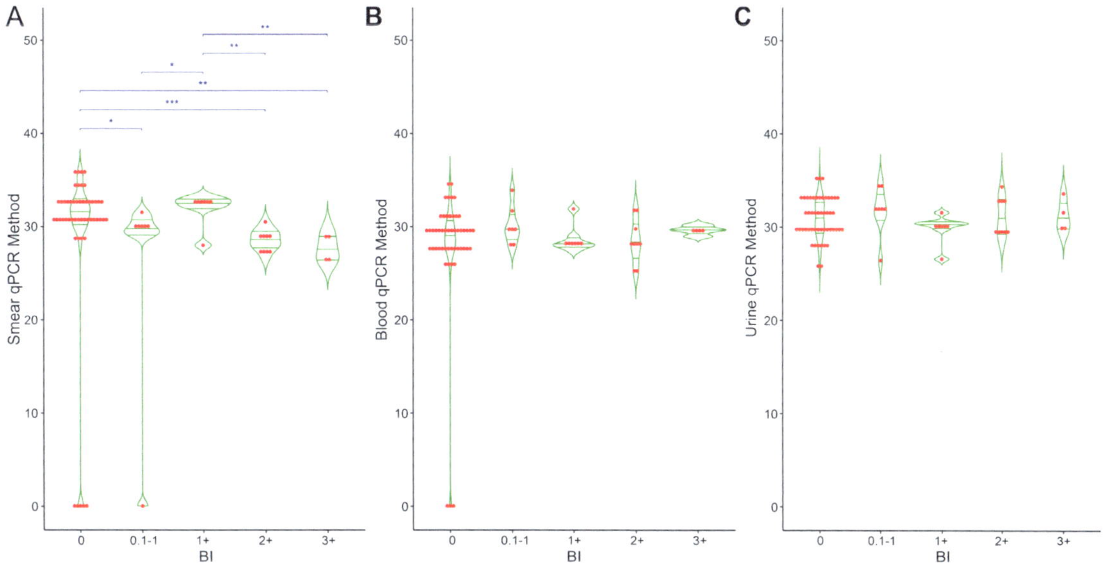

Figure 5.8. Polymerase chain reaction (PCR) procedure in leprosy.

Source: Diana D and Harish MC (2024) qPCR detection of Mycobacterium leprae DNA in urine samples of leprosy patients using the Rlep gene target. Front. Mol. Biosci. 11:1435679. doi: 10.3389/fmolb.2024.1435679

5.3. Imaging Techniques

Tech progress has reshaped what tools we have to diagnose infections like leprosy. Nowadays, non-invasive imaging gives us a quick peek at how tissues change without needing a biopsy. Ultrasound, for instance, lets us see peripheral nerves in action, showing things like nerve swelling and signs of inflammation, features that usually hint at leprosy's neuropathic effects. This kind of imaging helps not only in catching the disease early on, but also checks how well treatments are working. In most cases, even methods like echocardiography and bioelectrical impeinteraction, which you'd typically tie to other tropical ailments—might support evaluations of broader complications related to leprosy (Faisal et al., 2015). Some newer optical imaging methods are already pushing past the limits of traditional histology. Techniques such as nonlinear optical microscopy, and its cousin second-harmonic generation (SHG), give us a fresh look at what's happening inside skin lesions caused by leprosy. Basically, these approaches let us assess how collagen and other body structures rearrange—an aspect especially noticeable in the tuberculoid variant of the disease. While the classic staining techniques stick to the basics, SHG imaging pulls in much richer details about the extracellular matrix. Sure, figures like optical density and entropy, on their own, might not seem too groundbreaking; but when mixed with standard histopathology data, they help differentiate leprosy from other similar granulomatous conditions, like sarcoidosis (Utinoet al., 2018). Integrating imaging with new technology, for example, artificial intelligence, is starting to change the rules for diagnosing leprosy. Generally speaking, AI-powered systems can sift through bulky imaging data faster and with more pinpoint accuracy, detecting nerve and skin issues before they escalate. There's also exciting progress with lab-on-chip and microfluidic platforms that come with optical detectors, which can make a difference in places with limited resources where leprosy is common. These biomedical engineering innovations support quick screening, real-time checks, and even allow for custom-tailored treatment strategies, all of which contribute to better patient care. In a way, stepping beyond our traditional clinical approaches and combining in modern computational tools is gradually turning leprosy diagnosis into a more objective, reproducible science (Faisal et al., 2015) (Figure 5.9).

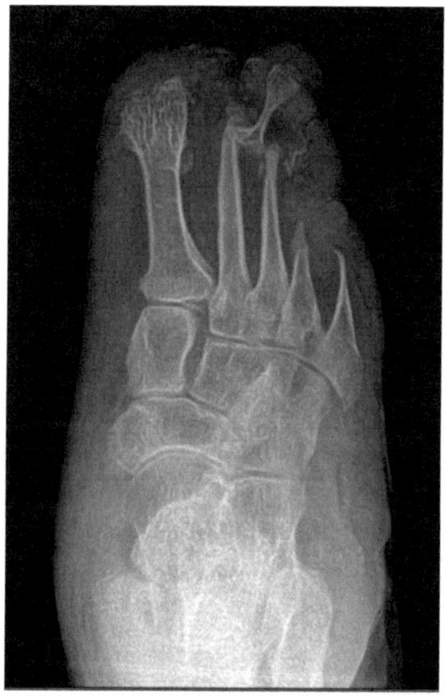

Figure 5.9. Imaging techniques.

Source: Radiopaedia. (n.d.). *Leprosy Radiographic Image.*

5.3.1. Role of Radiography in Leprosy Diagnosis

Imaging has long been a key player in detecting infectious diseases, offering a non-invasive window into what's happening inside the body. When it comes to leprosy, radiography steps up—providing a direct look at how *Mycobacterium leprae* alters bones and soft tissues. You might see on an X-ray that bones seem to be receding, show signs of inflammation (osteitis), or even display damage to the phalanges; these recurring details help doctors figure out if leprosy is present, especially in cases where the disease is advanced or hasn't been treated—since just observing clinical symptoms generally isn't enough. In many cases, combining radiographic evidence with physical exams and lab tests offers a more tangible picture of disease progression. This mixed approach not only speeds up early diagnosis but also improves treatment planning, which is pretty important given leprosy's complex nature and its heavy socio-epidemiological impact on communities with limited resources (Perez et al., 2024). Radiography, however, does more than simply capture images. It helps assess how severe leprosy is and even distinguishes it from other conditions that cause similar bone problems. Studies often point out that certain X-ray markers tend to align with the immune response seen in leprosy, ranging broadly from milder, paucibacillary cases to the more pronounced multibacillary forms. For instance, erosions and noticeable bone loss are generally more marked in lepromatous leprosy, reflecting a heavier bacterial load and more extensive tissue damage. Radiographs also have the neat ability to catch early skeletal involvement, often before irreversible deformities set in, thereby paving the way for timely intervention. That said, it's important to remember that flat, two-dimensional images come with limitations, especially in anatomically complex areas. Newer imaging advances like 3D techniques and micro-CT have, in most cases, proven to offer superior consistency and a finer view of subtle bone microarchitecture changes, potentially opening the door to more precise diagnosis and improved monitoring of skeletal lesions in leprosy (Morgan et al., 2014) (Figure 5.10).

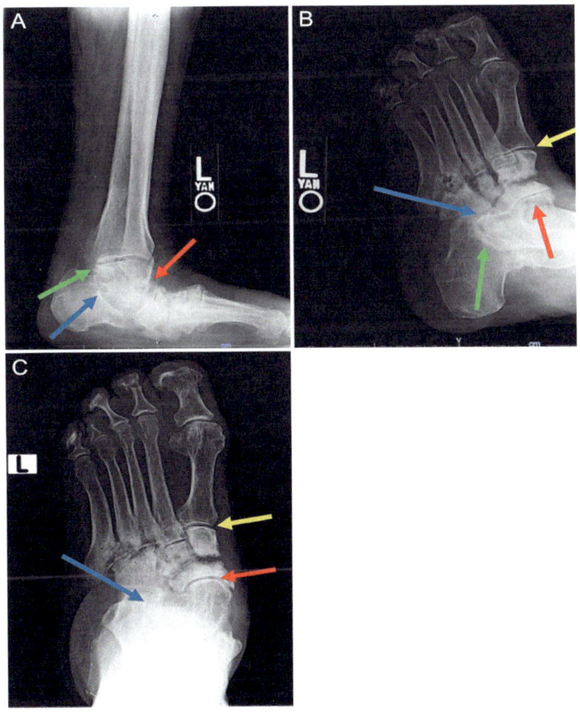

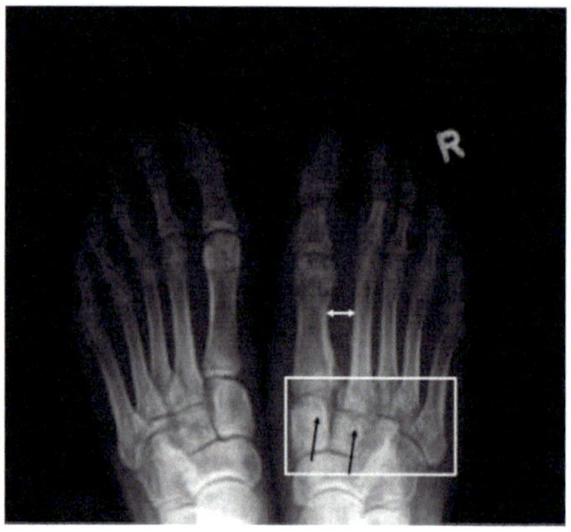

Figure 5.10. Signs of early-stage neuro-osteoarthropathy (Charcot foot) on conventional dorsoplantar (D–P) radiograph, showing changes in the midfoot, including osteopenia (white box), cartilage fragmentation at the tarsometatarsal (TMT) joints I and II and the cuneiform I and II bones (black arrows). An increased joint space between metatarsal bones I and II (white arrow) is observed, indicating Lisfranc dislocation with lateral displacement of the metatarsal (MTT) bones.

Source: Kress G T, Swerdlow M, Shin L (May 30, 2024) Lepromatous Leprosy and Charcot Neuroarthropathy of Insensate Feet: A Case Report. Cureus 16(5): e61362. doi:10.7759/cureus.61362

5.3.2. Magnetic Resonance Imaging (MRI) and Its Applications

MRI is now a key tool for detecting various infectious conditions. In leprosy, it gives a closer look at peripheral nerves – pretty much a signature of the disease. High-res images from MRI can pick up nerve thickening, swelling, and inflammation even before obvious signs show up, which means doctors might step in sooner to stop lasting damage. Although ultrasound or simple blood tests often take center stage, MRI's tendency for showing exactly how nerves are affected is important, especially when paired with fresh bioengineering ideas (Faisal et al., 2015). MRI doesn't just fill in for a clinical exam, it covers the gaps left by standard tests. For instance, while blood tests offer useful immune markers, they frequently miss the precise anatomical details needed for planning treatment. In many cases, MRI's non-invasive view of deep nerve issues – the kind that you can't feel by touch – makes a big difference. It even helps differentiate leprosy from other nerve problems, like those related to diabetes or compression, reinforcing its role by repeating those key points. Its sensitivity to subtle soft tissue changes also means it can highlight nerve abscesses or fibrosis, and that naturally guides therapy (Faisal et al., 2015). Even though ultrasound shines when it comes to tropical diseases such as lymphatic filariasis and visceral leishmaniasis, MRI still hasn't found its footing in leprosy diagnosis – a fact partly due to cost and access issues. Generally speaking, as technology advances and more affordable MRI options roll out, the chance for broader use in low-resource settings goes up. When you compare ultrasound procedures, like FASH and FASE, MRI offers crisper spatial details and better contrast, which are critical for catching those slight nerve shifts in leprosy cases. Mixed in with clinical insights and on-the-spot imaging, MRI helps stage the disease more precisely and track treatment response in ways that even seem a bit unpredictable at times. With ongoing technical improvements and some specialized training, MRI might soon become a regular part of diagnosing leprosy, boosting early detection and patient care in the regions that need it most (Figure 5.11).

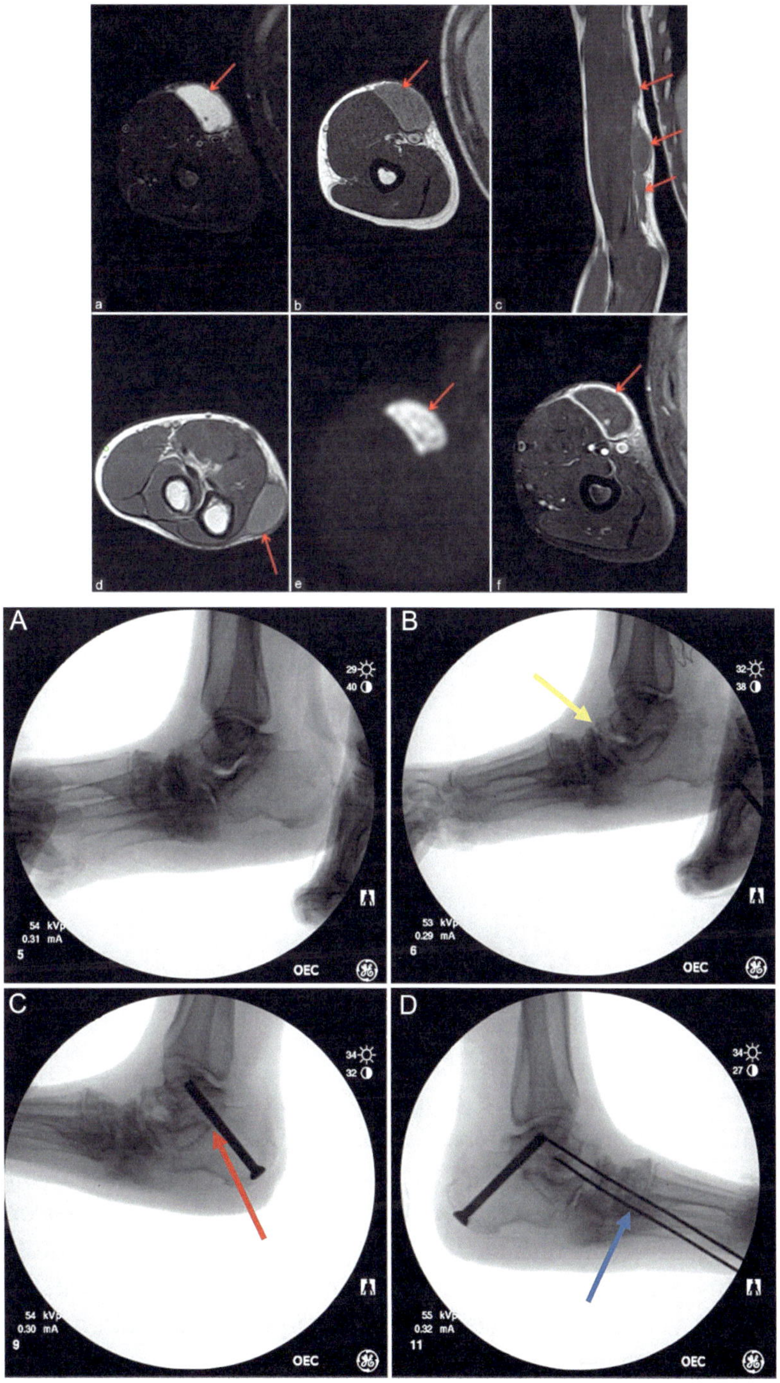

Figure 5.11. Lepromatous Leprosy and Charcot Neuroarthropathy of Insensate Feet.

Source: Kress G T, Swerdlow M, Shin L (May 30, 2024) Lepromatous Leprosy and Charcot Neuroarthropathy of Insensate Feet: A Case Report. Cureus 16(5): e61362. doi:10.7759/cureus.61362

5.3.3. Ultrasound in Assessing Leprosy-Related Complications

Medical imaging has come a long way, especially now when diagnosing infections in places lacking resources feels like an uphill battle. Ultrasound stands out—not only is it portable and relatively inexpensive, but it also gives real-time images that come in handy in these settings.

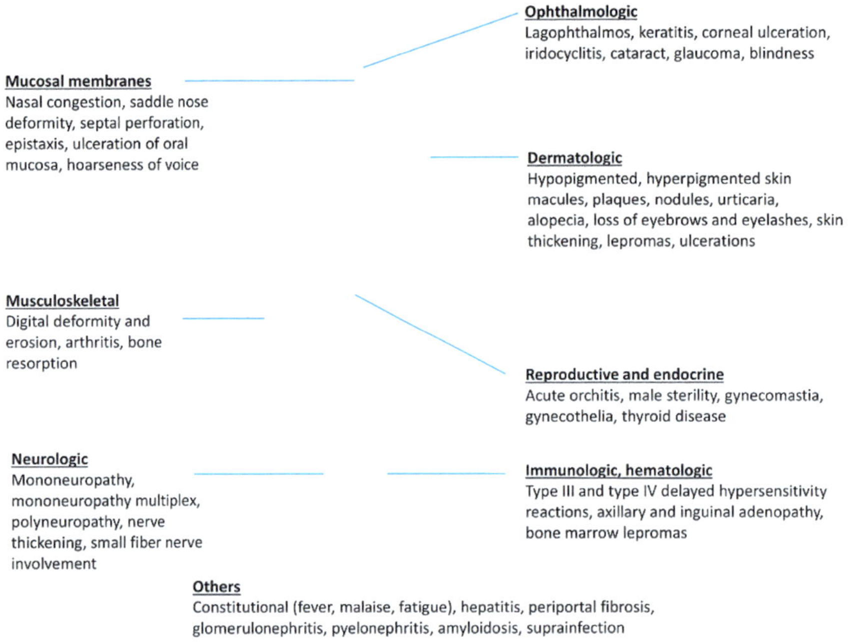

Figure 5.12. Manifestations.

Source: Benlamkadam S, Errahmany A, Raymond K, et al. (April 01, 2024) Hansen's Disease: A Practical Update on a Neglected Globally Significant Infection. Cureus 16(4): e57374. doi:10.7759/cureus.57374

Take leprosy, for instance; this disease, which tends to interefere with the nerves and muscles, now gets a non-invasive scan that shows nerve swelling, thickening, and even subtle shifts in nearby tissues. Catching these hints early can help doctors fine-tune treatments before any irreversible damage sets in. Further, point-of-care ultrasound routines, borrowing ideas from approaches used for other tropical infections, point to how this tool may fill in critical diagnostic gaps (Bélard et al., 2016). It's interesting that ultrasound can spotlight soft tissue alterations and musculoskeletal changes that matter a lot when dealing with leprosy complications. Patients sometimes develop a kind of neuropathic arthropathy—something akin to Charcot neuroarthropathy seen in diabetes—that comes with inflamed joints, bone wear, and misalignments. In many cases, ultrasound manages to pick up early signs like synovitis, tiny fluid buildups, and even bone erosions, which can lead to prompt differentiation from other causes of joint swelling. While a good clinical exam remains the cornerstone, adding ultrasound into the mix helps uncover these almost hidden changes that might predict a progression toward more severe deformities and disability. Generally speaking, this fits with studies that support comprehensive imaging analysis to help guide offloading techniques and targeted therapies (Vella & Cachia, 2008). Still, ultrasound's potential in leprosy care is a bit of a work in progress, with many experts stressing that more research is needed to fine-tune protocols that truly address leprosy-specific issues.

Training healthcare providers to use ultrasound effectively in these cases is crucial, particularly in regions where resources are limited. The fact that early nerve and tissue changes are so subtle means that only high-resolution equipment paired with skilled interpretation can do the job. Some are even suggesting that focused ultrasonography, much like what's successfully done for other tropical diseases, might eventually move from a supplementary role to a primary diagnostic tool in leprosy management. Addressing present limitations through both technology enhancements and capacity building might just transform ultrasound into the frontline method in leprosy care (Bélard et al., 2016) (Figure 5.12).

5.4. Emerging Diagnostic Methods

Biomedical research has pushed forward new ways to catch complex diseases early. Leprosy, caused by *Mycobacterium leprae*—is a clear case; our usual tests often miss it until the signs are loud and clear, which then helps it spread. New techniques now hunt for a combination of immune signals that generally tie back to how far an infection has spread and what flavor it takes. Instead of leaning on just one marker, these methods look at several cues, showing that we're beginning to grasp the complex interaction between our bodies and the microbes. This progress is key for better screening in areas hit hardest by the illness, helping us tell apart who might be quietly infected from those who aren't, and what kind of clinical picture they show—guiding treatment and easing the overall burden. In the quest for simpler and more reliable tests, LFAs have grabbed attention because they're straightforward and work well—even in spots with few resources. Recent work has even bundled the search for several immune markers like anti-PGL-I antibodies, IL-10, CCL4, and IP-10, which capture bits of both humoral and cellular responses to *M. leprae*, into a single assay. Generally speaking, getting a broad snapshot of the immune response in one go fits well with leprosy's varied nature, as it can show up in either milder or more intense forms with their own characteristics.

This mixed approach not only lays out the body's diverse reactions but also helps spot an infection before obvious signs appear. Such advances open the door to large-scale screening programs and ongoing checks on treatment effectiveness in affected communities (Van Hooij et al., 2016). Looking at neglected tropical diseases like leprosy makes it clear that smarter testing tools are a must—ones that can flex with shifting populations, environmental twists, and even economic ups and downs. Leprosy's stubborn persistence, even with multi-drug treatments, points out gaps in current surveillance and testing setups. New viral outbreaks spread by insects have shown just how fast pathogens can bounce back and go global, which drives home the need for heightened diagnostic alertness. In most cases, mixcombining advanced immune diagnostics with broader public health efforts tailored for tropical regions seems like a promising route to catch infections sooner and act in time. These innovative approaches, fueled by ideas from many fields, aim to curb disease spread and ease the economic hit that comes with it (Rodriguez-Morales, 2019) (Figure 5.13).

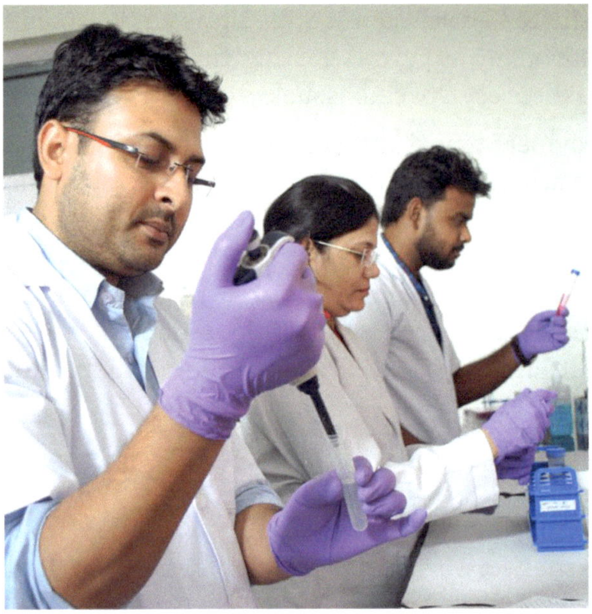

Figure 5.13. Emerging diagnostic methods.

Source: The Leprosy Mission International. (n.d.). *Emerging Diagnostic Methods.*

5.4.1. Novel Biomarkers for Leprosy Detection

Immunological research on leprosy has been shaking up our understanding of how hosts and pathogens interact – a kind of subtle interaction that points to the need for better markers to spot the disease early. The response to *Mycobacterium leprae* isn't one-size-fits-all; it shifts with host genetics, which is why you sometimes see cases that are paucibacillary and other times multibacillary. Traditional tests tend to bank on one marker, and that just doesn't cut it when you're dealing with such variety. In most cases, recent work has pushed a multiparametric approach into the spotlight, combining markers like anti-PGL-I antibodies, IL-10, CCL4, and IP-10 to cover innate, cellular, and humoral immunity all at once. Researchers, by using quantitative lateral flow assays that work on whole blood samples, have shown improved sensitivity and specificity when they try to tell apart infected individuals from healthy contacts or those in endemic areas (Van Hooij et al., 2016). This kind of multiplexed profile kind of paints a more detailed picture of disease status and transmission risk, especially in field settings where a fancy lab just isn't available. Biotechnological progress has, in a similar spirit, combined molecular and immunodiagnostic tools in innovative ways. Mapping the immunogenic antigens of *Mycobacterium leprae* has led to recombinant proteins and mimetic peptides , tools crafted to hit specific immune responses connected to the infection. These biomolecules show up as key parts of ELISA, offering a boost in detecting infection-related antibodies, often with better sensitivity. You also see lateral flow assays, along with optical and electrochemical biosensors, coming into play as rapid, portable and user-friendly devices. This mix lets clinicians sidestep elaborate sample processing without missing out on those all-important biomarkers, which is pretty critical when quick action is needed (Lima et al., 2019). In many ways, the merging of molecular biology with biosensor tech is steering leprosy diagnostics into a new era of easier access and high-throughput screening. Even with these encouraging strides, rolling out new biomarker-based assays to everyday clinics is still a bumpy ride. Generally speaking, the varied immune responses demand large-scale validation to pin down robust marker combinations that can sort patients over different geographic and genetic backgrounds. Cost-effectiveness and simple deployment are big hurdles too, especially in resource-limited areas where leprosy sticks around. Ongoing research is thus focused on altering assay sensitivity and cutting down on false positives and negatives, with extra attention given to those early stage, even sometimes asymptomatic, cases. There's real promise in coupling multiplexed biomarkers with lateral flow devices, backed by miniaturized biosensors for real-time, point-of-care tests; such advances might just help break transmission chains and lead to earlier, more precise detection than what conventional tests offer (Van Hooij et al., 2016; Lima et al., 2019).

5.4.2. Advances in Rapid Diagnostic Tests

Rapid diagnostic tests have shifted how we tackle infectious diseases, especially in places where resources are scarce. Biotech breakthroughs have led to the creation of handy, portable tools that spot pathogens quickly even when fancy labs aren't around. For instance, early testing for illnesses like leprosy can drastically cut transmission and boost patient care. LFAs are now making a buzz for offering rapid results in the field—they mix low cost with high precision in ways that fill some obvious gaps in current strategies. Testing right at the point of care, in many cases, links up efficiently with broader public health aims to fight neglected tropical diseases (Rodriguez-Morales, 2019). To summarize, these advances help ramp up disease surveillance and speed up treatment initiation. At the same time, fresh molecular and immunodiagnostic methods have upped our ability to pinpoint *Mycobacterium leprae*—the microbe behind leprosy, with greater sensitivity and specificity. The ELISA is widely used to catch infection-related antigens, pushing diagnosis beyond just a clinical check. Interestingly, scientists have been working with mimetic peptides that mirror key bits of *M. leprae*, offering a flexible alternative to natural antigens; these peptides, by echoing important immunogenic regions, add another layer of accuracy to serological tests. Pairing these molecular approaches with rapid formats like optical or electrochemical biosensors further streamlines the whole process, giving quick, reliable results that are easy to deploy in labs with limited access (Lima et al., 2019).

In many cases, these biotechnological strides not only help with detection but also play a role in monitoring disease trends and steering public health actions. Broadly speaking, combining rapid diagnostic tools into existing healthcare systems calls for continuous innovation and some on-the-ground validation. Future research seems set to fine-tune biosensor technology and develop multiplex assays that can, all at once, detect several markers related to leprosy—thus bumping up diagnostic precision. Also, adapting point-of-care devices to work in various field conditions tackles some of the socioeconomic and geographical barriers faced in leprosy-endemic areas. Generally speaking, these developments align with the World Health Organization's drive for improved diagnostics and surveillance to control neglected tropical diseases. By leaning on new biotech platforms like lateral flow assays and cutting-edge molecular methods, healthcare providers can setstart treatment earlier, track infection dynamics more accurately, and ultimately reduce the disease burden. In this light, these promising innovations clearly underscore the central role of rapid diagnoses in modern leprosy control strategies (Lima et al., 2019; Rodriguez-Morales, 2019) (Figure 5.14).

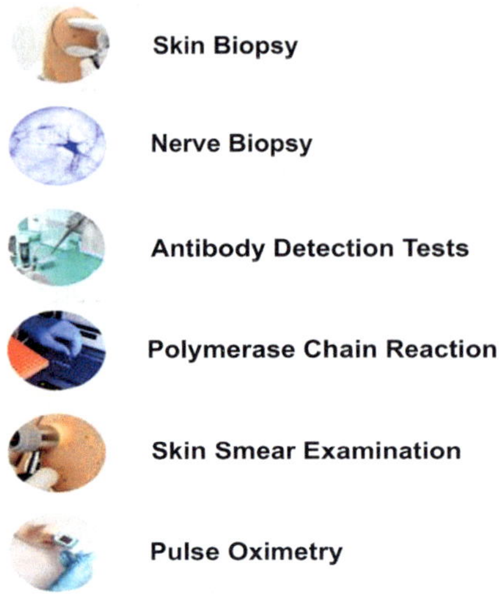

Figure 5.14. Rapid leprosy diagnostic tests.

Source: Drlogy. (n.d.). *Rapid Leprosy Diagnostic Tests.*

5.4.3. Use of Artificial Intelligence in Diagnosis

Modern tech in medicine has turned things upside down when it comes to handling infections like leprosy. AI now jumps right into the mix, churning through huge piles of patient records, images, and biomarkers instead of relying solely on old-fashioned lab tests and clinical observations. Sometimes it picks up those tiny details that a human might overlook, speeding up early detection in ways that could lead to timelier treatment and less chance of spreading disease. Biomedical engineering that combines these AI tools has even been tried out for tropical diseases in general, hinting at a more hands-on, cross-angled push for better health outcomes (Faisal et al., 2015). Generally speaking, this kind of leap in technology isn't just about fancy machines, it's about rethinking how we catch and manage complex diseases. Recent studies have put a spotlight on AI's tendency for diagnosing both viral and bacterial infections. In most cases, hepatitis research has shown that AI can sort and predict different disease variants with a surprising level of detail (John-Otumu et al., 2020). This matters a lot when you consider conditions like leprosy, where detecting slight differences among its many clinical presentations is key. Tools like microfluidic setups, lab-on-chip devices, and AI-powered clinical support systems hint at fast, non-invasive, point-of-care solutions that might ease the load on clinicians. Combining these smart techniques could cut down on our dependence on highly specialized experts and broaden screening in areas where help isn't always close at hand, even if it means facing hurdles like gathering enough quality data and fitting new AI tools into current healthcare routines. Some researchers have even tried combining different machine learning models into hybrid systems, which has worked well for other diseases (John-Otumu et al., 2020). In most cases, though, making these systems work in everyday settings will depend on teamwork among doctors, data individuals, and policymakers to ensure the tools are reliable, easy-to-use, and culturally sensitive. Overall, while the future of AI in leprosy diagnosis looks pretty promising, there's still a lot to sort out before these digital advances can reshape everyday healthcare.

A CLOSER LOOK

NERVE IMAGING IN LEPROSY

In the early stages of leprosy, large nerves exhibit a normal appearance on US and MR images. This can be explained by the fact that the nerve damage mostly occurs at the intradermal level and does not affect the main trunks extensively. In the limbs and extremities, the occurrence of nerve shape changes, and echo textural abnormalities do not correlate with the disease duration but seem to have a direct relationship with the number and severity of acute reactional episodes (reversal reactions) that the nerve has suffered during the disease. In general, the more and more severe episodes of reversal reactions undergone in the past, the more extensively deranged the nerve echotexture. On the other hand, patients with long-standing disease who did not undergo reversal reactions show normally appearing nerves. No significant correlation has also been found between the nerve abnormalities visualized on US and MR imaging and the two main disease poles—paucibacillary and multibacillary: this indicates that the clinical types of leprosy cannot be separated based on imaging features. Both paucibacillary and multibacillary forms present borderline histopathologic features that are often overlapping. Abnormally swollen nerves are often found within or in proximity to osteofibrous tunnels, such as the cubital tunnel for the ulnar nerve, the carpal tunnel for the median nerve, the area of the fibular head and neck for the peroneal nerve and the tarsal tunnel for the tibial nerve. In most instances, the abnormal segment of a nerve is more extended longitudinally than one can expect in case of compressive neuropathy and is typically located proximal and not distal to the tunnel. The nerve swelling can be quantified by measuring the nerve cross-sectional area or the caliber when the nerve size is too small for a reliable calculation of the area. Even if measurements obtained at specific levels are a valuable means to obtain better standardization, the nerve cross-sectional area should be sampled, in logical terms, at the site where the nerve is maximally enlarged and the histopathologic changes are, therefore, most relevant. The nerve area can then be used as a baseline reference to better perceive nerve size changes during follow-up studies. Two methods are used to measure the nerve cross-sectional area: the indirect method, based on calculating the nerve diameters by calipers and application of the ellipse formula (transverse diameter x anteroposterior diameter × $\pi/4$), and the direct method, based on manual tracing and automated calculation of the area. Both methods can be used depending on the examiner's preference and the equipment software available on US and MR devices. Abnormally swollen nerves may exhibit a preserved echotexture with fascicles that are enlarged but still visible as individual structures. If severe intraneural derangement occurs, the nerve assumes a more homogeneous pattern with loss of the fascicular structure on both US and MR imaging. No specific imaging signs exist to differentiate compression-related damage from histopathologic derangement pertaining to the underlying disease. The presence of an abrupt nerve caliber change at the entrance of an osteofibrous tunnel is the only finding that may suggest a concurrent compressive syndrome. In some instances, nerve abnormalities can be encountered in patients with normal neurophysiological findings, implying the concurrence of abnormal morphology with preserved nerve function in leprosy patients. Recently, sonoelastography has been tested in leprosy neuropathy with promising results, even if further validation on larger series of patients is required (Figure 5.15).

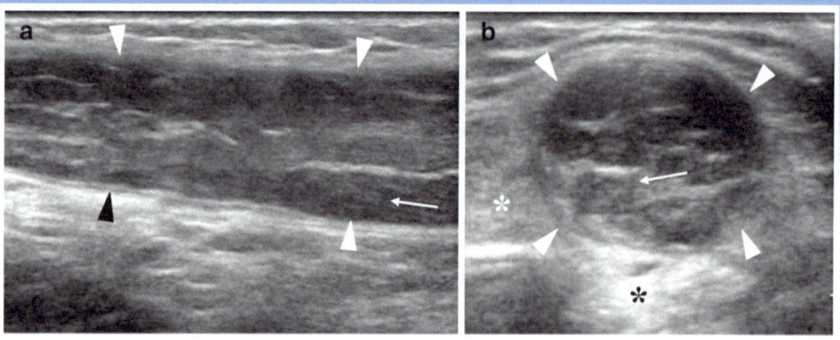

Figure 5.15. Ultrasonography (US) examination of the ulnar nerve at the elbow in a 32-year-old patient with borderline tuberculoid leprosy, presenting with long-standing symptoms and recent worsening of nerve function. Long-axis (a) and short-axis (b) 17–5 MHz US images show diffuse swelling of the ulnar nerve (arrowheads), characterized by markedly swollen fascicles (arrow) and poor visualization of the hyperechoic bands of the interfascicular epineurium.

Source: Springer Nature. (n.d.). Ultrasound Examination of Ulnar Nerve in Borderline Tuberculoid Leprosy.

SUMMARY

Diagnosing leprosy isn't a walk in the park. The disease shows up in so many different ways that even though we've got clinical checks and modern molecular tests helping catch it early, there are still plenty of bumps in the road, especially in areas that lack the latest tools. In many cases, combining traditional clinical exams with newer lab techniques seems to offer the best shot at detecting *Mycobacterium leprae* reliably, even though high-tech methods often run into issues with cost and access. This kind of combined, multidimensional approach not only helps in nailing an early, accurate diagnosis but also plays a key role in keeping the disease from spreading further in communities that are hard hit, ultimately boosting public health efforts. It's hard to stress enough how important it is to pinpoint exactly which species is causing the damage and to understand the way the disease behaves. You see, different patients can end up with very different outcomes and responses to treatment – a fact that underscores the need for precise detection, something molecular diagnostics are steadily improving. Think about similar challenges seen with diseases like cutaneous leishmaniasis, where even the best high-tech tests sometimes struggle in low-resource spots (Henry et al., 2022). Addressing these gaps generally means putting energy into creating diagnostic tools that are not only affordable and easy on the patient, but also simple enough to use in the field. Further, ramping up the training for healthcare workers and making sure that these diagnostic resources are readily available still remains crucial for cutting delays, preventing disabilities, and hitting disease elimination goals. Then there's the broader picture, which often gets overlooked. Social and psychological factors, like stigma and patient isolation—can seriously interefere with how and when people decide to seek help and even affect whether they stick with treatment plans (as seen with some quarantine challenges in managing infections (Samantha et al., 2020)). Ultimately, if we want diagnostic approaches to work well, they need to be paired with supportive measures that tackle these human issues. In most cases, combining technological progress with an understanding of resource limits and social challenges makes a big difference. This kind of comprehensive strategy not only improves leprosy control efforts but also works wonders for patient well-being over the long haul.

Accurate leprosy diagnosis is crucial. Instead of following a rigid checklist, doctors begin by looking for common skin patches and checking nerves—signs that usually hint at leprosy but don't always give the full picture. In many cases, a hands-on examination is paired with tests like skin smears and biopsies that let lab techs spot those acid-fast bacilli under the microscope. Histopathology, which examines tissue patterns like granulomatous inflammation and nerve changes, also helps sort out the various forms of the disease. This mixed approach, in most cases, improves how precisely the condition is diagnosed and helps set up treatment that fits each patient's needs. Still, since cases with very few bacteria (paucibacillary types) sometimes evade detection, extra tests are often needed to catch the illness early enough to prevent further spread and disability. New molecular tests have taken center stage by shifting the focus right to the DNA of *Mycobacterium leprae* found in patient samples. PCR assays, for instance, zoom in on specific genetic sequences and generally offer enhanced sensitivity and specificity—even when the bacterial load is low. This means that active versus latent infections can sometimes be teased apart sooner than before. Advances in nanotechnology have also introduced platforms using materials like gold nanoparticles which make the detection process both speedy and accurate. All of these innovations work together with older methods, potentially even enabling tests to be performed on the spot in areas where leprosy is common (Daraee et al., 2014). There are also blood tests designed to pick up antibodies against the bacterium's antigens, with those targeting PGL-I often noted for their high specificity. While these serological tests provide a non-invasive and relatively quick screening option, their sensitivity can vary based on the form of the disease and the bacterial count, so they rarely stand alone. As a result, clinicians typically mix these tests with thorough clinical exams and molecular methods to boost overall diagnostic confidence. In addition, emerging imaging techniques and immune-response assays are being looked at to better understand disease states and monitor how well treatment is working. In short, combining clinical observations with microbiological, molecular, and immunological tools creates a well-rounded strategy that supports timely treatment and keeps control measures on track (Haworth et al., 2017).

KEY TERMS FROM THIS CHAPTER

- Bacteria's genetic code
- Buruli ulcer
- Diabetic neuropathy
- Disease identification
- Enzyme-linked immunosorbent assay
- Histopathological methods
- Immune-based assays
- Leprosy detection
- Biosensors
- Chronic neurological issues
- Diagnosing leprosy
- Electrodiagnostic tests
- Health equity
- Hypogonadism
- Lateral flow assays
- Sensory loss

References

1. Bélard, S., Tamarozzi, F., Bustinduy, A. L., Wallrauch, C., Grobusch, M. P., Kuhn, W., Brunetti, E., Joekes, E., & Heller, T. (2016). Point-of-Care Ultrasound Assessment of Tropical Infectious Diseases--A Review of Applications and Perspectives. *The American journal of tropical medicine and hygiene*, *94*(1), 8–21. https://doi.org/10.4269/ajtmh.15-0421 (accessed on 10th May 2025).
2. Steinmann, P., Dusenbury, C., Addiss, D., Mirza, F., & Smith, W. C. S. (2020). A comprehensive research agenda for zero leprosy. *Infectious diseases of poverty*, *9*(1), 156. https://doi.org/10.1186/s40249-020-00774-4 (accessed on 10th May 2025).
3. van Hooij, A., Tjon Kon Fat, E. M., Richardus, R., van den Eeden, S. J., Wilson, L., de Dood, C. J., Faber, R., Alam, K., Richardus, J. H., Corstjens, P. L., & Geluk, A. (2016). Quantitative lateral flow strip assays as User-Friendly Tools To Detect Biomarker Profiles For Leprosy. *Scientific reports*, *6*, 34260. https://doi.org/10.1038/srep34260 (accessed on 10th May 2025).
4. Beissner, M., Huber, K. L., Badziklou, K., Halatoko, W. A., Maman, I., Vogel, F., Bidjada, B., Awoussi, K. S., Piten, E., Helfrich, K., Mengele, C., Nitschke, J., Amekuse, K., Wiedemann, F. X., Diefenhardt, A., Kobara, B., Herbinger, K. H., Kere, A. B., Prince-David, M., Löscher, T., ... Bretzel, G. (2013). Implementation of a national reference laboratory for Buruli ulcer disease in Togo. *PLoS neglected tropical diseases*, *7*(1), e2011. https://doi.org/10.1371/journal.pntd.0002011 (accessed on 10th May 2025).
5. Nsagha, D. S., Bamgboye, E. A., Assob, J. C., Njunda, A. L., Kamga, H. L., Zoung-Kanyi Bissek, A. C., Tabah, E. N., Oyediran, A. B., & Njamnshi, A. K. (2011). Elimination of leprosy as a public health problem by 2000 AD: an epidemiological perspective. *The Pan African medical journal*, *9*, 4. https://doi.org/10.4314/pamj.v9i1.71176 (accessed on 10th May 2025).
6. Brooks, S. K., Webster, R., Smith, L., Woodland, L., Wessely, S., Greenberg, N., & Rubin, G. J. (2020). The psychological impact of quarantine and how to reduce it: Rapid review of the evidence. *The Lancet*, *395*, 912–920. https://doi.org/10.1016/s0140-6736(20)30460-8 (accessed on 10th May 2025).
7. Fabri, A.daC., Carvalho, A. P., Vieira, N. F., Bueno, I.deC., Rodrigues, R. N., Monteiro, T. B., Correa-Oliveira, R., Duthie, M. S., & Lana, F. C. (2016). Integrative literature review of the reported uses of serological tests in leprosy management. *Revista da Sociedade Brasileira de Medicina Tropical*, *49*(2), 158–164. https://doi.org/10.1590/0037-8682-0226-2015 (accessed on 10th May 2025).
8. Cachia, M. J., & Vella, S. (2008). *Charcot Neuroarthropathy: Pathogenesis, Diagnosis and Medical Management.* Malta Medical Journal. 2008, Vol.20(3), p. 13-19 https://core.ac.uk/download/46602192.pdf (accessed on 10th May 2025).
9. Cattamanchi, A., Martin, A., Soto, A., Tamhane, A., Bah, B., et al. (2012). Performance of the 2007 WHO algorithm to diagnose smear-negative pulmonary tuberculosis in an HIV prevalent setting. *PLoS ONE*, *7*(12), e51336. https://core.ac.uk/download/pdf/10674396.pdf (accessed on 10th May 2025).
10. Utino, F. L., Garcia, M., Velho, P. E. N. F., França, A. F. E. D. C., Stelini, R. F., Pelegati, V. B., Cesar, C. L., de Souza, E. M., Cintra, M. L., & Damiani, G. V. (2018). Second-harmonic generation imaging analysis can help distinguish sarcoidosis from tuberculoid leprosy. *Journal*

of biomedical optics, *23*(12), 1–7. https://doi.org/10.1117/1.JBO.23.12.126001 (accessed on 10th May 2025).

11. Perez, R. L., Chase, J., & Tanner, R. (2024). Shared challenges to the control of complex intracellular neglected pathogens. *Frontiers in public health*, *12*, 1423420. https://doi.org/10.3389/fpubh.2024.1423420 (accessed on 10th May 2025).
12. Daraee, H., Eatemadi, A., Abbasi, E., Fekri, A. S., Kouhi, M., & Akbarzadeh, A. (2014). Application of gold nanoparticles in biomedical and drug delivery. *Artificial Cells, Nanomedicine and Biotechnology*, *44*, 410–422. https://doi.org/10.3109/21691401.2014.955107 (accessed on 10th May 2025).
13. Dayal, R. (2015). *Diagnosis of Childhood Leprosy – Changing Trends.* Ann Natl Acad Med Sci (India), 51(4): 178-193, 2015 https://core.ac.uk/download/pdf/287211130.pdf (accessed on 10th May 2025).
14. De Vries, H. J. C., & Schallig, H. D. F. H. (2022). Cutaneous leishmaniasis: A 2022 updated narrative review into diagnosis and management developments. *American Journal of Clinical Dermatology*, *23*, 823–840. https://doi.org/10.1007/s40257-022-00726-8 (accessed on 10th May 2025).
15. Ibrahim, F., Thio, T. H., Faisal, T., & Neuman, M. (2015). The application of biomedical engineering techniques to the diagnosis and management of tropical diseases: a review. *Sensors (Basel, Switzerland)*, *15*(3), 6947–6995. https://doi.org/10.3390/s150306947 (accessed on 10th May 2025).
16. Farro, M., & Podgorny, I. (2015). "PRE-COLUMBIAN MOULAGES". HUACOS, MUMMIES AND PHOTOGRAPHS IN THE INTERNATIONAL CONTROVERSY OVER PRECOLUMBIAN DISEASES, 1894-1910. *Medicina nei secoli*, *27*(2), 629–651. (accessed on 10th May 2025).
17. Nandwani, R. R., Totade, S. K., Gupta, U., & Jain, M. (2017). Role of fine needle aspiration cytology in diagnosing leprosy: in a tertiary care hospital. *International Journal of Research in Medical Sciences*, *3*(3), 749–756. Retrieved from https://www.msjonline.org/index.php/ijrms/article/view/1369 (accessed on 10th May 2025).
18. Haworth, C., Banks, J., Capstick, T., Fisher, A. J., Gorsuch, T., Laurenson, I. F., Leitch, A., et al. (2017). British Thoracic Society guidelines for the management of non-tuberculous mycobacterial pulmonary disease (NTM-PD). *Thorax*, *72*, ii1–ii64. https://doi.org/10.1136/thoraxjnl-2017-210927 (accessed on 10th May 2025).
19. Hella, J. (2019). *Understanding the Epidemiology and Transmission of Tuberculosis Among Adults in Rural and Urban Tanzania*. https://core.ac.uk/download/511532396.pdf (accessed on 10th May 2025).
20. John-Otumu, A. M., Ogba , G. U., & Nwokonkwo, O. C. (2020). A survey on artificial intelligence based techniques for diagnosis of hepatitis variants. *Journal of Advances in Science and Engineering*, *3*(1), 43-56. https://doi.org/10.37121/jase.v3i1.83 (accessed on 10th May 2025).
21. Ingrid Sousa Lima M, Caroline dos Santos Moraes E, Diniz Pinho J, Henrique Corrêa Soares G, Vinícius Cantanhêde Santos Í. Molecular and Biotechnological Approaches in the Diagnosis of Leprosy [Internet]. Hansen's Disease - The Forgotten and Neglected Disease. IntechOpen; 2019. Available from: http://dx.doi.org/10.5772/intechopen.75506 (accessed on 10th May 2025).

22. Morgan, J. A. (2014). *The Methodological and Diagnostic Applications of Micro-CT to Palaeopathology: A Quantitative Study of Porotic Hyperostosis*. https://core.ac.uk/download/61643529.pdf (accessed on 10th May 2025).

23. J. Rodriguez-Morales, A. (Ed.). (2019). Current Topics in Neglected Tropical Diseases. IntechOpen. doi: 10.5772/intechopen.73918 (accessed on 10th May 2025).

24. Richens J. (2004). Genital manifestations of tropical diseases. *Sexually transmitted infections*, *80*(1), 12–17. https://doi.org/10.1136/sti.2003.004093 (accessed on 10th May 2025).

*25. Mycobacterium leprae*Diana D and Harish MC (2024) qPCR detection of *Mycobacterium leprae* DNA in urine samples of leprosy patients using the Rlep gene target. Front. Mol. Biosci. 11:1435679. doi: 10.3389/fmolb.2024.1435679 (accessed on 10th May 2025).

26. Van Den Bergh, P., Van Doorn, P. A., Hadden, R. D. M., Avau, B., Vankrunkelsven, P., Allen, J. A., Attarian, S., et al. (2021). European Academy of Neurology/Peripheral Nerve Society guideline on diagnosis and treatment of chronic inflammatory demyelinating polyradiculoneuropathy: Report of a joint task force—Second revision. *European Journal of Neurology*, *28*, 3556–3583. https://doi.org/10.1111/ene.14959 (accessed on 10th May 2025).

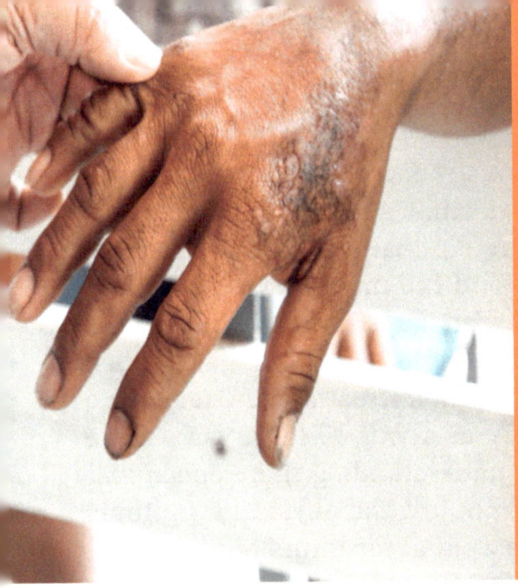

Chapter 6

TREATMENT OPTIONS FOR LEPROSY

Contents

Introduction

Leprosy—commonly called Hansen's disease, has troubled communities worldwide for ages, combining both medical and social issues in ways that aren't always clear-cut. The way it spreads and develops has led to a lot of confusion and unjust stigma over time. Science, bit by bit, has shed light on the microbe behind it, *Mycobacterium leprae*, and how it interacts with our bodies. Its signs can be all over the map, mostly hitting the skin and peripheral nerves, yet treatment methods have evolved a lot over the past century. In most cases, knowing how to treat it well matters not only for controlling the disease but also for easing its heavy social impact. Modern treatments paint a very different picture from those older, less reliable methods—even if some complications still emerge. Multi-drug therapy (MDT) protocols, backed by global health groups, have changed the game by cutting down infectivity and keeping disabilities at bay. Still, dealing with extra infections like tuberculosis, which often show up in leprosy patients, can complicate treatment outcomes. Even though reports of co-infection are less common these days, we still have not fully wrapped our heads around the immune genetics and how these microbes interact, which might shift treatment plans as time goes on. To summarize, these overlapping challenges mean that ongoing research and careful, nuanced care are needed to cover every angle for those affected (Rawson et al., 2014). Beyond the medical side, handling leprosy also gets complex with broader social and cultural factors that shape patient experiences. In many regions—South Asia being a big example—the condition still carries a heavy stigma, which often affects whether individuals decide to seek help or stick with their treatment. There have even been cases where people convert to religions like Christianity as a way to forge new, more positive identities and rebuild community bonds. It turns out that understanding these social and religious layers is key for designing treatment programs that tackle not just the physical symptoms but also the mental and social hurdles. This whole-picture view is essential for lifting both medical outcomes and social wellbeing for those living with the condition (Staples et al., 2014) (Figure 6.1).

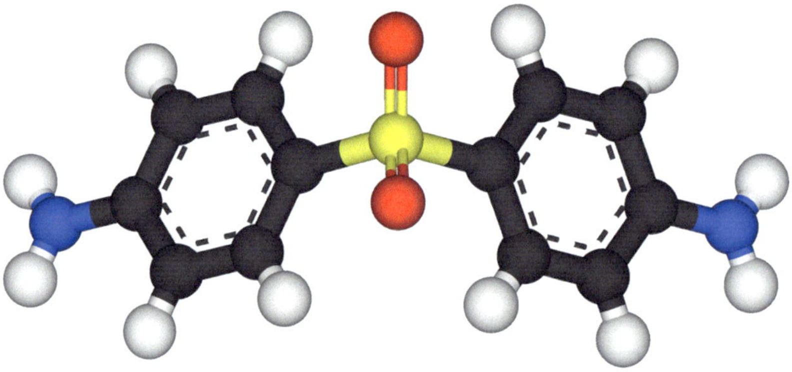

Figure 6.1. The treatment options for leprosy.

Source: By Fvasconcellos - Own work, Public Domain, https://commons.wikimedia.org/w/index.php?curid=1312292

6.1. Multidrug Therapy (MDT)

Mycobacterium leprae, the microbe behind leprosy, has long been a stubborn health issue, especially in regions where new cases emerge every year. Simple symptom relief isn't enough; truly tackling the disease means going after the microbe itself while keeping drug resistance at bay. MDT has become the go-to treatment, combining a few antibiotics to attack the bacteria from different angles. Usually, this cmbination includes dapsone, rifampicin, and clofazimine; each one plays its part by hitting different bacterial pathways to clear out the infection thoroughly. Even though MDT has proven its worth, getting rid of the bacteria can be a slow road, and patient immune responses often vary. In most cases, doctors are now testing extra therapies that boost the body's own defenses alongside MDT (Kimberly et al., 2024). Adding clofazimine into the mix shows off both the treatment perks and the real-world challenges of managing leprosy. This drug not only targets mycobacteria, lowering the bacterial load when used with other antibiotics, but it also seems to stimulate the immune system, a small help for the patient's natural defenses. Still, its wider use runs into issues like limited production and high costs in resource-poor settings, which means access isn't always easy. And yes, even if side effects aren't common, they do emerge enough to force careful monitoring so patients stick with their regimen. Yet, research generally indicates that clofazimine's role in MDT boosts cure rates and cuts down on resistance, underlining its key importance in a full-scale leprosy treatment plan (Dotsenko et al., 2013). Researchers are now exploring if adding extra immune boosters to standard MDT might optimize leprosy care. These additional agents are designed to enhance the body's immune response – something that's crucial for keeping *Mycobacterium leprae* under control and speeding up bacterial clearance. For example, compounds like levamisole, thalidomide, and even essential vitamins (A, D, E, and C) have shown immunostimulatory properties that could work hand-in-hand with MDT to lower the bacterial burden and reduce the risk of relapse. This more integrative approach, which combine antimicrobial therapy with immune support, hints at ways to cut down both the length and severity of the disease. To summarize, these new developments help cover the gaps left by MDT alone and look set to improve patient outcomes while bolstering long-term control over leprosy (Kimberly et al., 2024) (Figure 6.2).

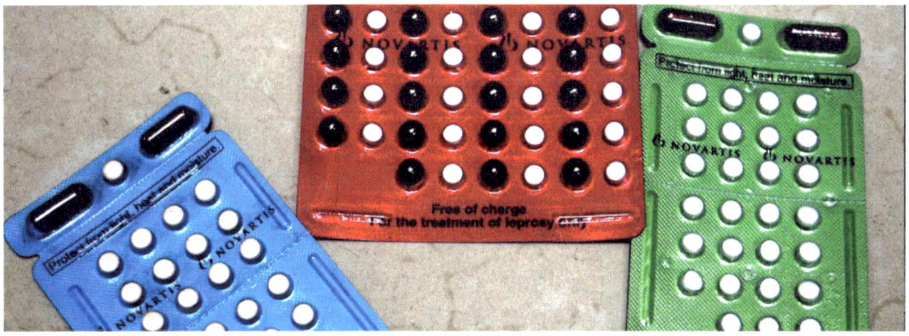

Figure 6.2. Multidrug therapy (MDT) for leprosy disease.

Source: The Leprosy Mission Trust India. (n.d.). *Multidrug Therapy (MDT) for Leprosy Disease.*

6.1.1. Components of Multidrug Therapy (MDT)

Leprosy treatment has changed a lot over the years—MDT now sits at the center of modern care. Rather than a single antibiotic, MDT brings together a combination that targets *Mycobacterium leprae*, the microbe causing the disease, and works to keep drug resistance at bay. Typically, you'll find dapsone, rifampicin, and clofazimine in the mix. Dapsone acts to keep bacterial growth in check, rifampicin goes in hard, and clofazimine has a dual role, in handling both microbes and inflammation. All these drugs, when combined, seem to work in tandem, cutting down treatment time and lessening the chance of spreading the infection—a real win considering new cases still emerge around the world (Kimberly et al., 2024). Compared to the old single-drug approaches, this careful balancing of dose and schedule marks a big leap forward for patient care and public health. Still, even with this progress, MDT doesn't answer every problem. It's clear that while the antibiotics do a fine job eliminating the bacteria, they don't completely tackle issues like nerve damage and the body's unpredictable immune responses. Recent studies generally show that adding treatments designed to modulate the immune system—think of agents like thalidomide or even some vitamins—might help reduce those damaging inflammatory reactions and nerve issues. In most cases, supplementing MDT with these extra measures seems likely to improve bacterial clearance and lower the risk of severe reactions, potentially decreasing disability rates overall

(Kimberly et al., 2024). It turns out that treating leprosy effectively might need a two-pronged approach: one that attacks the microbe directly, and another that helps the body handle its own immune responses. On an even broader scale, the push to remove leprosy as a public health concern emphasizes how crucial it is to keep improving MDT within wider strategies. Global initiatives have stressed that treatment isn't just about clearing bacteria—it's equally about reducing new infections and preventing disabilities. Sure, MDT is fundamental, but it works best when coupled with early case detection, strong patient follow-through, and robust healthcare support. Researchers are continuously tinkering with the individual components, altering doses and treatment durations to fit different needs while trying to cut down on side effects. In a nutshell, fitting MDT into larger health policies is essential for keeping up the fight against leprosy and achieving those World Health Organization targets for 2030. Combining traditional antibiotic work with fresh diagnostic tools and supportive immune therapies could be just the holistic shift needed to fully control and eventually wipe out the disease.

6.1.2. Effectiveness of Multidrug Therapy (MDT) in Treatment

Leprosy treatment has come a long way—MDT shifted the game for patients. Before MDT, treatments mainly stuck with one drug at a time, and that often meant running into issues like drug resistance and not fully wiping out *Mycobacterium leprae*. Now, the mix of rifampicin, dapsone, and clofazimine is combined together in a way that quite effectively tackles the bacteria while keeping resistance risks lower. This combo not only slows down the disease's progress but also cuts its contagiousness, which helps curb spread in communities. Even though it's generally effective in clearing active infections, recent studies flag up some challenges, like when tuberculosis shows up alongside, which can complicate treatment plans in endemic regions. Clearly, this overlap calls for further probing to fine-tune MDT and manage any complications from co-infections (Rawson et al., 2014). MDT does a solid job curing leprosy, yet it doesn't completely seal the deal when it comes to stopping transmission, meaning extra preventive measures are needed. Recent systematic reviews, in most cases, show that adding a single dose of rifampicin as post-exposure prophylaxis can drop incidence rates by roughly 50%–60% among high-risk groups.

This approach works hand in hand with MDT, targeting those latent asymptomatic carriers and breaking up transmission chains in affected areas. Further, pairing these prophylactic tricks with vaccination efforts, like using the Bacillus Calmette–Guérin (BCG) vaccine—seems to boost overall protection. So, while MDT remains the backbone for treatment, combining in these additional strategies is pretty crucial for a wider public health impact and lasting leprosy control (Asyura et al., 2021). When it comes to cost-effectiveness, MDT along with its preventive partners is key, especially in resource-limited settings. Economic analyses suggest that implementing MDT on a large scale—alongside rifampicin post-exposure prophylaxis—can generate substantial savings over time by cutting down both leprosy-related illness and its spread. These savings matter a lot for endemic countries that often juggle tight healthcare budgets. At the same time, making MDT work optimally means tackling hurdles like drug resistance, treatment adherence, and managing side effects—issues that become complex with added infections. By addressing these challenges through ongoing research and smart policy moves, MDT can keep its strong standing as the primary choice for managing leprosy (Rawson et al., 2014; Asyura et al., 2021) (Figure 6.3).

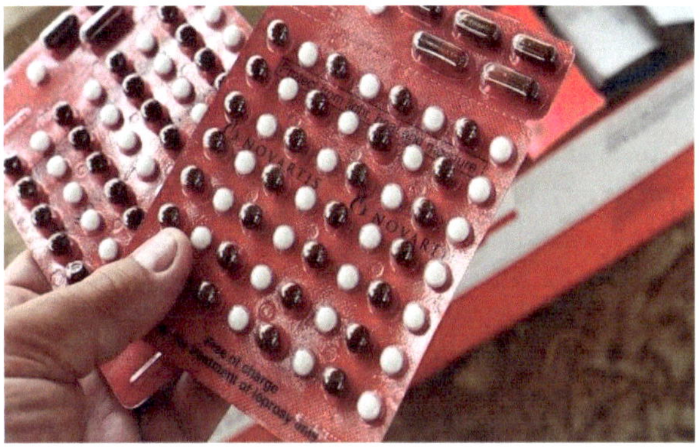

Figure 6.3. Leprosy disease: Complication and effectiveness of multidrug therapy (MDT).

Source: Imgur. (n.d.). *FTlb76e. https://i.imgur.com/FTlb76e.jpg.*

6.1.3. Duration and Adherence to Multidrug Therapy (MDT)

Timely diagnosis matters when dealing with leprosy – delays let the disease sneak up and often worsen disabilities. MDT, as most individuals call it, uses a combination of dapsone, rifampicin, and clofazimine for tougher, multibacillary cases, and just dapsone with rifampicin for the milder, paucibacillary ones. In most cases, the whole idea is that this cocktail clears out the bacteria pretty well. Still, sticking to the full treatment schedule—about six months for PB and at least 12 months for MB cases—proves complex. Missing doses or cutting therapy short can let the infection stick around and even open the door to resistance. Some studies even suggest that when patients understand the side effects – like dapsone's link to anemia , and the value of not breaking the therapy chain, adherence improves. Supporting patients to manage these side effects, even if it means a few hiccups along the way, often helps them finish treatment without any major changes, keeping disease complications lower (Nariya et al., 2019). A long treatment plan means that patients and healthcare providers usually end up in a kind of long-term arrangement. Regular visits become normal, and keeping track of medications and side effects feels like a day-to-day task. Generally speaking, the duration of the therapy and factors like socio-economic conditions and health system challenges both play a role in how well people stick to their treatment. The introduction of MDT brought more careful monitoring and helped build stronger ties between patients and their care teams. Combining leprosy services into general health care may even cut through stigma and make care easier to get, so maintaining a supportive network and frequent follow-ups is key to preventing dropouts and ensuring the microbes are completely eliminated (Nariya et al., 2019).

On top of all that, there's been some buzz about adding extra therapies – think immunomodulators – to the mix in hopes of boosting treatment results. For example, agents such as levamisole along with vitamins A, D, E, and C might give the immune system a hand in clearing the bacteria, possibly even shortening the treatment time or easing the disease's impact. While the standard MDT usually does the job, these add-ons could reduce the burden of long-term treatment by making it a bit lighter on the patient. Still, it's important to note that more research is needed—safety, effectiveness, and whether patients can manage a combined regimen are still up for discussion before such approaches become the norm.

6.2. Alternative Treatment Options

Medical research has come a long way recently, opening up a variety of treatment options for chronic and infectious conditions that go well beyond the old standard drug plans. Take leprosy, for example—it's become pretty clear that new approaches are needed since patients react differently, resistance can emerge, and the usual therapies sometimes come with harsh side effects. Some emerging ideas focus on keeping patients on board with their treatment while cutting down on whole-body toxicity. Sometimes, combining in targeted agents or selective receptor modulators like those seen in other areas might just induce similar breakthroughs in leprosy care. Even though the exact details, like pharmacodynamics and pathogen-specific targets, aren't exactly the same, figuring out what works elsewhere can generally guide future research toward treatments for leprosy that deliver better results with fewer drawbacks (Gilbert et al., 2025).

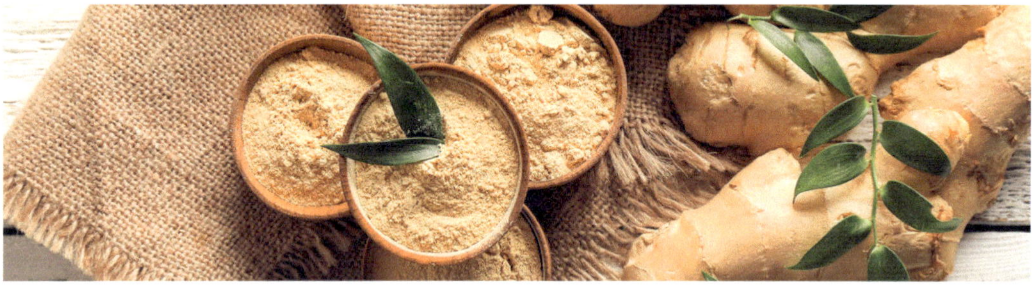

Figure 6.4. Ginger as a medicinal ingredient in the treatment of leprosy.

Source: By Photograph: Frank C. Müller, Baden-Baden - Self-photographed, CC BY-SA 3.0, https://commons.wikimedia.org/w/index.php?curid=4129876

To summarize, these insights push us to look beyond the traditional multidrug approaches. Less invasive procedures have also changed the scene when it comes to treating infections and inflammatory conditions. Advanced endoscopic methods, such as endoscopic retrograde appendicitis therapy (ERAT) (Zhang et al., 2024), clearly show how technology can help focus treatment exactly where it's needed, all while preserving organ function in a way that feels almost effortless. Sure, leprosy primarily hits the skin and peripheral nerves, but there's a chance that ideas from these minimal-touch techniques might be reworked into strategies that lower the bacterial load or handle inflammation in a more local, targeted way. Reducing overall immune suppression and systemic toxicity can do wonders for patient outcomes, especially for those who can't tolerate standard systemic treatments. It's interesting how successes in one medical area can inspire fresh innovation for another. Personalized medicine now also plays a big part in exploring these alternative treatments, especially for a complex disease like leprosy. Hormonal alters and receptor-based therapies, which have already been combined to treatment systems in other tissue-specific conditions, offer one possible blueprint to tackle issues such as nerve irritation and damage to the skin or mucous membranes, all while avoiding some of the side effects seen with broader treatments (Gilbert et al., 2025). On top of that, individual lifestyle factors and other health concerns naturally have to be considered when choosing a treatment, making sure that any alternative fits the patient's needs and safety. In most cases, future therapies will likely mix these tailor-made approaches with sharper early diagnosis and more hands-on monitoring, promoting a more comprehensive way to manage leprosy that goes way beyond just antibiotics. This shift should ultimately raise quality of life and help keep the disease in check over the long haul (Figure 6.4).

6.2.1. Role of Immunotherapy

MDT has long been the main approach for treating leprosy – using multiple drugs to hit *Mycobacterium leprae* head-on. Still, sometimes the body's own defenses just don't do enough, leaving some infections to persist or even worsen. In such cases, boosting the immune response has started to look promising. Immunotherapy, instead of trying to knock the bacteria down directly, works by stimulating the host's immune system to better clear the infection and protect the nerves; this could mean fewer long-term disabilities. It highlights how crucial cell-based immunity is, suggesting that standard MDT might benefit from some extra immune support (Kimberly et al., 2024). Immunomodulators come into play as agents that help strengthen natural defenses. Drugs like levamisole and thalidomide, along with micronutrients such as zinc and selenium, have been noted to kick the immune system into action – sometimes in unexpected ways. They tap into different immune pathways, affecting both the innate and adaptive systems so that macrophages can more efficiently mop up the bacteria. When used with MDT, these agents might boost overall treatment success and even trim down the therapy duration. In addition, supplements like vitamins A, D, E, and C are tossed into the mix as further immune-system enhancers, supporting a multi-layered strategy for handling both the infection and its complications (Kimberly et al., 2024). Looking at the bigger picture, the idea of immune-based treatments isn't limited to leprosy. Take psoriasis, for example , a condition where fine-tuning the immune response is key to managing symptoms. Generally speaking, balancing the immune reaction is complex but holds promise for innovative vaccines or targeted immune boosters against *Mycobacterium leprae*. Such strategies could lower relapse rates and improve the overall quality of life, though it's important to tread carefully so as not to induce harmful immune overreactions. In most cases, any new immunotherapy should be designed to work in tandem with existing regimens rather than complicate the treatment process.

6.2.2. Use of Herbal and Traditional Remedies

In many parts of the world where modern healthcare isn't always within reach, people end up relying on time-honored local remedies, especially when it comes to challenges like leprosy. Individuals here lean on a combination of traditional herbal treatments—not just because of deep-rooted cultural beliefs, but also because economic hurdles and far-off clinics leave them with few other options. Local healers, who command a special kind of trust and authority, shape how people seek help and stick with a treatment plan. You might say these practices go way beyond being just an "alternative" form of care; they're woven into the fabric of local health solutions, offering a bridge to modern treatment approaches that could fill some serious gaps in care and boost community involvement (Macfarlane et al., 2005). A growing chunk of botanical research suggests that herbal remedies might have something to offer when it comes to softening the harsh symptoms of leprosy. Many plants used in traditional medicine have properties, like fighting off microbes, reducing inflammation, and even giving the immune system a stimulate—that could work hand in glove with standard MDTs. Yet even though these natural approaches are widely popular, they still face a lack of rigorous clinical trial support, which makes their formal inclusion in treatment protocols a bit of a challenge. Variations in how they're prepared, dosed, and administered by different healers further complicate the issue when it comes to standardizing these remedies. Still, by acknowledging the potential of these plants as handy complements to modern treatments, we might be onto a promising way to boost overall care, especially in situations where conventional drugs are either hard to come by or plagued by side effects and cost issues (Balogun et al., 2019). Combining herbal methods with modern leprosy treatments isn't some quick fix—it calls for careful, ongoing research and smart policy moves that balance scientific discipline with cultural sensitivity. A good starting point would be systematically recording indigenous knowledge, setting up quality checks, and training practitioners so they can work safely alongside biomedical health providers. Early projects in places like PNG hint that even a small, well-considered step toward integration—rather than a wholesale merging—can open doors to mutual trust, shared resources, and broader outreach without putting treatment safety at risk. Generally speaking, a successful combination of these systems depends on supportive government policies, proper resource allocation, and regular evaluations to keep things ethical and effective in the long run (Macfarlane et al., 2005) (Figure 6.5).

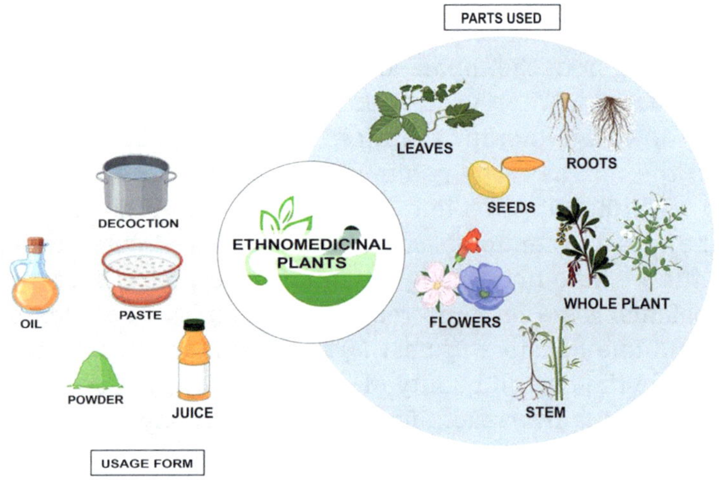

Figure 6.5. Diagram illustrating the plant parts utilized and the forms in which ethnomedicinal plants are used.

Source: Kimta N, Majdalawieh AF, Nasrallah GK, Puri S, Nepovimova E, Jomova K and Kuča K (2024) Leprosy: Comprehensive insights into pathology, immunology, and cutting-edge treatment strategies, integrating nanoparticles and ethnomedicinal plants. Front. Pharmacol. 15:1361641. doi: 10.3389/fphar.2024.1361641

6.2.3. Investigational Drugs and Clinical Trials

Experimental treatments for tough infections often rely on testing new drugs that, after enduring pretty intense clinical trials, might someday become the norm. Take leprosy, for instance – multidrug therapy has cut down the number of cases, yet stubborn resistant strains force researchers to look for new options. Clofazimine, first used for leprosy, now pops up with wider anti-mycobacterial capabilities, and there's even speculation it might help with multidrug-resistant TB. Even though it appears promising in fighting these resistant microbes, issues like limited global supply, high cost, and low manufacturing output mean that its use isn't widespread. In most cases, clinical trials show that clofazimine has a low rate of serious side effects – roughly on par with first-line treatments , which generally encourages more evaluation and possibly expanded use in leprosy and similar infections (Dotsenko et al., 2013). This whole scenario underlines the need to balance how easy a drug is to get with the real clinical benefits it offers. Switching gears a bit, research isn't stopping at clofazimine; scientists have been poking around for other agents that might tackle both infection and inflammation, especially since leprosy can bring on immune complications. Dapsone is one example – it was taken from treatments of other inflammatory issues and is now being reconsidered because it might handle bacterial infections while reducing inflammation. Clinical studies have even highlighted dapsone's potential when conventional treatments just don't cut it, hinting at its role as either an add-on or an alternative therapy. For example, its use in familial Mediterranean fever, where it helped control sudden attacks in some patients, kind of shows its anti-inflammatory strength, which might be useful in managing leprosy reactions and related nerve problems. These kinds of findings, generally speaking, push forward more trials to fine-tune treatments that combine antimicrobial with immune-modulating actions. On a broader note, advancing investigational drugs through robust, if sometimes unpredictable, clinical trials provide a framework for checking how effective, safe, and properly dosed they are – all of which are key to better leprosy treatments. Methodologically sound studies, in most cases, give data that can alter multidrug regimens, especially for patients who either develop resistance, experience intolerances, or have adverse reactions to standard drugs. Such research also helps researchers pinpoint who might benefit most, decide on treatment lengths, and flag potential drug interactions while keeping an eye on long-term outcomes and shifts in resistance patterns. This ongoing, sometimes complex, process of clinical evaluation not only reinforces a drug's clinical strength but also its real-world feasibility in varied healthcare settings, ultimately paving the way for more effective, accessible and patient-centered therapies that are absolutely vital for global leprosy control programs.

6.3. Management of Leprosy Complications

Even after the bacteria are gone, leprosy leaves behind plenty of challenges that need careful handling. Nerve damage, for instance, can hit hard leading to sensory loss, visible deformities, and disabilities that can change a person's life. In most cases, detecting nerve involvement early and jumping on treatments like corticosteroids or similar immunosuppressive drugs is key to calming down inflammation and avoiding lasting damage. Besides that, regular physiotherapy and even the use of specialized footwear can slow down the progression of disability by preserving function and helping to ward off extra injuries. Patients, too, play a big part; learning basic self-care and recognizing early warning signs is absolutely crucial for reducing long-term effects. Integrating these approaches into primary healthcare, especially where resources are limited, ensures that care remains as comprehensive as possible (Akshay et al., 2009). Then there are other hurdles, take the flare-ups known as erythema nodosum leprosum (ENL) reactions. These sudden, inflammatory episodes can worsen nerve problems and induce systemic symptoms, making the clinical picture even murkier. Typically speaking, such situations are managed with immunomodulatory drugs like corticosteroids and thalidomide, though these treatments must be handled delicately to keep side effects in check. In settings where leprosy care is woven into primary healthcare, it becomes extra important for health workers to stay sharp in identifying and managing these reactions promptly. Early intervention at the first signs of a reaction is essential to slow nerve damage and ultimately boost the quality of life for those affected (Akshay et al., 2009). Of equal importance is addressing the broader, more personal needs of those dealing with leprosy complications. The stigma that follows physical deformities and disability can hold someone back from social and emotional recovery. As a result, community-based rehabilitation and even vocational training programs can go a long way by empowering individuals, fostering economic independence, and breaking down social barriers. Moreover, surveillance efforts within primary care help catch relapses or new complications early, ensuring that treatment isn't delayed and disability rates are kept in check. Even though multidrug therapy remains the main force in clearing the bacteria, pairing it with strong management of these additional challenges creates a well-rounded strategy that's crucial for long-term disease control and eradication efforts (Akshay et al., 2009) (Figure 6.6).

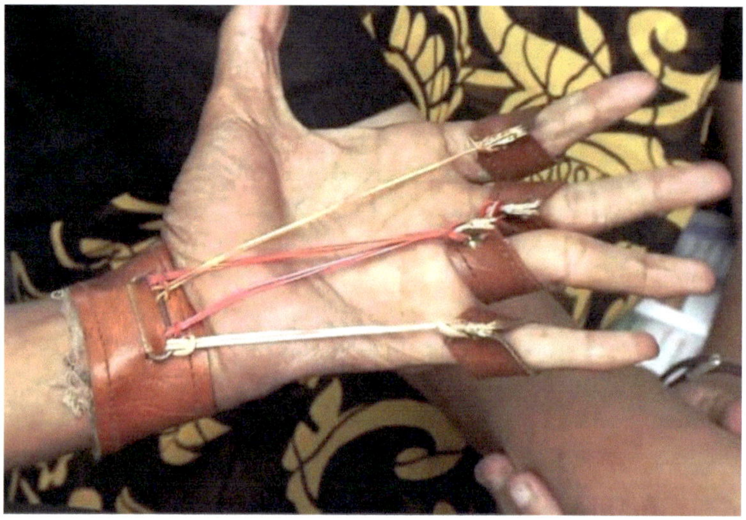

Figure 6.6. The management of leprosy complications.

Source: Paras Hospitals. (2018). *The Management of Leprosy Complications.*

6.3.1. Physical Rehabilitation Strategies

Physical rehabilitation plays a major role in managing leprosy complications—it isn't just about treating a body; it's about tackling nerve damage head on. Early on, routines like physiotherapy and occupational therapy jump into action to help restore function, keep people mobile, and ward off disabilities. You see, techniques such as muscle strengthening, sensory reeducation, and even splints are used to protect affected limbs and help stop deformities before they set in, especially when nerve sensation is compromised. Often these plans get tailored to match how severe a patient's impairment is, so the treatment remains both effective and lasting. Health professionals also spend time showing patients self-care basics, which, generally speaking, keeps long-term daily functions from slipping away. Rehabilitation goes beyond just physical fixes; it tends to open doors socially too. People with leprosy can face stigma—visible deformities often lead to isolation and added emotional stress. That's why, in most cases, physical therapy is teamed up with vocational coaching and some psychosocial support to boost one's job prospects and independence. This mixed approach sometimes helps individuals find a pathway back into the workforce, breaking the cycle of poverty commonly connected to disability (Cornell University, World Health Organization, and World Bank, 2011). Creating environments that truly welcome persons with disabilities not only brings about bodily recovery but also helps restore dignity and social participation, lessening the long-term socioeconomic impact of the disease. Even though physical rehab mainly focuses on fixing the body's structure and function, newer methods and community-based initiatives are changing the game. Local support groups and hands-on, tailored interventions are bridging the gap between clinical care and everyday living, empowering patients in unexpected ways. Innovations like mobile health apps now allow for remote check-ins and ongoing guidance, making continuous care possible even in areas short on resources (Bonkass et al., 2024). Adding elements like counseling or cognitive behavioral techniques to the usual physical therapy mix addresses mental health too, helping reduce stigma along the way. To summarize, this broadened, almost holistic, approach, which sometimes even involves a bit of redundancy in reminders about self-care—seems to signal a promising future for truly sustainable, inclusive leprosy rehabilitation.

6.3.2. Psychological Support and Counseling

Treating leprosy isn't just about fixing the body—it's also about facing the heavy, often overlooked mental toll that comes with it. Stigma makes life harder by pushing people into loneliness, triggering bouts of depression and anxiety that can stall their healing and make returning to everyday life tougher. In most cases, doctors now see that simply curing physical symptoms won't cut it; a broader plan that mixes in counseling, some basic education, and even cognitive behavioral therapy can help ease the mind's distress.

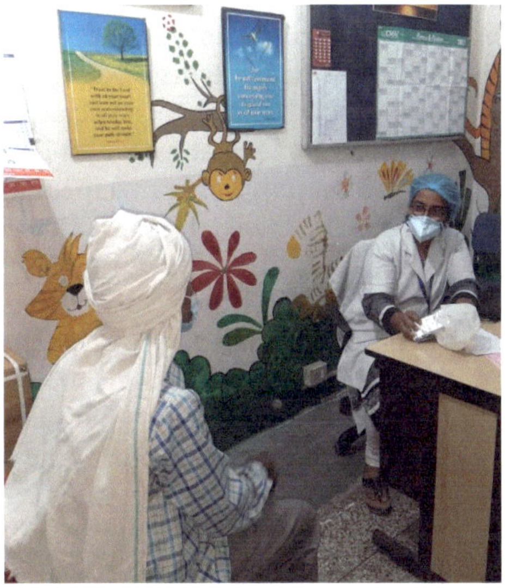

Figure 6.7. Counsellor motivates the patient counseling of leprosy care and health services.

Source: TLM Shahdara. (2021). *Counselor Motivates the Patient: Leprosy Care and Services.*

These steps give patients better tools to cope and, in turn, help them stick with their treatment plans for improved health and a warmer welcome back into society (Bonkass et al., 2024). Counseling, for example, plays a big role in lightening the load of chronic conditions like this. Research from other illnesses shows that when patients get clear information and honest emotional support, both their body and spirit tend to improve. Sometimes a simple chat can lower stress levels and lift someone's mood, working alongside medicine as a non-drug way to address that complex mind-body mix that comes with long-term disease. Generally speaking, when people understand more about what they're dealing with, and when someone is there to guide them—they tend to manage their symptoms better and feel a bit less overwhelmed by fear. It all ends up helping them move toward a smoother, more sustainable recovery (J et al., 2017). A key part of all this is making sure the psychological help fits local customs and situations. In places like India, where leprosy is common and mental health services might be lacking, it becomes extra urgent to tailor support so it resonates with local beliefs and traditions. When these care methods mesh with cultural norms, they tend to work better. Further, using new tech solutions or community support networks can push these services further, especially in areas with limited resources. In many cases, policy shifts that fold mental health care into leprosy programs—along with grassroots awareness efforts—can impact the stigma and give people the confidence to ask for help without worry. To summarize, a treatment plan that weaves together both the medical and the personal sides of care seems to be the best bet for easing leprosy's many burdens (Bonkass et al., 2024) (Figure 6.7).

6.3.3. Addressing Social Stigma and Discrimination

Stigma and discrimination still interfere with how well leprosy treatments work. It isn't just a battle against *Mycobacterium leprae* - often, the very places where patients live make it hard to get diagnosed on time or stick with a multi-drug treatment plan. Many end up isolated, which, quite frankly, makes them hesitate to seek help; as a result, the illness tends to worsen and jump from one community to another. You need a broad, sometimes complex strategy - like public campaigns that bust old myths and clear up confusion about leprosy. When awareness is boosted and empathy starts to take root, fear and social exclusion drop, and patients feel more open to following treatment plans. To summarize, combining these social fixes with the clinical side shows that handling leprosy means dealing with both medical issues and everyday social vibes (Craig et al., 2018). Overcoming stigma isn't a one-person job. Generally speaking, it takes a team effort among doctors, community figures, and the patients themselves. Medical staff must get solid training so they can spot and push back on discriminatory attitudes both in clinics and out in the wider world. Using communication methods that genuinely respect cultural differences helps people feel safe enough to share their own stories - breaking the long-held silence about leprosy. Communities playing an active role is huge too; they help make the condition less of a taboo and support those in treatment. Sometimes, using tools similar to those in tuberculosis care to measure stigma can shine a light on just how well these efforts are working. With some systematic, if not perfectly neat, checks in place, approaches can be altered to fit local realities, which tends to boost treatment adherence and overall health outcomes (Craig et al., 2018). In short, combining social insight with clinical know-how feels like a strong step forward. Beyond local efforts, combining perspectives from different fields cranks up our ability to ease the stigma for leprosy patients. Observations from other diseases—ones with similarly complex, intracellular microbes—show that biology and social factors are pretty complex when it comes to how an illness impacts someone and how well treatments do their job (Perez et al., 2024). Such points highlight why getting researchers and community groups together is so key; they need to look at cultural, economic, and even deeper structural issues feeding into discrimination. When we combine medical treatment efficiently with social justice moves, policies end up better protecting patient rights and, oddly enough, create fairer access to healthcare. Ultimately, facing stigma and bias head-on is absolutely critical if leprosy treatments are ever going to work fully, because social acceptance is the foundation upon which lasting medical progress is built.

6.4. Global Health Initiatives

Global health efforts have stepped up the fight against leprosy by getting effective treatments out more evenly. In many communities hit hardest by poverty, where healthcare is hard to reach, the pain persists much longer. For instance, when Novartis donates multidrug therapy, it shows how a public-private mix can boost drug supplies in the very regions where leprosy is common. Instead of just focusing on treatment, these strategies often look for early signals of illness and work to lessen long-term disabilities, which in turn cuts down both complications and the stigma individuals face. Strengthening local health systems in poorer countries generally helps spread the word and keeps treatment going steadily—even if there are still hurdles like gaps in healthcare worker training and hurdles with routine screening and referrals.

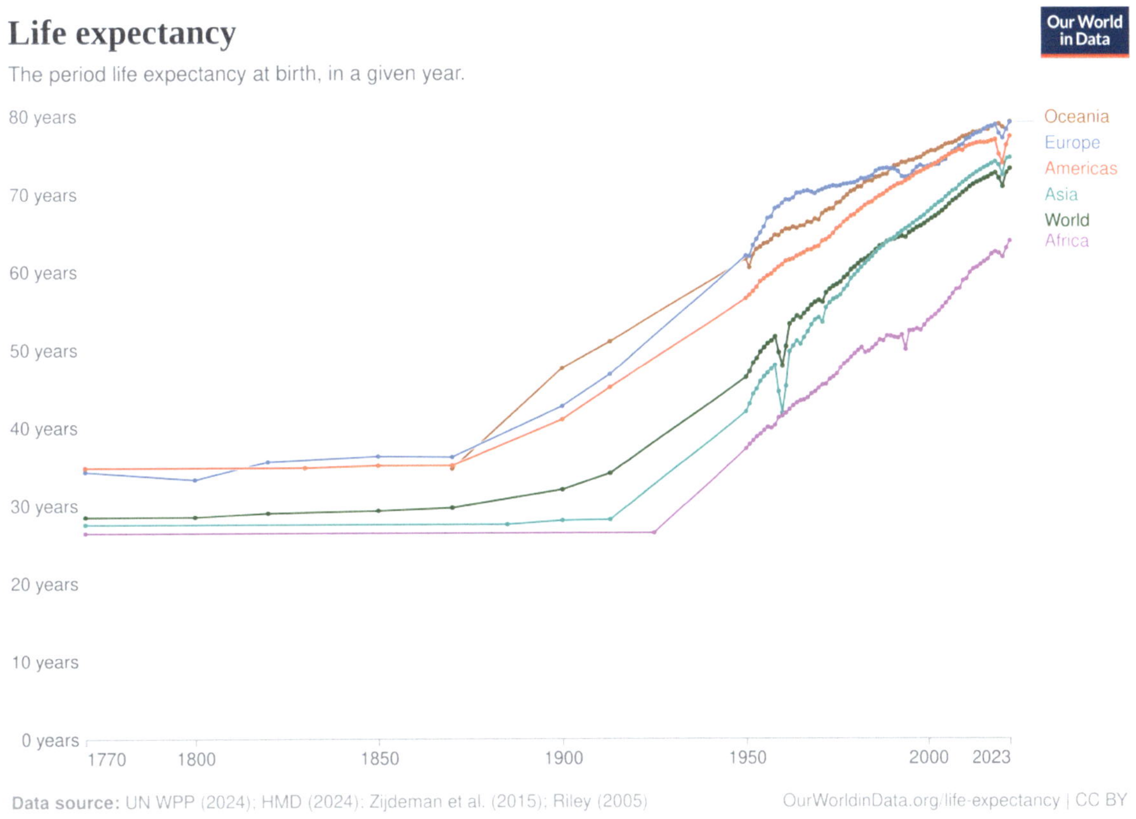

Figure 6.8. Global health initiatives.

Source: By Max Roser - https://ourworldindata.org/life-expectancy, CC BY 4.0, https://commons.wikimedia.org/w/index.php?curid=83546093

Tackling these issues is key if we're to expand treatment and keep on the path toward leprosy elimination. More than just handing out drugs or updating treatment methods, many global programs now combined efforts to tackle several neglected tropical diseases (NTDs), leprosy being a big part of that mix. By setting leprosy facts against the bigger project of NTD control, these initiatives can make better use of their resources and bring communities more into the fold. Look at large-scale preventive treatments for issues like lymphatic filariasis and onchocerciasis—they show that coordinated mass drug campaigns can pull their weight. This kind of integrated model works by using existing health tools to deliver multidrug therapy for leprosy alongside care for other NTDs, boosting cost-effectiveness and overall results. Further, there's an ever-growing understanding that you need to team up both medical treatment and social or environmental strategies to turn down transmission and stigma (Savioli et al., 2006). Even though there's been some promising progress, the long-term and wider reach of these global initiatives still hinge on fixing persistent gaps in healthcare delivery and funding. While drug donations offer fast relief, the bigger problem is making sure that solid treatments finally reach those most left behind, often people in remote or socially isolated areas. Limited resources mean that widescale screening and quick diagnosis sometimes just aren't feasible, even though these are vital for early care. It's pretty clear that training for health workers and extra systemic support is needed (reports note that many providers simply don't have enough time or updated know-how to properly screen for associated conditions). On top of that, global policies must juggle funds between developing new treatment options and putting current ones in full use, ensuring today's patients keep benefiting while innovation moves forward (Savioli et al., 2006). All of these layered challenges will shape whether leprosy control improves all over the world (Figure 6.8).

6.4.1. World Health Organization (WHO)'s Role in Leprosy Control

Global advances in treating leprosy owe a great deal to the work done by the WHO. They saw early on that leprosy hit communities hard – both in health and in economic ways , and decided to shake things up by standardizing how patients are treated. For instance, they pushed the use of a combination therapy (MDT) that mixes rifampicin, dapsone, and clofazimine, which has helped simplify regimens and cut down on drug resistance. Their guides even break down the details like weight-based dosing and treatment lengths for both the milder paucibacillary and the more intense multibacillary cases, making sure that treatment fits each patient's needs. This sort of steady, standardized method has proven pretty reliable around the world, especially in regions where medical resources might be thin (Thangaraju et al., 2022). Generally speaking, by keeping an eye on treatments regularly, WHO keeps these protocols tightly aligned with broader global health targets, helping to bring down instances of the disease and improve outcomes for those affected. Taking things further than just treatment, the WHO also steps in when complications or unexpected reactional states arise in leprosy care. Issues like ENL and type 1 lepra reactions complicate managing the illness, meaning doctors often have to adjust therapies on the fly. Their guidelines suggest using corticosteroids and clofazimine in a thoughtful way to ease these reactions while keeping side effects in check. In most cases, there's even support for exploring new options—research into repurposing drugs like metformin highlights their willingness to combine the old with the new in managing inflammation. This kind of adaptive approach shows how WHO isn't stuck in one mode but continuously alters its methods based on the latest scientific insights. Further, by pushing for leprosy control to be part of broader health programs, they help ensure there's ongoing monitoring, earlier detection, and faster treatment – all key steps for breaking the cycle of transmission and reducing long-term disabilities (Thangaraju et al., 2022). The COVID-19 pandemic threw yet another curveball, underscoring just how essential WHO's guidance can be when multiple public health challenges collide. Their prompt distribution of evidence-based advice helped clinicians deal with the extra complications arising when patients on immunosuppressive therapies for leprosy reactions encountered SARS-CoV-2. WHO maintained a cautious approach, urging health workers to stick with the proven multidrug regimens even as they explored safer, alternative immunomodulatory options when needed. They also teamed up closely with national health programs to adjust care delivery so that, despite lockdowns and stretched resources, leprosy patients could keep receiving treatment uninterrupted. This balancing act – holding on to the fundamentals of leprosy control while navigating new risks posed by COVID-19 – highlights WHO's flexible, considered approach, one that aims to build resilience in overall health care systems and keep the global drive toward leprosy elimination moving forward.

6.4.2. Community-Based Programs and Outreach

Managing leprosy well goes further than just giving medicines. In places where clinics are few and far between, tapping into local know-how counts. Community efforts pull together neighbors and local networks to spot cases early, lessen shame, and keep individuals on their multidrug courses. Local health workers, often acting as community connectors—help clear up what leprosy truly is, bust myths, and catch issues quickly. When care is woven right into everyday life, it not only benefits the patient but also builds social acceptance.

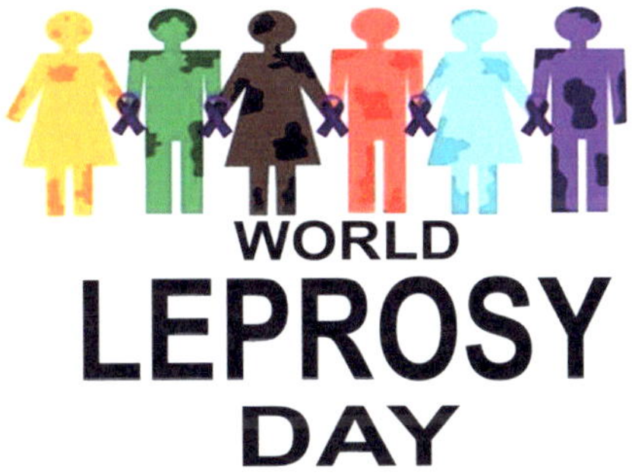

Figure 6.9. World Leprosy Day.

Source: VALIDATE Network. (n.d.). *World Leprosy Day.*

Tailored outreach that fits the local scene proves more effective across different cultures and economic backgrounds (Rodriguez-Morales, 2019). Further, as these community initiatives grow, they make leprosy treatment more reachable and lasting in underserved areas. Looking back, the fight against leprosy shows that fresh, innovative outreach is needed to tackle nagging problems like disability risks and discrimination. Even though multidrug therapy made huge leaps, new cases have settled into a plateau, hinting that community involvement might need a reboot. Recent plans generally speak of combining up disease tracking, patient lessons, and stigma busting by way of grassroots action. These mixed efforts often combine digital tools with practical mapping of where leprosy pops up, helping target help so it hits home. When national groups join hands with local partners, the extra boost of post-exposure prophylaxis and disability support comes through, creating a more well-rounded approach to battling the disease. Bringing research together with everyday practice lets teams adjust to both the clinical and social dimensions of leprosy—a key part of global visions aiming for zero transmission (Steinmann et al., 2020). This sort of teamwork, in most cases, is vital for keeping progress steady and one day wiping out the disease. It's clear that ongoing support and community-driven projects are a must for reaching the bold goals set in global leprosy elimination plans. The World Health Organization's targets for 2030 remind us of that urgent local partnerships and grassroots inclusion are the way forward. By involving communities directly and pooling resources, trust builds up and treatment stays sensitive to cultural needs. Also, letting local programs grow makes it easier to shuffle new research—think fresh diagnostic tools or even vaccine breakthroughs—into everyday practice, bridging that awkward gap between discovery and help (Steinmann et al., 2020). To summarize, combining community outreach with a combination of approaches not only ensures thorough care and eases the disease's grip but also stimulates us steadily toward finally erasing leprosy (Figure 6.9).

6.4.3. Funding and Resource Allocation for Leprosy Treatment

Effective leprosy care isn't just about the latest medical breakthroughs—it's also about having the right mix of funds and supplies. MDT once shifted the balance by sharply reducing leprosy cases and changing the fight against the disease. But, as you might expect, keeping those gains going means a steady flow of money to back national programs and community outreach. Cases have mostly leveled off, so tapping into new, sometimes creative, funding methods becomes key for challenges like cutting disability rates and easing stigma. Boosting health setups and firing up local health workers matters too, since these elements directly shape how services perform. Without smart and fair cash distribution, even top-notch treatments might not be fully used, ultimately hindering efforts to lower transmission and disability rates (Iteba et al., 2007). In many low-resource settings, performance-based financing models have started to show promise in stretching available resources further. These models tie incentives to clear, measurable targets so that health workers and clinics work harder on following treatment protocols and checking in with patients—crucial for managing long-term conditions. Strengthening local systems to track leprosy cases and outcomes also plays a big role here. Generally speaking, linking funds to performance not only boosts accountability and spurs local problem-solving but also supports programs that often struggle with sporadic funding (Iteba et al., 2007). Even with these positives, noticeable funding gaps still persist, especially for research, boosting preventive measures, and tackling broader issues like stigma and discrimination. The Global Partnership for Zero Leprosy, for example, shows just how important international alliances can be when it comes to pooling resources and coordinating efforts to hit lofty targets by 2030. In most cases, putting more money into fresh research and building program capacity means not just purchasing drugs but also funding integrated services like rehabilitation and community education. A long-term commitment from governments and donor organizations remains vital, with transparent fund distribution helping to ensure fair access to treatment. Clearly, giving equal focus to clinical care and broader social support is essential to break the cycle of infection and genuinely improve lives (Steinmann et al., 2020).

A CLOSER LOOK

CLOFAZIMINE DRUGS USED TO TREAT LEPROSY

Clofazimine is an aminophenazone dye, which preferentially binds to mycobacterial DNA, both inhibiting mycobacterial growth and exerting a slow bactericidal effect on *M. leprae*. Clofazimine also has anti-inflammatory properties and is therefore used in type 2 reactions at higher (200–300 mg daily) and divided doses, acting as a steroid-sparing agent and allowing use of lower doses of steroids. Reports of resistance to clofazimine are extremely rare (Figure 6.10).

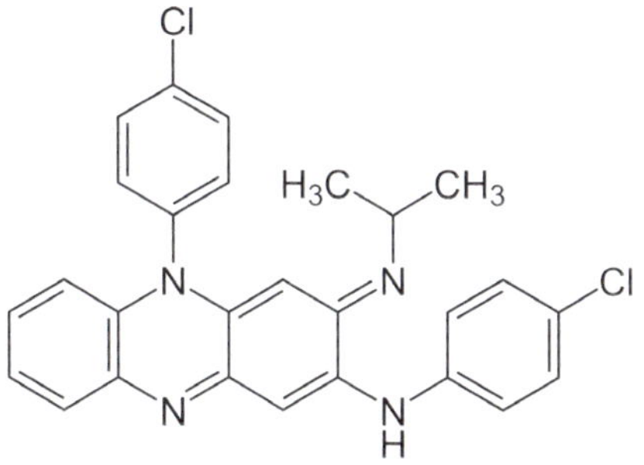

Figure 6.10. Clofazimine drugs used to treat leprosy.

Source: IndiaMART. (2023). Clofazimine Drugs Used to Treat Leprosy.

Adverse Effects

Clofazimine is extremely well tolerated at the dosages used in leprosy MDT regimens, that is, 300 mg monthly and 50 mg daily for adults. However, it does commonly cause darkening and dryness of the skin, particularly within leprosy lesions. The conjunctivae are also affected. Darker skin colors are more susceptible to the hyperpigmentary effects of the drug. Skin discoloration tends to develop from the third month of treatment but clears within 6–12 months of treatment discontinuation. Clofazimine is also excreted through breast milk and can cause mild discoloration of the skin of the infant. Prolonged use of high-dose clofazimine produces more significant skin pigmentation and ichthyosis and rarely severe gastrointestinal side effects due to crystal deposition in the intestinal tract.

Pharmacology

The pharmacokinetics of clofazimine is complex. Oral absorption is highly variable. It has a long half-life of approximately 70 days. Clofazimine is widely distributed throughout the reticuloendothelial tissues. It tends to bind to lipids and is stored in the body and slowly released. Therefore, the loading dose of 300 mg, which is subsequently given monthly, ensures that an optimal amount of clofazimine is maintained in the body tissue even if patients occasionally miss their daily dose. Clofazimine is largely unmetabolized. Its major route of excretion is through bile, and less than 1% is excreted in urine.

Drug Interactions

Dapsone may inhibit the anti-inflammatory activity of clofazimine. Concurrent administration of clofazimine with aluminum- or magnesium-containing antacids must be avoided because this leads to decreased absorption of clofazimine. Clofazimine in combination with phenytoin will lead to a reduction in efficacy of phenytoin.

SUMMARY

Leprosy treatment has changed a lot over time – it's not just about the drugs anymore. Nowadays, the focus includes how patients stick with their treatment and exploring new ways to keep the disease from coming back. It isn't simply about the medication; the way care is given plays a big role too. Giving people a say over where and how they get treated can boost their commitment and overall satisfaction, which seems to help cure the illness and stop relapses. Still, there are parts of this approach that fall short, like not enough clear communication or teaching for both patients and those who support them. Generally speaking, better training and closer oversight of healthcare workers is essential if we want to keep those good outcomes going (Mkopi et al., 2013). There's growing evidence that a one-time dose of rifampicin after exposure – known as SDR-PEP – can add a lot to traditional multidrug treatments. Some studies from various controlled trials suggest that this approach might drop new leprosy cases by about 50%–60%, especially when it's paired with vaccinations such as the Bacillus Calmette-Guérin shot. This layered approach not only seems to improve how individuals fare but also tackles public health concerns by breaking the chain of transmission. Further, when you look at the cost side of things, this method appears affordable enough to scale up within national health programs, offering a hopeful way forward toward controlling, and eventually eliminating, leprosy (Asyura et al., 2021). Looking at what we know today, a combined strategy that brings together multidrug therapy, patient-focused care, and post-exposure prevention is pretty much key for the future of leprosy control. Merging these ideas calls for a steady commitment from healthcare systems: they need to adjust everyday practices, boost how they educate patients, and set up strong support networks. In many cases, doing so can lead to more consistent treatment adherence and lighten the overall impact of the disease on society. Ongoing research along with national-scale trials remains crucial to fine-tune these interventions to fit local health trends and cultural characteristics, ultimately moving us closer to the global goal of leprosy eradication (Mkopi et al., 2013; Asyura et al., 2021).

Antibiotic therapy is the backbone of treating leprosy, essential for curing the infection and stopping its spread. For ages, doctors have relied on a combination of drugs—dapsone, rifampicin, and clofazimine in what's called multidrug therapy—to hit *Mycobacterium leprae* hard. But it's not all about the pills. How treatment is given can be just as important for how patients recover and how communities stay healthy. Some studies out of Australia's Kimberley region show that approaches like directly observed therapy (DOT) sometimes fall short in addressing the cultural and social realities of those affected. In most cases, this points to the need for care systems that are centered around the person and that feel culturally right, helping patients stick with and complete their treatment (Oliver, 2022). Besides that, these more holistic strategies also work to lessen the old stigma attached to leprosy care. New ideas now hint that adding therapies focused on nerve repair could nicely complement the usual antibiotics. Leprosy often leaves patients with nerve damage and lost myelin, so treatments aimed at protecting nerves and even rebuilding myelin are gathering interest as new ways to improve recovery. Recent research, for example, spotlights the Klotho protein, an epigenetic player that might boost mitochondrial health and help mend myelin. While most current drugs aim straight at wiping out the bacteria, combining agents that encourage nerve regeneration might change the game for patients facing neuropathic issues. Generally speaking, this dual strategy shows a broader grasp of the disease and highlights the pressing need to deal with both the infection and its fallout (Moos et al., 2020). To sum it up, handling leprosy today means combining trusted multidrug antibiotic methods with fresh ideas for nerve healing. Successful treatment isn't just about clearing bacteria; it also calls for care models that respect cultural nuances and individual situations, which in turn boosts treatment adherence and offers social support (Oliver, 2022). At the same time, weaving in cutting-edge biological approaches aimed at nerve repair, and, say, even combined with traditional methods—marks a shift in how we deal with the disease's disabling sides (Moos et al., 2020). All these parts together underline a treatment plan that melds infection control, symptom relief, and personalized support—key steps for better outcomes and for moving closer to finally eliminating leprosy.

KEY TERMS FROM THIS CHAPTER

- Clinical trials
- Dapsone
- Harmful immune overreactions
- Immunosuppressive drugs
- Medical research
- Pathogen-specific targets
- Clofazimine
- Drug resistance
- Heavy stigma
- Levamisole
- Microbe
- Personalized medicine

References

1. *Guidance* Craig, G., Meershoek, A., Zwerling, A., Daftary, A., Citro, B., Smyth, C., Lewis, D., Ni Cheallaigh, D., Byrne, E., Mitchell, E. M. H., Leimane, I., Malar, J., Levy, J., van der Land, J., Macintyre, K., Johnston, L. G., Ferris France, N., Engel, N., Mumba, O., ... Nair, T. (2018). *TB STIGMA – MEASUREMENT GUIINTERACTION*. CHALLENGE TB. https://doi.org/10.18745/PB.20489 (accessed on 10th May 2025).
2. Steinmann, P., Dusenbury, C., Addiss, D., Mirza, F., & Smith, W. C. S. (2020). A comprehensive research agenda for zero leprosy. *Infectious diseases of poverty*, *9*(1), 156. https://doi.org/10.1186/s40249-020-00774-4 (accessed on 10th May 2025).
3. Oladunni Balogun F, Omotayo Tom Ashafa A, Sabiu S, Ayokun-nun Ajao A, Palanisamy Perumal C, Idowu Kazeem M, et al. Pharmacognosy: Importance and Drawbacks [Internet]. Pharmacognosy - Medicinal Plants. IntechOpen; 2019. Available from: http://dx.doi.org/10.5772/intechopen.82396 (accessed on 10th May 2025).
4. Akarsu S, Avcı C. A Review of Possible Triggering or Therapeutic Effects of Antimicrobial Vaccines on Psoriasis [Internet]. An Interdisciplinary Approach to Psoriasis. InTech; 2017. Available from: http://dx.doi.org/10.5772/67691 (accessed on 10th May 2025).
5. Timothy Miles Rawson, Vaseem Anjum, Jasmin Hodgson, A Kameswara Rao, Krishna Murthy, Pss Sundar Rao, Jonnalagada Subbanna, PV Ranganadha Rao; Leprosy and tuberculosis concomitant infection: A poorly understood, age-old relationship; Leprosy Review; 2014; 85; 4; 288-295; DOI: 10.47276/lr.85.4.288 (accessed on 10th May 2025).
6. HABIBALLA AHMED, M. M., ANURADHA, and P. WADHWA. "A REVIEW ON AGENTS FOR THE TREATMENT OF LEPROSY INFECTION". *Asian Journal of Pharmaceutical and Clinical Research*, vol. 14, no. 3, Mar. 2021, pp. 25-29, doi:10.22159/ajpcr.2021.v14i3.40373. (accessed on 10th May 2025).
7. Asyura, M. M. A. Z., Wijaya, I. R., Toshukowong, T., & Wang, R. S. (2021). Effectiveness Analysis of Single Dose Rifampicin-Post-Exposure Prophylaxis (SDR-PEP) as A Preventive Intervention for Leprosy Transmission: A Systematic Review of Randomized Controlled Trials. Journal of Public Health for Tropical and Coastal Region, 4(2), 35-43. https://doi.org/10.14710/jphtcr.v4i2.10794 (accessed on 10th May 2025).
8. Bonkass A-K, Fastenau A, Stuetzle S, Boeckmann M, Nadiruzzaman M (2024) Psychosocial interventions for persons affected by Leprosy: A systematic review. PLOS Ment Health 1(3): e0000091. https://doi.org/10.1371/journal.pmen.0000091 (accessed on 10th May 2025).
9. Perez, R. L., Chase, J., & Tanner, R. (2024). Shared challenges to the control of complex intracellular neglected pathogens. *Frontiers in public health*, *12*, 1423420. https://doi.org/10.3389/fpubh.2024.1423420(accessed on 10th May 2025).
10. Moos, W. H., Faller, D. V., Glavas, I. P., Harpp, D. N., Kanara, I., Mavrakis, A. N., Pernokas, J., Pernokas, M., Pinkert, C. A., Powers, W. R., Sampani, K., Steliou, K., Vavvas, D. G., Zamboni, R. J., Kodukula, K., & Chen, X. (2020). Klotho Pathways, Myelination Disorders, Neurodegenerative Diseases, and Epigenetic Drugs. *BioResearch open access*, *9*(1), 94–105. https://doi.org/10.1089/biores.2020.0004 (accessed on 10th May 2025).
11. Cornell University, World Health Organization, & World Bank. (2011). *World Report on*

Disability, Chapter 8: Work and Employment. https://core.ac.uk/download/5131044.pdf (accessed on 10th May 2025).

12. Donders, G. G. G., Akinosoglou, K., Massie, Z., & Özçelik, A. S. (2025). Review of current and emerging estrogen receptor agonists for vaginal atrophy. *Expert opinion on pharmacotherapy, 26*(3), 249–255. https://doi.org/10.1080/14656566.2025.2451150(accessed on 10th May 2025).
13. Dotsenko, S., Falzon, D., Hwang, T. J., Jafarov, A., et al. (2013). Safety and availability of clofazimine in the treatment of multidrug and extensively drug-resistant tuberculosis: Analysis of published guidance and meta-analysis of cohort studies. *BMJ Open, 4*(1), e004143. https://core.ac.uk/download/28945497.pdf (accessed on 10th May 2025).
14. Kimberly, Kesya; Ferina, Siti Aisha Nabila; and Esti, Prima Kartika (2024) "Immunomodulators in leprosy: A narrative review," *Journal of General - Procedural Dermatology & Venereology Indonesia*: Vol. 8: Iss. 1, Article 10. DOI: 10.7454/jdvi.v8i1.1123 (accessed on 10th May 2025).
15. Sweta Nariya, Madhvi Kareliya, Ajita Pillai, Neela Bhuptani;
16. An evaluation of adverse drug reactions, adherence to treatment and quality of life in patients with leprosy receiving multidrug therapy in a tertiary care teaching hospital; Leprosy Review; 2024; 95; 3; e2024015; DOI: 10.47276/lr.95.3.2024015 (accessed on 10th May 2025).
17. Iteba, N., Mapunda, M., Minja, G., Mukasa, A., et al. (2007). *Performance-Based Financing: Report on Feasibility and Implementation Options Final September 2007.* https://core.ac.uk/download/pdf/11307103.pdf (accessed on 10th May 2025).
18. Mkopi, A., Range, N., Amuri, M. *et al.* Health workers' performance in the implementation of Patient Centred Tuberculosis Treatment (PCT) strategy under programmatic conditions in Tanzania: a cross sectional study. *BMC Health Serv Res* **13**, 101 (2013). https://doi.org/10.1186/1472-6963-13-101 (accessed on 10th May 2025).
19. Siddiqui, M. R., Velidi, N. R., Pati, S., Rath, N., Kanungo, A. K., Bhanjadeo, A. K., Rao, B. B., Ojha, B. M., Krishna Moorthy, K., Soutar, D., Porter, J. D., & Ranganadha Rao, P. V. (2009). Integration of leprosy elimination into primary health care in orissa, India. *PloS one, 4*(12), e8351. https://doi.org/10.1371/journal.pone.0008351 (accessed on 10th May 2025).
20. Kumar, B., Narang, T., & Dogra, S. (2020). Response to: Management of leprosy patients in the era of COVID-19. *Dermatologic therapy, 33*(6), e14052. https://doi.org/10.1111/dth.14052(accessed on 10th May 2025).
21. Macfarlane, J. (2005). The relationship between cultural beliefs and treatment-seeking behavior in Papua New Guinea: Implications for the incorporation of traditional medicine into the health system. Curtin Thesis; https://core.ac.uk/download/195631402.pdf (accessed on 10th May 2025).
22. V Kaufman-Shriqui, H Factor, O Perets, Knowledge, attitudes, and barriers of dietitians toward screening patients for food insecurity, *European Journal of Public Health*, Volume 33, Issue Supplement_2, October 2023, ckad160.1089, https://doi.org/10.1093/eurpub/ckad160.1089 (accessed on 10th May 2025).
23. Oliver, S. J. (2022). From Isolation to Inclusion: Embracing Local Perspectives in Examining the Treatment Model of Care for Aboriginal Persons Affected by Tuberculosis or Leprosy in

the Kimberley Region, North Western Australia [Doctor of Philosophy (College of Medicine)]. The University of Notre Dame Australia. https://researchonline.nd.edu.au/theses/386(accessed on 10th May 2025).

24. Savioli, L., Engels, D., Daumerie, D., Jannin, J., Alvar, J., Asiedu, K., Gastellu-Etchegorry, M., Simarro, P., & Mariotti, S. P. (2006). Response from Savioli and colleagues from the Department of Neglected Tropical Diseases, World Health Organization. *PLoS medicine*, *3*(6), e283. https://doi.org/10.1371/journal.pmed.0030283(accessed on 10th May 2025).

25. Shanmugapriya, J., & Sathesh, K. S. (2017). *A Prospective Study on Quality of Life in Patients with Urinary Calculi*. Asian J Pharm Clin Res, Vol 10, Issue 8, 2017, 191-193 https://core.ac.uk/download/477853023.pdf (accessed on 10th May 2025).

26. Staples, J. (2014). *Putting Indian Christianities Into Context: Biographies of Christian Conversion in a Leprosy Colony*. JAMES STAPLES Brunel University, Uxbridge, Middlesex, UB8 3PH Email: James.staples@brunel.ac.uk ; https://core.ac.uk/download/29140363.pdf (accessed on 10th May 2025).

27. Thangaraju, P., Ty, S., & Venkatesan, S. (2022). Repurposing of drugs for non-responding erythema nodosum leprosum cases – A perspective. *Journal of Young Pharmacists*, 2022; 14(3):266-267

28. Editorial | doi:10.5530/jyp.2022.14.53(accessed on 10th May 2025).

29. Zhang, A., Fan, N., Zhang, X., Guo, H., Zhou, Y., Zeng, L., Lin, Y., & Jiang, X. (2024). Endoscopic retrograde appendicitis therapy. *Therapeutic advances in gastroenterology*, *17*, 17562848241275314. https://doi.org/10.1177/17562848241275314 (accessed on 10th May 2025).

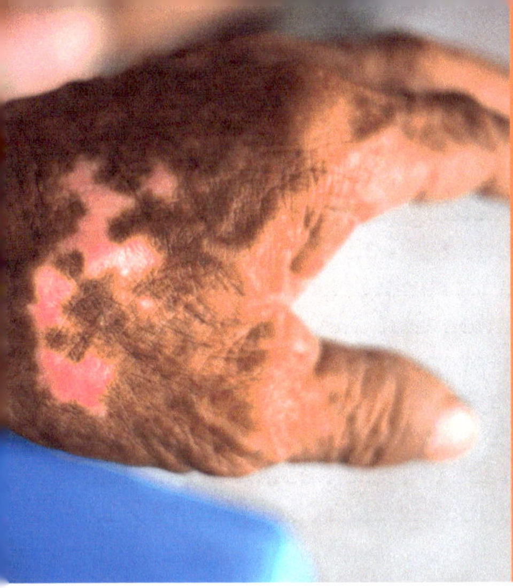

Chapter 7

LEPROSY COMPLICATIONS

Contents

Introduction

Leprosy is a persistent infectious illness that carries a combination of physical and social challenges. Caused by *Mycobacterium leprae*, it has been a long-time source of both medical complications and community struggles. Even though antibiotics have generally slashed its global presence, many people, especially in areas where early detection or proper healthcare is hard to find, still suffer from its side effects. Nerve damage, gradual disability, and other issues often follow a late diagnosis, making treatment complex. It's not just about clinical care; these complications deeply affect someone's everyday life (Newport & Myrvang, 2009). The social side of leprosy adds another layer of complexity, even where the disease is uncommon. In places like the Netherlands, for instance, where leprosy hardly ever makes an appearance, it still shows up among migrants from formerly high-prevalence regions. People hit by leprosy frequently end up wrestling with feelings of shame and isolation, which in turn drive them to keep their condition secret. This secrecy then reduces their participation in society and can even harm their mental well-being. Many times, healthcare pros might not fully grasp the extent of this internal stigma, simply because leprosy is so rare in their setting (De Groot et al., 2011). Often, the role of the healthcare system itself gets called into question. When diagnosis drags on for years, nerve damage and disfigurements can take a harsh toll, underlining the need for greater awareness and a more attentive clinical eye. Patients regularly mention that they struggle not just with the physical effects but also with getting accurate information, proper rehabilitation services, or a supportive network to lean on. In most cases, treating leprosy goes well beyond medicine, it calls for educational outreach, psychosocial support, and efforts to reintegrate these patients back into their communities. Such a combined approach may do a lot to lessen both the physical hurdles and the social isolation that come with the condition (De Groot et al., 2011) (Figure 7.1).

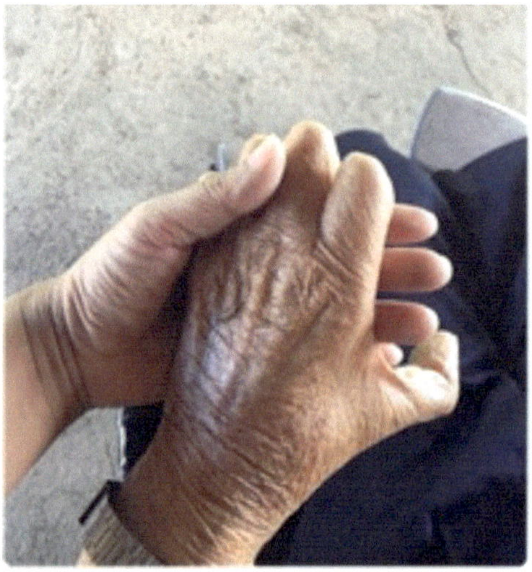

Figure 7.1. Leprosy complications.

Source: Shutterstock. (2017). *Leprosy Complications.*

7.1. Physical Complications

Leprosy isn't just a skin problem, it often brings along a complex mix of issues that weigh heavily on someone's daily life. Peripheral nerve damage, for instance, tends to rob people of feeling and muscle strength, which eventually can lead to real disabilities. These nerve problems might also hide injuries until they get infected, sometimes spiraling into stubborn ulcers and even crooked deformities. In some cases, the type of leprosy that spreads out (commonly known as lepromatous leprosy) also messes with hormone balance, triggering things like hypogonadism and other genital issues, such as epididymo-orchitis. You might notice that these genital signs sometimes look a lot like common sexually transmitted infections—, though, generally speaking, their roots are both parasitic and mycobacterial, conditions you'd mostly find in tropical regions. All of this jumble of symptoms means that doctors have to be extra careful when distinguishing leprosy-related issues from other illnesses found in similar climates. When you break it down, quick action is essential not only to stop permanent damage but also to ease the social stigma that comes with visible changes (Richens, 2004). Caring for people with leprosy goes far beyond just killing off the bacteria. The treatment process is more like a long journey involving not only initial tests and therapies but also continuous support long after the medicines have done their stuff. Even after leaving the treatment center, many individuals still battle with persisting problems like neuropathy or deformities that call for regular check-ups and help boosting their functional abilities. And it's not just medical issues on the table—cultural factors and public health setups play a huge part, too, by influencing how easily someone can jump back into follow-up routines or get the kind of tailored care they need. In most cases, combining these elements into health policies is a key move to lessen the heavy challenges that come with leprosy and ensure that patients receive care that truly covers all bases (Pinheiro et al., 2019). There's also a bad mix of musculoskeletal damages to consider. Chronic nerve issues along with the body's own inflammatory overreactions can end up causing deformities like contractures, a claw-like hand, or even a foot drop that makes moving around a real struggle. Sometimes, the immune system's angry responses—what doctors refer to as Type 1 and Type 2 lepra reactions—add fuel to the fire by further damaging the nerves, which then forces a quick switch to anti-inflammatory treatments. On top of that, numb areas often fall victim to secondary bacterial infections that speed up tissue damage and, in some advanced cases, push patients toward needing surgery. All these complications carry a hefty economic and emotional toll, underscoring the fact that early detection and a team-based, multidisciplinary care approach do matter. Tackling these physical fallout issues is as much about better clinical outcomes as it is about fighting the deep-rooted stigma and social exclusion that many affected people still face today (Figure 7.2).

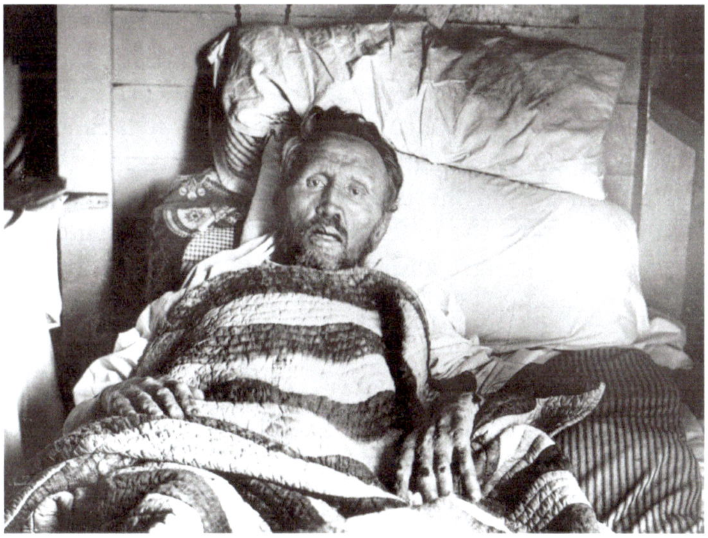

Figure 7.2. Physical complications.

Source: By Sydney B. Swift - http://www.tremelo.be/projects/gtremelo2/pictures//1247663387702/orig_Damiaan_sterfbed_2.jpg, probably from Sacred Hearts Archives or Hawaii State Archives, Public Domain, https://commons.wikimedia.org/w/index.php?curid=15838607

7.1.1. Skin Lesions and Their Effects

Leprosy sets off a wide range of skin marks caused by *Mycobacterium leprae* that throw a real curveball into patient care. You might see these signs show up as light patches or reddish spots that sometimes look like small bumps, plaques, or macules. These physical hints not only serve as signals for diagnosis but also tend to echo the unpredictable way the immune system is behaving. Nerve damage is a big part of the story too, when feeling is lost, tiny injuries can fly under the radar and later morph into nasty infections. In many cases, such nerve-related issues help keep the skin problems stubborn and more severe. And lesions on delicate or visible parts of the body often stir up deep emotional distress, fueled by social stigma. This combination of physical and mental challenges makes fighting leprosy in areas where it's common all the more demanding, calling for care that looks after body and mind alike. Peeling back another layer, the complications aren't just skin-deep. Often, the lesions create pathways to more serious damages, digging into the tissue beyond what you can see on the surface. For example, tropical diseases, leprosy included, can sometimes cause ulcer-like wounds or wart-like patches in even the genital area, which might be mistaken for a sexually transmitted infection. These skin marks may also tag along with wider bodily issues like lowered hormone levels (hypogonadism, notably in some lepromatous cases), showing just how complex the relationship is between what appears on the skin and overall health. Generally speaking, when these lesions hang around and diagnosis or treatment is delayed, the path leads to irreversible physical changes and disabilities. After all, any break in the skin can be an invite for further infections and immune reactions that only add fuel to the tissue damage fire. It seems clear that thorough skin care and prompt, ongoing intervention are musts for managing the evolving complications in leprosy patients (Richens, 2004). On the longer side, skin lesions linked to leprosy can bring about complex nerve problems that impact normal skin function. Take, for instance, the rather rare trigeminal trophic syndrome, here, peripheral nerve injury results in odd sensations like numbness and tingling, along with persistent ulcers that plague the face. This kind of neuropathy can sneak up after surgical interventions or directly from nerve damage caused by the infection itself, making the clinical picture even more complex. Those stubborn ulcers tend to keep the cycle of tissue injury and delayed healing in motion, which can lead to more pronounced facial disfigurement and functional issues. In most cases, doctors handling facial or maxillofacial treatments need to keep a keen eye on these nerve-related complications, as even well-intended surgeries might inadvertently worsen them. Recognizing and addressing these nerve issues early is key to easing their debilitating impact and, ultimately, improving the quality of life for those battling this complex disease (Di Luca et al., 2017) (Figure 7.3).

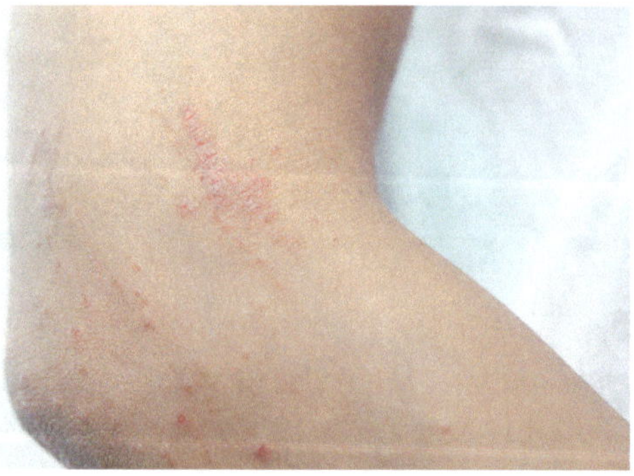

Figure 7.3. Skin lesions and their effects.

Source: Valley County Health System. (n.d.). *Skin lesions. https://www.valleycountyhealthsystem.org/assets/site/images/Skin%20Lesions.png.*

7.1.2. Nerve Damage and Sensory Loss

Leprosy isn't just about obvious skin spots – it quietly messes with the nerves, too. The infection sneaks in, mainly hitting Schwann cells so that the protective myelin sheath gets stripped away and the nerve fibers themselves suffer injury. As a result, normal nerve function breaks down and the affected regions lose their ability to sense pain or temperature. This loss in feedback means that even small bumps or burns may go unnoticed, which over time can spiral into chronic ulcers, misshapen limbs, and recurring infections. In most cases, these issues pile up, meaning early treatment is generally key to stopping permanent nerve damage. Managing these nerve complications usually calls for medical plans aimed at slowing further harm and, if possible, reviving some function. Corticosteroids are often the first choice since they help lower inflammation and soothe the immune system's attack on the nerves. Interestingly, while some randomized trials suggest that steroids might not always boost long-term outcomes in patients with long-established nerve issues or only mild sensory loss, treatments stretching about five months tend to show better results than shorter courses. This timing, coupled with how long the treatment lasts, appears to play a crucial role in balancing recovery and avoiding side effects like diabetes or new ulcers (Van Veen et al., 2009). Such findings underscore the complex nature of nerve repair in leprosy and point to the need for treatments that fit each patient's specific situation. There's also been interest in using surgery to ease nerve pressure. Decompressive procedures aim to physically free up trapped nerves and improve their function, yet current controlled trials generally indicate that adding surgery to corticosteroid treatment doesn't bring clear benefits, especially when nerve damage is less than six months old. Although the concept is to relieve pressure, the reports on long-term outcomes and potential side effects remain sketchy. Clearly, the absence of a strong edge for surgical options means we still have to wait for more robust studies to confirm their role. Until then, corticosteroids remain the cornerstone for handling nerve damage and sensory loss connected to leprosy (Van Veen et al., 2009) (Figure 7.4).

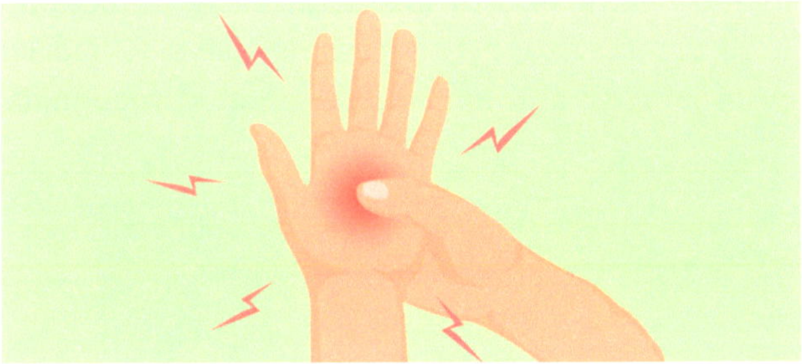

Figure 7.4. Nerve damage.

Source: BuzzRx. (n.d.). *What Are Common Nerve Damage Symptoms?*

7.1.3. Musculoskeletal Deformities

Leprosy tends to worsen in ways that go far beyond skin issues. When the disease moves into its multibacillary stage, it often brings along a host of complications, musculoskeletal problems are quite common and leave patients debilitated. *Mycobacterium leprae* sneaks into the peripheral nerves, triggering inflammation that eventually causes a loss of feeling and hampers movement. This nerve damage, over time, leads to muscle weakness and wasting, especially in the hands and feet, which in turn make injuries and extra infections more likely. Before long, this chain reaction of nerve injury and muscle decline shows up as joint contractures, clawed hands, and even foot drop, all of which can severely restrict how much someone moves. Oddly, in many areas where leprosy is widespread, these issues often fly under the radar despite their dramatic impact on quality of life and everyday social interactions—clearly calling for thorough clinical care and rehab efforts. Late diagnosis and slow treatment have a huge role in why so many leprosy patients end up with these musculoskeletal deformities. Research generally shows that people receiving treatment well into the disease tend to have more advanced deformities, thanks to prolonged nerve damage and a lack of early help. In several studies coming out of endemic regions, even the newest multibacillary cases ended up with disabilities—more than half had some level of impairment, and many even reached Grade 2 status, where the deformities become clearly visible (Rodriguez-Morales, 2019).

These severe issues not only mark the natural course of the disease but also expose deeper problems like poor public awareness, persistent social stigma, and gaps in access to care. And during flare-ups of the disease, when acute inflammation sets in, nerve function is hit even harder. In most cases, catching the disease early, educating patients properly, and starting treatment right away are key to stopping irreversible damage. Beyond the immediate medical damages, the social and economic fallout from these deformities is huge. People with visible signs of the disease often face stigma and exclusion, which pile on top of the physical challenges they already endure. This not only cuts down their ability to work but also keeps communities locked in cycles of poverty, especially in tropical and subtropical areas where leprosy is still common (Rodriguez-Morales, 2019). There's also evidence showing that family members of affected individuals seem to be at higher risk for the more severe forms, emphasizing why proactive screening and prevention are so important (Rodriguez-Morales, 2019).

Tackling these musculoskeletal issues demands a combination of strategies: combining direct medical treatment with public health efforts aimed at early detection, focused rehab services, and robust social support. To summarize, by addressing these varied challenges, health systems can better ease the burden of leprosy and help those affected reconnect with their communities (Figure 7.5).

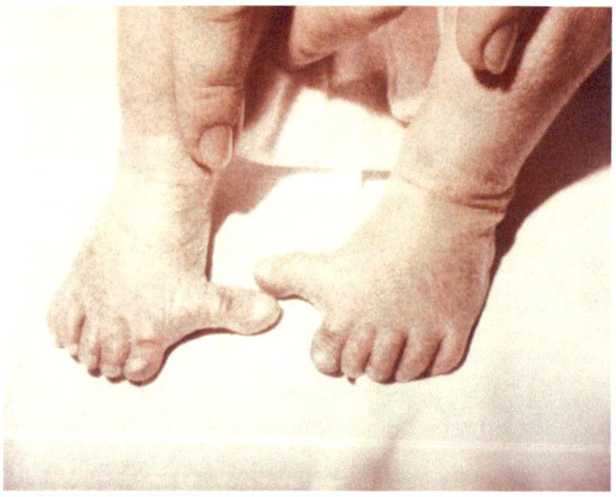

Figure 7.5. Musculoskeletal deformities.

Source: UNSW Embryology. (n.d.). *Polydactylia.*

7.2. Psychological Complications

Leprosy not only affects the body but also takes a heavy toll on how people feel inside. Many patients experience relentless, neuropathic pain that complicates their treatments and adds extra strain to their daily lives. This constant ache makes it hard to manage everyday tasks and can trigger bouts of depression and anxiety. In many cases, the stigma and loneliness that follow the disease only make matters worse, chipping away at quality of life. Research out in areas where leprosy is common shows that quite a few patients suffer from moderate to severe pain—an issue that closely connects with higher levels of disability and a drop in mental health (Santos et al., 2016). Clearly, treating leprosy means taking care of both physical symptoms and the mental challenges that come along with the disease. Rejection and discrimination are huge roadblocks when it comes to the mental health of those living with leprosy. Communities sometimes push people with the disease to the sidelines, which only feeds a cycle of stigma. Many end up feeling isolated and even worthless, with these harsh feelings persisting long after the medical problems are managed. Studies looking into the quality of life have uncovered striking differences in mental well-being between patients and those who have not been affected by the disease (Githui et al., 2022). In most cases, it seems the unmet need for mental health help and social programs that encourage reintegration only deepens the problem. So, creating community-based support networks that include both health care and social inclusion is key to turning things around. The mental challenges linked to leprosy often get worse when additional health issues or economic hardships are involved. For example, people dealing with other conditions like tuberculosis or HIV generally report poorer mental outcomes compared to some who struggle with different chronic illnesses. Interestingly, patients fighting metabolic issues like diabetes sometimes have a slightly better mental quality of life, perhaps thanks to more coordinated healthcare approaches. These mixed results point to a picture where psychological struggles aren't uniform; instead, they're shaped by a jumble of biological and social factors (Githui et al., 2022). Ultimately, targeting these varied influences with tailored interventions, and combining traditional treatments with genuine psychosocial support—is vital for improving long-term mental well-being (Figure 7.6).

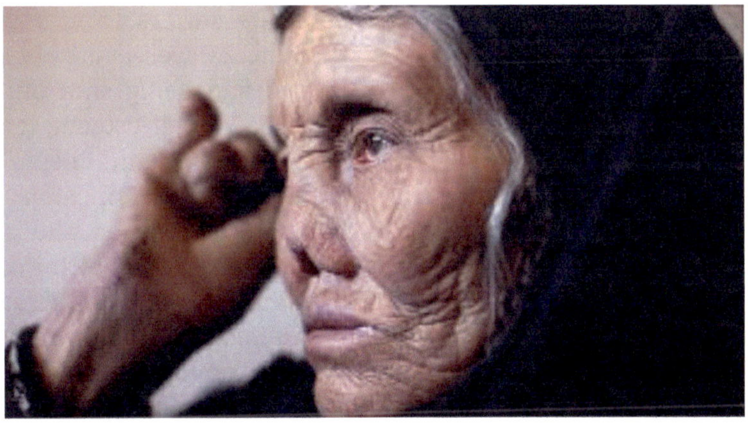

Figure 7.6. Leprosy mental health.

Source: By Vinzenz von Beauvais - Miniatur aus einer Handschrift des Vinzenz von Beauvais, Public Domain, https://commons.wikimedia.org/w/index.php?curid=7668457

7.2.1. Stigma and Social Isolation

Leprosy doesn't just attack the body, it digs into the mind and social life, leaving marks that run deep. Many who live with it feel an overwhelming mix of shame and self-doubt, so much so that they hide their condition and gradually lose confidence in themselves. This hidden burden tends to shrink their social world, sometimes even when outright discrimination isn't obvious. In places such as the Netherlands, where leprosy is nearly unheard of, individuals coming from former colonies often face late diagnoses and a surprising lack of awareness among local healthcare providers. All of these factors mix together, making isolation and social exclusion even more likely, and they point clearly to the need for dedicated psychological and community support (De Groot et al., 2011). Where a person with leprosy finds themselves can significantly shape how much stigma they experience. In cramped settings like prisons, for instance, close quarters and limited privacy push any existing prejudice to the forefront. Studies of incarcerated individuals show a complex web of negative feelings—despair, rejection from family, and that ever-present societal bias. Cultural ideas sometimes even frame the disease as a kind of divine punishment, adding another layer of separation. Generally speaking, it's not just a medical issue; the environment and ingrained beliefs call for educational and psychological strategies that truly address these unique challenges (Lira et al., 2014). Addressing the stigma connected to leprosy requires more than just treatment for the physical symptoms. Medical professionals, who often don't realize how deeply the social side effects patients, need better training to pick up on these cues. Support groups and the spread of clear, accurate information can restore confidence and help people find their way back into a social life. In areas where leprosy rarely appears, like non-endemic countries, these efforts become even more crucial because there's little institutional experience in handling such stigma. In most cases, combining medical care with thoughtful social and emotional support is key to improving long-term outcomes for those affected (De Groot et al., 2011) (Figure 7.7).

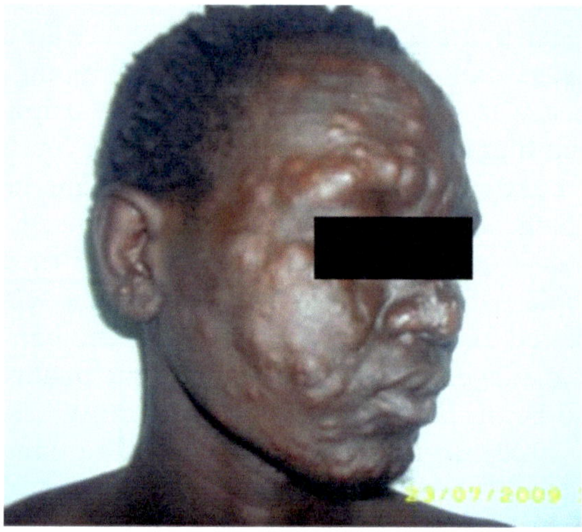

Figure 7.7. Understanding the stigma of leprosy.

Source: South Sudan Medical Journal. (2010). *Understanding the Stigma of Leprosy.*

7.2.2. Mental Health Issues Associated with Leprosy

Chronic illness isn't just about hurting physically – it messes with people's minds too. When someone suffers from a disease like leprosy, their mental well-being often takes a heavy blow. Stigma and being shut out by society tend to wear down self-esteem, leaving those affected feeling isolated and unsure of themselves. This emotional strain, in many cases, spirals into bouts of depression and anxiety that further block them from getting the help they need. Community myths and unfounded fears only add to the mix, keeping those fighting leprosy even more locked away from proper support. Clearly, treating leprosy well means looking beyond just the physical symptoms and adding real psychological care into the picture (Newport & Myrvang, 2009). Digging a little deeper, the mental struggles of people with leprosy get even more complicated when you consider the visible physical changes that sometimes come with the illness. Disabilities or disfigurements, which often emerge when the disease goes untreated or advances, can amplify the stigma and, as a result, heighten the psychological pressure on the individual. Living with these outward signs can lead to ongoing stress, anxiety, and even episodes that remind one of post-traumatic stress disorder. In many regions where leprosy still persists, getting access to mental health services isn't easy, leaving clear gaps in care. A combination of community education, supportive counseling, and peer groups can, generally speaking, help empower patients and cut down on the relentless judgment (Mtui et al., 2011). On top of all that personal struggle, the mental health burdens connected to leprosy create serious challenges for public health systems in places where the disease is common. It becomes a complex situation where money and resources have to be carefully managed to cover these deep-seated issues. Strategies that work to lower stigma, like community awareness programs—can sometimes ease the psychological side of things. Yet, investments aimed at training healthcare workers to spot and treat mental health damages as a normal part of leprosy care still fall short, often because of tight budgets. Cost worries tend to limit how widely these comprehensive approaches are used, so there's a pressing need for more funding and smarter policies. Recognizing mental health as a key part of treating leprosy could improve lives while easing the overall weight that this long-overlooked disease puts on society (Newport & Myrvang, 2009; Mtui et al., 2011) (Figure 7.8).

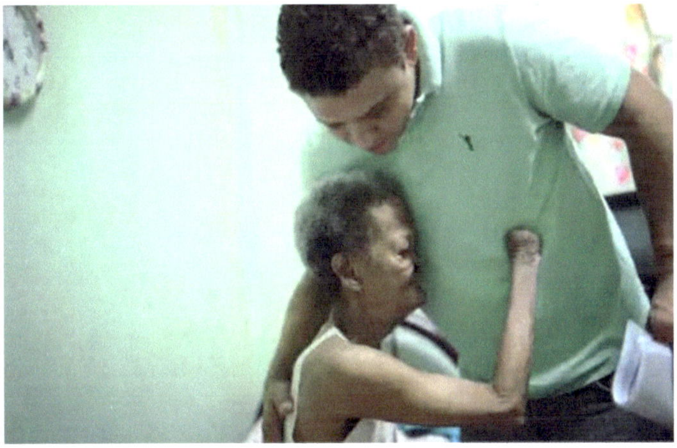

Figure 7.8. Mental health issues associated with leprosy.

Source: ET HealthWorld. (2022). *Mental Health Services to Leprosy Patients.*

7.2.3. Coping Mechanisms and Support Systems

People facing long-term health issues deal with more than just physical pain; social stigma, money damages, and mental strain all mix together. Leprosy complications, for instance, push individuals to find coping skills that become essential survival tools. Often, patients come up with a mix of practical alters, like rearranging daily routines to suit physical limits, and simple emotional fixes, such as reaching out for company when loneliness creeps in. Peer support groups and local outreach projects emerge unexpectedly, offering a kind of belonging and shared strength. In many cases, these everyday strategies not only lift one's quality of life but also impact the social barriers that complicate matters further. Generally speaking, recognizing these adaptive behaviors sheds light on care models that combine holistic support with traditional medical treatment (Baba et al., 2020). In settings where healthcare resources are stretched thin, for example, in rural or conflict-hit regions—informal networks suddenly carry a lot of weight. Health workers, community volunteers, and even family members step in to cover the gaps that formal systems leave behind. When government backing is either limited or completely missing, people often rely on small-scale activities like farming or local trades to keep their families afloat. At the same time, training local caregivers and traditional birth attendants expands the community's ability to deliver basic services, indirectly supporting those with leprosy problems by boosting overall health know-how. These grassroots approaches clearly underscore the need for interventions that fit naturally with everyday coping practices and local social dynamics (Baba et al., 2020). Beyond the immediate fixes, the wider effects of leprosy-linked stigma hit hard on both financial stability and mental well-being. Generally, the isolation and discrimination connected to the condition not only deepen economic hardship but also steal away a person's sense of dignity. The capabilities approach, for example, shows how disabilities and stigma often slit open opportunities for a meaningful life, stressing the need for measures that restore autonomy and encourage social participation. Support systems that weave together education, vocational training, and community engagement can break the cycle of poverty that leprosy complications tend to trigger, helping patients regain both stability and self-respect. In this light, combining stigma reduction with empowerment efforts within rehabilitation programs becomes, arguably, essential to address the full range of leprosy's impacts on individuals and their families (Figure 7.9).

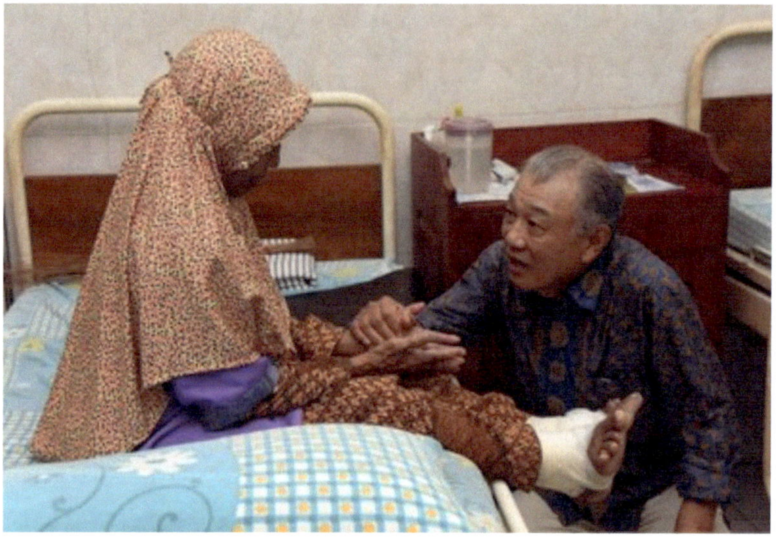

Figure 7.9. The coping mechanisms and support systems.

Source: The Laotian Times. (2025, January). *Image_1-4. https://laotiantimes.com/wp-content/uploads/2025/01/image_1-4.jpg.*

7.3. Economic Impact

Leprosy complications hit people in more ways than one. Many individuals dealing with the disease not only face steep medical bills but also struggle to keep up with regular work due to physical limitations and the sting of social rejection. People often find that their ability to maintain a steady income wavers, trapping them in cycles of poverty that deeply affect their families. On top of that, even when a surgery,say, one to clear up cataracts, generally restores vision and functionality, the overall price tag, including post-surgery care and rehab, adds up fast (Tabassum et al., 2024). These extra expenses slowly nibble away at household budgets, making the fiscal side of leprosy care an issue that public health planners can't simply ignore. When you zoom out to look at the whole health system, the costs connected to leprosy management show just how tight funding can get. Treatments and interventions, while tackling immediate health problems, often come with hefty price tags that strain budgets, particularly in low-income areas. Newer surgical techniques and better care standards—though a definite step forward—can push overall healthcare spending even higher. It turns out that decisions on treatment approaches or tech adoption can shift health budgets quite a bit, sometimes representing a large slice of total expenditures (Mtui et al., 2011). In most cases, finding that sweet spot between targeted treatment and broad prevention efforts becomes crucial, even if the choices are anything but straightforward. Beyond the obvious medical bills, there's an even bigger picture here. The long-term disabilities associated with leprosy send indirect costs rolling in, costs like the extra strain on social support systems and the loss of contribution from those who can't work at full capacity. That's why national strategies for battling neglected tropical diseases need to fold in detailed cost analyses, planning for these hidden expenses over several years. Sound financial practices, like regular cost reviews, timely budgeting, and coordinated planning, help spot funding gaps before they balloon, keeping programs viable even when external funding is a major player (Mtui et al., 2011). In the end, understanding these economic ripples is key not only for patient care but also for building a more sustainable health system.

7.3.1. Cost of Treatment and Healthcare Access

Many issues in getting proper leprosy care come from deep-rooted problems in our health system that tend to hit marginalized individuals the hardest. A lot of the stumbling happens because many doctors simply don't have a good grasp on Hansen's disease—this lack of know-how can push back both diagnosis and treatment start times. That gap not only fuels old misunderstandings about contagiousness but also adds layers of stigma, making it even tougher for patients to seek help. In many cases, these issues leave people suffering longer and facing more serious complications, since treatment isn't provided quickly enough. What happens then is that delays force more costly, intricate interventions later on, showing just how health access and financial strain are connected together (Kuhns 2012). Money matters further complicate things, especially in regions where health services are underdeveloped. Patients often end up shouldering high out-of-pocket costs—traveling to specialized centers, sticking with lengthy medication routines, and even paying for rehabilitation. For low-income individuals, these added expenses frequently mean they either drop out of treatment or avoid starting it altogether, which in most cases leads to risks like irreversible nerve damage. Many health systems in developing countries just aren't equipped with the right resources to deliver steady, quality care, which restricts both the availability and affordability of treatments. These structural faults reveal broader public health issues where support and funding for groups dealing with leprosy just aren't enough (Rodriguez-Morales, 2019). Tackling these cost-related hurdles calls for an approach that mixes medical, social, and financial help. Policies aimed at broadening health coverage, boosting doctor training to ease stigma, and rolling out community programs for early detection and ongoing care are key. Empowering people through education and advocacy also plays a big part in keeping treatment on track and reducing social isolation. On top of that, international cooperation and funding to strengthen fragile health systems are vital for keeping treatments affordable over time. Without addressing these intertwined problems, the cycle of high costs and limited access will likely stick around, making it increasingly hard to beat leprosy as a public health challenge (Kuhns 2012; Rodriguez-Morales, 2019) (Figure 7.10).

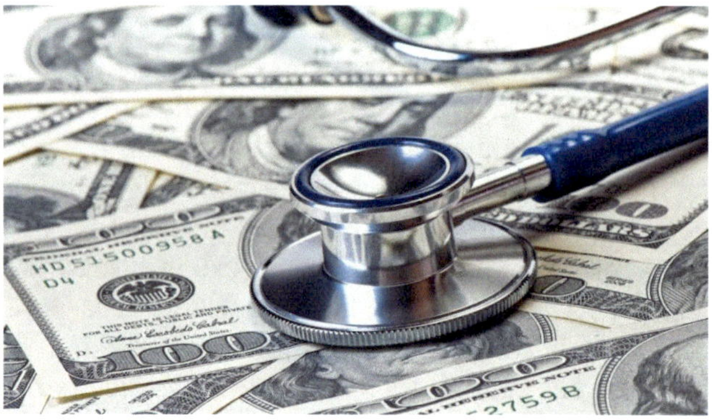

Figure 7.10. Cost of treatment.

Source: Exude, Inc. (2018). *Health Costs.*

7.3.2. Loss of Productivity Due to Disability

Leprosy doesn't just rack up medical bills; it degrades a person's ability to work and earn a living. The disease often leads to physical limitations—things like reduced mobility and diminished sensory skills—that can sap someone's capacity to hold down a job, especially roles that require lots of physical effort. In many cases, this drop in productivity sets off a vicious cycle where the loss of income spills over to affect not just the individual but their family and even the wider community. And then there's the extra weight of stigma, which tends to push people further into social isolation and fewer job opportunities, ultimately deepening both financial and human costs that don't get nearly enough airtime in global health debates (Wilsher, 2011). Taking a closer look at the efforts to stop these disabilities reveals plenty of challenges too, particularly in places that are already strapped for resources. Programs aimed at preventing disability, like those caring for nerve damage or even supplying protective footwear—try to keep people functioning so that they can continue earning a living. But honestly, the research out there on how cost-effective these interventions are often doesn't hold up well methodologically; as a result, it's tough to say which strategy is the best bet for keeping productivity afloat among those hit hardest by the disease. Further, the everyday self-care practices, which many believe help prevent further decline, aren't getting enough attention from an economic standpoint. Generally speaking, bolstering these prevention programs with stronger economic backing is key to using scarce resources wisely and cutting down on productivity losses (Van Veen et al., 2009). When you consider the many ways leprosy-related disability hits productivity, it becomes clear that we need to combine health and socioeconomic strategies if we're going to tackle this issue effectively. Traditional studies tend to zero in on mortality rates or immediate medical expenses, but they miss out on capturing how these disabilities knock away individuals' ability to lead fulfilling lives. In most cases, this isn't just about lost money, it's about losing the freedom to participate in society and contribute meaningfully. The double whammy of stigma and physical impairment not only brings down personal morale but also keeps communities from moving forward. To cut back on these long-term losses, comprehensive approaches are needed ones that push for reintegration into society, better access to prevention measures, and initiatives that empower affected individuals to regain both their economic footing and social standing (Wilsher, 2011).

7.3.3. Economic Burden on Families and Communities

Chronic illnesses can hit families hard, not just health-wise but by stretching their wallets thin in ways you might not expect. When complications emerge, take leprosy, for instance, the price tag for long-term care, ongoing medication, and consistent help can leap up quickly. It's not just about paying for the doctor; there's also the hidden hit of lost wages when someone can't work or has to spend time caring for a loved one.

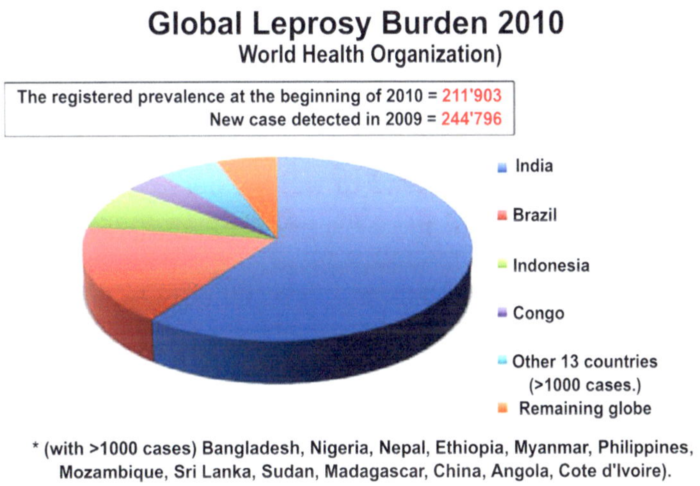

Figure 7.11. Global leprosy burden in 2010. Country-wise representation of the total number of leprosy cases registered globally at the beginning of 2010.

Source: Singh, P. (2016). *Global Leprosy Burden in 2010.*

In most cases, these rising costs force households to pour almost all their money into dealing with the illness, which chops away at funds needed for essentials like schooling, good food, or a stable living environment, setting off a vicious circle of financial stress and declining health outcomes (Yoder et al., 2024). At a community level, the burden spreads out in unexpected ways. Public health systems often find themselves scrambling, allocating hefty slices of their budgets to cover everything from initial diagnosis to treatment and even rehabilitation services. Generally speaking, when a lot of people face issues like leprosy, the knock-on effects include not only a slump in overall work output but also growing social exclusion, which further degrades the area's productivity. As a result, social services get pushed to their limits, economic expansion slows down, and more individuals lean on government or outside aid for support, as certain pandemic analyses have pointed out (Faramarzi et al., 2024). Dealing with the money crunch that comes with diseases like leprosy, therefore, calls for more than just medical fixes. It's about rolling out financial help, setting up safety nets, and crafting job-support programs that all work together to ease the shock on affected households. Often, making healthcare more affordable and detecting problems early can cut down on the worst complications, and their steep price tags. Community-led rehab and education also matter, as they help bust the stigma that sometimes keeps people from landing jobs or feeling part of society. In most cases, thinking about financial and social hurdles as part of the disease management picture enables policymakers to build resilient support systems. Studies have shown that these broad approaches can improve both health outcomes and overall economic stability (Faramarzi et al., 2024; Yoder et al., 2024) (Figure 7.11).

7.4. Treatment Challenges

Managing leprosy treatment is no small feat – it's complex up in both inner challenges and outside issues. One big hitch is that the multidrug therapy drags on for about six months to a year, which in most cases makes it tough for patients to stick with it; this often leads to drug resistance. The disease sneaks up slowly and shows itself in a combination of ways, so catching it early is complex delays mean treatment starts later and complications have room to grow. When *Mycobacterium leprae* stirs up immune responses, particularly those type 1 and type 2 lepra reactions, extra treatments are combined. These reactions tend to worsen nerve damage and then call for careful alters to the immune system, all to help prevent disability. In other words, treatment isn't just about clearing out the microbe—it's also about cooling down the inflammation and keeping long-term problems at bay, often requiring a team approach tailored to each patient's characterestics. Looking deeper, it's not only the drugs that complicate things; the complex molecular and cellular pathways add another layer of difficulty.

For example, signaling networks like the NF-κB pathway play a key role in controlling inflammation and innate immune responses during leprosy. When these signals misfire, tissue damage can get worse and strategies to lower inflammation without weakening the body's essential defenses become all the more complicated. Generally speaking, trying to target NF-κB, though promising, is a real balancing act because it's involved in so many normal functions. New treatments that attempt to modulate these pathways have to juggle fighting the disease with avoiding too many side effects. Understanding these underlying molecular tricks is crucial for developing the next generation of therapies that can ease immune-related issues while still keeping the infection in check (Guo et al., 2024). Overall, these hurdles highlight why we need more advanced research and precision approaches in leprosy care. There's also a promising digital twist to the story. Emerging health tech – think artificial intelligence, wearable gadgets, and telemedicine platforms – could help spot leprosy sooner, keep an eye on whether patients follow their regimens, and even offer real-time advice for managing flare-ups. Yet, in many resource-limited settings where leprosy is most common, challenges like spotty internet, cost issues, and limited user know-how hold these tools back. Drawing unexpected parallels with pandemic management, where IoT and AI made a real difference in monitoring and tracking diseases, one can see the potential for tackling chronic infections like leprosy. Combining these innovative tools with everyday medical practice might lead to more personalized care, better drug planning, and extra remote support when complications arise (Firouzi et al., 2021). Of course, for these advances to truly shine, overcoming infrastructural and economic hurdles remains a key piece of the puzzle.

7.4.1. Availability of Multidrug Therapy (MDT)

Access to treatment is key when it comes to handling leprosy and keeping its complications at bay. MDT has long been the go-to remedy, cutting down on transmission and warding off disabilities. Still, getting MDT to everyone isn't always easy; economic hurdles and fragile healthcare systems, especially in areas where neglected tropical diseases like leprosy still stick around—can get in the way. Global efforts try to bridge these gaps, but differences in treatment access persist, affecting many populations. Efforts from international groups and local programs have pushed MDT a long way, yet uneven distribution and lack of proper patient guidance continue to slow progress. Basically, making sure that MDT is available to everyone without interruption is vital for reducing the long-term issues seen in untreated or poorly managed cases (Amal et al., 2017). Leprosy brings on some pretty complicated challenges, particularly when sudden inflammatory reactions attack nerves.

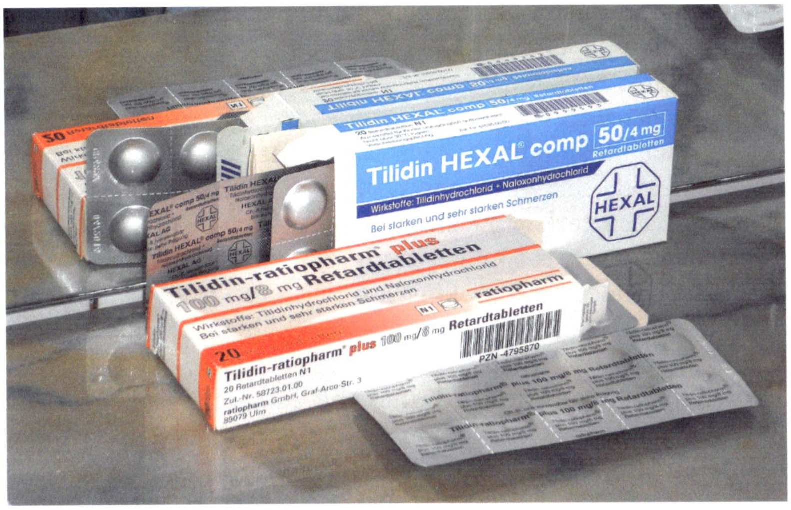

Figure 7.12. Leprosy MDT tablet.

Source: By Ralf Roletschek - Own work, CC BY-SA 3.0, https://commons.wikimedia.org/w/index.php?curid=20717356

Early use of MDT can lower bacterial counts, and that seems to lessen the chance and impact of these damaging episodes. However, the problem isn't just about handing out MDT—it's also about detecting and managing those flare-ups before they lead to irreversible harm. Some studies even suggest that immune biomarkers might flag these reactional states, helping clinicians step in quicker with the right treatments. Without prompt treatment with MDT, patients risk facing serious complications like nerve damage, deformity, and lasting disability; hence, pairing MDT with careful clinical monitoring remains a must to slow disease progression and keep life as normal as possible (Khadge et al., 2015). Keeping MDT accessible isn't just about its effectiveness but also about having robust healthcare systems and strong local and global commitments. It means training healthcare workers to notice early signs, ensuring steady drug supplies, and teaching patients to stick with the treatment plan. Since leprosy mostly affects marginalized communities, tackling stigma and boosting outreach efforts are just as critical, so individuals don't wait too long to get help. Although MDT has changed the game in leprosy control, ongoing infrastructure challenges and social factors still block a full end to its debilitating effects. Continued investment and thoughtful planning are needed to keep MDT programs growing, all with the hope of cutting down the worldwide burden of leprosy-related disability (Khadge et al., 2015; Amal et al., 2017) (Figure 7.12).

7.4.2. Adherence to Treatment Regimens

Managing leprosy well isn't just about having powerful antibiotics at hand—it's also about patients sticking to their treatment plans. When individuals miss doses or stop too soon, the pathogenic *Mycobacterium leprae* can hang around, leading not only to a persisting infection but, over time, to nerve damage and even disability. There's a jumble of things that impact whether someone stays on course—the lengthy, sometimes complex multi-drug regimens, those bothersome side effects, and various social and cultural hurdles. Especially among indigenous groups, standard approaches like Directly Observed Therapy (DOT) often fall short because of cultural mismatches and a lack of trust between patients and their healthcare providers. For that reason, many experts now suggest that tailoring treatments to fit a patient's real-life experiences and cultural backpack can help boost adherence and cut down leprosy-related illness (Phillips et al., 2020). It's also clear that sticking with treatment isn't only a matter of patient behavior; the system itself can trip people up too. For instance, treatments that involve painful shots like intramuscular injections can discourage continued use of needed medications—sometimes leading to treatment being dropped altogether. Recent work on related mycobacterial illnesses, such as Buruli ulcer, has generally shown that fully oral antibiotic regimens, often easier on the body and simpler to take—can lead to higher adherence. By reducing side effects and making life a bit easier, these approaches suggest there might be a way to ease the treatment burden of leprosy without sacrificing effectiveness (Phillips et al., 2020). This evidence reminds us that strong drugs alone aren't enough, how the treatment is designed counts, too. Building genuine trust and embracing cultural sensitivity remains crucial, particularly over long treatment spans. Indigenous communities often carry the weight of historical and ongoing inequities, which can foster understandable wariness toward conventional healthcare. In these cases, weaving family support and local cultural practices into treatment plans has shown promise in keeping patients engaged with their therapy. When doctors take the time for shared decision-making and explain, sometimes even repeatedly, why a treatment matters, what side effects might emerge, and the long-term health stakes, it lessens fears and clears up any confusion. In the end, creating a service where patients feel culturally safe not only meshes clinical goals with what matters to them but also helps prevent the setbacks that come from leaving treatment unfinished (Oliver, 2022).

7.4.3. Management of Drug-Resistant Leprosy

Tackling drug-resistant leprosy isn't as simple as sticking to the usual treatment playbook. Often, incomplete treatment routines—or even the crafty nature of *Mycobacterium leprae*'s genetics—lead to the failure of standard multidrug therapies. Doctors, generally speaking, have to be on high alert since leprosy tends to persist and mix unpredictably with the body's defenses. They run tests like molecular assays and check drug sensitivity early on, so they can fine-tune treatments as needed. Also, conditions like diabetes, which in many instances further complicate mycobacterial infections, call for care that looks at the whole patient, including regular metabolic check-ups (Faurholt-Jepsen et al., 2013). In short, taking a broad approach like this is key to cutting down relapses and keeping those resistant strains from spreading further—a tough but necessary hurdle in leprosy control programs. When it comes to managing resistant cases from a treatment standpoint, doctors often shift to second-line medicines and mix in extra therapies to both curb the bacteria and avoid heavy side effects. Drugs such as fluoroquinolones, macrolides, and minocycline have proven useful when rifampicin and dapsone, the usual go-to drugs, don't work anymore. That said, using these alternatives calls for extra caution; one must weigh risks like toxicity, potential drug clashes, and factors that vary from patient to patient—for example, co-infections like HIV, which can alter immune responses and drug behavior. Occasionally, if complications like nerve issues or abscesses arise, surgery might be needed (a bit similar to what happens with complex abdominal infections (Chalya et al., 2013)). Combining medicinal and surgical routes, therefore, adds an extra layer of promise in boosting outcomes and lessening long-term problems. Beyond changing up medications, effectively handling drug-resistant leprosy means ramping up public health initiatives too. Early detection, patient education, and helping individuals stick with their treatment plans are all crucial. Community programs that ease stigma and make treatment more accessible are vital in keeping therapy on track, since lapses can induce resistance. At the same time, solid surveillance systems help to track how resistance patterns evolve and whether treatments are doing the job—allowing adjustments as new challenges arise. Ongoing research into fresh drugs and immune-boosting methods shows promise, too. Lessons from dealing with other tough infections remind us that coordinated, multidisciplinary care—paying attention to things like nutrition and immune status—is key in managing diseases prone to resistance and complications (Chalya et al., 2013; Faurholt-Jepsen et al., 2013). All these combined efforts are essential to easing the burden of drug-resistant leprosy and its many challenges (Figure 7.13).

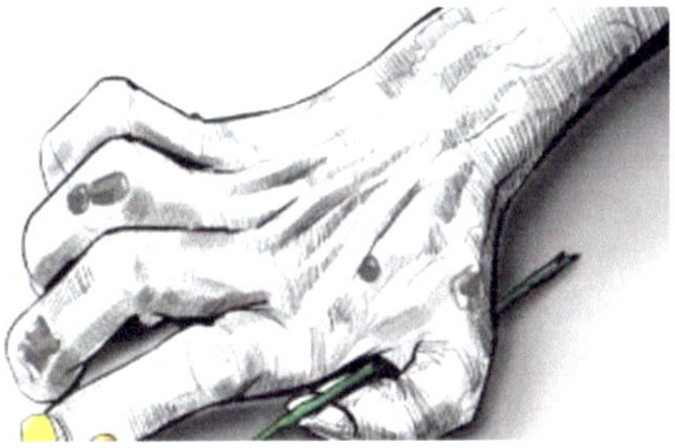

Figure 7.13. The management of drug-resistant leprosy.

Source: Google. (n.d.). *Skin condition. https://encrypted-tbn0.gstatic.com/images?q=tbn:ANd9GcS5J ahTG9PnBUjMsj4Iwkd5YyppjvmzQ9AMDg&s.*

A CLOSER LOOK

SKIN MANIFESTATIONS IN LEPROSY REACTIONS

Type 1 leprosy reaction does not usually raise the question of differential diagnosis, since it often occurs in patients under treatment and is clinically characterized by modifications of preexisting lesions which involve an acute inflammatory phenomenon. In some cases, the patient may seek medical attention, for the first time, during a type 1 leprosy reaction. This reaction must be differentiated from pathologies that begin acutely with inflammatory plaques, such as erysipelas and Sweet's syndrome. In these cases, the examination for AFB is negative. Diagnosis must be based on an investigation of neuropathy and histopathology (Figure 7.14).

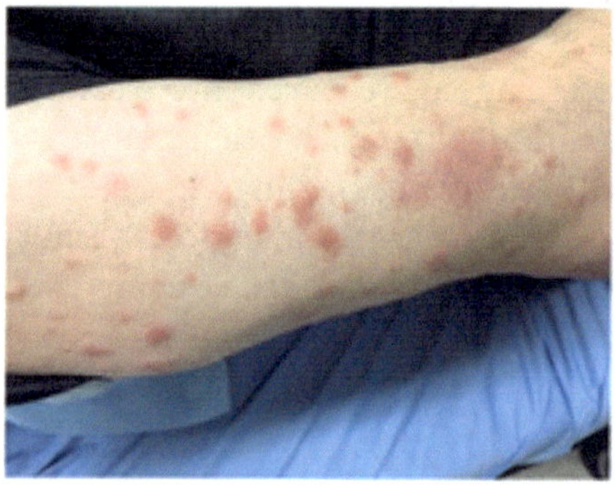

(a)

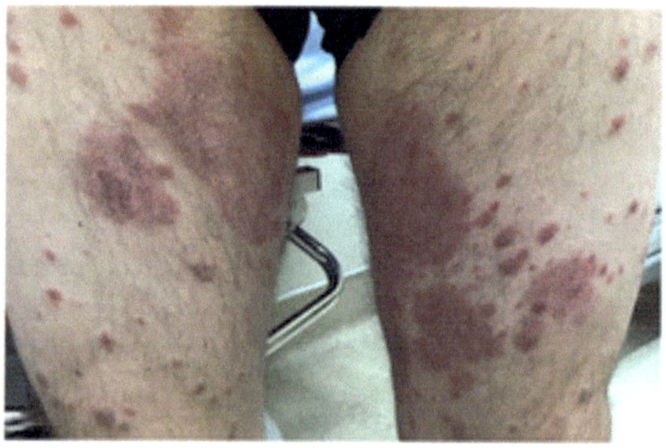

(b)

Figure 7.14. Skin manifestations in leprosy reactions.

SourceNaidu P, Sharma R, Kanji JN, Marks V, King A. Autochthonous North American Leprosy: A Second Case in Canada. Infectious Disease Reports. 2021; 13(4):917-923. https://doi.org/10.3390/idr13040083

Erythema nodosum leprosum (ENL), the main cutaneous expression of type 2 leprosy reaction, is characterized by acute eruptions of nodules. In BL, ENL may appear with plaques that are depressed in the center and becoming hyperpigmented. Differential diagnosis must be made with fixed drug eruption and nodular vasculitis, which have different etiology. Wheals caused by immunocomplexes can appear in type 2 leprosy reactions. In acute onset of leprosy, anamnesis and AFB investigation will help in diagnosis.

SUMMARY

Leprosy isn't just about an initial diagnosis or one-off treatment, it's a challenge that stretches far beyond the clinic visit. The condition brings with it a whole lot of complications, from nerve issues to the heavy burden of social stigma, meaning that individuals need ongoing help that's both medical and emotional. Health systems, generally speaking, must get set up for long-term support to ward off disability and keep quality of life intact. Regular check-ups after discharge and a bit of continuous monitoring work wonders in ensuring that no one gets left behind. Placing treatment within a broader frameset of community and policy lets care teams dodge some recurring hurdles, showing that keeping up with interventions is key (Pinheiro et al., 2019). It's clear that a swift end to treatment isn't the end of the story, such an approach demands steeper investments in both policy and community commitment. This way of looking at care reminds us that leprosy isn't simply a medical issue; it touches on larger public health challenges that need constant attention. At the same time, when medical societies and infectious disease experts team up, understanding and handling leprosy's fallout gets a real boost. Chatting casually at international meetups, for example, has helped mix hands-on experience with fresh research insights, inducing new ideas in both diagnosis and treatment strategies. Specialists in infectious diseases, along with those in tropical medicine, show just how much teamwork matters when coming up with flexible care plans. These collaborative moves, somewhat like a back-and-forth conversation, fuel the ongoing evolution of patient care (Newport & Myrvang, 2009). Often, such exchanges induce changes that ultimately ripple through even the most diverse healthcare settings. In wrapping it all up, dealing with leprosy means looking past just treating the obvious symptoms. Fast detection, continuous treatment, and extra support that stretches well beyond the hospital door are all part of the picture. It highlights how leprosy remains an ever-present public health puzzle, one that policies must address by ensuring everyone gets care at every stage of the illness. Recognizing that social and cultural angles play a role too, there's a call for a more holistic approach, one that weaves together medical and emotional support to cut down stigma and stall disability before it starts. Some existing research points to the need for tougher healthcare plans that link steady care with community rehab to ease long-term issues. In the end, facing leprosy head-on calls for long-term, team-driven efforts that respect patient dignity and help individuals reintegrate into everyday life (Pinheiro et al., 2019).

Leprosy complications hit everyday life and physical ability hard. A look back at a study from the Centre Hospitalier Régional Spécialisé in Guinea shows that many patients on multidrug therapy ended up dealing with things like plantar ulcers and other physical disabilities. Most of those affected were in the 25–59 age range, with men , often farmers , taking the brunt of it, which hints at some occupational risks mixed with age vulnerabilities. Over nearly 10 years, there was a noticeable drop in the number of leprosy reactions and related complications, suggesting that better management and community awareness might be doing some good. Still, the fact that foot wounds and lasting disabilities are still around confirms that, in many cases, leprosy's long-term effects remain a serious issue, especially in regions where early care and prevention just aren't as accessible (Hébélamou et al., 2024). The economic and social fallout from these complications seems to go hand in hand with delays in diagnosis and treatment, and that only makes the physical disabilities worse. Research out of Bangladesh, for example, shows that quite a few leprosy patients end up with Grade 2 disabilities—that is, clear deformities and loss of function. It's interesting, and generally speaking, men show up more in these stats, and people from poorer backgrounds tend to face an even bigger risk. The study even pointed out factors like the lack of sufficient funds and the somewhat painless nature of early symptoms as key reasons why patients delay seeking help, which then results in even more complications (Sinha et al., 2024). To summarize, these studies show that the challenges posed by leprosy stretch far beyond just clinical symptoms. Ulcers, deformities, and disabilities come not only from the bacterial infection itself but also from delayed treatment and insufficient patient education. While efforts to boost community awareness and improve healthcare provider training have made some inroads, there's still a lot of work to be done, especially for vulnerable individuals such as rural farmers and those with limited financial means. In most cases, combining early detection, effective treatment, and proactive disability prevention seems absolutely crucial for lessening leprosy's long-term impact and achieving better outcomes (Hébélamou et al., 2024; Sinha et al., 2024).

KEY TERMS FROM THIS CHAPTER

- Chronic nerve issues
- Deformities
- Emotional distress
- Epididymo-orchitis
- Genital issues
- Health policies
- Hormone balance
- Hypogonadism
- Immune reactions
- Lowered hormone levels
- Medical complications
- Muscle strength
- Neuropathy
- Peripheral nerve damage
- Social isolation
- Surgical interventions

References

1. G., Gateau, T., Chauty, A., Omollo, R., Ochieng Otieno, M., Egondi, T. W., Ampadu, E. O., Agossadou, D., Marion, E., Ganlonon, L., Wansbrough-Jones, M., Grosset, J., Macdonald, J. M., Treadwell, T., ... study team (2020). Rifampicin and clarithromycin (extended release) versus rifampicin and streptomycin for limited Buruli ulcer lesions: a randomised, open-label, non-inferiority phase 3 trial. *Lancet (London, England)*, *395*(10232), 1259–1267. https://doi.org/10.1016/S0140-6736(20)30047-7 (accessed on 10th May 2025).
2. Van Veen, N. H., Schreuders, T. A., Theuvenet, W. J., Agrawal, A., & Richardus, J. H. (2012). Decompressive surgery for treating nerve damage in leprosy. *The Cochrane database of systematic reviews*, *12*(12), CD006983. https://doi.org/10.1002/14651858.CD006983.pub3 (accessed on 10th May 2025).
3. Baba A, Theobald S, Martineau T, Sabuni P, Nobabo MM, Alitimango A, Raven J. 'Being a midwife is being prepared to help women in very difficult conditions': midwives' experiences of working in the rural and fragile settings of Ituri Province, Democratic Republic of Congo. Rural and Remote Health 2020; 20: 5677. https://doi.org/10.22605/RRH5677 (accessed on 10th May 2025).
4. van Veen, N. H., McNamee, P., Richardus, J. H., & Smith, W. C. (2009). Cost-effectiveness of interventions to prevent disability in leprosy: a systematic review. *PloS one*, *4*(2), e4548. https://doi.org/10.1371/journal.pone.0004548 (accessed on 10th May 2025).
5. Santos, V.S., Santana, J.C.V., Castro, F.D.N. *et al.* Pain and quality of life in leprosy patients in an endemic area of Northeast Brazil: a cross-sectional study. *Infect Dis Poverty* **5**, 18 (2016). https://doi.org/10.1186/s40249-016-0113-1 (accessed on 10th May 2025).
6. di Luca, A., Ralli, M., Hemied, S., de Vincentiis, M., & di Luca, N. M. (2017). An atypical case of trigeminal trophic syndrome: A legal medicine perspective in medical responsibility. *SAGE open medical case reports*, *5*, 2050313X17723548. https://doi.org/10.1177/2050313X17723548 (accessed on 10th May 2025).
7. Faramarzi, A., Norouzi, S., Dehdarirad, H., Aghlmand, S., Yusefzadeh, H., & Javan-Noughabi, J. (2024). The global economic burden of COVID-19 disease: a comprehensive systematic review and meta-analysis. *Systematic reviews*, *13*(1), 68. https://doi.org/10.1186/s13643-024-02476-6(accessed on 10th May 2025).
8. Faurholt-Jepsen, D. (2013). The double burden. *Danish Medical Journal.* https://core.ac.uk/download/pdf/16666765.pdf (accessed on 10th May 2025).
9. Firouzi, F., Farahani, B., Daneshmand, M., Grise, K., Song, J., Saracco, R., Wang, L. L., et al. (2021). Harnessing the power of smart and connected health to tackle COVID-19: IoT, AI, robotics, and blockchain for a better world. *IEEE Internet of Things Journal*, *8*, 12826–12846. https://doi.org/10.1109/jiot.2021.3073904 (accessed on 10th May 2025).
10. Githui, S., Kaguthi, G., Karugu, M., Kipruto, M., et al. (2022). A comparative study on the quality of life of leprosy patients in Kilifi and Kwale Counties in Kenya. *African Journal of Health Sciences, 35*(3). https://core.ac.uk/download/544237877.pdf (accessed on 10th May 2025).
11. Pinheiro, M. G. C., Lins, S. L. D. F., Gomes, B. R. D. S., Simpson, C. A., Mendes, F. R. P., & Miranda, F. A. N. (2019). Contextual analysis of health care at discharge in leprosy: an integrative review.

Análise contextual da atenção à saúde na alta em hanseníase: uma revisão integrativa. *Revista gaucha de enfermagem*, *40*, e20180258. https://doi.org/10.1590/1983-1447.2019.20180258 (accessed on 10th May 2025).

12. Guo, Q., Jin, Y., Chen, X., Ye, X., Shen, X., Lin, M., Zeng, C., et al. (2024). NF-κB in biology and targeted therapy: New insights and translational implications. *Signal Transduction and Targeted Therapy*, *9*. https://doi.org/10.1038/s41392-024-01757-9 (accessed on 10th May 2025).
13. Hébélamou, J., Grovogui, F. M., Manet, H., Povogui, L., Béavogui, I., Kourouma, K., Sow, A., & Delamou, A. (2024). Trend and Factors Associated with Medical-Surgical Complications in Patients Discharged from Leprosy Multidrug Therapy at the Specialized Regional Hospital in Macenta, Guinea, from 2012 to 2021. *Tropical medicine and infectious disease*, *9*(12), 290. https://doi.org/10.3390/tropicalmed9120290(accessed on 10th May 2025).
14. Khadge, S., Banu, S., Bobosha, K., van der Ploeg-van Schip, J. J., Goulart, I. M. B., Thapa, P., Kunwar, C. B., et al. (2015). Longitudinal immune profiles in type 1 leprosy reactions in Bangladesh, Brazil, Ethiopia and Nepal. *BMC Infectious Diseases*, *15*. https://doi.org/10.1186/s12879-015-1128-0 (accessed on 10th May 2025).
15. Kuhns, Kristen E., "What's to Know?: Navigating Knowledge Gaps of Hansen's Disease in the U.S.." Thesis, Georgia State University, 2012. https://scholarworks.gsu.edu/anthro_theses/66(accessed on 10th May 2025).
16. Tabassum, S., Kumari, M., Kujur, A., & Lakra, M. D. (2024). Cataract surgery in leprosy patients: visual outcomes and complications. *International Journal of Research in Medical Sciences*, *12*(5), 1497–1501. https://doi.org/10.18203/2320-6012.ijrms20241232 (accessed on 10th May 2025).
17. Lira, M. O. S. C. E., Mistura, C., Sarmento, S. S., Silva, R. A., et al. (2014). *Stigmata and Prejudice: Reality of Carriers of Leprosy in Prisional Units.* Revista de Pesquisa: Cuidado é Fundamental Online, 6 (2014) 2. DOI: https://doi.org/10.9789/2175-5361.2014.v6i2.493-506(accessed on 10th May 2025).
18. Mitra, A. K., & Mawson, A. R. (2017). Neglected tropical diseases: Epidemiology and global burden. *Tropical Medicine and Infectious Disease*, *2*, 36–36. https://doi.org/10.3390/tropicalmed2030036 (accessed on 10th May 2025).
19. Mtui, J., & Osoro, O. (2011). *Aggregate Cost Implications of Selected Cost-Drivers in the Tanzanian Health Sector*. Commissioned by: Ministry of Health and Social Welfare; Final Report 12/1/2011. https://core.ac.uk/download/pdf/11307328.pdf (accessed on 10th May 2025).
20. Newport, M. J., & Myrvang, B. (2009). Proceedings of a joint meeting between the Norwegian Society of Infectious Diseases and the Royal Society of Tropical Medicine and Hygiene, Oslo, 20 June 2008. *Transactions of the Royal Society of Tropical Medicine and Hygiene*, *103*(4), 321–324. https://doi.org/10.1016/j.trstmh.2008.11.010 (accessed on 10th May 2025).
21. J. Rodriguez-Morales, A. (Ed.). (2019). Current Topics in Neglected Tropical Diseases. IntechOpen. doi: 10.5772/intechopen.73918(accessed on 10th May 2025).
22. Van Veen, N. H., Nicholls, P. G., Smith, W. C., & Richardus, J. H. (2016). Corticosteroids for treating nerve damage in leprosy. *The Cochrane database of systematic reviews*, *2016*(5), CD005491. https://doi.org/10.1002/14651858.CD005491.pub3(accessed on 10th May 2025).
23. Oliver, S. J. (2022). From Isolation to Inclusion: Embracing Local Perspectives in Examining

the Treatment Model of Care for Aboriginal Persons Affected by Tuberculosis or Leprosy in the Kimberley Region, North Western Australia [Doctor of Philosophy (College of Medicine)]. The University of Notre Dame Australia. https://researchonline.nd.edu.au/theses/386(accessed on 10th May 2025).

24. Pavithra, G. (2017). *Clinico-Epidemiological Study of New Multibacillary Leprosy Patients Visiting a Tertiary Care Hospital: A Prospective Observational Study.* https://core.ac.uk/download/327695965.pdf (accessed on 10th May 2025).

25. Richens J. (2004). Genital manifestations of tropical diseases. *Sexually transmitted infections*, *80*(1), 12–17. https://doi.org/10.1136/sti.2003.004093 (accessed on 10th May 2025).

26. Chalya, P.L., Mchembe, M.D., Mshana, S.E. *et al.* Clinicopathological profile and surgical treatment of abdominal tuberculosis: a single centre experience in northwestern Tanzania. *BMC Infect Dis* **13**, 270 (2013). https://doi.org/10.1186/1471-2334-13-270 (accessed on 10th May 2025).

27. Sinha, S., Haq, M. A., Ahmad, R., Banik, S., Kumar, S., & Haque, M. (2024). Unmasking the Hidden Burden: A Delayed Diagnosis of Leprosy Patients With Grade 2 Disability and Its Effects on the Healthcare System in Bangladesh. *Cureus*, *16*(4), e58708. https://doi.org/10.7759/cureus.58708(accessed on 10th May 2025).

28. Social implications of leprosy in the Netherlands - stigma among ex-leprosy patients in a non-endemic setting; Leprosy Review; 2011; 82; 2; 168-177; DOI: 10.47276/lr.82.2.168 (accessed on 10th May 2025).

29. Wilsher, Emma, Jane (2011) *The impact of Neglected Tropical Diseases, and their associated stigma, on people's basic capabilities.* Masters thesis, Durham University.. https://etheses.dur.ac.uk/3301/(accessed on 10th May 2025).

30. Yoder, K., Burris, R., Gurunathan, S., Phillips, G., Perez, K., Habib, A. A., & Narayanaswami, P. (2025). The Economic Burden of Myasthenia Gravis (MG): A Survey of Affected People and Their Families. *Muscle & nerve*, *71*(2), 244–251. https://doi.org/10.1002/mus.28313(accessed on 10th May 2025).

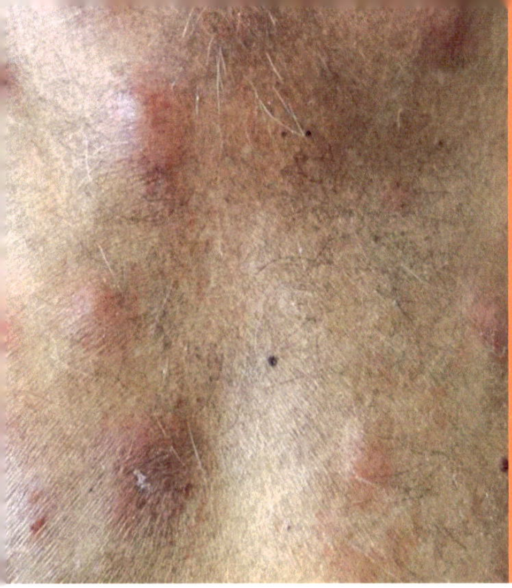

Chapter 8

LEPROSY REACTIONS AND THEIR MANAGEMENT

Contents

Introduction

Leprosy is still a big public health worry in many regions where it's common, mainly because it sticks around for a long time and can lead to serious complications. Even though we've seen some progress with antimicrobial drugs, doctors still wrestle with a variety of immune responses that can emerge unexpectedly—sometimes before treatment starts, sometimes during, or even afterwards, and these can end up causing nerve damage and disability if not detected quickly. The World Health Organization backs a treatment that mixes rifampicin, dapsone, and clofazimine in what's known as multi-drug therapy to help stop both the infection and its spread. Still, the side effects and the full range of these reactions turn the treatment process into a complex balancing act. For that reason, diving into alternative treatment plans and getting what's behind these immune issues is generally key to making long-term outcomes better for patients (Sivakumaran et al., 2024). The body's immune response in leprosy is a combined bag. Both cell-driven and blood-related (humoral) defenses set in, and you can see everything from a small, localized flare-up right up to widespread, systemic involvement. Two main reaction types tend to show up—a reversal reaction (Type 1) and another called erythema nodosum leprosum (Type 2), and these usually arise when the immune system goes a bit overboard reacting to *Mycobacterium leprae* antigens. This overreaction can sometimes interefere with the nerves in a big way. In most cases, managing this means carefully balancing immunosuppressive treatments to rein in the inflammation while also pushing ahead with antibiotics to clear the infection. It's a tough act that calls for treatment plans tailored to each patient's reaction type, its severity, and how well they respond to the medications. Honestly, nailing this balance is crucial for avoiding permanent damage and boosting quality of life for those with leprosy (Sivakumaran et al., 2024).

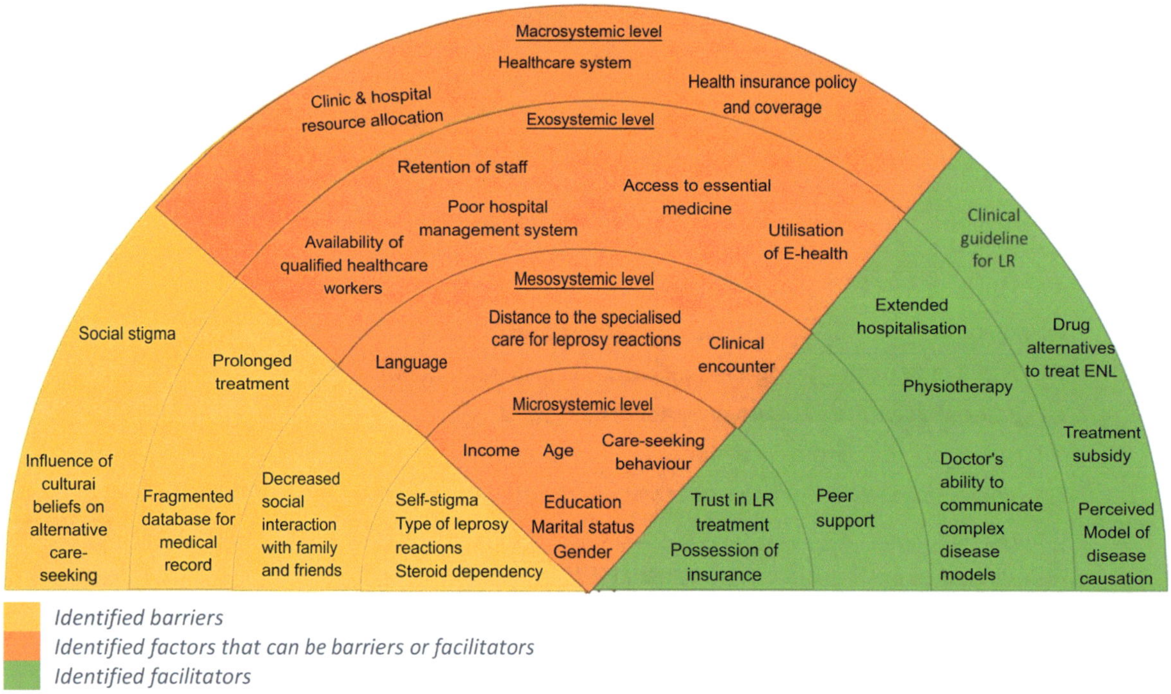

Figure 8.1. Leprosy reactions.

Source: Putri, A.I., Peters, R.M.H., De Sabbata, K. *et al.* A socio-ecological model of the management of leprosy reactions in Indonesia and India using the experiences of affected individuals, family members and healthcare providers. *BMC Health Serv Res* **25**, 196 (2025). https://doi.org/10.1186/s12913-025-12340-5.

Catching leprosy reactions early on is key, as early diagnosis and keeping an eye on drug-related side effects can make a noticeable difference. Lately, some alternative regimens, like using a monthly cocktail of rifampicin, ofloxacin, and minocycline (mROM), have come under the spotlight, especially in areas where leprosy isn't as widespread, because they seem to bring down toxicity and help patients stick with their treatment. Preliminary studies suggest that mROM not only cuts the bacterial load significantly but also comes with a milder safety profile compared to the traditional WHO multi-drug therapy, though reactions still emerge more often than one would hope. This means that doctors need to remain extra vigilant and adjust treatments as needed.

Ongoing research and clinical trials, in most cases, are essential to see if these new approaches can lower relapse rates and side effects while handling the immune challenges effectively; if they do, it could be a major boost to global efforts in controlling leprosy and reducing its long-term, disabling effects (Sivakumaran et al., 2024) (Figure 8.1).

Overview of Leprosy Reactions

Leprosy is a long-term infectious ailment caused by *Mycobacterium leprae* that often sets off a puzzling immune flare-up we call leprosy reactions. In many instances, you get sudden bouts of inflammation that toss a wrench into the ongoing progression of the disease, affecting nerves and sometimes leading to lasting disability. Generally speaking, there are two main kinds you see: one, often referred to as a reversal reaction (or type 1), where the body's cell-driven attack increases in areas already marked by the disease, and the other, Type 2 or erythema nodosum leprosum, where deposits of immune complexes trigger widespread symptoms, involving both the skin and nerves. Not to be overlooked, if these inflammatory episodes aren't spotted and managed quickly, they can take a toll on nerve function in an almost irreversible way. Getting a handle on these immune dysfunction is key since they form the backbone of clinical hurdles and guide how treatments are tailored for better patient outcomes.

		PNL	Other clinical forms	Total
No leprosy reaction		**46 (88.5%)**	33 (49.3%)	79
Leprosy reaction	Type 1 reaction	2 (3.8%)	**14 (20.9%)**	16
	Type 2 reaction	0	7 (10.4%)	7
	Neuritis	**3 (5.8%)**	2 (3.0%)	5
	Type 1 reaction with neuritis	1 (1.9%)	7 (10.4%)	8
	Type 2 reaction with neuritis	0	4 (6.0%)	4
	Total	52	67	119

PNL, Pure neural leprosy.

Figure 8.2. The overview of leprosy reactions.

Source: Pitta IJR, Hacker MA, Vital RT, Andrade LR, Spitz CN, Sales AM, Antunes SLG, Sarno EN and Jardim MR (2022) Leprosy Reactions and Neuropathic Pain in Pure Neural Leprosy in a Reference Center in Rio de Janeiro – Brazil. Front. Med. 9:865485. doi: 10.3389/fmed.2022.865485

On the biomedical side, the challenges of leprosy reactions multiply when you look at regions where the disease is common. In endemic areas, accessing quality healthcare gets complicated by money issues, patchy services, and shortfalls in specialized staff and essential medications, issues flagged in studies from Indonesia and India (Putri et al., 2025). Individuals in these regions often face a jumble of obstacles: delayed diagnoses, insufficient treatments, and cultural factors that shape how and when people seek help. In most cases, these layered challenges make managing the condition a much more nuanced affair, one that mixes medical, social, and even psychological insights. Recognizing this complex interplay isn't just academic—it's a vital step toward reshaping health policies and care models that better serve those affected. Handling leprosy reactions goes beyond simply prescribing corticosteroids; it demands a broader system that ensures people stick to their treatment regimes. You see, different healthcare setups can result in varied outcomes, Indonesia's public insurance program, for example, has increased care access despite struggles like sporadic medication availability and regulatory tangles, while India's targeted subsidy system delivers intensive, specialist care even though it's not without its own coverage and resource hiccups (Putri et al., 2025). Interestingly, advances in related areas, such as less invasive procedures in chronic pain management, point toward innovative ways to reduce disability and boost quality of life for many patients. Ultimately, combining smart clinical interventions with system-level reforms and a real focus on patient needs seems to be the comprehensive strategy required to curb nerve damage and pave a better path for long-term recovery (Figure 8.2).

8.1. Types of Leprosy Reactions

Leprosy is a complex condition, and diving into its clinical impact means noticing how the immune system sometimes overreacts, induceing what people call leprosy reactions. The body's fight against *Mycobacterium leprae* or *Mycobacterium lepromatosis* can go into overdrive, leading to sudden bouts of inflammation that alter the disease's course. Different reactions, which can stem from either a cell-driven process or from immune complexes, keep things unpredictable. In most cases, these variations hint at deeper immune dysfunction that call for custom treatments. Getting the right diagnosis is key—not only to ease inflammation but also to protect nerves and avoid disability; clear clinical and immunological checks are, generally speaking, a must in effective care. Think about Type 1, or the so-called reversal reaction. This one tends to emerge in borderline cases, when the immune response shifts suddenly to better spot and attack the bacteria. Often, existing skin spots get red and swollen and nerves may also puff up, if not managed well, acute neuritis could set in, damaging nerve function. Marked by a surge in pro-inflammatory cytokines, this reaction can ramp up local tissue damage even as it hints that the body is, in a way, rallying its defenses. Often, quick use of corticosteroids helps to calm the situation, reducing inflammation and keeping permanent nerve issues at bay (Putri et al., 2025). However, there's the Type 2 reaction, which covers events like erythema nodosum leprosum (ENL). Quite distinct, this reaction comes from immune complex deposits that trigger widespread inflammation throughout the body. Typically seen in lepromatous leprosy, it reflects a humoral immune hiccup, affecting the skin and nerves, and causing fever along with other systemic symptoms. In this case, circulating antigen-antibody complexes kick off a complex, multi-organ flare-up that complicates the disease, often needing long-term, varied treatment. While corticosteroids are still a go-to, new treatments aimed directly at the errant immune pathways are under exploration. Regional differences in healthcare often mean that diagnosing and treating these reactions can be hit or miss—underscoring that integrated care plans, matched to local resources and patient needs, are important (Putri et al., 2025).

8.1.1. Type 1 Reactions (Reversal Reactions)

The way our body handles leprosy has a huge impact on the kinds of symptoms and complications that show up. Type 1, or reversal reactions, tend to hit in those borderline cases - you can think of it as a sudden surge in the cell-based defense against *Mycobacterium leprae*. Sometimes old skin spots flare up with redness and swelling, and nerves get tender or puffy, which may quickly result in nerve issues. In reality, this immune jump isn't a clear win; while it may hint at a bounce-back in defense, it can also lead to stubborn nerve damage if the reaction isn't detected and managed quickly. Generally speaking, since the symptoms can show up in all sorts of ways, detecting these changes early is key to avoiding lasting disability and other problems (Aftab et al., 2016). When it comes to handling these Type 1 reactions, the main goal is to calm down the inflammation so the nerves stay safe, all while keeping up a solid antimicrobial fight against the infection. Prednisolone – a well-known corticosteroid – is often the go-to because it cuts down on inflammation and eases nerve pain and swelling during these episodes. In clinical settings, doctors usually mix and match the steroid dosage and treatment time to hit the right balance between effectiveness and avoiding the drawbacks of too-long steroid use. It's not unusual for this care to involve a team effort, with skin and nerve experts chipping in to sort out complications. Research even shows that patients with these reactions often wind up on multiple medication, underlining the need for a broad approach that takes on not just the infection, but also the body-wide inflammatory fallout (Aathawale et al., 2017) (Figure 8.3).

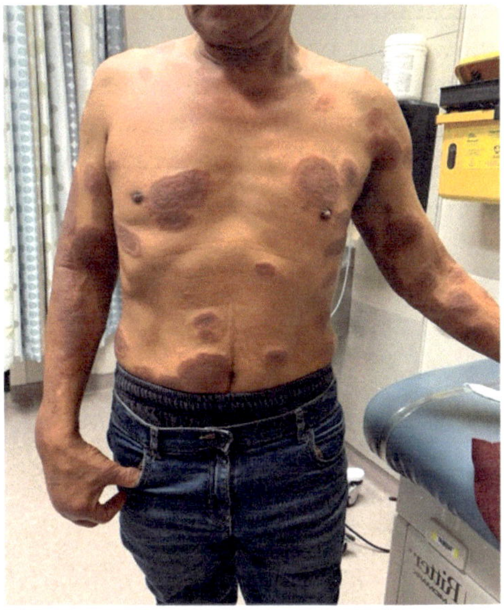

Figure 8.3. A type 1 leprosy reaction in a 50-year-old man with borderline lepromatous leprosy showing numerous asymmetric macules, papules, and plaques with infiltrative borders and central healing. The patient's skin lesions exhibit redness and edema due to the type 1 leprosy reaction.

Source: Canadian Medical Association Journal. (2024). *Type 1 Leprosy Reaction in Borderline Lepromatous Leprosy.*

8.1.2. Type 2 Reactions (Erythema Nodosum Leprosum (ENL))

Leprosy isn't just about the initial microbe—it gets complex once the immune system sets into overdrive during treatment. When treatment stumbles into unexpected immune reactions, patients, especially those with the lepromatous type—can face type 2 lepra reactions, also known as ENL. In most cases, about 90% of these situations emerge either during or shortly after starting multidrug therapy, often within two years. Patients experience painful, red bumps along with symptoms like recurring fever, joint aches, and nerve issues (mononeuritis multiplex), which cause real discomfort and can lead to lasting nerve damage. This response, generally speaking, points to an overactive immune reaction driven by immune complexes, making careful monitoring a must during treatment (Kumar et al., 2024). The presentation of ENL isn't uniform at all—it can swing from mild, sporadic episodes to severe and even unusual forms that throw off the usual pattern. One especially bothersome variant, erythema nodosum leprosum necroticans (ENN), sometimes shows up with ulcerative lesions and heavier systemic symptoms, often delaying diagnosis and upping the risk of further complications. Managing these reactions calls for a delicate balancing act: while corticosteroids typically serve as the front-line defense to calm inflammation, stubborn or intense cases may need an extra push from drugs like methotrexate. This kind of combination therapy can help lesions heal (though sometimes not without a few scars), underscoring the complex double-edged nature of both the condition and its treatment (Alfieri et al., 2024). Getting a handle on type 2 lepra reactions means detecting things early—whether it's those characteristic red nodules, systemic inflammation, or nerve damage—so that irreversible nerve damage can be avoided. Treatment plans need to be tailored to the severity and recurring nature of the reactions, juggling immunosuppressive medication with ongoing anti-mycobacterial therapy. This careful mix helps keep the infection in check without provoking an even stronger immune response. In most cases, the high stakes involved underline why a team-based approach, drawing in dermatologists, neurologists, and immunologists, is so vital. Ongoing research and vigilant follow-up during and after treatment are essential in mitigating these type 2 reactions and improving the quality of life for those affected (Alfieri et al., 2024; Kumar et al., 2024) (Figure 8.4).

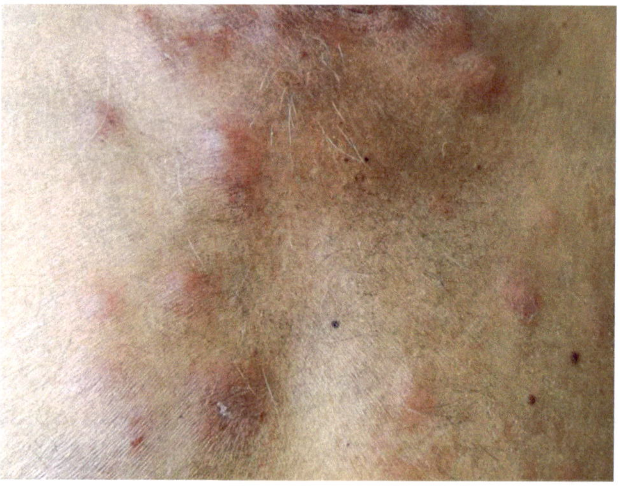

Figure 8.4. Type 2 lepra reaction: Erythema nodosum leprosum.

Source: WebPathology. (n.d.). *Type 2 Lepra Reaction: Erythema Nodosum Leprosum.*

8.1.3. Differences Between the Two Types of Reactions

Leprosy reactions come in two main flavors—Type 1 reactions (T1R) and ENL. Generally speaking, both kinds arise when the immune system sets in against *Mycobacterium leprae* antigens, yet they do so in different ways. Type 1 tends to be a delayed response, driven mainly by cell-based immunity that hits the borderline forms of leprosy. This reaction usually fires up inflammation in pre-existing skin marks and the peripheral nerves, sometimes leading to nerve problems. Then there's ENL.

This form, seen mostly in lepromatous leprosy, is more of a Type 2 hypersensitivity event, where immune complexes deposit in tissues and humoral responses take the spotlight. As a result, ENL often shows systemic signs—fever, painful nodules, and a general feeling of malaise—that set it apart from Type 1. Recognizing these nuanced immune differences is key to proper management and prognosis (Jain et al., 2024). The timing and overall pattern of the two are also quite different. Type 1 reactions usually emerge during or right after the start of multidrug therapy, signaling a shift in the cell-mediated arm of the immune system and induceing localized inflammation along with sudden nerve tenderness. In most cases, ENL is a bit more unpredictable—sometimes it comes back over and over or persists chronically. It typically brings along widespread pain from nodules, fever, and even swollen lymph nodes, all of which hint at broader, systemic involvement. This divergence in clinical presentations drives different treatment plans; corticosteroids are generally preferred to curb the nerve inflammation in Type 1, while ENL often demands agents like thalidomide or other immunomodulators to dampen the overall inflammatory response (Jain et al., 2024). Beyond the immediate clinical signs, both reactions bear deep psychosocial implications that further complicate patient care. While each type causes serious physical discomfort, the unpredictable and recurring nature of ENL often increases psychological stress, anxiety, and even social stigma. Patients with Type 1 may find their activity curtailed by nerve pain and sensory loss, which in time can lead to a gradual disability. In contrast, the systemic issues accompanying ENL not only knock on multiple functional doors—they can also push patients toward social isolation and economic difficulties due to missed work. Studies even reveal cultural twists, as seen in comparisons between Indonesian and Indian patients, where differences in openness, social interaction, and healthcare seeking come to light (Putri et al., 2022). To summarize, a well-rounded treatment plan that mixes clinical steps with psychological support is essential to tackle these multifaceted challenges.

8.2. Pathophysiology of Leprosy Reactions

Immune responses in leprosy show a wild interplay between our body's defenses and the bacteria behind the disease – mainly *Mycobacterium leprae* and *Mycobacterium lepromatosis*. Sometimes during the chronic phase, a reaction suddenly sets in, catching clinicians off guard with its abrupt start and unpredictable intensity. Type 1, or reversal, reactions tend to be driven by a boost in cell-based immunity; for example, a spike in interferon-gamma sets off interleukin-15 and even stimulates autophagy pathways along. This immune surge rouses inflammatory cells to roll into affected skin and nerves, leading to swelling and edema that, if left unchecked, may trigger irreversible nerve damage. In short, these cellular shifts point to the need for quick detection and timely intervention to protect nerve function and ease long-term disability. Digging a little deeper, one finds that leprosy reactions often upset the balance between T helper 17 (Th17) cells and T-regulatory (Treg) cells. In most cases, an overabundance of Th17 cells paired with fewer Treg cells alters cytokine levels – with lower amounts of tumor growth factor-beta and higher levels of interleukin-6 and interleukin-21 – which in turn fans the flames of inflammation and tissue injury. It's not merely a matter of antigen load; these changes reflect a more complex underlying process. Then there's ENL, a type 2 reaction, that seems to involve innate immune actors like neutrophils and myeloid-derived suppressor cells, along with sensors such as Toll-like receptor 9. All these intertwined immune threads help explain why the clinical picture can shift so unpredictably (Putri et al., 2025). Moreover, understanding these multifaceted dynamics is key to effective care. Studies from regions like Indonesia and India reveal that even when public health initiatives expand access to care, challenges like medication shortages, broken information systems, and communication gaps persist. In most cases, merging the microscopic insights with practical improvements in healthcare delivery is essential to curbing nerve damage and reducing disability over time (Putri et al., 2025) (Figure 8.5).

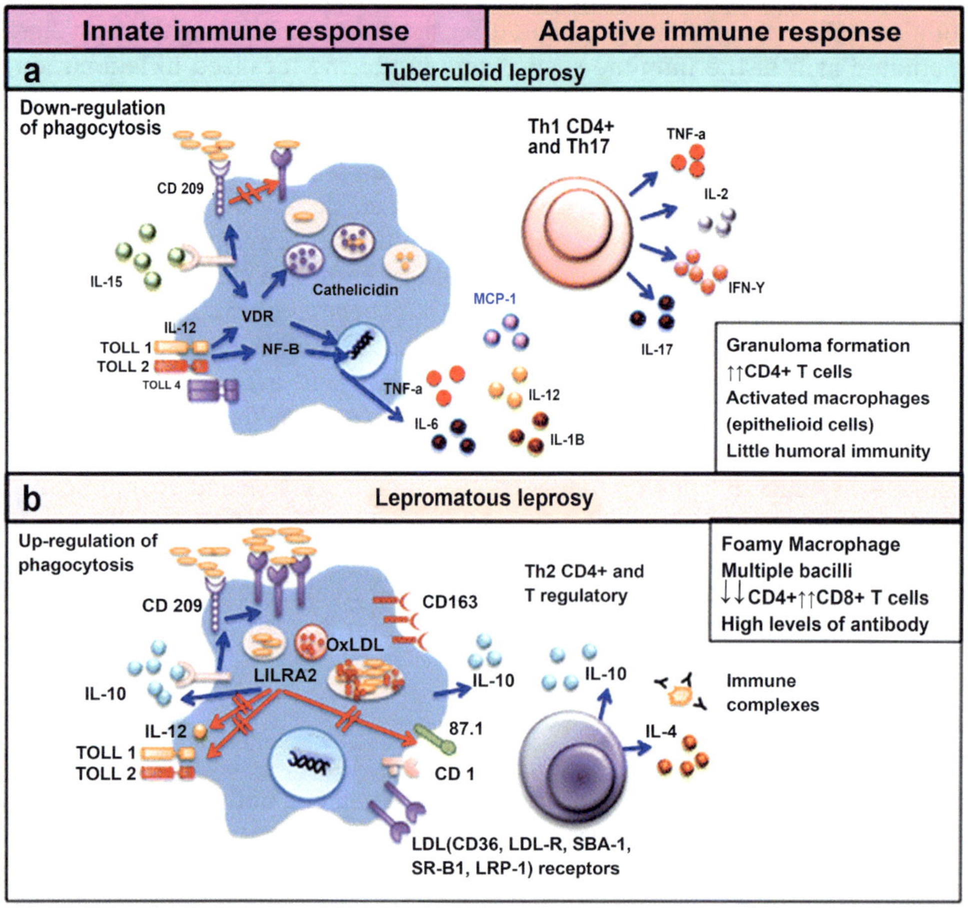

Figure 8.5. Diagram illustrating the immune response to *M. leprae* in Type 1 reaction that leads to erythema, oedema, and tissue injury.

Source: Fonseca, A.B.d.L., Simon, M.d.V., Cazzaniga, R.A. *et al.* The influence of innate and adaptative immune responses on the differential clinical outcomes of leprosy. *Infect Dis Poverty* **6**, 5 (2017). https://doi.org/10.1186/s40249-016-0229-3

8.2.1. Immune Response in Leprosy

Leprosy's course and its clinical outcomes hinge a lot on how each person's immune system reacts—a response that can be wildly different from one individual to the next. Some individuals show a strong cell-driven defense that pretty much keeps *Mycobacterium leprae* under control; in these cases, the infection stays limited to a few spots and is known as paucibacillary (PB) leprosy, meaning there isn't a heavy buildup of bacteria. On the other hand, when the immune system tips more toward a humoral or regulatory mode, the bacteria tend to multiply more freely, leading to multibacillary (MB) leprosy with more aggressive symptoms. Then there's the twist of leprosy reactions, sudden bouts of inflammation that arise when cytokines are thrown out of whack or immune complexes start depositing unexpectedly. Generally speaking, type 1 reactions involve too much cytokine release leading to local flares, whereas types 2 and 3 are marked by immune complex activity that can damage several organs (Héctor et al., 2024).

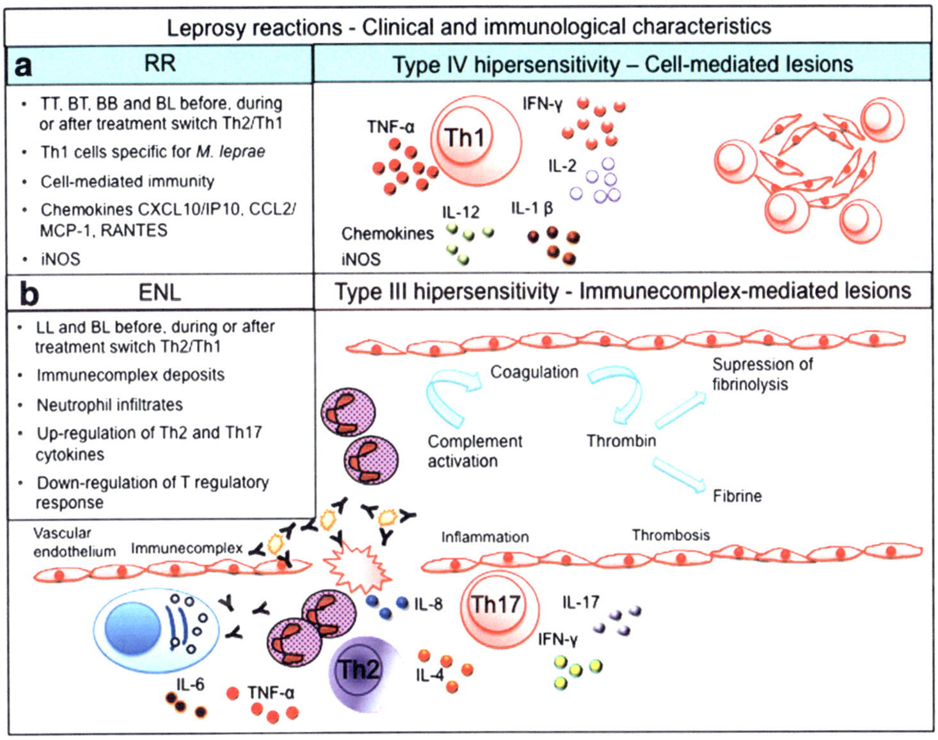

Figure 8.6. Diagram illustrating the immune response in type 1 reaction leading to neuritis and nerve damage.

Source: Fonseca, A.B.d.L., Simon, M.d.V., Cazzaniga, R.A. *et al.* The influence of innate and adaptative immune responses on the differential clinical outcomes of leprosy. *Infect Dis Poverty* **6**, 5 (2017). https://doi.org/10.1186/s40249-016-0229-3

Newer studies digging into the immune environment of leprosy patients have laid out a more nuanced picture of the circulating mediators that steer the disease process. Researchers using multiplex microbead immunoassays have noticed that, in most cases, PB patients tend to have a cytokine mix that leans towards regulation, possibly helping to keep both inflammation and bacterial spread in check. Meanwhile, MB patients often show a spike in pro-inflammatory markers, and that rise usually goes hand in hand with more severe disease. It's also interesting that even household contacts of leprosy patients sometimes have boosted levels of chemokines and cytokines, including IFN-γ, which might offer some protection against prolonged exposure to the bacteria. To summarize, this balancing act between various cytokines seems to not only affect who's likely to get the disease, but also how intense and risky the leprosy reactions might turn out to be (De Carvalho et al., 2024). Detecting these patterns is pretty important for flagging biomarkers that could warn us about impending disease progression or reaction episodes. When you step back and look at it, the immune response in leprosy is a real mixed bag—where both pro-inflammatory and regulatory components interact in unpredictable ways to shape the disease and its complications. Managing leprosy reactions successfully depends on recognizing these immune triggers, whether they stem from a hyperactive cellular response like in type 1 reactions or from immune complex issues seen in types 2 and 3.

In most cases, the key to tailoring treatment lies in understanding these immunologic nuances well enough to lower the inflammation, prevent disability, and generally help patients fare better. Recent advances in immune profiling have undoubtedly opened up promising paths for more targeted therapies, yet bringing these insights into everyday clinical practice still poses a challenge. Ultimately, a comprehensive grasp of immune dynamics remains essential for fine-tuning reaction management in broader leprosy control initiatives and for reducing the long-term consequences (De Carvalho et al., 2024; Héctor et al., 2024) (Figure 8.6).

8.2.2. Role of Cytokines in Leprosy Reactions

Leprosy reactions kick off a wild immune response that isn't as straightforward as one might hope. Even when treatments knock out *Mycobacterium leprae* effectively, the body's counterattack can sometimes go overboard and hurt its own nerves. Researchers looking at skin and nerve samples have noticed that levels of certain molecules, like TNF-α, TGF-β, and even the enzyme that makes nitric oxide—tend to spike. These markers, working in tandem, seem to fuel both the inflammation and the nerve damage; basically, the same system designed to protect ends up causing harm. High bacterial counts hanging around along with these surges in cytokines make it clear that there might be other factors at play. In most cases, trying to lower this excessive cytokine production could be a useful strategy to reduce nerve injury and improve patient outcomes (Lockwood et al., 2011). Over time, our ability to profile immune markers has opened up the conversation about what's going on in leprosy reactions. Recent studies using bead-based tests have found that the mix of plasma cytokines isn't one-size-fits-all. In many instances, for Type 1 reactions, molecules like CXCL10 and IL-6 seem to be on the rise, hinting at a more aggressive immune response. By contrast, Type 2 reactions show more of a combination—IL-6 still features prominently, but there are also boosts in IL-7 and PDGF-BB, and this suggests that each reaction type has its unique signature.

Basically, these cytokines are not only messengers in the disease process, but they might also serve as signals for diagnosis and keeping track of how patients respond to treatment (Moubasher et al., 2009). Knowing exactly how cytokines drive these processes is key for creating better management plans to stop irreversible nerve damage. The way pro-inflammatory and growth factor signals shift around seems connected to both the severity and look of the disease. Detecting causes like TNF-α, IL-6, and CXCL10 gives a solid reason to try therapies that can alter their effects. When doctors start checking cytokine levels routinely, treatments might be tailored more to each person's immune profile, hopefully fine-tuning the timing and choice of immunomodulators. To summarize, ongoing work into these cytokine pathways holds real promise for cutting down the damage associated with leprosy reactions and for boosting long-term outcomes (Moubasher et al., 2009; Lockwood et al., 2011) (Figure 8.7).

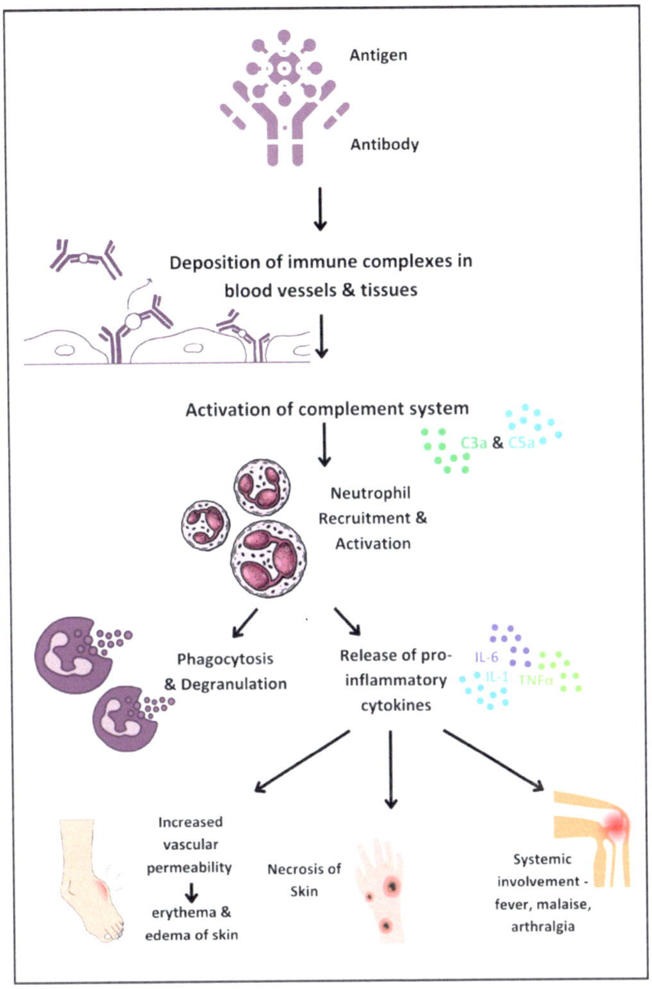

Figure 8.7. Diagram illustrating the immunopathogenesis of type 2 reactions.

Source: Indian Journal of Dermatology, Venereology and Leprology. (2024). *Immunopathogenesis of Type 2 Reactions.*

8.2.3. Impact of Leprosy Reactions on Nerve Function

Leprosy can trigger a tangle of reactions when the body fights off *Mycobacterium leprae*, and these events tend to interefere with nerve function in unexpected ways. You might see things split into two main types—Type 1, which individuals often call a reversal reaction, and Type 2, known as erythema nodosum leprosum. In most cases, the inflammation flares up suddenly, chipping away at the nerve's insulation and injuring its fibers. This immune-driven flare can lead to a loss of feeling, weak muscles, and even hiccups in the body's automatic processes. If the problem isn't detected and managed quickly, the damage might become permanent, raising the risk of deformities and disability. Generally speaking, the intensity and frequency of these episodes are a big deal in deciding the extent of nerve injury, making it essential to understand these reactions to develop long-term care plans (Calderone et al., 2024; Putri et al., 2025). Diagnosing problems stemming from leprosy reactions isn't always straightforward. Patients might first notice just a slight tingling or a bit of tenderness in a spot, only for symptoms to suddenly ramp up during a reaction. The mix of nerve swelling, poor blood flow, and fibrous tissue formation tends to complicate nerve signals, which further worsens the deficits. This slow-but-steady decline calls for quick intervention so further injury can be nipped in the bud. While corticosteroids are usually the go-to to ease the inflammation and try to keep the nerves working, some people still end up with persisting issues despite the best treatments. All these factors point to the need for treatment plans that are as individual as the patients themselves, with a close watch on those earliest signs of nerve damage, since they shape the overall outcome (Calderone et al., 2024). Beyond the immediate nerve damage, factors like how easy it is to access healthcare and how well patients know about their condition add another layer of complication. In many endemic regions, the way healthcare is set up—public insurance, resource availability, and even social support systems—can seriously influence how fast these reactions get spotted and treated. For example, if access to corticosteroids or other therapies is limited by resource allocation issues, nerve damage might run its course unchecked. On top of that, psychological and social hurdles sometimes delay people from seeking care, which can only make nerve impairment worse. Adjusting healthcare delivery to overcome these hurdles, with better patient counseling, earlier diagnoses, and care plans that mix medical and social support—seems pretty crucial for protecting nerve health during these reaction episodes (Putri et al., 2025) (Figure 8.8).

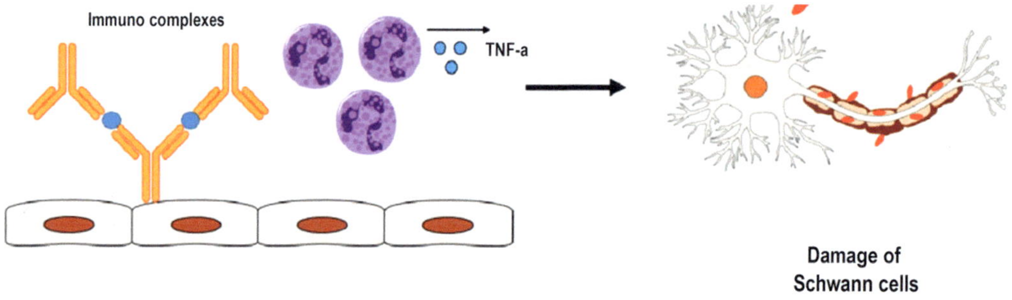

Figure 8.8. Type 2 leprosy reaction (T2LR) as an indirect mechanism of nerve damage.

Source: Cardona-Castro, N. (2018). *Type 2 Leprosy Reaction (T2LR) as an Indirect Mechanism of Nerve Damage*. ResearchGate.

8.3. Diagnosis of Leprosy Reactions

Identifying leprosy reactions quickly is crucial to prevent lasting nerve damage and help patients do better. Doctors usually rely on clinical checks; for example, a sudden flare in skin lesions or a noticeable shift in nerve sensitivity might signal an immune reaction. Systems like the Ridley-Jopling grouping, along with WHO standards, help outline the various disease stages and reaction types, guiding clinical decisions. In practice, tests such as slit-skin smears to spot *Mycobacterium leprae* are followed by checking for any loss of feeling, which offers signals about nerve involvement. Still, clinical indicators can sometimes be unclear, especially when disease progression or secondary infections complicate the issue. Generally speaking, recent advances in molecular tests seem promising by making early, subclinical detection more reliable. Combining these modern tools with time-tested methods often paves the way for starting multidrug and immunomodulatory treatments early, which is key to cutting down on disabilities (Tjouwardi & & Angelica, 2025). It's not just about lab tests, though. Even though clinical and bacteriological evaluations form the backbone of diagnosing leprosy reactions, real-world challenges often stand in the way of smooth diagnosis. In endemic areas like Indonesia and India, healthcare delivery is affected by fractured information systems, a scarcity of specialized professionals, and limited medication supplies—all factors that tend to delay diagnosis and worsen patient outcomes. People's habits when seeking care, influenced by cultural and socioeconomic factors, also add unexpected twists to the process. For instance, comparative studies from Indonesia and India show that public health insurance and subsidy programs can have variable impacts on access to proper evaluation and steady follow-up care. When you look at it, diagnosing leprosy reactions has to be seen in the context of broader healthcare hurdles and opportunities for improvement (Putri et al., 2025). Bringing together a full diagnosis of leprosy reactions means taking a multidisciplinary approach that weaves in both clinical and psychosocial elements. Early detection hinges on a healthcare system that can offer integrated care—prompt clinical checks paired with the right medications, like corticosteroids or other alternatives, are essential. A little counseling and patient education can work wonders, reassuring patients and helping them recognize the symptoms earlier, even if they repeat themselves in conversation. Setting up routine screening programs and training local health workers can further reduce delays and lessen the risk of permanent nerve damage. Financial assistance, such as targeted aid and expanded insurance coverage, also plays a role in ensuring timely diagnosis and better treatment results. In most cases, enhancing diagnostic methods for leprosy reactions isn't solely about clinical or technological advancements—it's also about smart health policy adjustments that consider local context and patient needs (Putri et al., 2025; Tjouwardi & & Angelica, 2025).

8.3.1. Clinical Assessment and History Taking

Doctors usually start out by asking lots of questions – not in a textbook order, but more like getting to know the story behind the symptoms. They ask when things began, how the changes unfolded, and what treatments had been tried before; all this turns out to be especially key in cases where leprosy triggers a reaction. The mix between a person's defenses and *Mycobacterium leprae* is anything but straightforward, so getting the timing and feel of the symptoms right can often hint at whether it's a Type 1 or even sometimes a Type 2 reaction (generally speaking, this makes a real difference). And it's not just about the now—doctors need to dig into any past experiences with medications, because managing leprosy often means juggling several drugs that each come with their own characteristics and side effects. In many instances, paying attention to skin problems caused by these drugs (Surekha et al., 2025) can help ensure nothing gets missed that might lead to a mistaken diagnosis or a wrong treatment alter. A good exam doesn't stop at asking questions – it goes hand in hand with a hands-on check-up. In practice, this means taking a close look at skin lesions, testing nerve responses, and being watchful for any signs of body-wide inflammation that might complicate things further. Sometimes, there may be subtle hints like issues in the mouth or other parts of the body that echo what's been observed in other immune-related skin issues (Surekha et al., 2025). Often, doctors will also check on a person's nutrition and basic metabolism, because these everyday factors can influence how a reaction shows up and how robust a patient might be. This scattered yet careful approach can then lead to a treatment plan that might include corticosteroids or even immunomodulators, all tailored to what's going on with the patient – trying to ease tissue damage and avoid long-term disability. It turns out that understanding a patient's history isn't only about symptoms and drugs - sometimes the environment and what someone eats can also stir up the situation. Even though leprosy is mainly about bacteria and the body's immune response, metabolic hiccups or not getting enough nutrients can sometimes push the reaction into a more complicated realm. You might even see a similar pattern in veterinary cases, where diet issues seem to trigger extra complications in animals. Bringing that idea into human care, it makes sense for doctors to ask casually about eating habits and any known metabolism problems - a broader look like this can uncover hidden influences and steer the care in a more rounded direction. To summarize, this mix of focused medical checks and a look at the everyday factors helps ensure that both the main disease and any secondary issues are addressed, boosting the overall management of the reaction and, ultimately, the patient's quality of life (Figure 8.9).

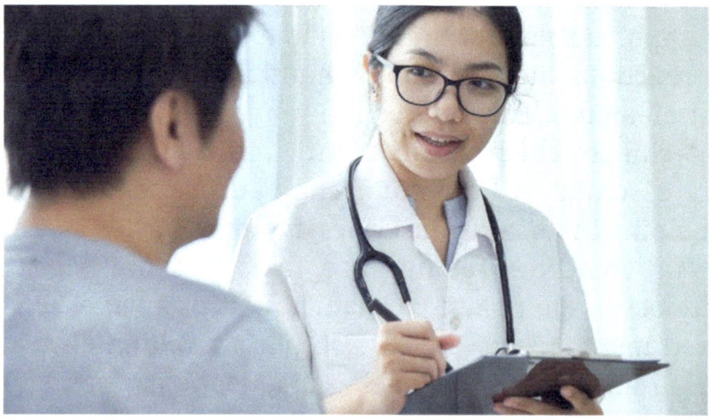

Figure 8.9. The clinical assessment and history taking.

Source: University of Reading. (n.d.). *The Clinical Assessment and History Taking.*

8.3.2. Laboratory Tests and Imaging Techniques

Timely lab tests make a difference when figuring out leprosy reactions. Quick results aren't just numbers—they show us what the immune system is up to and how inflamed a patient might be. Traditionally, tests like skin smears and histopathology have been front and center for detecting *Mycobacterium leprae*, but these days, extra markers such as acute phase reactants and cytokine profiles sometimes help us differentiate a reaction from a slow buildup of disease. These indicators, by flagging heightened immune activity, give signals about the severity of both Type 1 and Type 2 reactions, stimulating clinicians toward the right immunomodulatory treatments. Routine panels—complete blood counts and liver function tests, also come in handy for watching drug toxicity during multidrug therapy. Even so, lab results need to be read alongside a doctor's own judgment, because occasionally the immune shifts are so subtle that only a careful look, in the light of emerging therapies, will uncover their true meaning (Saccomanno, 2025). Imaging, on the other hand, adds its own flavor to the whole picture, especially when nerves are in the mix. Take ultrasonography or magnetic resonance imaging (MRI): they often bring to light nerve inflammation, edema, and even granuloma formation, all of which tend to show up in Type 1 reversal reactions and nerve abscesses. High-resolution ultrasonography, in particular, can track peripheral nerve thickening and changes in vascularization in a non-invasive way. This sometimes means catching things early—before nerve damage becomes permanent. In some instances, radiography even reveals bone resorption and deformities from chronic neuropathy, painting a fuller picture of tissue involvement. Not every leprosy patient gets these imaging studies, but when reaction episodes are suspected, such exams help nail down the degree of inflammation and guide decisions on using corticosteroids or immunosuppressives to ward off long-term disability (Saccomanno, 2025). Lately, there's been a push toward predictive models that combine clinical and lab data for a sharper forecast of inflammatory conditions; similar ideas could be applied to leprosy reactions. Machine learning tools, for example, have shown some promise by predicting disease severity and treatment outcomes early, often without needing a whole battery of tests. By combining basic patient traits with clinical details, these systems take a kind of personalized approach that could change early triage and management. Although most tests so far have been in conditions like acute pancreatitis, many believe that adapting these models for leprosy reactions might improve how risks are sorted, get resources allocated more wisely, and prompt faster therapeutic responses. This gradual shift towards data-driven decision-making hints at a future where lab tests, imaging, and patient history all join forces to boost patient outcomes (Figure 8.10).

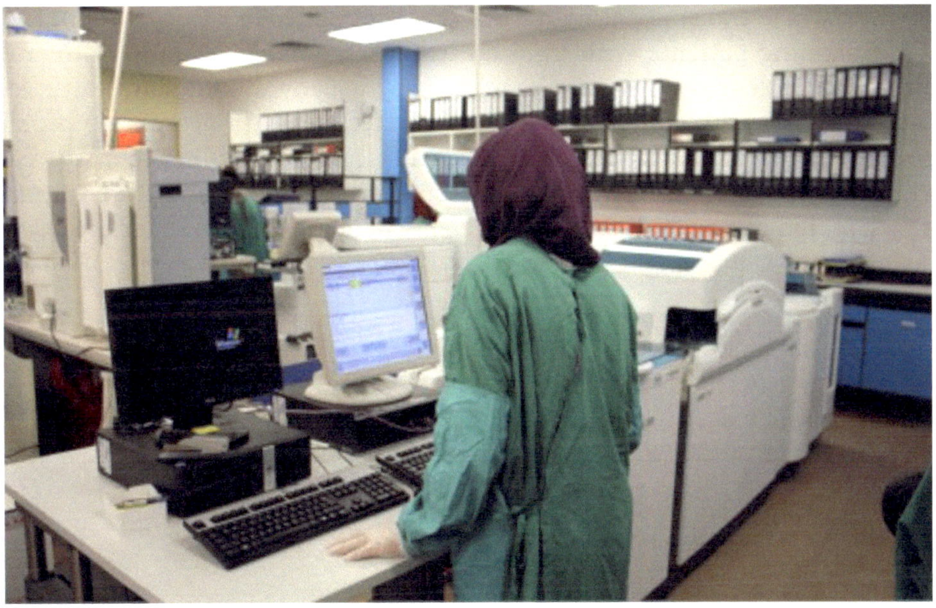

Figure 8.10. The laboratory tests and imaging techniques.

8.3.3. Differential Diagnosis of Leprosy Reactions

Leprosy reactions often prove to be quite a challenge to sort out from other skin and nerve problems. It's not a neat process, since, generally speaking, the reactions, like the reversal reaction (Type 1) or erythema nodosum leprosum (Type 2)—tend to show signs that mix together painful lesions, swollen nerves, and broad, systemic complaints. Sometimes the picture ends up looking a lot like infections such as tuberculosis, sarcoidosis, or even vasculitis, all of which share similar immune irregularities. The chronic nature of leprosy, in most cases, leads to delays in diagnosis, especially outside regions where the disease appears often—making it all the more important that doctors take a good look at a patient's history (including where they're from and any exposures) along with a detailed exam, to steer treatment before any irreversible nerve issues set in. Sometimes, the best way to untangle the mess is by peering into a biopsy. Tissue samples often provide signals, like clear hints of *Mycobacterium leprae*, clusters of granulomas, and signs of how the immune system is reacting at the site, which help in putting things in order. Typically, when a Type 1 reaction is going on, you see a ramped-up cell response, with granulomas coming together and some edema along for the ride; meanwhile, Type 2 reactions often show immune complex build-up and a rush of neutrophils. Still, digging through biopsy results isn't always straightforward since other issues like cutaneous tuberculosis or certain fungal infections might mimic these patterns. Increasingly, molecular and serological tests have stepped in as valuable helpers—detecting things like antibodies to phenolic glycolipid-I and other *M. leprae* markers—thus sharpening early diagnosis and helping differentiate leprosy reactions from other disorders (Fabri et al., 2016). The many faces of leprosy, with its varied immune responses, make it even more of a puzzle for clinicians. In many cases, immunological tests that pinpoint antibodies against particular *M. leprae* antigens step in as valuable tools to flag active disease and keep tabs on reactions, which is especially useful in regions where the disease transmits at high rates (Fabri et al., 2016). Doctors should be especially cautious when examining patients with unusual lesions, particularly those with travel histories or roots in places where leprosy is more common. They usually mix hints from the clinical exam, microscopic evaluations, and blood tests to rule out other similarly presenting problems such as lupus or rheumatoid arthritis. Ultimately, quickly and accurately telling leprosy reactions apart from similar diseases is key to preventing permanent nerve damage and ensuring that treatment is appropriately targeted calling for a collaborative effort among multiple specialists, which, frankly, isn't always as efficient as one might hope (Figure 8.11).

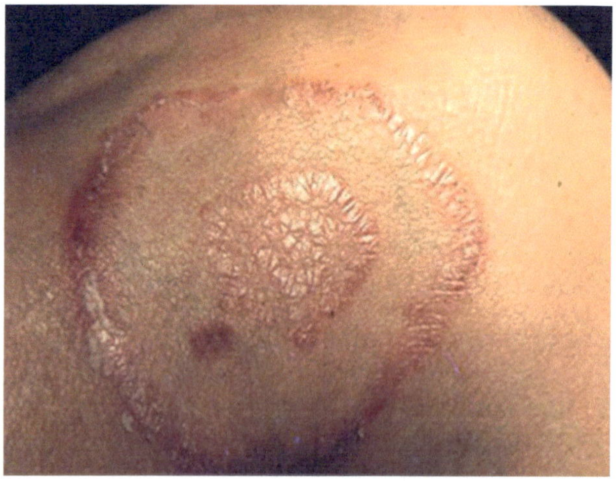

Figure 8.11. The differential diagnosis of leprosy reactions.

Source: Springer Nature. (n.d.). *The Differential Diagnosis of Leprosy Reactions.*

8.4. Management Strategies for Leprosy Reactions

Managing leprosy reactions isn't just about treating symptoms, it calls for a combination of clinical care with broader social and system-wide fixes. Patients sometimes hit real roadblocks in getting timely help, which can lead to delays and even permanent nerve issues. Healthcare infrastructure needs a boost, like steady drug supplies and better, more relaxed channels between providers and patients. Public health insurance, for instance, plays a big role in lessening the financial strain on individuals. A peek at Indonesia and India shows different angles: Indonesia tends to have wider insurance coverage that opens doors for many, whereas India tends to offer targeted subsidies for those who need it. All this points to the idea that combining money support, education, and simple logistics is key for managing these reactions in most cases (Putri et al., 2025). When it comes to medicines, corticosteroids are pretty much the go-to for calming inflammation and helping to avoid nerve damage. Still, long-term use of these medication stirs up worries about side effects and makes the push for alternative treatments. More and more, treatment plans are leaning on extra agents , aiming to spare corticosteroids, cut down on toxicity, boost how well patients stick to their regimen, and adjust to how severe or recurring the reactions might be. Continuous clinical monitoring remains crucial, too, since catching a reaction early means treatment can be adjusted on the fly. And it's not just about the drugs; combining in a dose of counseling and psychological support helps tackle the emotional and social challenges these patients face (Putri et al., 2025). New therapies and customized treatment plans offer hope, but they also come with their own set of complexities much like those seen in other chronic inflammatory issues. Take, for example, immunomodulatory agents such as Janus kinase inhibitors: they've shown promise for easing skin inflammation, yet they often require careful dosing and sometimes need backup therapies to avoid unwanted effects. Shifting these advances into leprosy care calls for a cautious, patient-tailored approach, one that weighs benefits against risks. Combining new pharmaceutical options with tried-and-true methods, along with supportive care, might just tip the scales toward better outcomes; however, ongoing research and vigilant clinical attention remain essential for fine-tuning these strategies.

8.4.1. Pharmacological Treatments

Timing is key when it comes to handling leprosy reactions. In most cases, doctors jump into action with medications that quickly calm the severe inflammation these patients face. Corticosteroids, for example, are the go-to option since they are powerful anti-inflammatory agents that help prevent nerve damage and reduce disability. Yet, getting these drugs isn't always straightforward—healthcare systems can complicate access, and patients sometimes struggle with sticking to their regimens. Look at Indonesia and India: in one place, a broad public insurance plan may spread the available treatments wide enough, even though occasional drug shortages can emerge; in another, targeted subsidies funnel resources to the most critical cases while a lack of specialized healthcare personnel holds back smooth delivery. It's clear that these differences, often under a complex web of systemic challenges, call for adapting drug strategies to the overall healthcare framework (Putri et al., 2025). Besides relying on corticosteroids, there's also growing interest in other medications that might give better overall results and carry fewer long-term side effects. Researchers are testing immunomodulatory drugs, like thalidomide and clofazimine, which seem to do a good job handling cases of erythema nodosum leprosum, the leprosy reaction that comes with painful skin bumps and a range of systemic symptoms. Generally speaking, developing extra therapies to target the immune system's weak spots could help, especially in cases where steroids just don't cut it. And when you consider that leprosy isn't only an immune problem but sometimes involves metabolic complications as well, new treatment paths suddenly appear. For instance, some recent work points to hypouricemic agents like Quercetin Phytosome™ (a drug usually used for cardiovascular and metabolic issues) as a potential partner in lowering harmful systemic inflammation—thanks to its antioxidant and anti-inflammatory traits. Researchers even propose that by pairing traditional therapies with these emerging drugs, we might break the ongoing cycle of chronic inflammation and unwanted side effects, potentially setting a new standard in treatment (Pierro et al., 2025). Rolling out these drug treatments means more than just having effective medications on hand; it also involves tackling deeper, systemic hurdles. It's not just the biology of the disease at play, but also factors like health insurance, doctor–patient communication, and culturally sensitive patient education that matter a ton. In Indonesia, for example, a broad insurance system does help improve access, but complex regulations and fragmented healthcare services sometimes make it tough to keep drug supplies consistent. Meanwhile, India's approach—prioritizing the most severe cases with targeted subsidies—is often hampered by a shortage of skilled healthcare workers to deliver specialized care. Taking on these broader challenges, along with offering timely counseling and patient guidance, can boost treatment success by detecting reactions early, getting therapy started fast, and helping patients stick with their plans. At its core, effective treatment is as much about building trust and clear communication as it is about the medicines themselves, and this dual strategy ultimately works toward reducing nerve damage and disability among leprosy patients (Putri et al., 2025) (Figure 8.12).

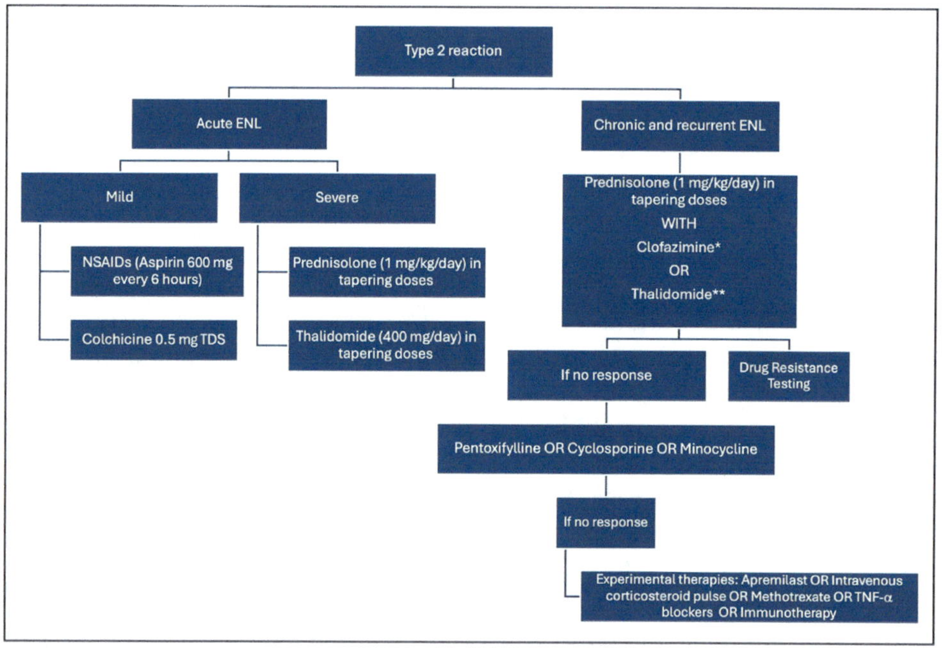

Figure 8.12. Management of type 2 leprosy reactions.

Source: Indian Journal of Dermatology, Venereology and Leprology. (2024). *Management of Type 2 Leprosy Reactions.*

8.4.2. Non-Pharmacological Interventions

Treating leprosy reactions isn't just about relying on drugs anymore. There's a growing shift where individuals now look at other ways to ease pain and inflammation, methods that have been kind of overlooked in the past. Physical activities, like a bit of guided exercise or simple physiotherapy, can keep nerves working well and might even ward off disability by boosting blood flow and easing stiffness in the limbs. Patient education, too, plays its part by helping people notice early warning signs and stick to their treatment plans, which may help dodge serious complications. To summarize, this more well-rounded approach not only tackles pain but also aims to improve everyday life and maybe even bring down some of those healthcare bills. Mind-body techniques are slowly slipping into everyday care for leprosy patients, as evidence keeps piling up about their help with pain and stress. Techniques like mindfulness meditation, guided imagery, and relaxation exercises are showing promise in easing both the mental burden and physical discomfort connected to flare-ups, and, generally speaking, they might even help balance the immune response, which is pretty important given the complex nature of these reactions. Doctors' support is key here, though sometimes limited training or a packed schedule can get in the way. Still, when these practices join forces with regular treatments, they can boost how well patients follow their plans and ease the severity of the reactions, leading to a more patient-centered approach (Barut et al., 2024). Changes in technology and global teamwork are also shaking up how we view non-drug treatments for chronic inflammation, leprosy reactions included. International research now hints that approaches like hydrotherapy and acupuncture, even a therapeutic dip or some targeted needling, could help ease nerve pain and inflammation without piling on more medications. For example, a session in a warm pool might reduce swelling and help joints move better, while acupuncture could offer a hand in managing neuropathic pain. Of course, more cross-border studies and a closer link between clinicians and researchers are needed to iron out standard protocols and get these methods working at their best. Embracing these mixed approaches could eventually shift care away from an over-reliance on drugs, addressing rehab needs that so often go unmet (Barut et al., 2024).

8.4.3. Importance of Multidisciplinary Care

Managing complex health problems isn't always a neat process. When a patient faces something as unpredictable as a leprosy reaction, you often need input from various corners of medicine—skin experts, nerve specialists, and immune system pros—to get a real handle on things. In many cases, bringing in different experts helps spot issues that might otherwise slip by unnoticed. Specialists pooling their views can often nail down the right diagnosis and even shape a treatment plan that feels personal. This kind of collaborative effort isn't just about ticking boxes; it means watching for hidden comorbidities and complications while staying flexible enough to adjust as the patient's condition changes. It even induces everyday learning among providers, as they pick up insights from one another, which eventually bumps up overall patient care quality (Srinivasan et al., 2024). Team efforts, often known as multidisciplinary teams (or MDTs), do more than care for patients directly—they increase entire ways of working in healthcare. Generally speaking, these groups come together in regular meetings to chat about test results and weigh different treatment options, reaching a consensus that's both evidence-based and patient-focused. Sometimes, in conditions like leprosy reactions where catching changes early can mean avoiding permanent nerve damage, these huddles help steer clear of unnecessary tests while zeroing in on the right interventions. In most cases, this shared strategy not only builds a safer, quicker response to disease but also sets up standardized care practices that keep things fair for everyone involved (Cui et al., 2024). Overall, the team's ongoing alters and improvements help refine both patient outcomes and how institutions run day-to-day. Leprosy reactions come with their own weight of challenges—stigma, disability, and a whole lot of emotional stress, which makes a team-based approach even more important. By looping in social workers, physiotherapists, and mental health professionals along with the medical crew, care becomes more than just treating symptoms; it's about supporting the whole person. Really, it's about making sure patients can move toward physical recovery while feeling more connected to their community, easing the heavy burden of disease-related stigma. In many cases, this also means detecting early on any hurdles to sticking with treatment and then shaping solutions that consider the patient's social and economic world. Hence, this kind of patient-focused method—despite a few rough edges and unexpected shifts in rhythm—captures the complex, real-life process of managing a condition, offering hope for more lasting and real-world health improvements (Cui et al., 2024; Srinivasan et al., 2024) (Figure 8.13).

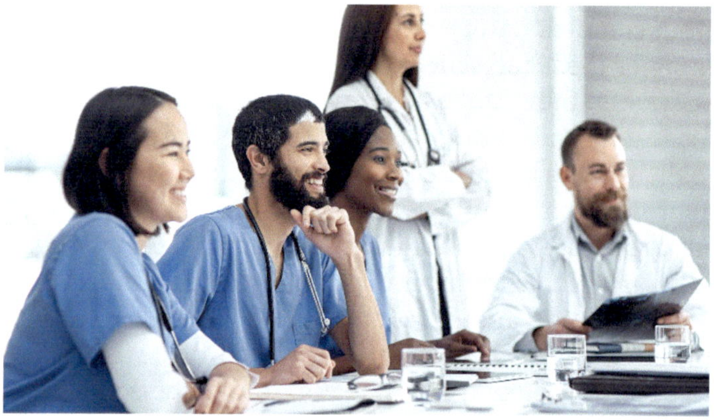

Figure 8.13. Multidisciplinary care.

Source: Partners of Self-Made. (2023). *POSM-June-8. https://posm.org/wp-content/uploads/2023/06/POSM-June-8.png.*

A CLOSER LOOK

LEPROSY NERVE DAMAGE

In leprosy nerve damage may occur at three levels:

- At the level of the cutis (skin) where nerve endings are affected;
- At the level of the subcutaneous nerves; and
- At the level of the nerve trunks.

The histopathology of reactional tuberculoid leprosy shows granuloma formation high in the dermis and dermal papillae. The granulomatous infiltrate sometimes seems even to erode the epidermis but obviously destroys the nerve endings in the papillae. It is not unlikely that the driving forces behind these damaging reactions are antigenic determinants in the epidermis and in the peripheral nerve endings which are similar to those of *M. leprae* antigens. The reaction could be an autoimmune phenomenon.

In borderline leprosy, the nerves of the lower dermis and especially those located around the adnexa are most often involved. Granuloma formation can be seen in and around these nerves together with a proliferation of Schwann cells in and around the perineurium. Damage can be attributed to compression and destruction of nerve fibers by the epithelioid granuloma. During the reactional episode, there is a further influx of immunocompetent cells with edema formation and expanding granuloma. This contributes further to nerve damage, especially when extracellular edema accumulates inside the thickened perineurial sheath, converting it into a rigid compressing tube compromising the axons inside.

The mechanisms that occur in nerve trunks and larger subcutaneous nerves are more complicated. At the tuberculoid end of the spectrum, these processes are similar to those in the skin, with massive granuloma formation with occasional colliquation and abscess formation. Further into the borderline range, these features are usually less distinct and often even absent. Frequently, only edema is observed.

Damage to cutaneous and subcutaneous nerves causes loss of sensation in the affected areas and loss of autonomic nerve function such as sweating and regulation of vascular tone. However, it is the damage to the peripheral nerve trunk which is the major consequence of T1R. This damage is partly caused by immunological reactions, but mechanical factors are also involved. During T1R, inflammation and consequently edema occurs in the nerve, as it occurs in the skin. The reaction leads to edema located within the interstitial tissues of the epi-, peri-, and endoneurium. Unlike the skin, the nerve cannot expand without limit. The perineurium, which is largely impermeable to fluids, forms a rigid compressing tube around the expanding endoneurium. This results in an increase in pressure within the nerve. As a result, the axons in the endoneurium are compressed by the increased pressure. As a consequence, there is a loss of conducting nerve fibers and thus loss of muscular strength, peripheral sensation and autonomic functions. The intra-axonal flow which brings nutrients from the cell to the peripheral nerve ending is interrupted, and sooner or later, the peripheral nerve fiber dies off and is destroyed (Figure 8.14).

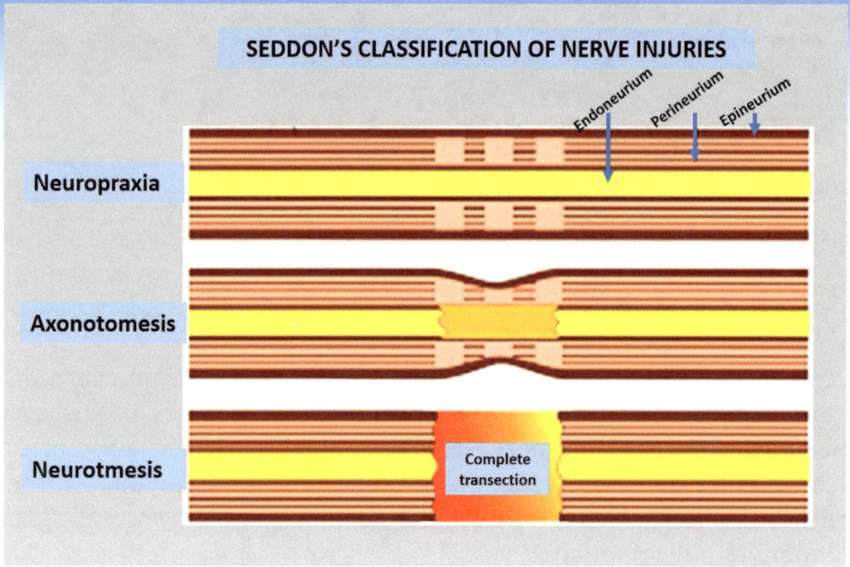

Figure 8.14. Mechanical nerve damage.

Source: By Davplast - File:Nerve_injuries_Armenian.jpg, CC BY-SA 4.0, https://commons.wikimedia.org/w/index.php?curid=73037258

When the pressure and the tension along and within the perineurium increase due to an increase in pressure in the endoneurium, there is an increase in the pressure exerted on the blood vessels which transverse obliquely through the perineurium. These blood vessels are then compressed. The venules with relatively low pressure are compressed more than arterioles with higher pressure. The compression of the venules will lead to higher pressure in the capillaries of the endoneurium, which may start "leaking" and thus increase the pressure in the endoneurium. This "venostatic edema" can maintain itself even when the immunological events subside.

In the histopathology of nerve in T2R, an increase in neural cell adhesion molecules (N-CAM) can be observed, and N-CAM-positive $CD8^+$ cells can be isolated from the tissues. *In vitro* it was shown that, during active T2R, when peripheral blood mononuclear cells (PBMC) were exposed to *M. leprae*, there was an increase in cytolysis of N-CAM-expressing Schwann cells by $CD8^+$ N-CAM-positive cells. It is interesting to note that IL-15 is capable of inducing N-CAM expression and that IL-15 mRNA is increased in leprosy tissues.

In T2R, the mechanisms leading to tissue destruction, which is the activation of granulocytes, also contribute to damage of nerve fibers and endings. It also has been shown that TNF-α, which seems to be a major cytokine involved in T2R, can demyelinize nerve fibers. Demyelination seems to be a major factor in nerve damage due to multibacillary leprosy as shown by nerve conduction studies. The damage in multibacillary leprosy can also be caused by lipoarabinomannan which on its own may lead to demyelination by complement activation and membrane attack complex (MAC) formation when in contact with the Schwann cell. Moreover, in the large nerve trunks, the immunological processes may give rise to venostatic edema with compression of axons as described for T1R.

SUMMARY

Managing leprosy reactions isn't just about the clinical things—you also have to deal with systemic issues and money problems that shape patient outcomes. Many times, treatment means not only testing patients quickly and giving them the right medication, but also making sure they get real, hands-on advice to help lessen nerve damage and disability. Look at what happens in different countries: Indonesia, for example, generally provides wide-ranging public insurance but still wrestles with bureaucratic hold-ups and logistical snags, while in India the care is more focused and specialized for those in deep need, even though it often suffers from resource shortages and insurance gaps (Putri et al., 2025). Sometimes it feels like there's always another layer of challenge added onto the basic clinical issues. Addressing the mental and educational side of treatment is just as important as the medicine itself. The stigma, plus other social hurdles, can discourage people from seeking help early, which only makes complications worse. In most cases, encouraging education that respects cultural backgrounds and fostering honest, relaxed conversations between healthcare individuals and patients can help break down these barriers. Even though you might expect inflammatory markers like IL-6 to show how severe a case might be, recent studies have not found a solid link, instead, a thoughtful look at the patient's history and a good physical exam still hold the most weight (Putri et al., 2024). There's a subtle reminder here that relying too much on one type of data might miss the bigger picture. To summarize, handling leprosy reactions means using a kind of all-around approach that mixes both the medical and socio-economic angles. It calls for better access to care, more reliable availability of medications, and a boost in the abilities of the healthcare workforce, all while adding systems of support that address mental and social needs. Patient education and fighting stigma are key because they help people step forward for treatment sooner and stick to their therapy longer. Future work should watch these different parts come together, with researchers and policy makers teaming up to test new ideas. In the end, crossing these hurdles in varied healthcare settings should lead to better outcomes for patients and lessen the long-term effects of leprosy reactions worldwide (Putri et al., 2025).

Grasping leprosy reactions isn't just academic—it matters for treatment and patient well-being. These reaction bursts, which individuals usually split into Type 1 (reversal reactions) and Type 2 (erythema nodosum leprosum), can emerge before, during, or even after starting multidrug therapy. In most cases, each one calls for a different kind of fix, so nailing the right diagnosis early on becomes key. For instance, corticosteroids typically back Type 1 events, while thalidomide and its kin become the go-to for Type 2, and sometimes you simply can't ignore the need to keep symptoms in check and nerves safe from long-term damage—Further, that balance helps keep disabilities at bay and lifts quality of life. All this pushes a patient-first style that weighs treatment upsides against possible side effects, aligning with today's trends in clinical care and management of complex diseases (Spilnichenko et al., 2024). It isn't enough to just dispense medications; managing these reactions also means keeping a close eye on patients and offering solid support. Detecting a flare-up quickly is fundamental to stopping irreversible nerve damage (which, let's face it, is the most common culprit behind leprosy's long-term harm). In many cases, multidisciplinary teams adjust treatment plans based on how severe the case is and what risks each person carries—pretty much mirroring best practices seen in other conditions, like nosocomial pneumonia, where personalized care and sticking to guidelines work wonders (Rademacher et al., 2024). And don't forget that teaching patients to recognize early signs and stick to their treatment helps keep the disease in check, all while we remember that the social and psychological ups and downs of leprosy must be part of the conversation. When you break it down, managing leprosy reactions turns into a balancing act between careful observation, targeted drug use, and overall patient support. Research generally points to steroids and immune modulators as the heavy hitters, yet it also hints that more work is needed to refine these strategies and curb side effects. Observations drawn from other areas of medicine show that a combination of teamwork and graded evidence can sharpen our treatment decisions (Rademacher et al., 2024). At the same time, newer ways of organizing care are calling for flexible systems that can alter their approach as disease trends and available resources shift—sometimes even in ways that feel a bit improvisational. Ultimately, truly understanding and managing these reactions combines clinical know-how, a focus on individual needs, and a broader health system outlook, ensuring patients get timely, effective, and yes, compassionate care (Spilnichenko et al., 2024).

KEY TERMS FROM THIS CHAPTER

- Alternative treatment plans
- Anxiety
- Cytokines
- Enzyme
- Erythema nodosum leprosum necroticans
- Infection
- Multiplex microbead immunoassays
- Reaction episodes
- Antimicrobial drugs
- Clinical presentations
- Disease progression
- Erythema nodosum leprosum
- Immunomodulators
- Multibacillary (MB) leprosy
- Paucibacillary (PB) leprosy
- Reversal reaction

References

1. Aathawale, S., Kulkarni, M., & Patil, A. (2017). Retrospective analysis of prescriptions in the management of lepra reactions: Results of a single center study from tertiary hospital in Maharashtra. *Asian. J. Pharm. Clin. Res., 10*(5), 191–193. https://core.ac.uk/download/477852811.pdf (accessed on 10th May 2025).
2. Aftab, H., Nielsen, S.D. & Bygbjerg, I.C. Leprosy in Denmark 1980–2010: a review of 15 cases. *BMC Res Notes* **9**, 10 (2016). https://doi.org/10.1186/s13104-015-1768-6(accessed on 10th May 2025).
3. Lockwood, D. N., Suneetha, L., Sagili, K. D., Chaduvula, M. V., Mohammed, I., van Brakel, W., Smith, W. C., Nicholls, P., & Suneetha, S. (2011). Cytokine and protein markers of leprosy reactions in skin and nerves: baseline results for the North Indian INFIR cohort. *PLoS neglected tropical diseases*, *5*(12), e1327. https://doi.org/10.1371/journal.pntd.0001327 (accessed on 10th May 2025).
4. Fabri, A.daC., Carvalho, A. P., Vieira, N. F., Bueno, I.deC., Rodrigues, R. N., Monteiro, T. B., Correa-Oliveira, R., Duthie, M. S., & Lana, F. C. (2016). Integrative literature review of the reported uses of serological tests in leprosy management. *Revista da Sociedade Brasileira de Medicina Tropical*, *49*(2), 158–164. https://doi.org/10.1590/0037-8682-0226-2015 (accessed on 10th May 2025).
5. Calderone, A., Aloisi, M. C., Casella, C., Fiannacca, S., Cosenza, B., Quartarone, A., & Calabrò, R. S. (2024). The neurological impact of leprosy: Manifestations and treatment approaches. *Neurology International*, *16*, 1492–1508. https://www.semanticscholar.org/paper/d47dd289d20848d4de16396e3f9938aaec84e087 (accessed on 10th May 2025).
6. de Carvalho, J. C., Pascoal-Xavier, M. A., Araújo, M. G., Teixeira-Carvalho, A., Martins-Filho, O. A., Peruhype-Magalhães, V., Coelho-Dos-Reis, J. G. A., & Araújo, M. S. S. (2024). Different profiles of chemokines, cytokines and cell growth factors in plasma samples from patients with leprosy, leprosy reactions and households contacts. *Memorias do Instituto Oswaldo Cruz*, *119*, e230129. https://doi.org/10.1590/0074-02760230129(accessed on 10th May 2025).
7. Cui, P., Blanshard, P., Campos-Partera, M. T., Moucquot, A., Naqvi, S. H. R., Dellamonica, D., & Moses, H. (2024). Enhancing multidisciplinary team processes in lung cancer care: A self-assessment toolkit and best practices. *Journal of Clinical Pathways*. J Clin Pathways. 2024;10(1):19-25. doi:10.25270/jcp.2024.01.02(accessed on 10th May 2025).
8. Cygrymus, E. R., & Lent, R. W. (2025). The Roles of Identity-Affirming Behaviors and Self-Efficacy in Coping With Weight Stigma in the Workplace: A Social Cognitive Perspective. *Journal of Career Assessment*, *0*(0). https://doi.org/10.1177/10690727251325855(accessed on 10th May 2025).
9. Dabas, Ravi, Siraj Ansari, Mayur M. Jadav, Vinita Rajpurohit, Asha Yadav, and Yogesh Soni. 2024. "Osteodystrophy Fibrosa in a Goat Kid: Clinical Assessment and Management". *UTTAR PRADESH JOURNAL OF ZOOLOGY* 45 (18):26-29. https://doi.org/10.56557/upjoz/2024/v45i184419.(accessed on 10th May 2025).
10. Deps, P. D., Yotsu, R., Furriel, B. C. R. S., de Oliveira, B. D., de Lima, S. L., & Loureiro, R. M. (2024). The potential role of artificial intelligence in the clinical management of Hansen's disease (leprosy). *Frontiers in medicine*, *11*, 1338598. https://doi.org/10.3389/fmed.2024.1338598(accessed on 10th May 2025).

11. Di Pierro, F., Rabbani, F., Tareen, M., Nigar, R., Khan, A., Zerbinati, N., Tanda, M. L., Cazzaniga, M., Bertuccioli, A., Falasca, P., Damiani, G., & Villanova, N. (2025). Potential pharmacological effect of Quercetin Phytosome™ in the management of hyperuricemia: results from real-life clinical studies. *Frontiers in nutrition*, *12*, 1519459. https://doi.org/10.3389/fnut.2025.1519459(accessed on 10th May 2025).

12. Jain, S., Chhabra, S., Dogra, S., Yadav, R., Chatterjee, D., & Narang, T. (2024). Comparative efficacy of *Mycobacterium indicus pranii* and *bacille Calmette–Guérin* as immunotherapeutic adjuncts in multibacillary leprosy: A clinical and molecular randomized controlled trial. *British Journal of Dermatology*. https://www.semanticscholar.org/paper/766f685660e8563721ae955a0293862f73612478 (accessed on 10th May 2025).

13. Kumar, H., Kumar, S., Mahato, S., & Singh, H. (2024). Erythema nodosum leprosum (type 2 reaction) in a patient with Hansen's disease from a tertiary care hospital in Jharkhand: A case report. *Biomedical and Pharmacology Journal*. https://www.semanticscholar.org/paper/9f49db338f4f9e300ec8e708d2e9b70c7e95d616 (accessed on 10th May 2025).

14. Mehta H, Jain S, Narang T, Chhabra S, Dogra S. Leprosy reactions: New knowledge on pathophysiology, diagnosis, treatment and prevention. Indian J Dermatol Venereol Leprol. doi: 10.25259/IJDVL_915_2024(accessed on 10th May 2025).

15. Moubasher, A. D., Andersson, A. K., Sousa, A. L., Sousa, A. L. M., Bandeira-Melo, C., Milne, C. D., Surh, C. D., et al. (2009). *Potential Plasma Markers of Type 1 and Type 2 Leprosy Reactions: A Preliminary Report*. https://core.ac.uk/download/pdf/8296881.pdf (accessed on 10th May 2025).

16. Niyonkuru, E., Iqbal, M. A., Zhang, X., & Ma, P. (2025). Complementary Approaches to Postoperative Pain Management: A Review of Non-pharmacological Interventions. *Pain and therapy*, *14*(1), 121–144. https://doi.org/10.1007/s40122-024-00688-1(accessed on 10th May 2025).

17. Paganini, C., Mortato, E., Tofani, L., Belcastro, A., Talamonti, M., Di Raimondo, C., Bianchi, L., & Galluzzo, M. (2025). Rosacea-like eruptions associated with upadacitinib in atopic dermatitis: two case reports and management strategies. *Dermatology reports*, 10.4081/dr.2025.10193. Advance online publication. https://doi.org/10.4081/dr.2025.10193(accessed on 10th May 2025).

18. Putri, A. I., de Sabbata, K., Agusni, R. I., Alinda, M. D., Darlong, J., de Barros, B., Walker, S. L., Zweekhorst, M. B. M., & Peters, R. M. H. (2022). Understanding leprosy reactions and the impact on the lives of people affected: An exploration in two leprosy endemic countries. *PLoS neglected tropical diseases*, *16*(6), e0010476. https://doi.org/10.1371/journal.pntd.0010476(accessed on 10th May 2025).

19. Putri, A.I., Peters, R.M.H., De Sabbata, K. *et al.* A socio-ecological model of the management of leprosy reactions in Indonesia and India using the experiences of affected individuals, family members and healthcare providers. *BMC Health Serv Res* **25**, 196 (2025). https://doi.org/10.1186/s12913-025-12340-5(accessed on 10th May 2025).

20. S. N. Putri, F. E. P. Mundhofir, R. Yuniati, N. Wijayahadi, and Y. Nindita, "Correlation between Degree of Leprosy Disability and Serum IL-6 Levels in Patients with Leprosy Reactions: An Observational Study at the Donorojo Jepara Leprosy Hospital Center," *Jurnal Kedokteran Diponegoro (Diponegoro Medical Journal)*, vol. 13, no. 3, pp. 162-166, Jun. 2024. https://doi.

org/10.14710/dmj.v13i3.45004(accessed on 10th May 2025).

21. Rademacher, J., Ewig, S., Grabein, B., Nachtigall, I., Abele-Horn, M., Deja, M., Gaßner, M., et al. (2024). Key summary of Microbean national guideline for adult patients with nosocomial pneumonia—Update 2024: Funding number at the Federal Joint Committee (G-BA): 01VSF22007. *Infection*, *52*, 2531–2545. https://www.semanticscholar.org/paper/fd2fd8362db900b6c698b6030623c22e8b7c6ade (accessed on 10th May 2025).

22. Rashidi, M., Pitton Rissardo, J., Byroju, V. V., Fornari Caprara, A. L., Rashidi, F., Prathiraja, O., Moharam, H., Elendu, C. C., Bahar, M., & Jayasinghe, M. (2025). Exploring the Neurological Manifestations of Leprosy: Clinical Insights and Implications. *Cureus*, *17*(1), e77799. https://doi.org/10.7759/cureus.77799(accessed on 10th May 2025).

23. Saccomanno S, et al. Extrapyramidal Reactions Induced by Dopamine Antagonists: Clinical Management and the Protective Role of Clear Aligners: A Case Report. J Dental Health Oral Res. 2025;6(1):1-6.(accessed on 10th May 2025).

24. Serrano-Coll, H., Wan, E. L., Restrepo-Rivera, L., & Cardona-Castro, N. (2024). Leprosy reactions: Unraveling immunological mechanisms underlying tissue damage in leprosy patients. *Pathogens and disease*, *82*, ftae013. https://doi.org/10.1093/femspd/ftae013(accessed on 10th May 2025).

25. Shields, J., Clough, A., Valenti, E. R., McWhirter, G., Kelley, M. J., & Passero, V. A. (2024). JCO Oncol Pract 20, 111-111(2024).

26. DOI:10.1200/OP.2024.20.10_suppl.111(accessed on 10th May 2025).

27. Sivakumaran, P., Barros, B., Antonio Dias, V. L., Lockwood, D. N., & Walker, S. L. (2024). A retrospective cohort study of monthly rifampicin, ofloxacin and minocycline in the management of leprosy at the Hospital for Tropical Diseases, London, United Kingdom. *PLoS neglected tropical diseases*, *18*(12), e0012699. https://doi.org/10.1371/journal.pntd.0012699(accessed on 10th May 2025).

28. Spilnichenko, V. K., & Kol'tsova, D. I. (2024). Retrospective analysis of approaches to organization management. *Science and Art of Management / Bulletin of the Institute of Economics, Management and Law of the Russian State University for the Humanities*. https://www.semanticscholar.org/paper/1b8f2f26b94d7d3ead8f9758cdaba1a53b0c9d5e (accessed on 10th May 2025).

29. Srinivasan, A. V.[1]; Dureja, G. P.[2]; Banerjee, Tapas Kumar[3]; Chaudhuri, Jaydip Ray[4]; Benny, Rajesh[5]; Archik, Shreedhar[6]; Mascarenhas, Amrithlal A.[7]; Marthala, Pradeep Reddy[8]; Agarwal, Amit Kumar[9]; Shah, Dhara[10]; Rajgopal, Jayesh[11]. Best Practices for the Evaluation and Management of Low Back Pain in Primary Care: A Multidisciplinary Expert Consensus. Indian Journal of Pain 38(1):p 40-50, Jan–Apr 2024. | DOI: 10.4103/ijpn.ijpn_35_23(accessed on 10th May 2025).

30. Surekha, Avvaru[1]; Babu, M. Niranjan[2]; Thejaswini, K.[2]; Vishnupriya, A.[2]; Vishnupriya, Bukke[2]; Yugesh, S.[2]; Kushma, T.[1]. A prospective study of clinical patterns and assessment of causality and severity of cutaneous adverse drug reactions in a tertiary care hospital. Journal of Clinical and Scientific Research ():10.4103/jcsr.jcsr_229_23, March 17, 2025. | DOI: 10.4103/jcsr.jcsr_229_23(accessed on 10th May 2025).

31. Tjouwardi, A. N., & Angelica, V. (2025). THE ANALYSIS STUDY OF DIAGNOSIS AND MANAGEMENT OF LEPROSY: A COMPREHENSIVE SYSTEMATIC REVIEW. *Journal of Advanced Research*

in Medical and Health Science (ISSN 2208-2425), *11*(4), 11-20. https://doi.org/10.61841/e79ews70(accessed on 10th May 2025).

32. Taninokuchi Tomassoni, M., Braccischi, L., Russo, M., Adduci, F., Calautti, D., Girolami, M., Vita, F., Ruffilli, A., Manzetti, M., Ponti, F., Matcuk, G. R., Mosconi, C., Cirillo, L., Miceli, M., & Spinnato, P. (2024). Image-Guided Minimally Invasive Treatment Options for Degenerative Lumbar Spine Disease: A Practical Overview of Current Possibilities. *Diagnostics (Basel, Switzerland)*, *14*(11), 1147. https://doi.org/10.3390/diagnostics14111147(accessed on 10th May 2025).

33. Van Den Bergh, P., Van Doorn, P. A., Hadden, R. D. M., Avau, B., Vankrunkelsven, P., Allen, J. A., Attarian, S., et al. (2021). European Academy of Neurology/Peripheral Nerve Society guideline on diagnosis and treatment of chronic inflammatory demyelinating polyradiculoneuropathy: Report of a joint task force—Second revision. *European Journal of Neurology*, *28*, 3556–3583. https://doi.org/10.1111/ene.14959 (accessed on 10th May 2025).

34. Villasante, S., Fernandes, N., Perez, M., Cordobés, M. A., Piella, G., Martinez, M., Gomez-Gavara, C., Blanco, L., Alberti, P., Charco, R., Pando, E., & Pancreatia Study Collaborators (2024). Prediction of Severe Acute Pancreatitis at a Very Early Stage of the Disease Using Artificial Intelligence Techniques, Without Laboratory Data or Imaging Tests: The PANCREATIA Study. *Annals of surgery*, 10.1097/SLA.0000000000006579. Advance online publication. https://doi.org/10.1097/SLA.0000000000006579(accessed on 10th May 2025).

35. Zidane, Z., Chahine, C., Mohtadi, K., Chakroun, A., Saïle, R., Bousfiha, A. A., Rkain, M., Chaer, S. E., Gueddari, Y. E., Hbibi, M., Daoudi, L. T., Benhsaien, I., Elhafidi, N., & Alj, H. S. (2024). An overview of a preliminary multicenter retrospective study on food and drug allergies in Moroccan pediatric population. *The Pan African medical journal*, *47*, 24. https://doi.org/10.11604/pamj.2024.47.24.41038(accessed on 10th May 2025).

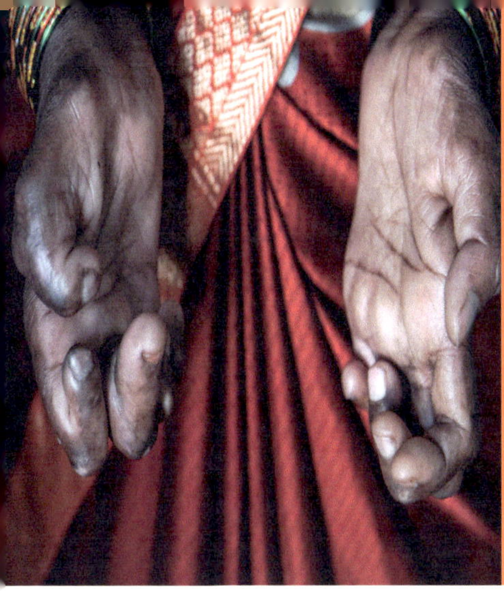

Chapter 9

PUBLIC HEALTH ASPECTS OF LEPROSY

Contents

Introduction

Hansen's disease, better known as leprosy, is a persistent infection from *Mycobacterium leprae* that for ages has been shrouded in stigma and left many struggling with disabilities. Even though modern medicine and public health measures have come a long way, this illness still sticks around, especially where healthcare doesn't run smoothly. Its hidden nature, with a long delay before clear symptoms show up, often means diagnosis and treatment lag behind, which in most cases just makes the spread and resulting disabilities worse. If you look at the global picture, you find that leprosy isn't spread evenly; there are stubborn hot spots in some countries—India, for instance, sees over 100,000 new cases each year. This lopsided distribution hints at deeper social, environmental, and healthcare gaps, pointing to the real need for strategies that are as unique as the communities they serve. Tackling leprosy properly means getting ahead of it with early checks, solid treatment plans, cutting down on the stigma, and preventing disability (Katoch, 2024). India's story with leprosy shows big leaps forward mixed with persistent hurdles. Its battle against the disease is a combination of ancient healing traditions and modern breakthroughs, such as the early use of multi-drug therapy (MDT) that, since the 1980s, has slashed the number of cases by almost 97%. Yet new cases seem to have hit a plateau—an indication there are still cracks in the system like weak surveillance and delays in detecting the disease early on. And, as if that weren't enough, antimicrobial resistance has started to creep in, putting current treatments in jeopardy and stressing the need for a more connected plan that ties clinical care efficiently to public health policies. In most cases, because health challenges vary so widely across regions, the fixes need to be custom-made—boosting health systems, getting communities more involved, and experimenting with fresh diagnostic and preventive tools (Katoch, 2024). When you look at leprosy's impact, it isn't just a clinical concern—it spills over into social, economic, and even environmental realms. The continuing stigma often forces affected individuals to stand apart from society, which makes them hesitant to seek help. Vulnerable groups, especially those living in cramped quarters with poor sanitation, end up paying the heaviest price. On top of that, we still don't have a complete grasp of how environmental factors and transmission routes play their part, which only complicates the issue for eradication efforts. So, a smart public health approach has to step away from a purely medical mindset and start addressing the social factors too—think better education, boosting community support, and policy alters that cut down discrimination. In the end, beating leprosy means pulling a lot of different strands together: early detection, cautious use of antimicrobials, disability prevention, and keeping the public informed through ongoing awareness campaigns—all moving us steadily toward a leprosy-free future (Katoch, 2024) (Figure 9.1).

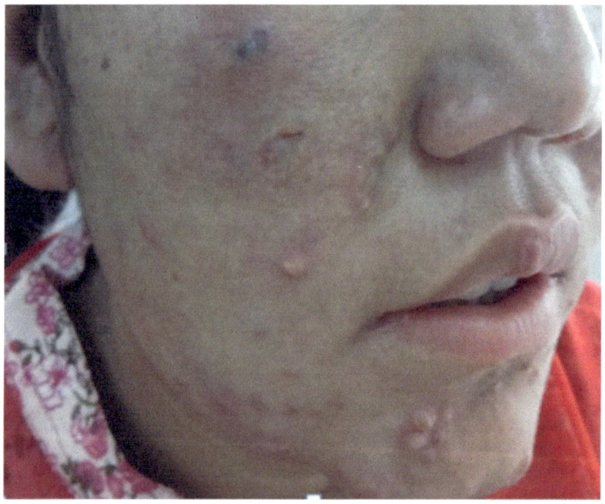

Figure 9.1. The public health aspects of leprosy.

Source: Physio-pedia. (n.d.). *Erythematous Papules Seen in the Face of Patient with Lepromatous Leprosy.* Physio-pedia.

9.1. Symptoms and Clinical Manifestations

Leprosy often shows up in a very understated way—almost as if it's trying not to be noticed. Subtle skin changes, like pale or slightly reddish patches that lose feeling, come first; these sensory gaps happen because the bacterium *Mycobacterium leprae* has a tendency for getting into the peripheral nerves, interfering with how pain and temperature are felt. You might also see those certain nerves, for example, around the ulnar, median, or even the back part of the leg—seem a bit thicker than normal. Left unchecked, that enlargement can eventually lead to deformed limbs and muscle weakness, a reminder that the disease can cause lasting harm. Generally speaking, catching these hints early is key for public health efforts to break the cycle of transmission and kick off timely multidrug therapy that stops the condition from worsening. The ways leprosy pops up vary a lot, and that depends on how the body's immune system reacts. On one end, there's the tuberculoid type, which usually brings along just a few, well-outlined lesions and marked nerve issues, but a strong cell-based immune response helps keep the bacteria from spreading too fast. Then there's the lepromatous form—this one often comes with many symmetric lesions (nodules, plaques, even more diffuse skin changes) and a weaker immune response that lets the bacteria run amok. In many cases, patients with lepromatous leprosy even face problems that go beyond the skin, like issues with mucous membranes and eyes, sometimes leading to complications such as blindness. All these diverse signs mean that diagnosing the disease isn't always straightforward, so health workers need to watch out for even the odd, atypical patterns. In most cases, understanding this broad range of immune responses is crucial when planning public health strategies that truly tackle the complex, unpredictable nature of leprosy (Faurholt-Jepsen et al., 2013). If you look past just the skin and nerve issues, leprosy's effects can be systemic and influence long-term treatment and community health programs. For example, coexisting conditions like diabetes seem to make infectious diseases worse by dulling the body's immune responses—much like what's been noted in the tuberculosis-diabetes link, and it wouldn't be surprising if similar interactions occur with leprosy (Faurholt-Jepsen et al., 2013). Peripheral neuropathy and the resulting disabilities can bring not only physical challenges but also serious social stigma and financial burdens, sometimes making it tougher for patients to stick with multidrug treatments. Further, there's the issue of reactional states—a sudden, inflammatory flare unique to leprosy, which can speed up nerve damage and push the risk of disability even higher if it isn't treated right away. All of these factors set up major hurdles for both individual patient care and wider public health efforts. Generally, a combination of early diagnosis, thorough clinical assessments, and ongoing monitoring is needed to keep the disease from spreading further and to help improve the quality of life for those living in affected areas (Faurholt-Jepsen et al., 2013).

9.1.1. Early Signs and Symptoms

Understanding the first signs of leprosy can change the game for public health. Early on, when patients notice slight changes, often small, hardly painful patches of skin that are lighter or a bit reddish—they may not think much of them. These lesions, which come with a loss of sensation thanks to peripheral nerve involvement, set leprosy apart from other skin issues. In most cases, a low-key early presentation means that doctors and community members might not connect the dots until serious deformities or nerve problems show up, and when that happens, treatment is delayed, allowing the infection to spread further and increasing the stigma associated with more severe cases (Van Haaren et al., 2016). So, catching these subtle signals early is a cornerstone in controlling the disease. Diagnosing early leprosy isn't as straightforward as it might seem, partly because the symptoms creep in so quietly and partly due to the complex social issues involved. Patients often miss the significance of a slight loss of feeling or subtle skin changes, sometimes even brushing them off, leading to underreporting. At the same time, some health professionals may stress the potential stigma or the severity of outcomes more than patients experience in early stages, which can mix up the way they talk about or handle the condition (Van Haaren et al., 2016). Additionally, depending on the type of leprosy, early signs can vary a lot, which makes thorough clinical training and a heightened sense of diagnostic care essential, especially in areas where the disease is common. Educational efforts and responses that respect cultural differences help fill these gaps, stimulating people to seek help sooner and easing the emotional and physical load when the disease does progress. When it comes to the bigger picture, detecting leprosy early is key in halting the spread and preventing lasting harm. A delay in diagnosis means *Mycobacterium leprae* gets more time to multiply and move from person to person, keeping the cycle alive in vulnerable communities (Hambridge, 2024). That's why health strategies often zero in on individuals with initial skin patches or nerve damages, using active case-finding and careful checking. Quick multi-drug therapy not only cures the individual but also cuts down how contagious they are. By involving community health workers, and even employing models that pinpoint high-risk populations—public health programs can work more efficiently. This proactive approach is solid in reducing both the cost of the disease and its deep social impacts, aligning with the global push to phase out advanced, hard-to-treat cases (Figure 9.2).

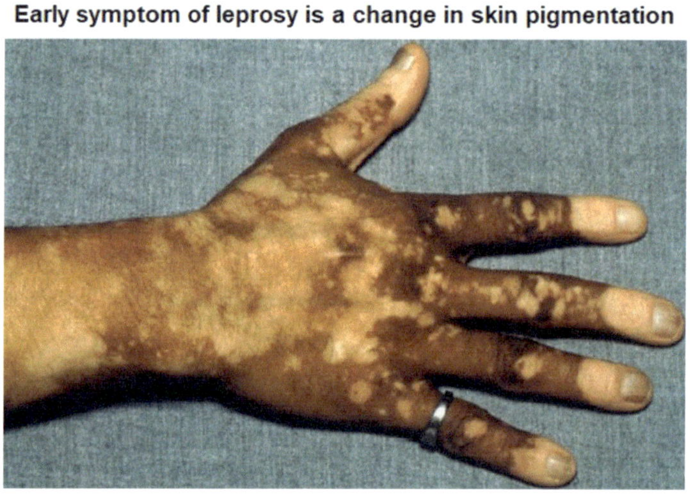

Figure 9.2. Early symptom of leprosy.

Source: Microbiology Notes. (2021). *Early Symptom of Leprosy.*

9.1.2. Long-Term Effects of Untreated Leprosy

Skipping proper treatment for leprosy can lead to a whole host of problems that stretch far past the initial infection. Without early care, the disease slowly works its way into the nerves, especially those on the outskirts, which erases feeling and leaves muscles weak. This fading sensitivity often means injuries go unnoticed, and before you know it, nerve damage can twist hands into a claw shape or even cause a drop-in foot support. When pain isn't there to warn you, small wounds and ulcers (commonly on the limbs) can become infected and worsen, eventually causing a chronic state of disability. Over time, these persisting issues impact mobility and self-care, lowering life quality while also opening the door to social stigma. In many cases, delaying treatment stokes not only individual health damages but also raises the overall public health burden by potentially increasing disability rates in communities. Often, the complications from untreated leprosy get compounded by extra infections and ongoing inflammation that work together to damage tissue further. Without early diagnosis and a proper multi-drug plan, *Mycobacterium leprae* tends to stick around and trigger repeated, painful inflammatory episodes, sometimes called erythema nodosum leprosum or type 2 lepra reactions. These bouts can speed up the damage to both nerves and skin, making the condition far tougher to manage. Further, as these physical changes become more obvious, people often face a combination of social and economic setbacks: discrimination at work, social exclusion, and even a vicious cycle that ties poverty to limited access to healthcare. Generally speaking, such outcomes underline the pressing need for early detection and effective treatment strategies that can prevent irreversible harm and ease the overall community burden (Nahid et al., 2019). Looking at the issue from a wider public health angle, leaving leprosy untreated sets up many challenges in controlling the disease in endemic areas.

Long-term untreated cases can essentially act as reservoirs, quietly fueling further transmission and interfering with efforts to eliminate the disease. Moreover, dealing with all these complications demands more complex and prolonged care—a burden that strains healthcare systems already working with limited resources. This problem is even more noticeable in environments with poor sanitation and weak antibiotic management, where factors like multidrug resistance and other infections only add to the crisis (Christy et al., 2018). In many instances, addressing these long-term effects calls for a combination of strategies, early detection, prompt treatment, community education, and better surveillance, to help reduce disability rates and transmission, all while supporting global efforts to ease both the social and health impacts of leprosy (Figure 9.3).

Effects of Leprosy

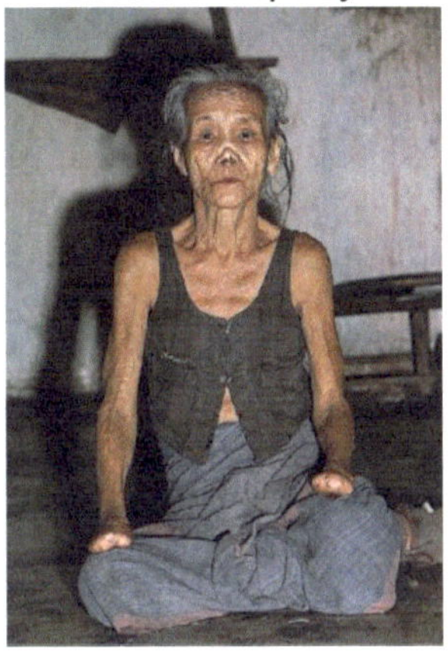

Figure 9.3. Absence of fingers and sunken nose as a result of severe effects of leprosy.

Source: Microbiology Notes. (2021). *Effects of Leprosy.*

9.1.3. Differentiation from Other Skin Diseases

Diagnosing leprosy in public health can be complex – the condition ends up looking a lot like other skin problems. You see conditions like psoriasis, eczema, and even some fungal infections showing up with red plaques, scaling, and changes in skin color; all of which make an initial diagnosis a real challenge. What sets leprosy apart is that it tends to interefere with the peripheral nerves, causing loss of sensation and even some muscle weakness – though these signs can be quite subtle at first glance. A closer look at how the pathogen interacts with the skin's normal bacteria and the body's immune response can help us narrow things down. In controlled studies, researchers have noticed that changes in skin microflora associated with leprosy differ from those seen in other dermatoses (Gall et al., 2025). This kind of insight is key, not only for better treatment plans but also for keeping the social stigma that sometimes comes with a misdiagnosis at bay. Digging further into the nerve-related damage, one finds even more signals that help set leprosy apart from other skin issues. Leprosy is, essentially, a chronic infection caused by *Mycobacterium leprae* that seems to target peripheral nerves and Schwann cells, rather than just sticking to the outer layers of the skin. In most cases, the degree of nerve damage directly links to clinical disabilities and long-term problems, which makes catching these signs early all the more important. Researchers, for example, have been looking at immunohistochemical markers like Krox-20, as well as measuring levels of nerve growth factor (NGF), neuregulin 1 (NRG1), protein zero (P0) and peripheral myelin protein 22 (PMP22) , all of which appear to flag the early nerve impairments unique to leprosy (Widasmara & Menaldi et al., 2019). These molecular hints essentially give a sort of fingerprint that distinguishes leprosy from other skin conditions that just don't show the same nerve-specific damage, ultimately helping to catch the disease sooner and improve outcomes in the community setting. Beyond just the clinical and molecular bits, the broader epidemiological picture plays a big role too. Unlike common skin ailments that often result from environmental irritants or autoimmune triggers, leprosy carries its own set of signals – think about its unique transmission dynamics, variable incubation periods, and distinct geographical spread. Generally speaking, identifying leprosy isn't just about detecting symptoms; factors like extended contact with untreated cases and socioeconomic conditions that foster endemicity are crucial parts of the puzzle. A misdiagnosis might not only lead to the wrong treatment but could also limit broader disease control efforts. That's why public health protocols often mix clinical checks, molecular diagnostics, and a careful look at epidemiologic data. This more holistic, albeit sometimes slightly complex, approach helps ensure quicker interventions, fewer cases of disease spread, and less of that tough social backlash connected to misdiagnoses – all of which are key for strengthening global strategies against leprosy (Widasmara & Menaldi, 2019; Gall et al, 2025) (Figure 9.4).

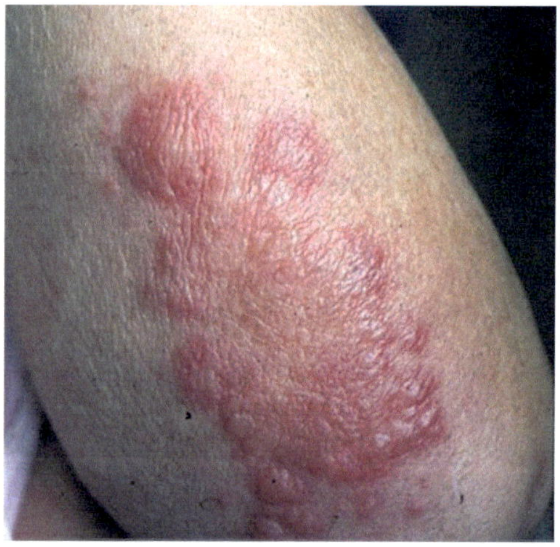

Figure 9.4. Differentiation from other skin diseases.

Source: Springer Nature. (n.d.). *Differentiation from Other Skin Diseases.*

9.2. Public Health Strategies for Control

Control of leprosy means tackling both its medical and social sides. In many underprivileged communities with scarce healthcare options, leprosy sticks around because people often don't have the right information—Further, the stigma barely helps. One way to mix things up is to treat leprosy along with other skin issues, a method that seems quite handy in places short on resources. Local health workers, trained to spot common skin problems as well as leprosy, can often catch the disease sooner and steer clear of treatments that miss the mark. There are even programs using telemedicine and training tools based on algorithms that appear to sharpen diagnosis and care, easing the overall disease load. Bundling leprosy care in with other skin conditions might also help cancel out some of the stigma, stimulating individuals to seek help without fear (Schmid-Grendelmeier et al., 2023). In effect, a patient-focused approach that makes the best out of limited means fits well with WHO's gradual shift toward embracing public health strategies that keep stigma in check, especially for neglected tropical diseases. Modern drug regimens like multidrug therapy have changed the game in leprosy control across the globe and induced hope for finally putting the disease in its place. Still, even these treatments can't fully stop the spread of *Mycobacterium leprae*, which shows just how complex the problem is. Issues like drug resistance, relapses, or patients not sticking to the plan underline the need for reliable tracking and follow-up care. Public health efforts now need to dig into epidemiological details to find out where the disease persists and how it hops between communities. And it isn't enough to just hand out medications; dealing with the complications and disabilities of leprosy calls for rehab and social support that go well beyond simple antimicrobial therapy. Even with fewer cases overall, the ongoing transmission hints that control measures remain delicate and must be kept sharp by combining medical care, social support, and vigilant public health monitoring (Gonçalves, 2013). It's also vital to look at the social roots that let leprosy endure and impact everyday lives. Factors like poverty, cramped living conditions, and a lack of education often lead to late diagnoses and poorer treatment results. That's why public health plans should break out into community outreach, education, and empowerment initiatives that help cut down on stigma and bust myths about the disease. Successful programs mix in health-promotion efforts that invite community involvement, ensuring patients don't get isolated but rather find the support they need among their neighbors. Moreover, by using existing health setups and linking leprosy control with efforts against other neglected tropical diseases, we can boost both efficiency and long-term results. Recognizing leprosy as a combination of health and social challenges, rather than just a lone medical problem, is key to building solutions that encourage early detection, steady treatment, and ultimately, social reintegration (Gonçalves, 2013; Schmid-Grendelmeier et al., 2023).

9.2.1. Early Detection and Diagnosis

Catching leprosy early is crucial, especially since the disease spreads in such a complex way and can hide for a long time before symptoms show up. People might be carrying *Mycobacterium leprae* for years without any obvious signs, which leaves doctors scrambling to spot it in time. In most cases, early diagnosis means not only getting the right multidrug treatment started but also stopping nerve damage that might otherwise lead to lasting disability. In Central Florida, for example, where leprosy used to be almost unheard of, low clinical suspicion often results in misdiagnoses or delays that boost both transmission risks and worse outcomes for patients. A bit more attention during check-ups, along with community education efforts, could bridge this gap, highlighting the need for stronger surveillance and improved diagnostic training to recognize even the faintest hints (Nazir et al., 2023). A complete skin and nerve exam stands out as the go-to move for early detection. Doctors keep an eye out for unusual patches on the skin, sometimes lighter, sometimes tinged with red, especially when these marks come with numbness or the feel of thickened nerves. Often, a simple acid-fast bacilli test on a skin smear or a biopsy helps confirm the infection, giving clear evidence of what's going on. In many cases, extra tools like nerve conduction studies or even some pretty advanced imaging techniques step in to objectively show how much the nerves are affected, which is key for preventing permanent damage. Further, splitting cases into either the paucibacillary or multibacillary type usually helps decide how long and how strong the treatment should be. To summarize, nailing the diagnosis early with these varied methods helps stop the disease from progressing and plays a big role in broader public health efforts (Nazir et al., 2023). Addressing early detection challenges calls for a combination of public health actions that stress awareness, education, and easy access to care. The persisting stigma around leprosy often stops people from seeking help early, which means they end up with more advanced stages of the disease. Generally speaking, public health campaigns need to work on destigmatizing the condition and informing both healthcare workers and the community about those early signs and how the disease spreads. It also makes sense to mix leprosy screening into routine health services and community outreach, especially in areas with limited access—so that cases get spotted sooner. The best results come from a combination of hands-on clinical care, strengthened health systems, and a bit of social support; together, these approaches help cut down on disability and improve life quality while easing the overall disease burden (Nazir et al., 2023) (Figure 9.5).

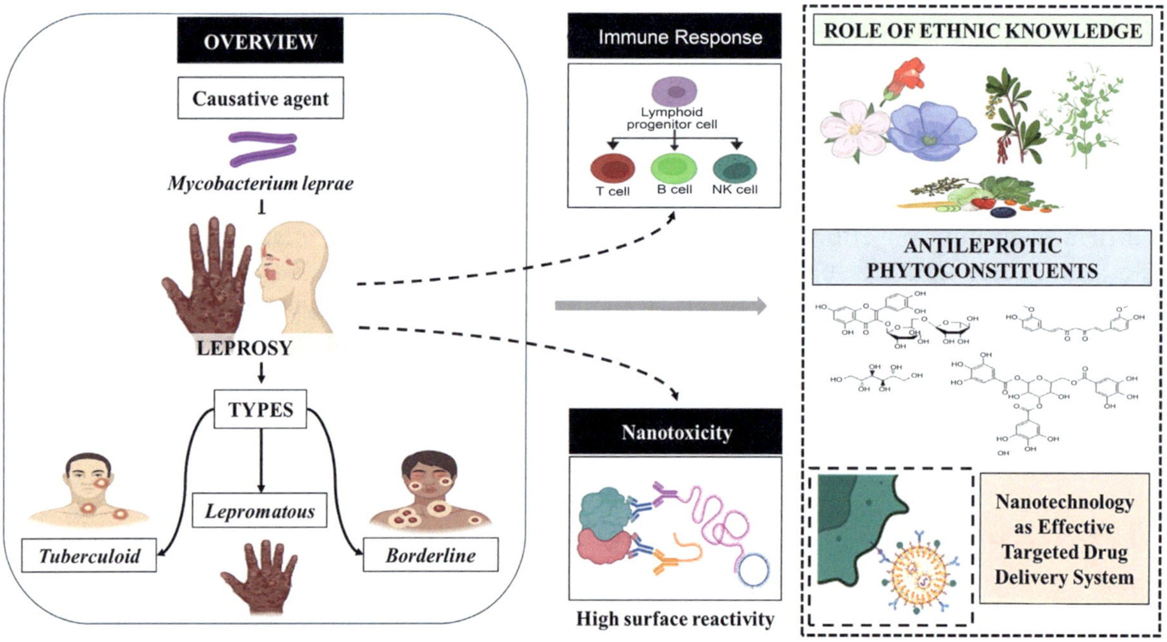

Figure 9.5. Early detection and appropriate intervention are the need of the hour to completely eradicate leprosy.

Source: Kimta N, Majdalawieh AF, Nasrallah GK, Puri S, Nepovimova E, Jomova K and Kuča K (2024) Leprosy: Comprehensive insights into pathology, immunology, and cutting-edge treatment strategies, integrating nanoparticles and ethnomedicinal plants. Front. Pharmacol. 15:1361641. doi: 10.3389/fphar.2024.1361641

9.2.2. Treatment Options and Protocols

Early diagnosis and sticking with a set treatment plan form the very backbone of fighting leprosy. Getting things going early not only helps cure the illness but also halts its spread. Multi-Drug Therapy (MDT), which means using a combination of antibiotics to target *Mycobacterium leprae* while keeping drug resistance at bay—is the mainstay worldwide. National programs often offer MDT free of charge, making sure that patients can finish their treatments.

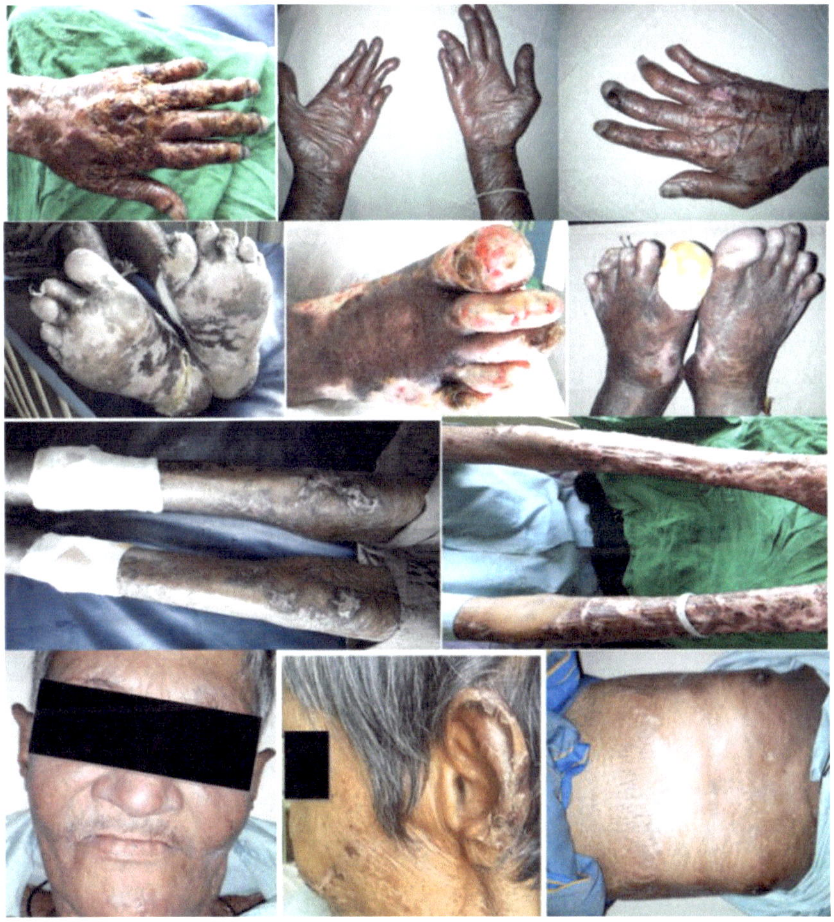

Figure 9.6. The treatment options and protocols.

Source: Herath, S., Navinan, M.R., Liyanage, I. *et al.* Lucio's phenomenon, an uncommon occurrence among leprosy patients in Sri Lanka. *BMC Res Notes* **8**, 672 (2015). https://doi.org/10.1186/s13104-015-1671-1

Besides the drugs, keeping an eye out for complications like nerve damage is key to lessening long-term disabilities. To summarize, combining ongoing checks, case tracking and treatment routines builds a rounded attack against the disease; this mix of personalized care with broader public measures is central to reducing leprosy rates and calming public health worries (Weekly Newsletter for the Center for Acute Disease Epidemiology of the Iowa Department of Public Health, 2017). The scene gets even messier when sociocultural factors step in, especially among Indigenous and marginalized groups where a long history and community dynamics shape health outcomes. Take the Kimberley region of Australia, for example—colonial health legacies and persisting social stigmas make it hard for patients to stick with treatment. In such settings, pushing for care that's culturally respectful and focused on the individual helps build real trust between healthcare providers and patients. Methods like directly observed therapy (DOT), and case management are used nationwide to boost adherence, but these approaches sometimes miss the mark culturally, which curbs their effectiveness. Involving the community more directly and adjusting treatment plans to honor local identities can not only improve completion rates but also boost overall well-being and community resilience (Oliver, 2022). Looking at the bigger picture, both historical challenges and current hurdles in leprosy treatment signal the need for fresh, equitable methods that mix solid biomedical results with cultural sensitivity. Generally speaking, paying attention to family history, keeping an eye on medication safety, and even linking leprosy care with other common health issues might improve outcomes a lot. It comes down to clearly stressing why treatment matters, working together on decisions, and building support systems that naturally respect cultural values. All these bits collectively help with better adherence to MDT, cut down on disease spread, and ease social stigmas. In public health terms, altering our treatment models to cover these many angles offers promising paths toward eliminating the disease and boosting life quality for those affected (Oliver, 2022) (Figure 9.6).

9.2.3. Community Education and Awareness Programs

Community effort and sharing correct information form the backbone of many public health moves. Take leprosy, for example—local learning plays a big role in easing stigma and stimulating early detection. Programs like these often try to clear up common myths by talking about what causes the disease, its signals, and how it spreads, even if some misconceptions stubbornly persist. In most cases, a friendly yet clear approach pushes affected individuals to get help sooner, which in turn cuts down on spreading and long-run damage. Educating people in this way connects efficiently with broader strategies aimed at prevention and behavioral change, showing real benefits over time. This method not only lifts health know-how but also makes community members active in public health, building trust between locals and health services (Mtui et al., 2011). Ethiopia's run with neglected tropical diseases, leprosy included, underscores how key local education and awareness can be in a broad fight against illness. Even though the nation reached its leprosy elimination target, stubborn issues like stigma and gaps in knowledge still emerge. In many instances, integrated education campaigns have worked wonders by breaking down social barriers—sometimes in ways that feel a bit all over the place, but effective, nonetheless. Efforts that mix mapping studies and hands-on research into joint intervention plans, as part of larger neglected tropical disease programs, show that combining medical care with community learning is a must. Overall, targeted awareness seems to boost acceptance of health interventions and fires up local action, which is especially crucial in areas where leprosy sticks around alongside other diseases (Deribe et al., 2012). When it comes to spending on community education within health systems, money matters a lot. Health analyses generally suggest that prevention programs—including outreach to educate communities—can bring far more benefits than simply pacing treatment budgets, because they drop future costs by keeping both new cases and severe outcomes at bay. It becomes essential for planners to weave costing exercises and resource checks into early program planning, ensuring things are both realistic and lasting. Coordinating education efforts with broader health strategies can also raise overall efficiency and help avoid doubling up on efforts—key when every dollar counts. Treating education as a central piece of leprosy control not only brings in funding and political support but also combines community engagement with public services in ways traditional methods simply don't manage to, ultimately strengthening control in a sustainable manner (Mtui et al., 2011).

9.3. Socioeconomic Impact of Leprosy

Infectious diseases can hit communities in areas ways that go well beyond just physical symptoms – they seep into daily life and affect economic well-being. Leprosy, for instance, isn't only a long-term health problem that might lead to disfigurement or disability; it also brings a heavy social and economic cost. People dealing with this disease often find themselves sidelined by stigma, which can cut them off from job opportunities and essential resources. Such exclusion ends up trapping families in poverty, with fewer chances to get an education or a stable job, making it extra hard to get back into the fold. In many places with limited access to good healthcare, diagnosis and treatment get delayed – extending the time the disease can cause harm and piling on further complications and expenses for everyone involved. All these mixed health and social issues point to the need for public health plans that work on both treatment and helping patients rejoin society (Nazir et al., 2023). The burden isn't carried by individuals alone – whole communities feel the strain when leprosy is around. Rising healthcare expenses and a drop in worker productivity have a knock-on effect in areas already struggling with low income and poor sanitation. Local health systems, already short on resources, often have a tough time keeping up with a disease that takes a while to show up and demands ongoing treatment. It isn't just about paying for a visit to the doctor; indirect costs like travel to clinics, lost income when someone becomes disabled, and extra caregiving within families add up quickly. Further, the persisting stigma may even stop people from seeking early help, which only pushes the problem further and makes overall costs climb. In effect, leprosy weaves itself into the cycle of poverty, making it clear that medical care must be combined with social and economic support (Nazir et al., 2023). Additional challenges emerge when coinfections and health system disruptions join the mix – challenges that have only grown during public health crises like the COVID-19 pandemic. Programs meant to control neglected tropical diseases, such as mass drug campaigns, often get interrupted, making it harder to keep the disease in check and preserve local stability. Vulnerable groups, sometimes dealing with other parasitic infections along with leprosy, face extra risks because treatments or the coinfections can weaken their defenses, sometimes inducing severe complications that spike healthcare needs. These overlapping issues tend to deepen existing social and economic gaps, especially when local healthcare facilities are on shaky ground. To summarize, these interwoven health and social challenges call out for coordinated, well-rounded public health actions that not only stay on track with leprosy control but also tackle broader issues like poverty, crowded living conditions, and limited healthcare access.

9.3.1. Stigmatization and Discrimination

Diseases do more than touch the body—they stir up reactions in society that can upend lives. Leprosy, long wrapped in fear and a tangle of old misunderstandings still suffers from deep stigma and bias. People often hold on to mistaken ideas about how easily it spreads or moral judgments that wrongly mark those affected, pushing them away from their own communities. This kind of rejection not only causes stress and anxiety but also makes individuals delay getting needed care, which can keep the infection going. In a lot of cases, the way society treats an illness totally shapes efforts to control it, so getting to grips with these mixed-up origins is key to breaking down harmful behavior and building a more welcoming path back into everyday life. Taking on the stigma means doing more than just handing out medicine—it calls for a broad public health plan that dives into the social and mental side of things too. Generally speaking, when we stick to overly simple or misinformed stories about a condition, we see real fallout like isolation, hurt feelings, and even money issues. Weight bias, for example, shows how a complicated view of a health issue can feed discrimination and block both better health and fair treatment (Gligorijevi et al., 2024). For those dealing with leprosy, swapping out messages of fear for lessons that stress how treated cases are not contagious, and that modern care can lead to full recovery, can deflate the stigma. Health workers, ideally, get trained to treat people with genuine respect, which keeps dignity intact while lowering the hurdles to receiving care; such people-first methods acknowledge the complex social realities behind each case. Everyday acts of discrimination against stigmatized groups can come in small, uneven doses but add up to serious damage to health and wellbeing. Research with groups like American Indian and Alaska Native communities shows that exclusion, stigma, and biases even at work are common and stir up a combination of intense feelings and coping struggles (Rene et al., 2024). In many ways, individuals coping with leprosy face similar challenges—dealing with social shunning, occasional harassment, and that heavy weight of internal shame. These experiences impact mental health and often block the sort of economic and social chances that are so vital for bouncing back. Public health efforts, then, must weave in culturally aware strategies that get these social pressures while also helping build healthier ways to cope. More awareness and education among both everyday individuals and healthcare providers may just ease these biases over time, improving health outcomes and knitting communities a bit closer together; addressing these deep-rooted issues is indispensable for a full, holistic approach to leprosy care (Figure 9.7).

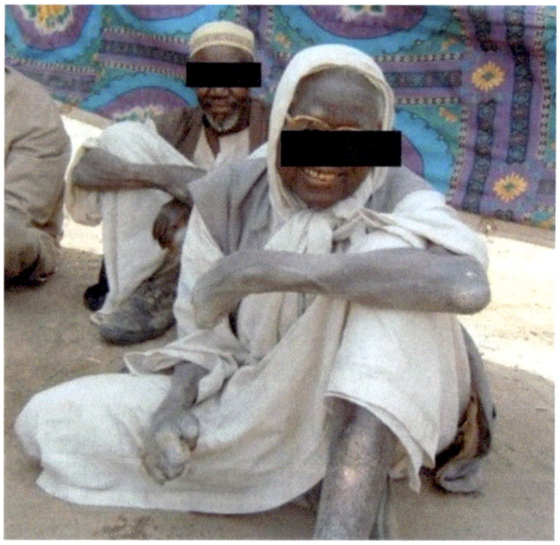

Figure 9.7. Stigmatization.

Source: South Sudan Medical Journal. (2010). *Stigma Related to Leprosy.*

9.3.2. Economic Burden on Affected Individuals

Leprosy still carries a heavy burden of stigma. People tend to shun those suffering from it, and this social exclusion can make everyday money problems even worse. The illness isn't just about physical pain; it also blocks access to regular work and steady income, which wrecks someone's financial footing. Treatment costs pile up—not only the bills for medicine and doctor visits but also expenses for traveling to care centers, lost days at work, and long-term support for disabilities. In many low-resource areas, aging healthcare systems only add to these expenses, trapping families in a cycle of poverty. Sometimes, extra complications like other diseases or infections extend the time needed for recovery, showing that the struggle goes well beyond basic clinical treatment (Christopher et al., 2022). Interruptions in health or social services during broader crises further complicate things. Take, for example, the COVID-19 pandemic: when funds and efforts shifted away from neglected tropical diseases like leprosy, routine drug programs were put on hold. This left many people even more strained financially, especially those depending on support to manage their condition or stave off disability. Lockdowns and social distancing also changed how people live and work, often in unexpected ways—leaving many marginal communities in areas endemic regions with fewer job chances and higher costs for care. In most cases, these sudden shifts raise the overall expenses and risk rolling back what little progress had been made in controlling the disease and helping patients (Danilo et al., 2021). When leprosy collides with other infections and deep-rooted social disadvantages, regaining financial stability becomes a steep challenge. Many individuals with leprosy-related disabilities need constant help, like regular check-ups and special devices, yet these supports are frequently too pricey or simply hard to find. The persistent stigma can even make it tough for them to land a decent job, pushing former workers into uncertain, informal gigs or outright unemployment. This economic isolation reinforces poverty by cutting off access to nutritious food, good schooling, and proper healthcare—all of which are essential for recovery and avoiding further disability. Generally speaking, public health programs should not focus solely on clinical care. They'd do well to include economic aid and local rehabilitation efforts so that, over time, individuals can gradually reclaim both their health and their economic independence (Christopher et al., 2022; Danilo et al., 2021).

9.3.3. Impact on Families and Communities

Leprosy doesn't just affect the person diagnosed, it also shakes up family ties and the way communities get along. Families end up shouldering a lot of emotional and social weight, dealing with both the day-to-day stress of caregiving and the isolation that often comes with being judged harshly. Often, this stigma pushes people away, leaving those affected feeling ashamed and abandoned. Misunderstandings about the disease stir up fear even among relatives, sometimes fracturing relationships or leading to outright rejection. When families lose their close-knit support, it becomes a real struggle to handle the illness, slowing down recovery and making it tougher for everyone to bounce back (Dako et al., 2017). Around town, the impact of leprosy is felt similarly. Historical ideas linking the disease with uncleanliness and contagion have led to widespread fear, and people often find themselves on the wrong side of judgment. This kind of treatment can cut off opportunities for jobs, healthcare, and even just making friends. In most cases, such exclusion not only drains the community of valuable human energy but also keeps the cycle of delayed treatment and underreporting alive, which in turn feeds a harsh loop of poverty and declining health outcomes. Tackling these challenges usually means coming up with public health strategies that are both culturally sensitive and bold enough to dismantle these outdated beliefs (Dako et al., 2017).

Public health efforts, then, have to go beyond just handing out medicine. They need to spread clear, easy-to-grasp information—after all, knowing that leprosy is treatable and less frightening than it once seemed is a game-changer. Tailored educational programs can turn families and neighbors into early detectors and steadfast supporters for those in need. In most cases, combining routine medical care with a dash of mental health support helps fight that self-inflicted isolation and builds a bit of resilience. Overall, these mixed approaches—raising awareness, encouraging early help, and addressing mental well-being—seem to be the key to easing the heavy public health load that leprosy brings and to helping communities move forward (Figure 9.8).

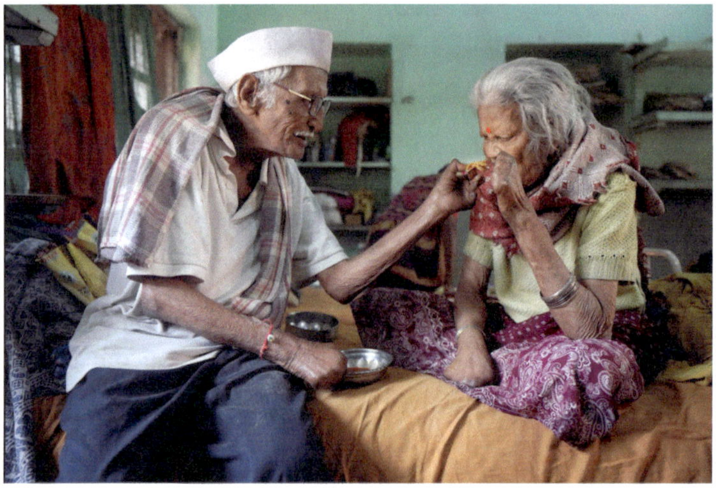

Figure 9.8. The impact on families and communities.

Source: Pulitzer Center. (n.d.). *Leprosy in India.*

9.4. Global Initiatives and Collaborations

Leprosy's fight has taken some unexpected turns over the past few decades. In the '80s and '90s, a short course multidrug therapy brought down case numbers dramatically—but then progress stalled, and everyone had to rethink their approach. Health organizations, governments, and research labs began working together, realizing that only a united effort could address the ongoing spread, the persisting disabilities, and the deep-seated social stigma connected to the disease. In 2018, the creation of the Global Partnership for Zero Leprosy (GPZL) highlighted this shift. It gathered voices from many parts of the world, combining research and practical strategies in a less-than-formal mix of expertise. By merging know-how in sometimes unexpected ways, these groups are tackling both scientific puzzles and stubborn logistical challenges, showing that global teamwork remains central to the push for leprosy elimination (Steinmann et al., 2020). Leprosy brings with it a combination of health challenges that go far beyond just medical treatment. It isn't only about better diagnostics and new treatments, but also about crafting policies that actively challenge discrimination and boost disability prevention while empowering those affected. In most cases, global collaborations help share everything from new technologies to evidence-based, everyday practices and culturally tuned frameworks that work in different socioeconomic settings. Especially in developing regions where health systems can be fragile or underfunded, efforts that mix law, advocacy, financing, and even stigma reduction become essential. These all-in-one public health strategies aim to spread fairness and make sure that communities often left on the fringes finally get the right kind of care (Rodriguez-Morales, 2019). At the heart of these worldwide actions is a need to align short-term fixes with long-term visions. Take GPZL's approach, for example, they cover diagnostics, build epidemiological models, dabble in digital tech, and even pursue vaccine development, in a move that shows how beating leprosy means trying new ideas in lots of fields. Generally speaking, there's also a focus on folding research directly into local health practices. Studies on post-exposure prophylaxis and similar interventions remind us that turning findings into real-world impact is key. Securing enough funds and solid political backing remains vital if we're to keep up the momentum towards the 2030 WHO targets. In many cases, international partnerships double as hubs for advocacy, capacity building, and sharing of local know-how—underlining that achieving zero leprosy is a shared global goal requiring steady, coordinated action (Steinmann et al., 2020).

9.4.1. WHO's Role in Leprosy Control

Over the years, people have worked hard to fight neglected tropical diseases by coming together from all over, and the WHO has been a key player in pushing new ideas for leprosy control. They run programs that try to cut down on cases and ease the disabilities caused by *Mycobacterium leprae*. Rather than sticking to just one fix, they mix things up, a heavy dose of drugs paired with local health talks and rehab sessions, for example.

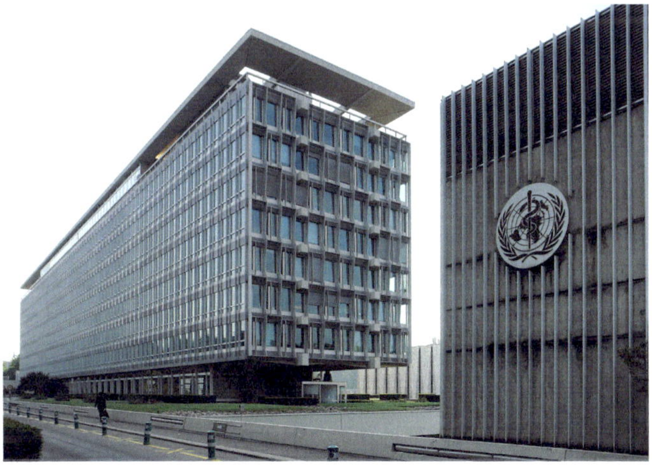

Figure 9.9. World Health Organization (WHO) urges governments to prioritize leprosy elimination.

Source: By I, Yann, CC BY-SA 3.0, https://commons.wikimedia.org/w/index.php?curid=2367501

This isn't only about medicine; it's about fighting stigma and handling real-life social issues too. In most cases, WHO even brings in social and environmental thoughts to shape community care practices that go well beyond basic treatments (Ackley et al., 2021). Leprosy isn't just a physical challenge—it hits communities through stigma, isolation, and even poverty. Generally speaking, the WHO's approach sees that reducing the spread means tackling these deeper problems as well. They involve the individuals affected as real partners rather than just patients, which kind of brings out a grassroots feel. This way, people aren't only treated but are also given a chance to regain a sense of dignity and independence, connecting health with bigger matters like poverty and personal growth. In a combination of treatments and supportive measures such as education, rehab and reintegration, the overall effort ends up slowly breaking the cycle of illness and hardship (Wilsher, 2011). On a wider level, WHO keeps pushing global policies that mix leprosy action with strategies for other tropical diseases. They focus on basics like clean water and good hygiene as much as on medicine—because prevention often beats just trying to cure. Clearly, WHO cares about what "community" means, making sure local voices get a say in how health ideas are put into practice. This hands-on style—sometimes a bit rough around the edges—relies on local health workers and makes room for everyday challenges while aiming for lasting improvements. It's a practical combination of targeted care and broad social support that keeps hope alive in places where leprosy still takes its toll (Ackley et al., 2021) (Figure 9.9).

9.4.2. Partnerships with NGOs and Local Governments

Public health work isn't a one-man show—usually, it takes a combination of different players banding together to make a real difference. Take leprosy, for instance. Local governments and NGOs often team up in ways that don't follow a strict blueprint. NGOs bring specialized know-how, street-level connections, and a touch of real-world insight that jives with the regulatory frameworks local bodies set up. This kind of loose, collaborative effort helps spread medical treatments and slowly erode the social stigma that hangs around like an unwelcome guest. When these groups join forces, they can launch quick-hit awareness drives, pick up on symptoms early, and set up community rehab programs that matter for vulnerable individuals. Integrating NGOs into local health circles usually ends up creating a combined approach to fighting leprosy. Generally speaking, it's about handling both treatment and the everyday issues that keep a community sick. This dual approach—combining leprosy care into standard health services while also having specific programs for those hit hardest—has shown promise in preventing long-term disabilities and even easing poverty in some cases. Government plans get a boost when NGOs add their own community-tailored projects, and enough of these small mismatches in style seem to work in keeping overall policy steady. It's a strategy reminiscent of what major development agencies have been trying out, suggesting that aligning everyday healthcare with targeted fixes could yield both practical and moral wins (Thomas et al., 2004). Looking at other infectious disease programs can shed some light on the potential of NGO-government teamwork for leprosy control. For example, in many developing regions, efforts to beat tuberculosis have gotten a serious lift from NGOs working hand in hand with government plans—showing, in most cases, that cohesive services and genuine community engagement are key. The BRAC model in Bangladesh, with its grassroots energy complementing official strategies, sort of builds a "value chain" in disease management. Adapting some of those ideas for leprosy might boost early detection, help patients stick with treatment, and even ease their journey back into society. To summarize, leaning into these more cooperative, sometimes complex approaches could make leprosy control more sustainable and effective, underscoring the vital role of NGO and local government partnerships (Ravichandran, 2004).

9.4.3. Research and Funding for Leprosy Initiatives

Ongoing progress in fighting neglected illnesses hangs on the mix of focused research and enough funds. Leprosy, though it can be cured, keeps troubling many communities that often slip through the cracks. Nowadays, local know-how and academic insight are being jumbled together in unexpected ways to tackle these issues. A lot of times, simply getting people involved shines a light on how diseases spread and where our healthcare efforts might be falling short. This hands-on style often ends up inducing fresh ways to spot diseases early, boost treatment follow-through, and even impact long-held stigmas. Steady funding, in most cases, ends up being the lifeblood that fuels both laboratory work and community projects, pushing forward evidence-based policies and scaling real-world fixes—steps seen as critical to pushing leprosy toward extinction (Aragon et al., 2023). Technology and interdisciplinary research have been shaking up our response to complex issues like leprosy. Combining tools from engineering, software know-how, and healthcare ideas, new methods are emerging that kind of reimagine what cost-effective care should be. For instance, the invention of low-cost telepresence robots shows how a dash of tech-savvy with a focus on public health can open up access to care for individuals in tough spots. These gadgets provide remote checks and even real-time chats, lowering the hurdles to getting proper treatment on time. It's a reminder that funding these cross-field projects isn't just about creating cool new devices—it's also about testing and rolling them out where they matter most, underscoring that tech-driven healthcare can lift treatment outcomes in resource-strapped settings. Looking ahead, keeping leprosy control programs effective means building a framework that mixes ongoing research with solid financial backing. Decision-makers, generally speaking, need to balance basic science with clinical trials, community health moves, and even a bit of social research. Further, leaning on community insights ensures these efforts dig deep into issues like poverty and spotty healthcare access. Bringing together governmental groups, NGOs, and universities often stirs up not only extra resources but also fresh ideas, which can speed up lowering leprosy cases and preventing disabilities. Funding models that push for better community ties and wider research involvement might well be the induce needed for comprehensive, lasting solutions. In the end, keeping a steady flow of resources paired with evidence-based strategies and a splash of technological innovation remains absolutely key to fair healthcare outcomes and our global push to eliminate leprosy (Aragon et al., 2023) (Figure 9.10).

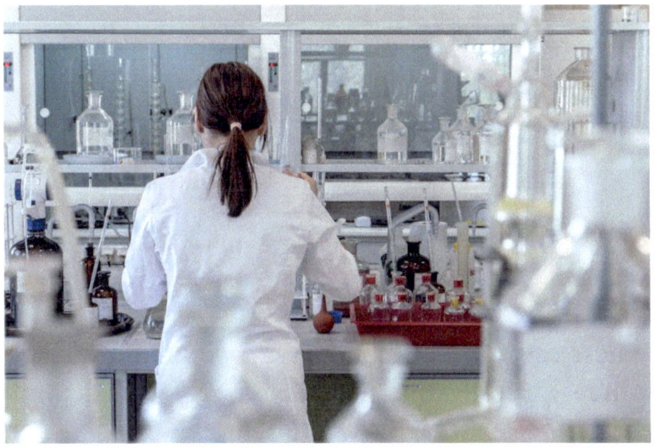

Figure 9.10. Leprosy research initiative.

Source: Leprosy Research Initiative. (n.d.). *Laboratory Research on Leprosy.*

A CLOSER LOOK

GEOGRAPHICAL DISTRIBUTION AND TRENDS OF NEW CASE DETECTION OF LEPROSY BY WORLD HEALTH ORGANIZATION (WHO) REGION AND SELECTED COUNTRIES

Leprosy, or Hansen's disease, is still a global health concern, with a significant number of new cases detected annually. Most new cases are concentrated in specific WHO regions and countries. India, Brazil, and Indonesia account for a large proportion of global new cases.

Global Situation in the Year 2019

The global number of new cases of leprosy detected in 2019 was 202,185. Their distribution by WHO region is reported in (Figure 9.11). Leprosy is still an important public health problem in three regions, namely, Southeast Asia, the Americas, and Africa. The Southeast Asian region reports the highest number with 143,787 new cases. They represent 71% of the global total. In this region India reports the highest number in the world with 114,451 cases; they represent 80% of the regional and 57% of the global new case detection (NCD). No data are available for the European region.

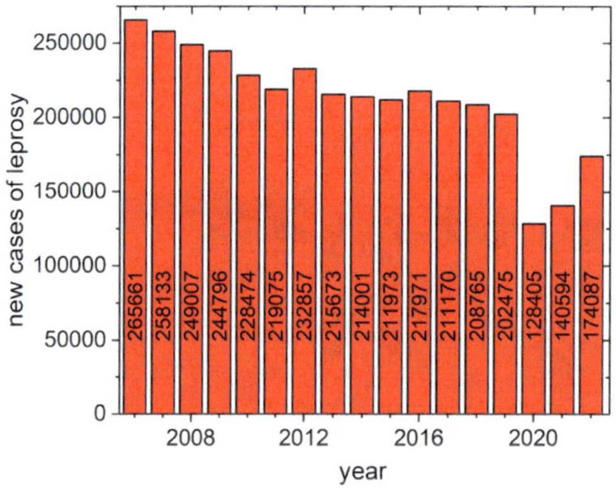

Figure 9.11. Global leprosy new case detection *Source:* By Pseudoneu Anondeux Zweitnamensmann - Own work, CC BY-SA 4.0, https://commons.wikimedia.org/w/index.php?curid=148154892

Global Trend

Ministries of Health from endemic countries report NCD of leprosy to WHO yearly. The number of countries reporting varies making comparisons between one year and another unreliable. However, the numbers of new cases detected and reported to WHO are the main indicator of the global leprosy burden and also the main indicator of disease incidence. At the global level, data are available from 1985–2019. The analysis of the global annual NCD of leprosy shows that this indicator has been relatively stable between the years 1985 and 1997 varying between 550,000 and 700,000 cases. Two major peaks were reported in 1998 and 2001. Between 2001 and 2005, there was a sharp decrease (strongly influenced by the Indian figures). Since 2006 this indicator of global NCD of leprosy excluding India is gradually, but slightly, declining.

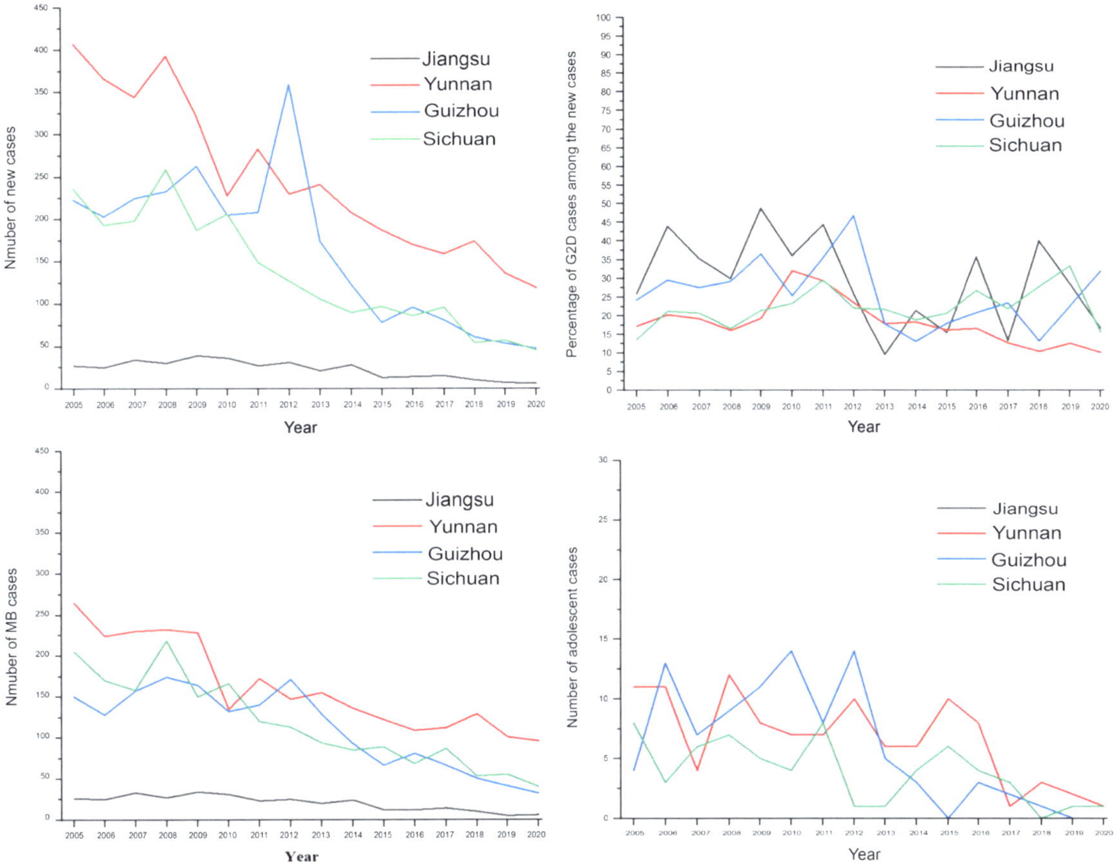

Figure 9.12. The comparison of the epidemiological features of new cases between Jiangsu, Yunan, Guizhou, and Sichuan. The gray line represents Jiangsu province, the red line represents Yunnan province, the blue line represents Guizhou province, and the green line represents Sichuan province.*Source:* Li X, Jin G, Yang J, Li Y, Wei P and Zhang L (2023) Epidemiological characteristics of leprosy during the period 2005–2020: A retrospective study based on the Chinese surveillance system. Front. Public Health 10:991828. doi: 10.3389/fpubh.2022.991828.

The number of new cases indicates the degree of continued transmission of infection. Global statistics showed in 2015 that 94% of new leprosy cases were reported from 14 countries reporting more than 1000 new cases each and only 6% of new cases were reported from the rest of the world. Pockets of high endemicity still remain in some areas of many countries, including countries reporting less than 1000 new cases. Some of these areas show very high notification rates for new cases and may still witness intense transmission (Figure 9.13).

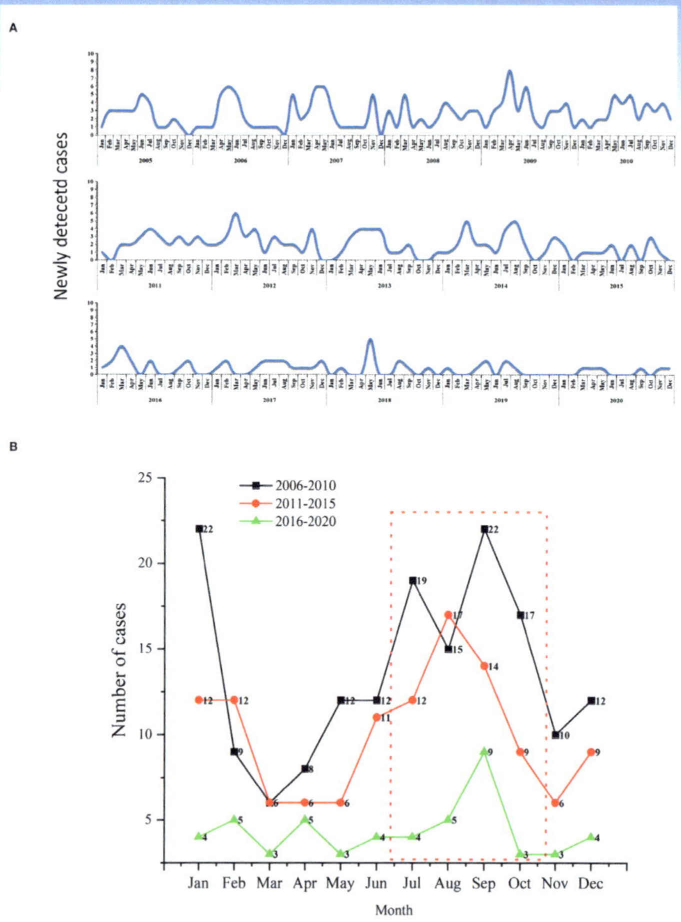

Figure 9.13. The temporal distribution of newly detected leprosy cases in Jiangsu Province, 2005–2020. **(A)** Monthly detection rate of the new cases; **(B)** Comparison of monthly detection rates per 5 years.

Source: Li X, Jin G, Yang J, Li Y, Wei P and Zhang L (2023) Epidemiological characteristics of leprosy during the period 2005–2020: A retrospective study based on the Chinese surveillance system. Front. Public Health 10:991828. doi: 10.3389/fpubh.2022.991828

Regional Trends: Southeast Asia

Annual regional data are available from 1991–2019. The Southeast Asian region's annual trend is very similar to the global one. Two major peaks occurred in 1998 and in 2001. Since then, a steady decrease took place up to 2006, and then the indicator leveled off. Figure 9.14 shows the annual leprosy NCD trend in India. Here too there are two major peaks reported in 1998 and 2001, a steady decrease up to 2006 and then the levelling off of the indicator.

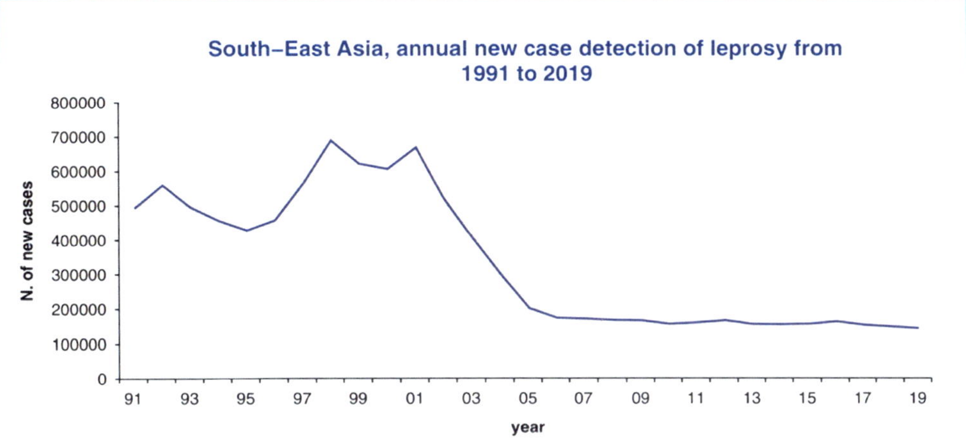

Figure 9.14. Southeast Asia – Annual new case detection (NCD) of leprosy from 1991–2019.

Source: Springer Nature. (n.d.). *Southeast Asia Leprosy NCD.*

It is the trend in India that has determined the shape of the Southeast and global graphics. In leprosy, something "exceptional" has happened in India between 1996 and 2006. The increase in NCD between 1996 and 2001 and the decrease reported from 2001–2006 are faster than expected for a chronic disease like leprosy. Among the many operational factors that may have determined this particular trend are increased, "exceptional," efforts in case of detection activities with clearance of the backlog cases (proportion of cases with onset of the disease in previous years). These could explain the fast increase in NCD, the fast decrease of the indicator, and it's levelling off to values nearer to the true incidence of the disease in the 2006–2019 period (Figure 9.15).

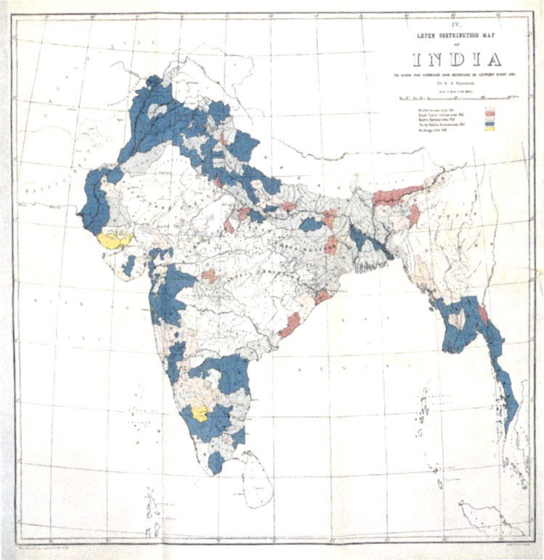

Figure 9.15. India – annual new case detection*Source:* https://commons.wikimedia.org/wiki/File:Map_showing_the_distribution_of_Leprosy_in_India_Wellcome_L0039112.jpg

Regional Trends: Americas, Africa, Western Pacific, and Eastern Mediterranean

- In the American region, the annual NCD of leprosy has been relatively stable between the years 1996 and 2009 varying between 40,000 and 50,000 cases; figures are now decreasing. In this region 92% of the cases are in Brazil (Figure 9.16).

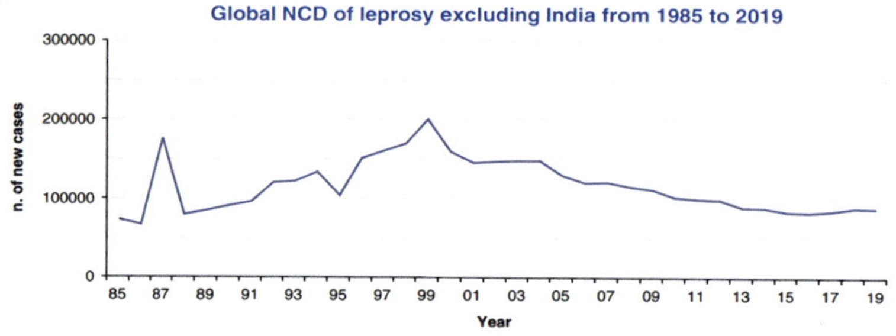

Figure 9.16. Americas – Annual new case detection of leprosy from 1991–2019.

Source: Springer Nature. (n.d.). *Americas Leprosy NCD.*

- In the African region, the last peak with 48,248 cases was reported in 2002; then figures started decreasing till 2011, and since then more or less stable (Figure 9.17).

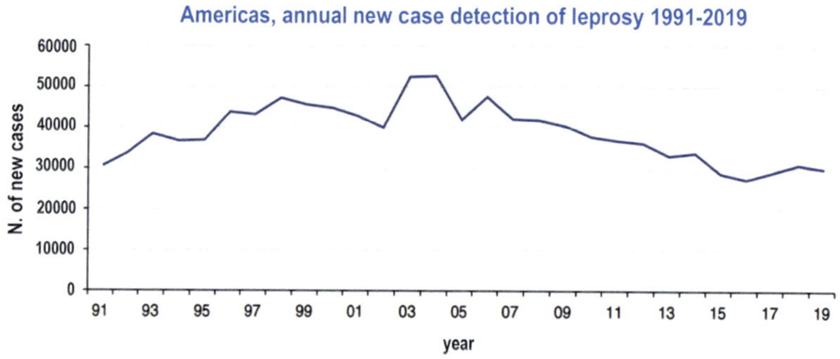

Figure 9.17. Africa – Annual new case detection (NCD) of leprosy*Source:*

- In Western Pacific region, a peak of new case detection of leprosy, with 7137 cases, was reached in 2005; since then, the indicator is declining.
- In Eastern Mediterranean, the annual number of new leprosy cases has been around 3000–4000 cases annually since 2003 but varies rather widely.

SUMMARY

Leprosy isn't just about physical symptoms, it seeps into everyday life in ways you might not expect, touching on how people feel, how they're treated, and even their finances. Instead of focusing solely on the bacterium, public health efforts need to tackle the heavy labels and unfair treatment that often-hit women and other vulnerable groups the hardest. Research generally points out that easing these social pressures calls for targeted actions, think community education mixed with healthcare that gets what local individuals need. Pairing treatment with some genuine emotional and social support might just help create friendlier, more welcoming spaces. In short, boosting primary care and adjusting policy frameworks could be the key to lowering both the number of cases and the wider fallout from the disease (Mendes et al., 2024). Fighting leprosy goes well beyond battling a microbe; it means looking closely at our surroundings and their role in health. Many studies suggest that environmental factors, like the quality of air in crowded, under-resourced areas, can worsen the impact of the disease. For instance, research on pollutants (consider traffic-related air fumes, for example) shows that external risks further complicate health challenges in communities already facing a lot. While the bacterium is the direct cause, living conditions and environmental stressors often determine how well someone can bounce back or get the care they need. Basically, addressing leprosy means layering direct medical care with broader public health policies designed to improve everyday living and access to services (Debelu et al., 2024). To summarize, beating leprosy calls for a long-term, united effort that bridges the gaps among medical treatment, social support, and solid public policy. Early detection, ongoing treatment, and vigilant monitoring are all vital if we hope to keep the disease at bay. Equally, knocking down the stigma via education, and yes, sometimes a bit of grassroots advocacy, helps empower patients and ease their return to normal life. Melding leprosy care into everyday primary health services not only makes treatment more accessible but also a lot more humane. Strengthening research and fine-tuning policies for those at the highest risk, particularly women can ramp up the effectiveness of these interventions. To summarize, comprehensive public health measures like these are needed, and fast, to cut down leprosy's widespread impacts (Mendes et al., 2024).

Leprosy remains a significant public health concern, particularly where access to proper medical care is a problem and financial struggles just continue to accumulate. It's a chronic disease that likes to take its sweet time to present, with a lengthy incubation period and cruel symptoms that make rapid diagnosis and treatment quite difficult. Human beings typically become exposed to it over prolonged, intimate periods, which information us that early detection and staying vigilant is absolutely crucial. Combat against leprosy is not a one-trick pony either, there's a need to utilize antibiotic regimens, stage community discussions to erode stigma, and integrate leprosy care into the broader healthcare infrastructure. Further, you've got to look at the whole picture by addressing the social factors that leave some individuals more vulnerable, making sure that everyone gets fair access to care so the disease can't spread further. Generally speaking, antimicrobial resistance connected to leprosy has become a growing worry on top of everything else. Despite multidrug therapy remaining effective for the majority of situations, caution is needed because silently erosion by resistance undermines the efficacy of treatment for many infections worldwide. In poor locations, where laboratory infrastructure and surveillance networks are haphazard, even a handful of resistant strains could shift the scales, heightening the general leprosy burden. This reality, touching mortality and chronic health issues as much, implies that enhancing health infrastructure, improving diagnostics, and developing new treatments are more necessary than ever. In the vast majority of instances, acknowledging the connection between controlling leprosy and global antimicrobial resistance patterns is central to informing regional and international health policy capable of protecting treatment outcomes (Christopher et al., 2022). Stepping back from antimicrobial concerns, it's also notable that leprosy is grouped with other neglected tropical diseases that most afflict poor populations. These diseases tend to accumulate disability and social marginalization—calculated in disability-adjusted life years, or DALYs, which combine death and chronic suffering into one large image. Health initiatives, both national and global, have increased measures focused on containing and eliminating these conditions more comprehensively. These efforts rely on prevention measures, enhanced healthcare provision, and patient rehabilitation while attempting to reduce not just the prevalence of the disease but also the significant burden of public stigma. Overall, there is an international acknowledgment that combating leprosy is part of the puzzle for gaining greater overall health equity and improved overall outcomes in countries where the disease continues to rage unchecked (Amal et al., 2017).

KEY TERMS FROM THIS CHAPTER

- Autoimmune triggers
- Community education
- Early detection
- Fungal infections
- Molecular diagnostics
- Multi-drug plan
- Peripheral neuropathy
- Social exclusion
- Blindness
- Community health programs
- Eczema
- Healthcare gaps
- Mucous membranes
- Nerve growth factor
- Psoriasis

References

1. Ackley, C., Elsheikh, M., & Zaman, S. (2021). Scoping review of Neglected Tropical Disease Interventions and Health Promotion: A framework for successful NTD interventions as evidenced by the literature. *PLoS neglected tropical diseases*, *15*(7), e0009278. https://doi.org/10.1371/journal.pntd.0009278 (accessed on 10th May 2025).

2. Steinmann, P., Dusenbury, C., Addiss, D., Mirza, F., & Smith, W. C. S. (2020). A comprehensive research agenda for zero leprosy. *Infectious diseases of poverty*, *9*(1), 156. https://doi.org/10.1186/s40249-020-00774-4 (accessed on 10th May 2025).

3. Deribe, K., Meribo, K., Gebre, T., Hailu, A., Ali, A., Aseffa, A., & Davey, G. (2012). The burden of neglected tropical diseases in Ethiopia, and opportunities for integrated control and elimination. *Parasites & vectors*, *5*, 240. https://doi.org/10.1186/1756-3305-5-240(accessed on 10th May 2025).

4. Begay, R. L., Roland, M. J., Blair, I. V., & Brondolo, E. (2024). Discrimination among American Indian and Alaska Native people: implications for public health communication. *Frontiers in public health*, *12*, 1384608. https://doi.org/10.3389/fpubh.2024.1384608(accessed on 10th May 2025).

5. Perez, R. L., Chase, J., & Tanner, R. (2024). Shared challenges to the control of complex intracellular neglected pathogens. *Frontiers in public health*, *12*, 1423420. https://doi.org/10.3389/fpubh.2024.1423420 (accessed on 10th May 2025).

6. Dako-Gyeke, M., Asampong, E., & Oduro, R. (2017). Stigmatization and discrimination: Experiences of people affected by leprosy in Southern Ghana. *Leprosy Review, 88*, 58–74. https://doi.org/10.47276/lr.88.1.58 (accessed on 10th May 2025).

7. Debelu, D., Mengistu, D. A., Aschalew, A., Mengistie, B., & Deriba, W. (2024). Global Public Health Implications of Traffic Related Air Pollution: Systematic Review. *Environmental health insights*, *18*, 11786302241272403. https://doi.org/10.1177/11786302241272403(accessed on 10th May 2025).

8. Faurholt-Jepsen D. (2013). The double burden. *Danish medical journal*, *60*(7), B4673. (accessed on 10th May 2025).

9. Gall, L. S., & Riely, P. E. (2025). *Effect of Diet and Atmosphere on Intestinal and Skin flora: Volume II – Literature Survey*. https://core.ac.uk/download/pdf/85249155.pdf (accessed on 10th May 2025).

10. Gligorijević, J., Stevanović, S., & Stanković, V. (2024). Weight bias and stigmatization: Is it a matter of public health? *Proceedings of the International Congress Public Health – Achievements and Challenges – Zbornik Radova*. Book of Abstracts - International congress Public health – achievements and challenges - zbornik radova, p. 262-262 https://www.semanticscholar.org/paper/5ced0a91d0b483657b7cb40df3e71659b9ed8772 (accessed on 10th May 2025).

11. Hambridge, T. (2024). *Shortening leprosy case detection delay: Narrowing the window of transmission and disease progression*. [Doctoral Thesis, Erasmus University Rotterdam]. (accessed on 10th May 2025).

12. van Haaren MA, Reyme M, Lawrence M, Menke J, Kaptein AA. Illness perceptions of leprosy-cured individuals in Surinam with residual disfigurements – "I am cured, but still I am

ill". *Chronic Illness*. 2016;13(2):117-127. doi:10.1177/1742395316657398 (accessed on 10th May 2025).

13. Katoch, V. M. (2024). Eradication of leprosy from India: Reflections on past, present & future. *The Indian Journal of Medical Research, 159*, 1. https://doi.org/10.4103/ijmr.ijmr_64_24 (accessed on 10th May 2025).

14. Manyi-Loh, C. E., Mamphweli, S., Meyer, E. L., & Okoh, A. I. (2018). Antibiotic use in agriculture and its consequential resistance in environmental sources: Potential public health implications. *Molecules, 23*, 795. https://doi.org/10.3390/molecules23040795 (accessed on 10th May 2025).

15. Marešová, P., Javanmardi, E., Baraković, S., Baraković, H. J., Tomsone, S., Krejcar, O., & Kuča, K. (2019). Consequences of chronic diseases and other limitations associated with old age – A scoping review. *BMC Public Health, 19*. https://doi.org/10.1186/s12889-019-7762-5 (accessed on 10th May 2025).

16. Widasmara D, Linuwih Menaldi S. Demyelination in Leprosy [Internet]. Hansen's Disease - The Forgotten and Neglected Disease. IntechOpen; 2019. Available from: http://dx.doi.org/10.5772/intechopen.76892(accessed on 10th May 2025).

17. Mendes, D. S. G. J., Soares, F. S., Da Silva, M. V., Alves, S. M. C., & Montagner, M. I. (2024). As vulnerabilidades das mulheres na hanseníase: Uma revisão integrativa de literatura. *Cadernos Ibero-Americanos de Direito Sanitário*. https://www.semanticscholar.org/paper/3c07ae3929c4949dc2cd369e3e179eff8be715d2 (accessed on 10th May 2025).

18. Miguel, D. C., Brioschi, M. B. C., Rosa, L. B., Minori, K., & Grazzia, N. (2021). The impact of COVID-19 on neglected parasitic diseases: What to expect? *Trends in Parasitology, 37*, 694–697. https://doi.org/10.1016/j.pt.2021.05.003 (accessed on 10th May 2025).

19. Mitra, A. K., & Mawson, A. R. (2017). Neglected tropical diseases: Epidemiology and global burden. *Tropical Medicine and Infectious Disease, 2*, 36. https://doi.org/10.3390/tropicalmed2030036 (accessed on 10th May 2025).

20. Mtui, J., & Osoro, O. (2011). *Aggregate Cost Implications of Selected Cost-Drivers in the Tanzanian Health Sector*. Commissioned by: Ministry of Health and Social Welfare. Final Report 12/1/2011. https://core.ac.uk/download/pdf/11307328.pdf (accessed on 10th May 2025).

21. Murray, C. J. L., Ikuta, K. S., Sharara, F., Swetschinski, L. R., Robles, A. G., Gray, A. P., Han, C., et al. (2022). Global burden of bacterial antimicrobial resistance in 2019: A systematic analysis. *The Lancet, 399*, 629–655. https://doi.org/10.1016/s0140-6736(21)02724-0 (accessed on 10th May 2025).

22. Weekly Newsletter for the Center for Acute Disease Epidemiology of the Iowa Department of Public Health. *Epi Update for Friday, October 6, 2017*. https://publications.iowa.gov/id/eprint/25283; https://core.ac.uk/download/95086440.pdf (accessed on 10th May 2025).

23. Nahid, P., Mase, S., Migliori, G. B., Sotgiu, G., Bothamley, G., Brożek, J., Cattamanchi, A., et al. (2019). Treatment of drug-resistant tuberculosis: An official ATS/CDC/ERS/IDSA clinical practice guideline. *American Journal of Respiratory and Critical Care Medicine, 200*, e93–e142. https://doi.org/10.1164/rccm.201909-1874st (accessed on 10th May 2025).

24. Nazir, A., Zafar, M. F., Ishfaq, A., Bakhtiar, M., Ali, S. A., Afzaal, U., Ullah, A., et al. (2023). Leprosy on the horizon: An upward trend in Central Florida. *International Journal of Surgery Global Health, 6*. https://doi.org/10.1097/gh9.0000000000000328 (accessed on 10th May 2025).

25. Oliver, S. J. (2022). From Isolation to Inclusion: Embracing Local Perspectives in Examining the Treatment Model of Care for Aboriginal Persons Affected by Tuberculosis or Leprosy in the Kimberley Region, North Western Australia [Doctor of Philosophy (College of Medicine)]. The University of Notre Dame Australia. https://researchonline.nd.edu.au/theses/386(accessed on 10th May 2025).

26. Pradeep, M., Wang, M., & Pan, C. (2020). *Telepresence Robots for Healthcare Management: COVID-19 Experience (Preprint)*. https://www.semanticscholar.org/paper/ace1e2d569d9986132b00f6ae75d21562b620802 (accessed on 10th May 2025).

27. Ravichandran, N., 2004. "**Tuberculosis Control in developing countries: A Generalized Community Health Worker Based Model**," IIMA Working Papers WP2004-06-01, Indian Institute of Management Ahmedabad, Research and Publication Department. (accessed on 10th May 2025).

28. Schmid-Grendelmeier, P., Rapelanoro Rabenja, F., Beshah, A. M., Ball, M. D., Dlova, N., Faye, O., Flohr, C., Hsu, C., Mavura, D., Manuel, R. C., Ramarozatovo, L. S., Sendrasoa, F., Wollenberg, A., Ruiz Postigo, J. A., & Taïeb, A. (2023). How to integrate atopic dermatitis in the management of skin neglected tropical diseases in Sub-Saharan Africa?. *Journal of the European Academy of Dermatology and Venereology : JEADV*, 10.1111/jdv.19096. Advance online publication. https://doi.org/10.1111/jdv.19096(accessed on 10th May 2025).

29. Thomas, P. (2004). *DFID Policy Project: DFID and disability. A Mapping of the Department for International Development and Disability Issues, Disability Knowledge and Research Programme, 82 pp* (accessed on 10th May 2025).

30. Tomás, C., Oliveira, E., de Sousa, D. W. A., Chupel, M. U., Furtado, G. E., Rocha, C., Teixeira, A., et al. (2016). Proceedings of the 3rd IPLeiria's International Health Congress. *BMC Health Services Research, 16*. https://doi.org/10.1186/s12913-016-1423-5 (accessed on 10th May 2025).

31. Wilsher, Emma, Jane (2011) *The impact of Neglected Tropical Diseases, and their associated stigma, on people's basic capabilities.* Masters thesis, Durham University.. https://etheses.dur.ac.uk/3301/(accessed on 10th May 2025).

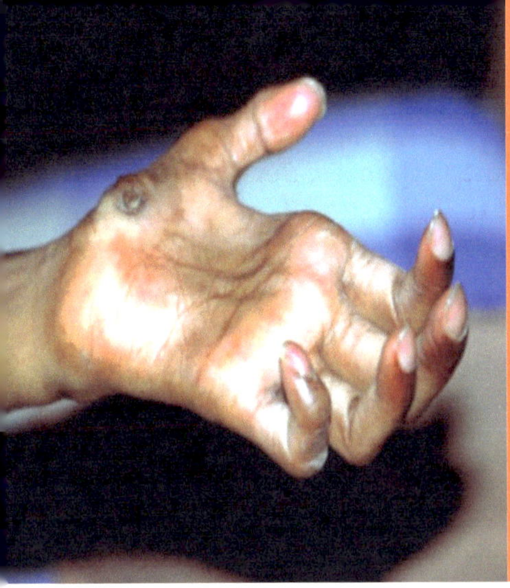

Chapter 10

UPDATES AND ADVANCEMENTS IN LEPROSY RESEARCH

Contents

Introduction

Infectious diseases have long steered how we think about public health and pushed scientific inquiry in new directions. Leprosy, or Hansen's disease as some call it, shows this vividly with its persisting symptoms, heavy stigma, and puzzling nature. It's caused by a tiny bacterium, *Mycobacterium leprae*, that meddles with the skin, nerves, mucous membranes, and even the eyes , leaving lasting marks and disability if not managed. Back in 1894, a modest place known as the Louisiana Leper Home opened in Carville, Louisiana, eventually growing into a national leprosarium by 1921. Even though that hospital closed in 1999, its influence still pops up in educational efforts and archives that capture both patient stories and medical progress (Turner, 2021). Over time, a deeper awareness of leprosy's effects has spurred fresh research into how the disease works, ways to catch it early, and even new treatments. Scientists today dive into the biological characteristics of *Mycobacterium leprae* as a way to crack its code. They're especially curious about the roles played by families of proteins, like the

PE/PPE bunch—that litter its genome and help it dodge our immune responses. Detailed looks at these proteins remain a hot topic as researchers try, in most cases, to understand how the disease moves forward and how the microbe interacts with its host. On top of that, the new MycobactERIal PE/PPE proTeinS (MERITS) database has popped up to fill a big gap. Packing over 22,000 non-redundant PE/PPE proteins, MERITS mixes details about their structural characteristics, chemical traits, where they settle inside cells, and even glimpses at their antigenic properties, all wrapped up in an interactive search tool. This tool offers a fresh way to zero in on diagnostic markers and potential therapy targets (He etal., 2024). Recent progress in the battle against leprosy feels like a jumble of past insights and modern smarts. The historical lessons from places like Carville still weigh in, lending context to today's clinical strategies and care models; meanwhile, tech advances like the MERITS database show how a bit of bioinformatics can help map out the complex interaction between a pathogen and its host. Generally speaking, combining old-school perspective with high-tech methods puts us on a promising track – not only for better individual care but also for advancing global efforts to spot the disease earlier, cut down its stigma, and ultimately bring its impact under tighter control (Figure 10.1).

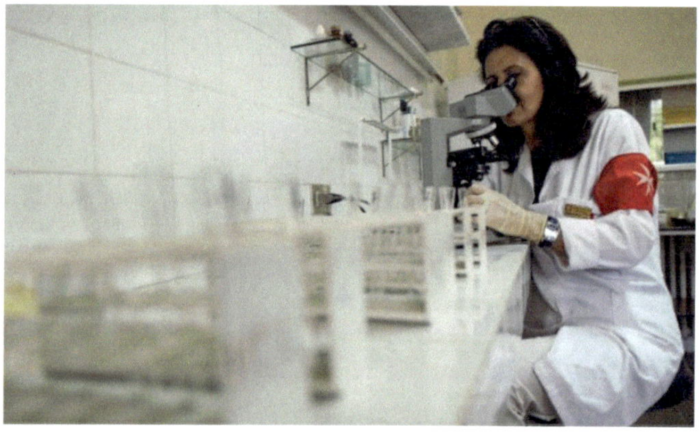

Figure 10.1. The order involved in significant developments in leprosy research.

Source: Sovereign Order of Malta. (2009, December 28). *Developments in Leprosy Research.*

10.1. Recent Diagnostic Techniques

New advances in diagnostics have taken on a important role when it comes to fighting complex infections like leprosy. Traditional tests that focus on a pathogen's shape and its serological traits often fall short, not always giving the detailed breakdown needed for specific treatment decisions; in many cases, they're simply too blunt. With mycobacterial infections—where the microbes grow so slowly that making a timely diagnosis becomes a challenge, researchers are turning to methods that, to be honest, seem to work better. For instance, by tagging amino acids like [35S] methionine and pairing that with advanced imaging, scientists have managed to come up with something akin to a "barcode" system that sorts out different mycobacterial species. Even though *Mycobacterium leprae* tends to be extra stubborn thanks to its lipid-rich cell wall and the hassles of metabolic labeling, looking at secreted proteins instead of the overall cell content still opens up new doors for identification (Furst et al., 1993). To summarize, this kind of approach could tip the scales toward earlier, more exact leprosy diagnoses, which in turn shapes treatment outcomes. Molecular techniques have also jumped into the mix, reshaping our view on diagnosing infectious diseases. Take polymerase chain reaction (PCR) methods—they're pretty much the frontrunners given their impressive sensitivity and tendency for isolating even minute traces of pathogen DNA. Although PCR has already been shown to be invaluable in illnesses like leishmaniasis, it carries just as much weight for leprosy research. By boosting species-specific DNA sequences, PCR sidesteps many of the pitfalls of older tests, like those painfully long culture times and often ambiguous serological results. This isn't just about catching an infection sooner; it's also about nailing down exactly which strain is at work, a point that matters a lot when it comes to both tailor-made treatments and keeping tabs on outbreaks (Ellis et al., 2022). Generally speaking, putting these molecular advances into practice in endemic regions could make a big difference in stopping leprosy in its tracks. On another front, researchers have started exploring bacterial metabolites and secreted compounds as natural hints for how to tell species apart. Mycobacteria, for example, churn out certain iron-binding substances—mycobactins—that vary from species to species, a clue that might just serve as a kind of biomarker. Recent alters in the way these mycobactins are extracted and labeled, such as using radioactive iron isotopes, have substantially boosted detection sensitivity, offering a faster and more reliable route to identification straight from clinical samples. This method, in a way, makes up for the characteristics of *Mycobacterium leprae*, which usually resists standard protein tagging approaches. When you mix these biochemical signals with both molecular and radiolabeling tools, you end up with a layered diagnostic framework that promises not only earlier intervention but also smoother patient management and sharper tracking of disease spread (Furst et al., 1993) (Figure 10.2).

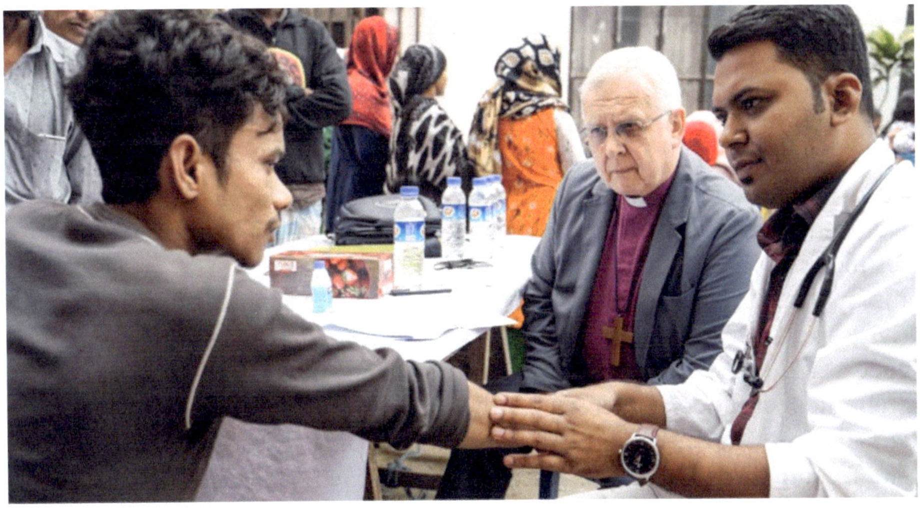

Figure 10.2. A five-minute finger prick test to diagnose leprosy.

Source: Leprosy Mission International. (n.d.). *Finger Prick Test for Leprosy Diagnosis.*

10.1.1. Molecular Methods for Detection

Microbiological identification has come a long way, especially when it comes to tracking infections like leprosy. Before, labs relied on looking at shapes through staining and running biochemical tests, which, honestly, just didn't always catch *Mycobacterium leprae* early enough. Nowadays, scientists are leaning on nucleic acid amplification to speed things up and clear away ambiguity in the diagnosis. Even methods that use radiolabeled protein synthesis, despite being complex with *M. leprae* due to its odd metabolism, have given us peek-worthy insights into how bacteria are grouped and why molecular tools are so necessary (Furst et al., 1993). To summarize, combining these new molecular diagnostics into everyday practice has reshaped both patient care and how we keep track of outbreaks. Recent breakthroughs in PCR technology have been pretty eye-opening too. Generally speaking, PCR can amplify those tiny amounts of genetic material that older staining methods often miss in leprosy cases where bacteria numbers are low. This means that not only can we get a more sensitive read, but PCR assays also help sort out different strains and detect even drug-resistant mutations—critical information for figuring out treatments and public health measures. Compared to past methods, PCR cuts the wait time and doesn't demand that the bacteria be alive, which is, in most cases, a major plus in places with limited resources. There's even evidence from similar infectious diseases, like leishmaniasis, that these techniques work well, and researchers have adapted those ideas to boost research and outcomes in leprosy too (Ellis et al., 2022). At the same time, emerging molecular techniques are shaking things up by homing in on pathogen-specific biomarkers with striking precision. The thick, lipid-rich cell walls of mycobacteria push researchers to get creative—focusing either on secreted proteins or on unique markers like mycobactins. For example, radiolabeling with isotopes such as 55Fe has shown promise in quickly telling apart different Mycobacterium species; this can be pretty important when fast diagnosis is key for keeping infections under control (Furst et al., 1993). Working alongside next-generation sequencing and real-time PCR variations, these methods paint a fuller picture of the microbe, helping tailor treatments and even track outbreaks in a more personalized way. In the end, the ongoing push to refine and standardize these molecular approaches not only drives leprosy research forward but also supports better practices in both clinical settings and public health responses against this long-neglected disease.

10.1.2. Serological Tests and Their Effectiveness

Advances in lab methods have transformed how we spot infectious diseases. Serological tests, for instance, are used to pick up antibodies or even antigens – little hints about what the body's fighting. In cases like mycobacterial infections such as leprosy, these tests offer a quick, noninvasive option that joins up with older techniques like microscopy and culture. It's worth noting, though, that the sensitivity and specificity of these tests can shift, often depending on which antigens are in play and what stage the disease is at. Modern strides in immunoproteomics and molecular biology have even uncovered fresh antigen candidates, which generally ups the chances of crafting better serodiagnostic tools, especially in those complex paucibacillary cases where the bacterial load is very low. To summarize, this progress is key to catching cases early and cutting down on transmission. Still, serological tests, despite their appeal, run into issues like cross-reactivity and the natural variability of immune responses among patients, which can complicate interpretation and clinical choices. A test's true value depends on its tendency for separating individuals who are truly infected from those who've merely been exposed but aren't showing disease, while also sorting out the different forms of the illness. Arguably, system-scale strategies combined with genome-scale data have been stepping up efforts to refine antigen selection, thus stimulating test performance upward. In many cases, combining serological assays with molecular techniques – like PCR – can help cross-check and validate results, boosting diagnostic accuracy, even if not perfectly. These methods, connected together loosely, help iron out previous issues with inconsistent sensitivity and specificity; hence, deploying them in regions where the disease is common could enhance screening programs, lead to earlier treatment starts, and ultimately improve patient outcomes (Ellis et al., 2022).

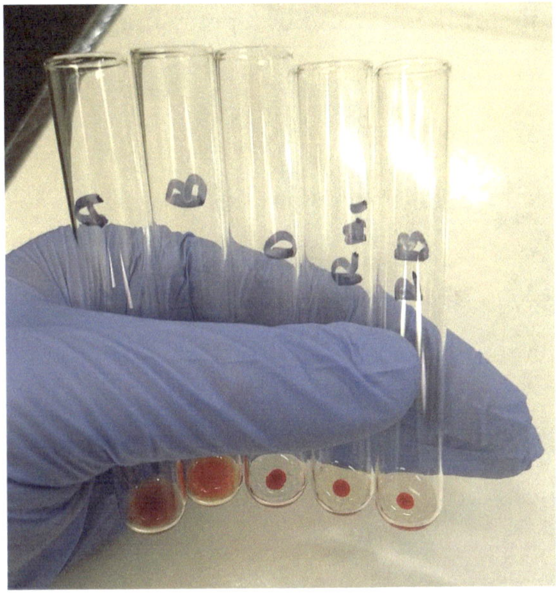

Figure 10.3. Serological tests.

Source: By SpicyMilkBoy - Own work, CC BY-SA 4.0, https://commons.wikimedia.org/w/index.php?curid=86499299

Expanding the view beyond leprosy, diseases like leishmaniasis show us both the promise and the limits of serological testing in tackling vector-borne infections. The sheer variety of Leishmania species and the many ways the illness can show up have pushed experts to use a combination of serological and molecular diagnostic tools—nowadays, PCR-based methods are often favored for their sensitivity and specificity. Insights from these other illnesses underline how combining serological tests with molecular diagnostics can help bypass the shortcomings of using them on their own. This idea carries direct implications for leprosy research as well, where catching the right pathogen signal remains a real challenge. Continued innovation—generally speaking, borrowing lessons from related fields—promises to fine-tune serological tests so they work better for early detection, treatment monitoring, and overall disease control strategies (Ellis et al., 2022). These crossover ideas offer a sort of roadmap for smoothing out leprosy diagnostics, which could ultimately boost global health outcomes (Figure 10.3)..

10.1.3. Imaging Techniques in Leprosy Diagnosis

Breakthroughs in diagnosing complex conditions like leprosy have changed how infections are handled. In many cases, doctors used to lean on clinical checks and histopathological confirmations, which, let's be honest, can take a while and sometimes throw up unclear results, especially when cases are new or borderline. Nowadays, imaging pops up as a non-invasive way to peek at nerve issues and tissue damage from leprosy. This fresh approach helps catch problems earlier, guiding treatment more exactly while lessening long-term setbacks. In a sense, combining in these visuals has opened up new insights that standard methods might miss. When you look closer, ultrasonography and MRI now play a starring role in detecting leprosy's signs. Ultrasound gives a real-time look at the peripheral nerves, showing changes like nerve thickening, shifts in vascularity, and even little spots that hint at inflammation or fibrosis. MRI, on the other hand, brings out the details by offering great contrast—letting doctors clearly map nerve involvement and soft tissue characteristics. This extra information can make it easier to tell whether a patient has active leprosy or is just dealing with leftover nerve damage, which is key for choosing the right treatment plan. Even though you need some specialized equipment and know-how to get these images, they mesh nicely with lab tests and help smooth out the overall approach to patient care. Still, challenges stick around. *Mycobacterium leprae* has its own characteristics—it's slow growth and tough cell wall, for instance, making standard lab techniques less reliable and highlighting the need for fresh diagnostic ideas (Furst et al., 1993). Advanced imaging, generally speaking, fills this gap by offering critical anatomical and pathological signals without invasive steps. Further, research into *M. leprae*'s metabolic profile and related biomarkers might eventually jive with imaging findings, boosting diagnostic accuracy and helping predict how treatments will pan out. With ongoing alters to imaging methods, teamed with collaborative research and tech advances, we're taking a big step forward in the evolving world of leprosy diagnosis and care (Health, 2018) (Figure 10.4).

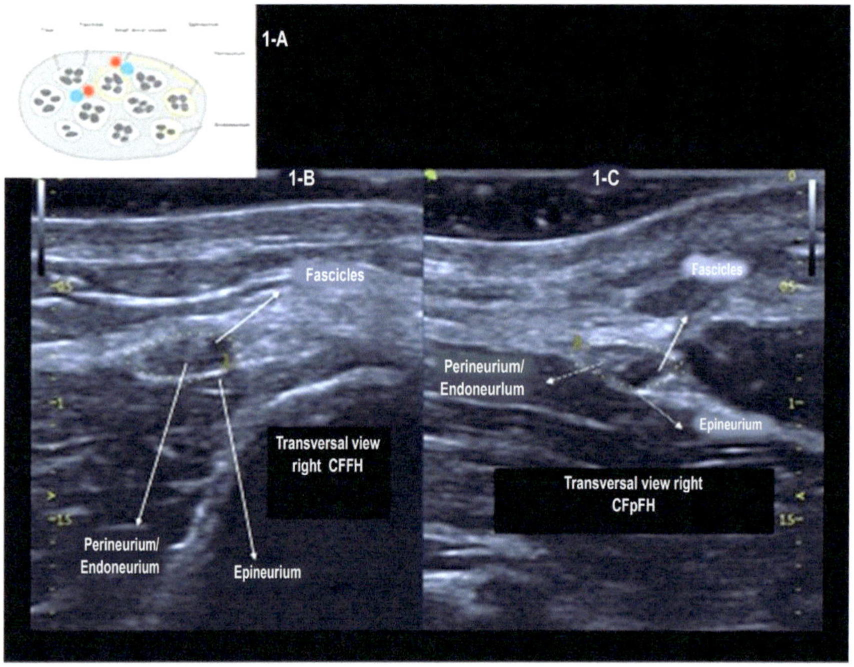

Figure 10.4. Point-of-care ultrasound of peripheral nerves in the diagnosis of Hansen's disease.

Source: Voltan, G., Filho, F. B., Leite, M. N., De Paula, N. A., Santana, J. M., Silva, C. M. L., Barreto, J. G., Da Silva, M. B., Conde, G., Salgado, C. G., & Frade, M. A. C. (2022). Point-of-care ultrasound of peripheral nerves in the diagnosis of Hansen's disease neuropathy. *Frontiers in medicine*, *9*, 985252. https://doi.org/10.3389/fmed.2022.985252

10.2. Advances in Treatment

Back when institutions like the national leprosarium in Carville, Louisiana first opened their doors, leprosy care mostly meant keeping patients separated and providing long-term support because there weren't any real cures. Today, the story looks quite different. Doctors now lean on multidrug therapy – a combination of dapsone, rifampicin, and clofazimine – which in most cases has turned treatment into something that aims to cure. Clinical research and deeper insights into the disease's microbiological and immunological characteristics have driven these changes; it's almost as if each new discovery peels away yet another layer of mystery about the disease. The early days, marked by both social and medical hurdles, now seem remote compared to modern public health strategies and drugs that work (Turner, 2021). In a sense, continual innovation remains key if we're to keep disease control on track. Diagnostic microbiology too has taken a wild-turn in refining treatment, even though earlier approaches – those relying on simple cell shapes and basic chemical tests , sometimes couldn't tell apart subtypes of *Mycobacterium leprae* from similar bacteria. With the advent of molecular biology techniques such as protein pattern analysis using radiolabeled compounds, and by tracking specific metabolic markers, tests have become faster and more precise. This helps doctors tailor treatments based on strain differences linked to drug resistance and virulence; strangely enough, sometimes repeating these markers feels like a broken record, yet it underlines their importance. There's even been promising work with mycobactins acting as species-specific indicators, it all comes together to ensure that patients get targeted help when they need it most (Furst et al., 1993). Still, challenges creep in, especially because *Mycobacterium leprae*'s slow growth and its thick, lipid-rich cell wall make both diagnosis and drug delivery a real headache. Researchers, in most cases, have had to get creative: working on analogs that mimic the bacterium's metabolic tricks has opened new drug ideas and ways to fight resistance. The days of large, isolated leprosaria are over, replaced by community-based treatment models that emphasize early diagnosis and strict adherence to multidrug therapy to prevent lasting disability. This gradual shift from seclusion to integrated care mirrors our evolving understanding of how best to manage the disease, ensuring that fresh scientific insights eventually benefit communities everywhere (Furst et al., 1993; Turner, 2021).

10.2.1. Multi-Drug Therapy (MDT) Updates

Recent breakthroughs in leprosy care have stirred up the long-used protocols of MDT. For decades, using a combination of dapsone, rifampicin, and clofazimine was the go-to, but now many are rethinking treatment lengths and drug choices. Researchers are tinkering with shorter courses and fresh alternatives—generally speaking, this could help ease side effects and slow down resistance. It's not a neat, linear process; sometimes patients in under-resourced areas still struggle with adverse drug reactions and issues with taking their medication consistently.

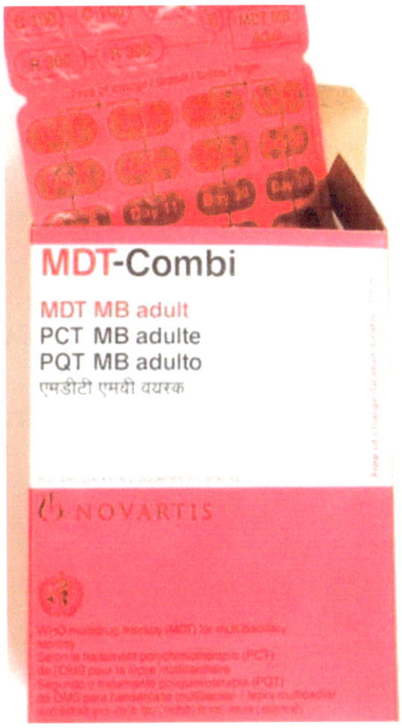

Figure 10.5. Multi-drug therapy (MDT) updates.

Source: Media Storehouse. (n.d.). *MDT Drug Combination Used in Leprosy Treatment.*

There's also a growing conversation about the tougher parts of MDT. Severe reactions, like immune-related damage that harms the skin and mucous membranes—pose a real challenge and sometimes throw a wrench in treatment plans. Recent studies hint at the value of adding immunomodulatory therapies alongside traditional drugs, a move that might help ease toxicity. In most cases, managing these complications means dermatologists, immunologists, and infectious disease specialists have to huddle together and come up with plans that not only improve tolerability but also support long-term care. Sometimes ideas echo across the team, even if the details don't always line up perfectly. International collaboration is picking up steam too, with global networks sharing clinical data and practical tips to tackle rare yet serious drug-related issues. These data-sharing platforms help with early detecting of complications and encourage a more flexible, patient-first approach. When experts from different corners of the world join forces, the focus naturally shifts toward boosting both clinical outcomes and overall quality of life. By pooling their collective knowledge, those in the leprosy research community keep stimulating forward the boundaries of treatment innovation while keeping patient safety front and center (Chang et al., 2020) (Figure 10.5).

10.2.2. New Pharmacological Agents in Development

Lately, there's been a growing buzz around the need for new treatments for infectious diseases, especially when it comes to neglected illnesses like leprosy. Traditional drugs do their job to a point but face problems—drug resistance, long treatment periods, and patients struggling to stick with tough regimens. This pushes the case for fresh pharmacological agents that can work better and lighten the treatment load. Some researchers aren't sticking to the usual antibiotic playbook; instead, they're checking out a combination of compounds with the potential to fight mycobacteria. For example, sutezolid has been showing some impressive strength that's on par with today's standards, inducing ideas of changing up how treatments are done. Then there's the side idea of using enzyme therapies, like lysins derived from mycobacteriophages, which might target bacteria more directly, possibly replacing older drugs and cutting down on issues like resistance and toxicity (Enriquez et al., 2025). Another interesting track in developing new drugs involves repurposing medications that we already trust for safety yet have not explored for battling mycobacteria. Statins, most often prescribed for cholesterol issues, seem to be doing more than just managing lipids. Recent studies hint that atorvastatin, simvastatin, and fluvastatin might also act against mycobacterial pathogens. Generally speaking, their extra antimicrobial effects could work hand-in-hand with first-line antibiotics; this kind of combo might even shorten the therapy duration and lessen the side effects that come from using high antibiotic doses. It's an approach that speeds up discovery since these drugs are already approved, and it offers a cost-effective strategy, especially in regions where leprosy still runs rampant (Enriquez et al., 2025). Then there's a whole other angle with nanotechnology that's starting to make waves. Advances in this field have led to the creation of biologically synthesized metallic nanoparticles (MNPs) that seem to pack a unique antimicrobial system. Using plant-based methods for synthesis not only boosts the effectiveness and compatibility of these nanoparticles but also tends to lower their environmental footprint and toxicity. Plants from biodiversity-rich spots, like parts of South Africa, provide natural reducing and stabilizing agents to produce silver, gold, and zinc nanoparticles that can attack bacteria whether by disrupting cell membranes or interfering with their metabolism. In many cases, these bioengineered nanomedicines might just revolutionize leprosy treatment by offering options that are both targeted and scalable, even though further validation is still on the horizon.

10.2.3. Challenges in Treatment Adherence

Managing leprosy relies a lot on patients keeping up with their multidrug therapy. There are several issues that can interfere with this, sometimes treatments drag on for six months or even longer, which can wear someone down, both physically and mentally. Side effects and adverse drug reactions often lead patients to skip doses or quit the regimen altogether. Then there's the heavy burden of social stigma and discrimination that makes people hesitant to seek the necessary care. Economic struggles and poor access to health facilities, particularly in rural areas hit hardest by leprosy, further complicate things. In most cases, handling this isn't only about medicine but also about addressing socio-economic and cultural challenges. New studies show that building integrated support systems can help boost treatment adherence (Enriquez et al., 2025). On the next front, even though breakthroughs in drug development offer solid hope against microbial resistance, patient compliance still proves to be a tough nut to crack. Recent work with novel antibiotics and therapeutic agents, similar to those being tested in Buruli ulcer treatment, points to simpler dosing schedules and lower toxicity levels as keys to improved adherence. You see, exploring adjuvant therapies and repurposing drugs, which might reduce treatment lengths and mitigate side effects, is looking pretty promising for leprosy too. Still, these scientific advances need to be paired with approaches that attend to mental health and the overall psychosocial wellbeing of patients. Research during the recent pandemic reminds us that psychological distress in communities with infectious diseases is common, suggesting mental health support is crucial for keeping patients on track (Shofner et al., 2021).

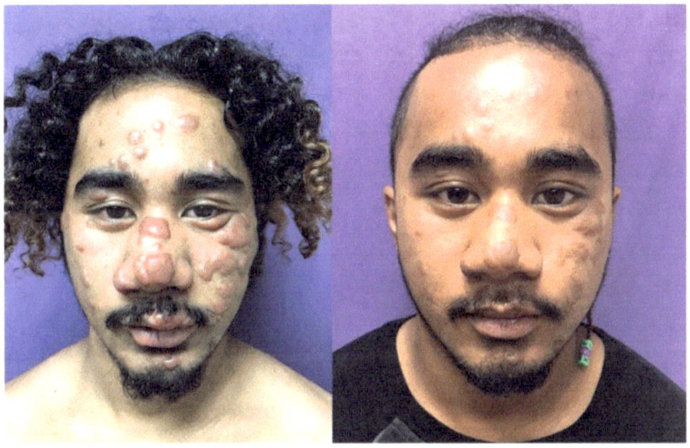

Figure 10.6. A 20-year-old male with multibacillary Hansen's disease (nodular lepromatous) treated with monthly rifampin, minocycline, and moxifloxacin and demonstrated rapid clinical improvement of skin nodules and plaques. This patient completed a 24-month course of monthly ROM with adequate adherence to the regimen and no adverse events without evidence of skin lesions or hyperpigmentation.

Source: Sage Journals. (2022). *Clinical Response to ROM Therapy in Hansen's Disease.*

Combining these fresh ideas with wider public health measures could ease the treatment burdens quite a bit. Long-term success against leprosy depends on looking at the full picture of patient experience and healthcare delivery. Educating individuals about how the disease spreads, the benefits of sticking with treatment, and coping with drug side effects can clear up many misconceptions and boost compliance. Still, building stronger community relationships and chipping away at stigma with effective awareness campaigns is just as important for encouraging timely diagnosis and regular therapy. Meanwhile, upgrading healthcare infrastructure in underserved areas helps ensure that medications are consistently available and follow-up care is in place. Even though new drugs play an important role, they won't cut it on their own without socio-behavioral support. A well-rounded approach that mixes modern treatment options with broad psychosocial care seems essential to overcoming adherence problems and pushing leprosy control forward (Enriquez et al., 2025; Shofner et al., 2021) (Figure 10.6).

10.3. Vaccine Research

Effective vaccine development has always been a complex business; the real challenge lies in getting the immune system fired up just right. Lately, tech breakthroughs have stimulated us into exploring fresh ways to uncover adjuvants that make vaccines work better. Old, standard adjuvants? They kind of fell short, offering little variety and making it hard to design strong vaccines for complicated foes like leprosy. Nowadays, AI steps in unexpectedly, combined to biomedical research and digs through huge biological datasets to flag potential compounds that can jumpstart a more tailored immune reaction. In most cases, combining AI with vaccine studies has sped up our hunt for next-generation vaccines that might change the game for infectious diseases and even cancer, pointing to a hopeful route for leprosy vaccine improvements (Zhang et al., 2024). Genomic and proteomic tools have flipped the script on how we see mycobacterial pathogens—those pathogenic microbes behind leprosy and similar issues. A big pile of genome-scale data now sits at scientists' fingertips, letting them look at the whole system and spot new antigen candidates that matter for vaccines. These "omics" methods let us dissect the different parts of a pathogen that set off immune responses, so designing vaccines becomes less guesswork and more about targeting specific, immune-triggering proteins. High-throughput screening, in its own rapid-fire way, chimes in by quickly sifting through loads of antigens, which speeds up picking the best potential candidates. Overall, these strides in computational biology and the new wave of immunoproteomics mark a major shift away from clumsy trial-and-error approaches, promising vaccines that are both more precise and effective against leprosy (Rana et al., 2018). Even with all this tech and data wizardry, there's still a mountain to climb before these findings shine in clinics. Candidates born from AI and "omics" must pass strict tests, proving they can stir a strong yet safe immune response without any nasty side effects. Leprosy itself, chronic and complex, means the vaccine shouldn't just block infection but also fine-tune ongoing immune reactions to lessen the disease's grip. Combining different angles, like running AI-driven searches for better adjuvants alongside system-wide antigen hunts—is pretty much the secret recipe for next-generation vaccines. Generally speaking, understanding the whole host-pathogen interaction and ensuring immune balance gives new hope for not just controlling but maybe even eradicating this very old disease (Rana et al., 2018; Zhang et al., 2024).

10.3.1. Current Status of Leprosy Vaccines

Recent progress in understanding mycobacterial foes has induced a fresh push to develop better vaccines for leprosy, a stubborn infectious illness that still leaves its mark worldwide. Scientists are now combining genome-wide insights with emerging omics methods, which lets them spot promising new antigen targets at a pace that old approaches just couldn't match. Computational biology teamed with immunoproteomics is combing through enormous datasets to flag molecular targets that might induce protective immune responses. These broad, system-level strategies hold the promise of designing next-generation vaccines rationally, even if traditional methods have, in most cases, struggled to curb transmission effectively. High-throughput technologies carry a special weight for leprosy, since older formulations like BCG tend to work only partially or vary a lot in their effectiveness. To summarize, leaning on this cutting-edge research framework seems to be a critical step forward in crafting a more effective preventive measure against the disease (Rana et al., 2018). Even with these exciting developments, real-life hurdles remain. Challenges in creating and rolling out new leprosy vaccines are complex up with wider social and health infrastructure problems typical of neglected tropical diseases (NTDs). Leprosy itself stands out as a prime example of an NTD suffering from low advocacy, inconsistent funding, and a lack of attention globally—even while it inflicts lifelong disability and harsh social stigma. Poverty and poor sanitation, often combined together in the worst-affected communities, make it even tougher to set up vaccination programs. To add to the mix, the COVID-19 crisis has interrupted ongoing immunization efforts and diverted precious resources, making progress toward the WHO's elimination targets even more elusive. This overall lack of sustainable funding and coordination emphasizes the need for strategies that mix vaccine innovation with better community education and disease monitoring (Butala et al., 2025). Current vaccine candidates under evaluation span a wide range, ranging from subunit vaccines that target specific mycobacterial proteins (unearthed using omics approaches) to modified whole-cell preparations that have been altered to boost immune responses. Several clinical trials have looked into these constructs in hopes of enhancing cell mediated immunity, which is crucial for fighting *Mycobacterium leprae* infections. Yet truly robust and widely accessible vaccines remain hard to come by, largely due to the pathogen's unique characteristics and the complicated nature of our immune responses. Future research must not only refine antigen selection—using insights from immunoproteomics—but also tackle the practical issues of getting vaccines to endemic areas. Combining scientific advances with thoughtful health policy seems vital for turning lab progress into real-world, preventive measures against leprosy, ultimately easing its burden on vulnerable populations (Butala et al., 2025; Rana et al., 2018) (Figure 10.7).

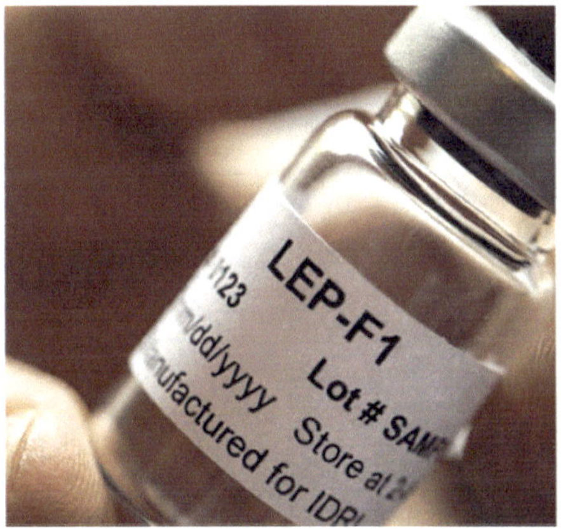

Figure 10.7. The leprosy vaccine.

Source: ILEP Federation. (2020). *The Leprosy Vaccine.*

10.3.2. Innovative Approaches in Vaccine Development

Scientists are leaning heavily on big genomic datasets paired with creative computer methods in vaccine work. Omics tools have turned the game around when it comes to detecting potential antigen targets for microbes like *Mycobacterium leprae*. Some labs now mix systems biology with immunoproteomics to dive deep into a pathogen's protein mix, uncovering candidates that older methods might simply miss. This marks a shift from guesswork towards a more focused, targeted approach—generally speaking, a promising way to bypass some long-standing vaccine hurdles. Genome-scale approaches seem to boost leprosy research by zeroing in on the tiny, essential molecular parts that keep bacteria alive and infectious, and that might even change how we handle prevention and diagnosis (Rana et al., 2018). AI is now joining the fray as an unexpected ally. Purpose-built platforms let researchers run huge screenings of vaccine components—including those all-important adjuvants that help fire up the immune system, even as new adjuvant ideas have trickled in only slowly over the years. In most cases, this mix of artificial intelligence with vaccine research broadens the discovery process, offering fresh ways to fine-tune these immune boosters that are key for fighting leprosy. Sometimes, the synergy between technology and biology opens up unexpected paths that might finally overcome some stubborn roadblocks in vaccine design (Zhang et al., 2024).

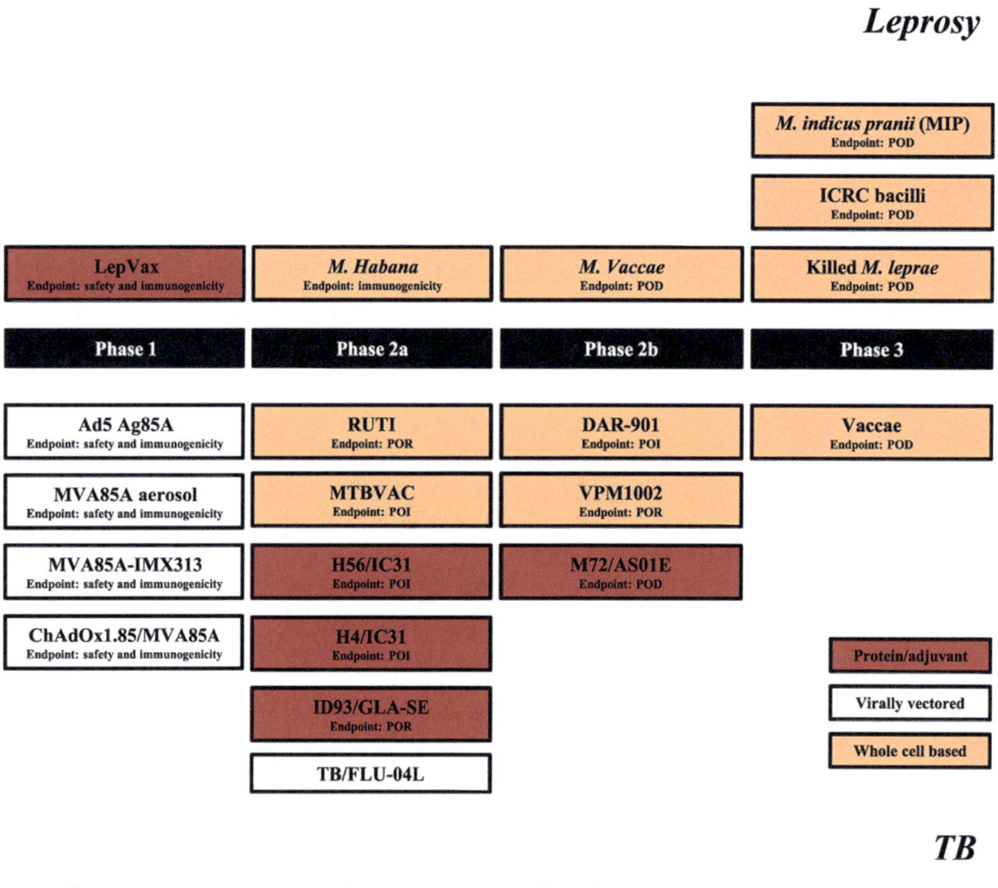

Figure 10.8. The innovative approaches in vaccine development.

Source: Coppola M, van den Eeden SJF, Robbins N, Wilson L, Franken KLMC, Adams LB, Gillis TP, Ottenhoff THM and Geluk A (2018) Vaccines for Leprosy and Tuberculosis: Opportunities for Shared Research, Development, and Application. Front. Immunol. 9:308. doi: 10.3389/fimmu.2018.00308

New techniques and tools are gradually piecing together a smarter plan against persistent diseases like leprosy. Bioinformatics exploits teamed with AI-driven adjuvant altering suggest that soon, vaccines may be more precise, safer, and longer lasting—even if tailoring them to varied genetic backgrounds and immune characteristics means a bit of extra work at first. This somewhat casual, yet innovative, approach not only speeds up early tests but also creates space for customizing vaccines to match diverse host responses. Overall, the merging of these advanced methods seems ready to fill in the existing gaps in leprosy vaccine efficacy, potentially shifting the whole landscape of disease control and elimination (Rana et al., 2018; Zhang et al, 2024) (Figure 10.8).

10.3.3. Potential Impact of Vaccines on Global Health

Vaccines have long shifted how we handle infectious diseases, cutting sickness and death around the globe. Look at leprosy, a disease that rarely gets the spotlight, which still spreads despite available multidrug therapies. People keep getting sick, which shows we need ways to stop the infection before symptoms even come on. The fact is that companies often ignore vaccine research for neglected tropical diseases like leprosy. It's a tough sell since affected individuals usually live in hard-to-reach, unstable areas, and the low profit potential leaves little incentive. These economic and social roadblocks slow vaccine progress and distribution, so creating creative partnerships becomes key for better health equity (Aerts et al., 2017). Integrating vaccines into everyday public health could change the game, breaking the chain of transmission and easing leprosy's wider economic and social strains. It's not all about the medicine, though; you also have to think about how different places work. Urban sprawl, rural layouts, political characteristics, and outdated infrastructure all play a part in who gets help. Generally speaking, the way city planning meshes with local governance can surprise you, making the need for flexible, interdisciplinary vaccination strategies all the more obvious (Talocci et al., 2022). Sometimes the details matter, and the puzzle only fits when things are adjusted on the fly. If leprosy vaccines catch on, they might even pave the way for tackling other overlooked diseases. In most cases, partnerships between public bodies and private companies can induce fresh ideas and better access in low-resource spots—even if the setup isn't perfect. Still, a lack of solid, on-the-ground studies has made it hard to scale things up. We need careful, real-world checks to show that vaccine programs do what they're supposed to and to guide policy for long-term success. To summarize, while the biomedical promise is clear, turning that promise into genuine global health improvements means building a whole system of support (Aerts et al., 2017) (Figure 10.9).

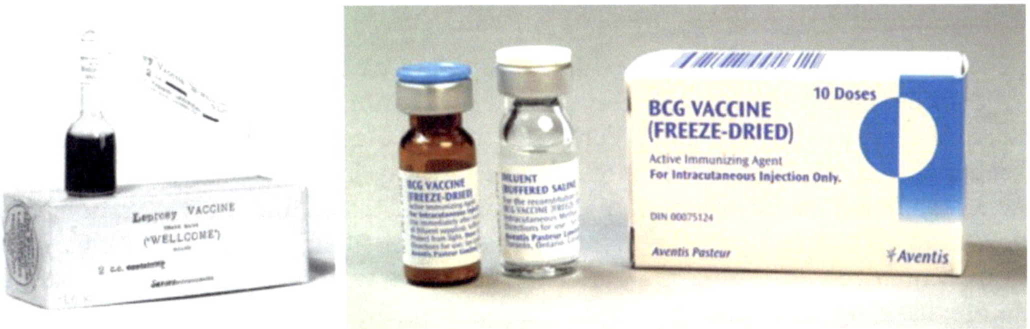

Figure 10.9. Photographs of vaccines. Left: a leprosy vaccine of unknown composition produced by the Wellcome Physiological Research Laboratories in London, United Kingdom, circa 1978. Right: a BCG vaccine to prevent tuberculosis, manufactured by Aventis Pasteur Canada in 2002.

Source: Springer Nature. (n.d.). *Leprosy and BCG Vaccine Images.*

10.4. Socioeconomic Factors

Infectious diseases combine with economic situations connects a pretty complex way that molds overall health. Looking back at old outbreaks like the 1918 flu, it's evident that people with low incomes tended to suffer more—poor nutrition, cramped living, and scarce medical help all piled up to increase risks (Van Doren, 2025). Leprosy, for instance, shows a similar pattern; communities struggling financially often deal with vulnerabilities that speed up disease spread and trip up treatment routines. In most cases, public health efforts have to reckon with more than just microbes, because the social and economic details work their own complex magic. This means that tackling leprosy smartly isn't only about biology, it's also about boosting living conditions, a decent diet, and easier access to health services in affected regions. Primary care is supposed to be the backbone when it comes to handling chronic infections, but its effectiveness hangs on socioeconomic factors. Studies in low and middle-income places reveal that hurdles like steep drug costs and a lack of preventive focus in policies hit the less privileged hardest (Dill et al., 2014). It's a complex scenario: early detection and sticking to treatment are crucial to avoid lasting damage, yet the limited resources and spotty patient education slow down progress. Generally speaking, when healthcare resources are thin and knowledge about how leprosy spreads isn't widespread, managing the disease becomes even complex. Addressing this requires a kind of reinvention in primary care—ramping up training, spicing up patient education, and bridging gaps left by economic inequities, all while trying to build community trust. Economic disparities don't just impact individual health; they also shape how leprosy plays out across different communities. Rural areas and underfunded urban neighborhoods often see higher rates of the illness, thanks to delayed diagnoses and scarce healthcare access (Van Doren, 2025). This trend isn't exactly new; history shows that isolated or neglected populations usually pay a heavier toll when epidemics strike. Many researchers now combine insights from anthropology with epidemiology to untangle the mix of cultural, historical, and economic forces that keep the disease around. In most cases, a tailored approach that increases social support, improves nutrition, and cuts down on stigma is seen as key to breaking the cycle of neglect and boosting health fairness in regions where leprosy stubbornly persists.

10.4.1. Impact of Stigma on Leprosy Patients

Looking back at history, the way people with leprosy were treated shows just how stubborn stigma can be. In Carville, Louisiana, for instance, there was a national leprosarium where patients were put aside from everyone else—a move born from both the desire to stop the disease spread and a deep-seated fear of what the illness might bring. In many instances, isolating those affected did help slow things down medically, yet it also reinforced exclusion and discrimination. The scars of such segregation still show up in the mental and social challenges that patients face even today. Carville's own archives (Turner, 2021) offer a observe how stigma morphed alongside modern medicine, emphasizing that healing isn't only about improved diagnosis but also about mending societal wounds. Stigma's reach, however, goes far beyond mere social alienation, it seeps into the very quality of life and mental well-being of those with leprosy. Feelings of shame, isolation, and low self-worth creep in, often making it harder for individuals to seek help when needed or stick to treatment plans. Such hesitancy, in turn, can help the disease persist longer within communities. Moreover, stigma complex with socioeconomic hardships means that people in marginalized groups, who sometimes have barely enough access to healthcare, suffer even more. Anthropological views, generally speaking, remind us that social inequalities only compound these health issues, turning every setback into a bigger challenge (Van Doren, 2025). Addressing stigma, then, calls for a combination of strategies, not just new medical breakthroughs, but also robust social support and education. Modern studies on leprosy now acknowledge that even the best biomedical advances can't wipe away the heavy burden of stigma by themselves. A more well-rounded plan is needed, one that combine medical care with psychological help and respects cultural nuances. Educational campaigns that bust old myths can ease public fear, creating friendlier settings for patients to accept and continue their treatments. Meanwhile, when patients join support groups or participate in counseling sessions, that ingrained stigma starts to lose its grip, slowly returning self-confidence and a sense of belonging. Researchers increasingly value personal narratives—stories preserved in national museums and archives serve as reminders of the actual human experience behind the statistics. To summarize, weaving together medical progress with real-life accounts (Turner, 2021) is key to breaking down long-held prejudice and opening the door to dignity and inclusion for everyone affected by leprosy (Figure 10.10).

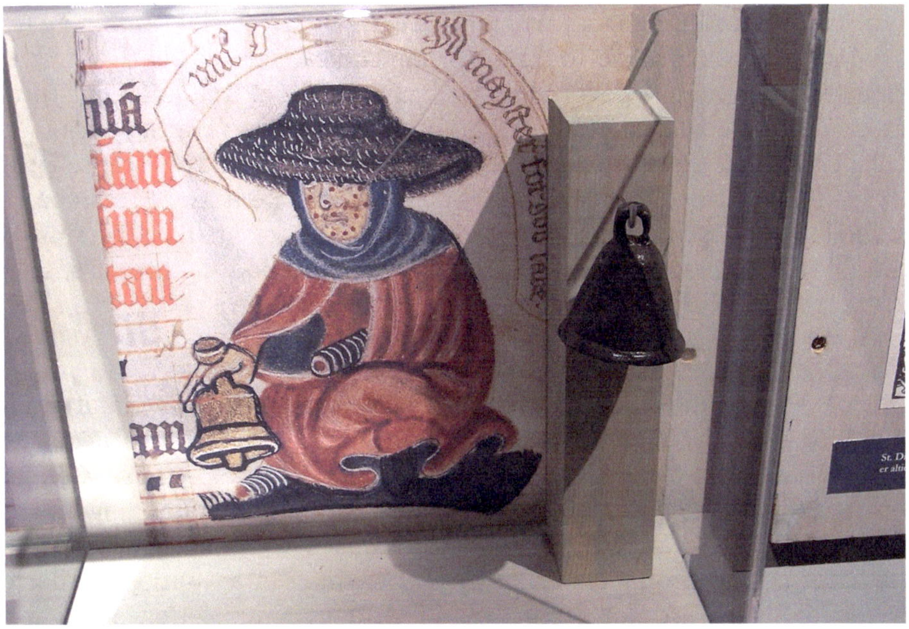

Figure 10.10. Facing the stigma of leprosy.

Source: By No machine-readable author provided. Cnyborg assumed (based on copyright claims). - No machine-readable source provided. Own work assumed (based on copyright claims)., CC BY-SA 3.0, https://commons.wikimedia.org/w/index.php?curid=173803

10.4.2. Access To Healthcare and Treatment

Boosting healthcare access for people with leprosy has taken on fresh forms as public health efforts have shifted toward fairness. In many places, especially where the disease has hit hard for a long time, care for leprosy isn't isolated—it's now nested in everyday health systems. Iran, for instance, built a widespread network of primary care that combines community input with smart planning. They set up both rural and urban centers to offer must-have services, which has slashed many hurdles for patients. This method leans on preventing illness and teaching individuals about health so that early signs are detected among vulnerable groups. Still, there are gaps, like the uneven quality between city clinics and those out in the countryside, reminding us that more work on better infrastructure and trained staff is needed (Aboutorabi et al., 2023). All of these shifts add up to a more inclusive, if not perfect, approach to managing leprosy. Old misunderstandings among healthcare providers can slow down the process of getting fast and proper leprosy treatment, especially in areas where the condition is rare or wrapped in stigma. In the US, for example, some studies suggest that doctors sometimes get the wrong idea about how easily leprosy spreads, which in turn delays care. That kind of misinformation often stokes unnecessary fear and discrimination, pushing patients into an awkward corner when they need help. The attitude of a provider isn't just about clinical skill—it also shapes whether patients feel welcome enough to show up for treatment. Interviews with clinicians treating Hansen's disease often reveal that they see themselves as the bridge over these knowledge gaps, chopping down stigma and smoothing out the treatment journey (Kuhns 2012). Without filling in these educational gaps, the push for timely, quality care remains uneven worldwide. Lately, new breakthroughs in leprosy research have been zeroing in on widening treatment access by combining traditional care with wider social support. Innovative ideas now pair clinical services with community outreach to tackle the intertwined issues of poverty, stigma, and isolation. One notable approach lets local health workers hand out medicines and check on patients up close, cutting back on the long trips to specialized centers. Even more, tying in leprosy care with broader disease programs means sharing resources in a way that makes overall patient management more rounded (Aboutorabi et al., 2023). To summarize, these advances promise not only better medical handling of leprosy but also stronger social inclusion and increased fairness for those battling the disease.

10.4.3. Role of Community Education and Awareness

Managing leprosy isn't just about handing out medical treatments; it's about sharing the right information among community members. People often get the wrong idea about how easily the disease spreads or how severe it might be—this, in most cases, leads to hesitation in seeking help promptly. Healthcare experts note that these widespread gaps in understanding often deepen social exclusion and cause delays in treatment. Sometimes, a focused, community-driven educational push can break these nasty cycles; simple efforts to debunk myths can encourage earlier diagnosis and steadier adherence to treatment plans. This mix of clear communication and practical care not only eases fears but also boosts the impact of overall public health strategies against leprosy. In fact, when nurses and other healthcare workers take time to pass on accurate information, they build a vital bridge over the chasm of ignorance (Kuhns 2012). Primary healthcare has changed over time, showing that local involvement plays a key role in fighting diseases like leprosy. Iran's spread of both rural and urban health centers, for example, gives a clear picture of how combining health education into everyday community life can make essential services easier to reach and even lift overall wellness. It isn't just about having the latest treatments—putting preventive care and awareness side by side empowers people to tackle health challenges together, even when things get a bit complex. The idea here is simple: aside from cool lab advances, robust health education within everyday care makes a difference in cutting down disease rates and harsh outcomes. Even as health systems keep evolving, stepping up outreach and education remains a driving force against leprosy and other often-overlooked illnesses (Aboutorabi et al., 2023). Keeping up steady support for community education turns scientific breakthroughs into real-world wins in leprosy research.

New methods in diagnosing and treating the disease only hit home once people understand and trust them, helping to smash the myths that keep isolation going. When communities are armed with solid knowledge, they build resilience and start standing up for their own health, taking part in prevention in ways big and small. This back-and-forth between fresh science and local know-how creates an approach that's just about essential for tackling the disease entirely. As research keeps moving forward, pairing it with clear, relatable education is indispensable for easing stigma, improving care use, and keeping leprosy under control in the long run (Kuhns 2012; Aboutorabi et al., 2023) (Figure 10.11).

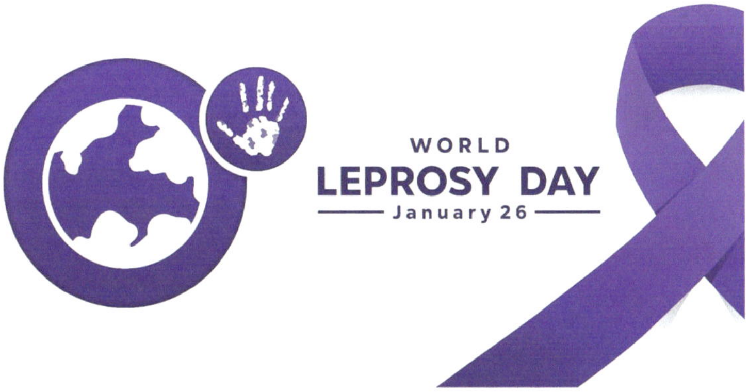

Figure 10.11. World leprosy day 2024: Awareness, prevention, and care strategies.

Source: Artemis Hospitals. (2024). *World Leprosy Day Awareness.*

A CLOSER LOOK

THE POTENTIAL ROLE OF ARTIFICIAL INTELLIGENCE (AI) IN HANSEN'S DISEASE (HD) (LEPROSY)

HD, commonly known as leprosy, is a contagious and chronic infectious disease. It experienced a resurgence in new cases after a reduction during the COVID-19 pandemic in 2020. Reflecting this shift, the number of countries reporting HD information increased from 143 in 2021 to 182 in 2022. Globally, 174,087 new cases were reported in 2022, representing a 23.8% increase compared to the 140,594 cases reported in 2021. The rise in newly detected cases in 16 of the 23 global priority countries in 2022 was attributed to improved leprosy services following the pandemic. While the overall increase in all priority countries was 25% compared to 2021, the growth varied from 3.4% in Micronesia to 107.4% in Myanmar.

HD is caused by *Mycobacterium leprae*; in some regions, *Mycobacterium lepromatosis* is also involved. The incubation period is long (average of five or more years). The bacillus is likely transmitted through droplets from the nose and mouth during prolonged close contact with untreated patients.

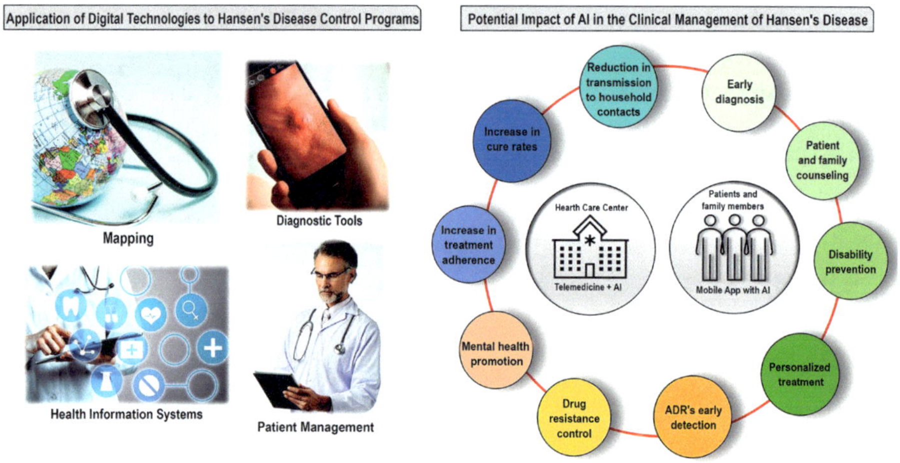

Figure 10.12. Integration of digital technologies and artificial intelligence (AI) in Hansen's disease (HD) management.

Source: Deps PD, Yotsu R, Furriel BCRS, de Oliveira BD, de Lima SL and Loureiro RM (2024) The potential role of artificial intelligence in the clinical management of Hansen's disease (leprosy). Front. Med. 11:1338598. doi: 10.3389/fmed.2024.1338598

The rapid progress of digital technologies offers great potential for transforming the approach to HD programs. At the International Federation of Anti-Leprosy Associations (ILEP) conference in 2020, various participants explored the application of new digital technologies to enhance HD services. ILEP members are adopting state-of-the-art technologies in mapping, diagnostics, health information systems, and patient management. This underscores the importance of staying updated on emerging technological trends to improve HD programs and ultimately enhance the well-being of individuals affected by the disease. Figure 10.12 illustrates the integration of digital technologies and AI in HD management.

Role of AI in Diagnosis of HD

The comprehensive strategy outlines decisive steps to combat HD worldwide, especially in regions with a shortage of specialized physicians. First and foremost, AI could be key in screening and diagnosing new HD cases, thus bridging this "expertise gap." This includes implementing initiatives to identify cases and contacts in regions with elevated HD detection rates, often referred to as HD hotspots, with prior education campaigns at community level. In addition, the evaluation of diagnostic tools such as antibody detection and molecular techniques is particularly valuable in identifying multibacillary cases, which account for approximately 69% of new HD cases globally.

Machine learning, a branch of AI, enables computers to learn from data and make decisions without explicit instructions. It is widely used in areas such as image recognition and speech processing. In healthcare, machine learning models can be trained to recognize skin lesions by analyzing images to identify disease patterns. Machine learning algorithms can also analyze patient data for diagnosis and risk prediction. These technologies, when validated and available in mobile apps, could significantly improve timely HD diagnosis.

AI algorithms to diagnose HD will initially classify people as suspected cases. However, a "human" doctor will make the final confirmation. AI can be a valuable tool for early detection and identification, helping medical experts make more accurate and efficient diagnoses. Finally, the availability of algorithms capable of diagnosing HD also signifies that an increasing number of new cases can be detected.

AI effectively recognizes the typical clinical presentations of HD, which experienced dermatologists or well-trained physicians can readily identify. However, laboratory tests can be invaluable for atypical clinical manifestations, asymptomatic individuals, or subclinical cases of HD, including SSS, skin or nerve biopsy, RLEP quantitative polymerase chain reaction (qPCR), and anti-PGL-I serology.

Treatment Personalization with AI

HD manifests differently among patients, requiring tailored treatment approaches for better outcomes and fewer complications. AI-driven personalized HD treatment starts with the comprehensive collection and combination of various patient data. This includes medical history, genetic information, clinical evaluations, past treatments, and socioeconomic background. The remarkable ability of AI to analyze this abundance of information offers a comprehensive view of the patient's situation, leading to more precise treatment decisions.

AI can contribute significantly to personalized HD treatment through two key aspects: risk stratification and prediction of individual response to therapy. By analyzing the collected data, AI algorithms can classify patients into risk groups based on factors such as HD type, bacterial load, and comorbidities. This risk stratification allows healthcare providers to allocate resources more effectively and prioritize high-risk patients who require closer monitoring and specialized care. In addition, based on a large dataset of treatment outcomes, AI can identify patterns and factors that influence the effectiveness of specific treatments for individual patients. Equipped with this predictive capability, healthcare providers can make informed decisions about drug selection and dosing, minimizing the risk of adverse effects, drug resistance, and treatment failure.

The role of AI is to go beyond the prescription phase and actively participate in the patient's treatment journey. AI-powered applications can provide real-time reminders and support and ensure that patients adhere to their treatment plans. This technology improves not only treatment outcomes but also the patient experience by providing personalized guidance and encouragement.

SUMMARY

Diagnostic technology has been changing over time, which in turn has reshaped how leprosy research is done. New molecular techniques, similar to those used for other infections—help us spot the bacteria much more precisely. Catching the disease early is key for cutting down transmission and avoiding serious complications. When these advanced methods get woven into everyday monitoring, they speed up finding new cases, and that can slow down how fast the disease spreads. Still, in most cases, these scientific breakthroughs need to go hand in hand with improved access and affordability to truly support communities hit hardest by both the disease and economic hardships (Ellis et al., 2022). Working together across different fields matters here, especially when social and economic challenges are part of the picture. Past experiences in community work and philanthropy remind us that pairing scientific progress with solid support systems can make a big difference. Historical trends show that strategic community engagement along with steady funding has been essential to overcome health crises (Tan & Prakash, 2015). When researchers, medical professionals, policymakers, and local communities join forces, leprosy programs tend to become more flexible and welcoming. This kind of mix not only helps patients stick with their treatments but also eases stigma and isolation, which often mess up effective leprosy care. At the end of the day, even though these new advances hold real promise for better detection, treatment, and prevention, real progress depends on ongoing commitment at many levels of society. The balance between innovative research and comprehensive social approaches will largely decide future elimination efforts. That means we constantly need to reexamine both our scientific approaches and the social-political structures that support them. In most cases, putting an emphasis on education, smart resource allocation, and policy improvements, while still pushing for new discoveries, will be key to overcoming the final hurdles. Ultimately, when all these efforts come together, they might not just control but eventually eradicate leprosy as a public health issue, marking a major step forward in both infectious disease research and global health fairness.

Leprosy research has made some big leaps in recent years. Scientists have dug deep into the inner workings of *Mycobacterium leprae* – the microbe behind the disease , and uncovered complex details at the molecular level. They found that groups of proteins, like the PE/PPE family, seem to interfere with both the microbe's attack plan and our body's defenses. A resource called MERITS is now on hand, offering loads of details about these proteins' shapes and roles, which naturally stokes new questions and ideas. This kind of work helps decode the complex back-and-forth between the host and its invader, setting the stage for clever new testing methods and treatments. It's a handy, user-friendly tool that fills in gaps about how the disease rolls out and how our immune systems respond (Agarwal et al., 2023). At the same time, while the lab results are promising, the overall support for leprosy studies remains a bit patchy. In places like India – a country long dealing with high leprosy numbers – research budgets and focus on linked oral health issues tend to fall short compared to global standards. Securing grants and dealing with tedious admin duties often hold back both dental and medical experts from chasing more groundbreaking work. Even so, there's a gradually emerging sense that steady investment in oral health research, including studies on leprosy complications, matters. Generally speaking, if these hurdles get smoothed over, a stronger research scene could induce fresh breakthroughs in diagnosis, treatment, and public health measures (Agarwal et al., 2023). Researchers aren't stopping at the biology either; they're also working on smarter ways to catch and fight the disease. By combining data from high-speed sequencing, structural studies, and immune system analyses, teams are pinpointing potential antigen targets that could flag the disease early and boost our natural defenses. Tapping into these robust datasets about protein signals and microbe interactions is opening up new paths for vaccine design that might sidestep past shortcomings. This shift toward a precision medicine approach means treatments can be altered to fit both the microbe's and the patient's unique genetic and immune profiles. To summarize, these advances underscore a determined—if sometimes imperfect—effort in the scientific community to outsmart leprosy with fresh, cross-disciplinary methods (He etal., 2024).

KEY TERMS FROM THIS CHAPTER

- Bioinformatics
- DNA sequences
- Genetic material
- Lipid-rich cell wall
- Microbiological identification
- Mycobacterial infections
- Polymerase chain reaction
- Serological tests
- Diagnostic markers
- Fibrosis
- Leishmaniasis
- Metabolic labeling
- Mycobacteria
- Pathogen-specific biomarkers
- Radiolabeled protein synthesis
- Ultrasonography

References

1. Chang, W. C., Abe, R., Anderson, P., Anderson, W., Ardern-Jones, M. R., Beachkofsky, T. M., Bellón, T., Biala, A. K., Bouchard, C., Cavalleri, G. L., Chapman, N., Chodosh, J., Choi, H. K., Cibotti, R. R., Divito, S. J., Dewar, K., Dehaeck, U., Etminan, M., Forbes, D., Fuchs, E., ... Carleton, B. C. (2020). SJS/TEN 2019: From science to translation. *Journal of dermatological science*, *98*(1), 2–12. https://doi.org/10.1016/j.jdermsci.2020.02.003 (accessed on 10th May 2025).
2. Aboutorabi, A., Darvishi Teli, B., Rezapour, A., Ehsanzadeh, S. J., Martini, M., & Behzadifar, M. (2023). History of primary health care in Iran. *Journal of preventive medicine and hygiene*, *64*(3), E367–E374. https://doi.org/10.15167/2421-4248/jpmh2023.64.3.3081 (accessed on 10th May 2025).
3. Aboyewa JA, Sibuyi NRS, Meyer M, Oguntibeju OO. Green Synthesis of Metallic Nanoparticles Using Some Selected Medicinal Plants from Southern Africa and Their Biological Applications. *Plants*. 2021; 10(9):1929. https://doi.org/10.3390/plants10091929 (accessed on 10th May 2025).
4. Aerts, C., Sunyoto, T., Tediosi, F., & Sicuri, E. (2017). Are public-private partnerships the solution to tackle neglected tropical diseases? A systematic review of the literature. *Health policy (Amsterdam, Netherlands)*, *121*(7), 745–754. https://doi.org/10.1016/j.healthpol.2017.05.005(accessed on 10th May 2025).
5. Agarwal, A., Das, M., Pradhan, S., Sharma, S., et al. (2023). *Funding Opportunities of Extramural Grants for Oral Health Researchers in India – A Prospective Approach*. https://core.ac.uk/download/588567199.pdf (accessed on 10th May 2025).
6. Zhijie He, Cong Wang, Xudong Guo, Heyun Sun, Yue Bi, Miranda E Pitt, Chen Li, Jiangning Song, Lachlan J M Coin, Fuyi Li, MERITS: a web-based integrated *Mycobacterial* PE/PPE protein database, *Bioinformatics Advances*, Volume 4, Issue 1, 2024, vbae035, https://doi.org/10.1093/bioadv/vbae035 (accessed on 10th May 2025).
7. Talocci, G., Brown, D., & Yacobi, H. (2022). The biogeopolitics of cities: a critical enquiry across Jerusalem, Phnom Penh, Toronto. *Planning Perspectives*, *37*(1), 169–189. https://doi.org/10.1080/02665433.2021.2019608 (accessed on 10th May 2025).
8. Butala, C. B., Cave, R. N. R., Fyfe, J., Coleman, P. G., Yang, G. J., & Welburn, S. C. (2024). Impact of COVID-19 on the neglected tropical diseases: a scoping review. *Infectious diseases of poverty*, *13*(1), 55. https://doi.org/10.1186/s40249-024-01223-2 (accessed on 10th May 2025).
9. Dill, A. (2014). *Primary Care Perspectives: A Descriptive Study of Primary Care Health Systems and Physicians Treating Cardiovascular Disease and Risk Factors in Karnataka, South India*. University of North Carolina at Chapel Hill; https://doi.org/10.17615/tpxq-qc13
10. (accessed on 10th May 2025).
11. Dominguez, E. J. P. (2025). *Treatment of Buruli Ulcer: Research, Development, and Repurposing of New Therapeutics Targeting Mycobacterium Ulcerans*. Universidade do Minho Escola de Medicina. https://core.ac.uk/download/650948436.pdf (accessed on 10th May 2025).
12. Dong, B. J., Chen, J. H., Coghi, P. S., Zhang, W. Y., Zheng, X. L., & Fan, X. X. (2024). *Revolutionizing Adjuvant Development: Harnessing AI for Next-Generation Cancer Vaccines*. https://core.ac.uk/download/628386033.pdf Zhang, W. Y., Zheng, X. L., Coghi, P. S., Chen, J. H., Dong, B. J., & Fan,

X. X. (2024). Revolutionizing adjuvant development: harnessing AI for next-generation cancer vaccines. *Frontiers in immunology*, *15*, 1438030. https://doi.org/10.3389/fimmu.2024.1438030 (accessed on 10th May 2025).

13. Gow, I., Smith, N. C., Stark, D., & Ellis, J. (2022). Laboratory diagnostics for human Leishmania infections: a polymerase chain reaction-focussed review of detection and identification methods. *Parasites & vectors*, *15*(1), 412. https://doi.org/10.1186/s13071-022-05524-z (accessed on 10th May 2025).
14. Furst, V. W. (1993). *Bacterial Taxonomy – Analytical Biochemical Methods with Special Reference to Mycobacteria*. https://core.ac.uk/download/326712128.pdf (accessed on 10th May 2025).
15. Kuhns, Kristen E., "What's to Know?: Navigating Knowledge Gaps of Hansen's Disease in the U.S.." Thesis, Georgia State University, 2012. https://scholarworks.gsu.edu/anthro_theses/66(accessed on 10th May 2025).
16. Loma Linda University Health. (2018). TODAY – March/April 2018. https://core.ac.uk/download/159479493.pdf (accessed on 10th May 2025).
17. Rana, A., Thakur, S., Kumar, G., & Akhter, Y. (2018). Recent Trends in System-Scale Integrative Approaches for Discovering Protective Antigens Against Mycobacterial Pathogens. *Frontiers in genetics*, *9*, 572. https://doi.org/10.3389/fgene.2018.00572 (accessed on 10th May 2025).
18. Shofner, Ashley D., "Exploring Mental Health & COVID-19: How a Pandemic Could Become America's Next Mental Health Crisis" (2021). Honors Theses. 834. https://encompass.eku.edu/honors_theses/834 (accessed on 10th May 2025).
19. Tan, P., & Prakash, R. (2015). *Philanthropy on the Road to Nationhood in Singapore: Philanthropy in Asia: Working Paper No. 1*. https://core.ac.uk/download/84911878.pdf (accessed on 10th May 2025).
20. Turner, Laura, "Stories from Both Sides of the Hedge: A History of and Digital Exhibit for the National Hansen's Disease Museum" (2021). *Electronic Theses and Dissertations*. 366. https://scholarworks.sfasu.edu/etds/366(accessed on 10th May 2025).
21. Van Doren, T. (2025). *Social Inequalities and Mortality During the 1918 Influenza Pandemic on the Island of Newfoundland*. Anthropology electronic theses and dissertations (MU). https://hdl.handle.net/10355/91637
22. https://doi.org/10.32469/10355/91637(accessed on 10th May 2025).

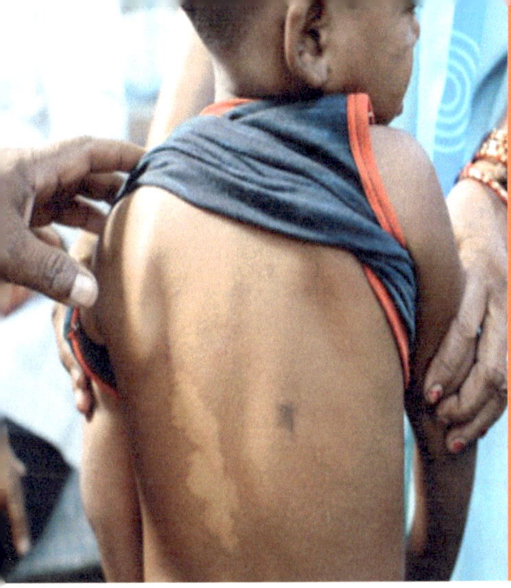

Chapter 11

PEDIATRIC LEPROSY

Contents

Introduction

Leprosy still sticks around as a real public health issue in some parts of the world, even with all the global efforts aimed at knocking it out. Caused by *Mycobacterium leprae*, this long-lasting infection shows up mainly on the skin and peripheral nerves, and if it isn't detected early, it can result in serious disabilities. Even though overall cases are generally down, the appearance of cases in kids tells us that transmission is still going on within communities. Children, with their still-maturing immune systems and extra vulnerability, provide key signals to how the disease spreads. Finding hidden infections among household contacts only highlights this secret burden and suggests we need better early detection methods and ongoing monitoring (Alves et al., 2013). Economic growth and better health care in many countries have cut the numbers for lots of neglected tropical diseases, yet leprosy remains a stubborn threat, especially for children in affected areas. Unlike some success stories like guinea worm or trachoma, leprosy keeps proving complicated, with delays in diagnosis, social stigma, and uneven access to care playing major roles. In most cases, pediatric leprosy cases flag that transmission is still active in the community, which means public health strategies must adapt to the unique risks that children face. Meanwhile, emerging health systems and mobile tech promise improvements in surveillance and management, though these tools need to be woven into broader, more comprehensive plans to truly battle pediatric leprosy alongside other neglected diseases (Hotez et al., 2019). Clinically, leprosy in kids often doesn't act the same way it does in adults, leading to a combination of unique challenges in diagnosis and disease progression. Early identification is crucial—not only to prevent long-term disabilities but also to break the chain of transmission. Recent studies using both serological tests and molecular approaches have shown, in most cases, that markers like nasal carriage detection can reveal hidden or subclinical infections among household contacts, a finding that is especially important for children at high risk. These diagnostic advances offer promising new paths for timely intervention and careful monitoring, which could ultimately help lessen both the burden and further spread of pediatric leprosy (Alves et al., 2013) (Figure 11.1).

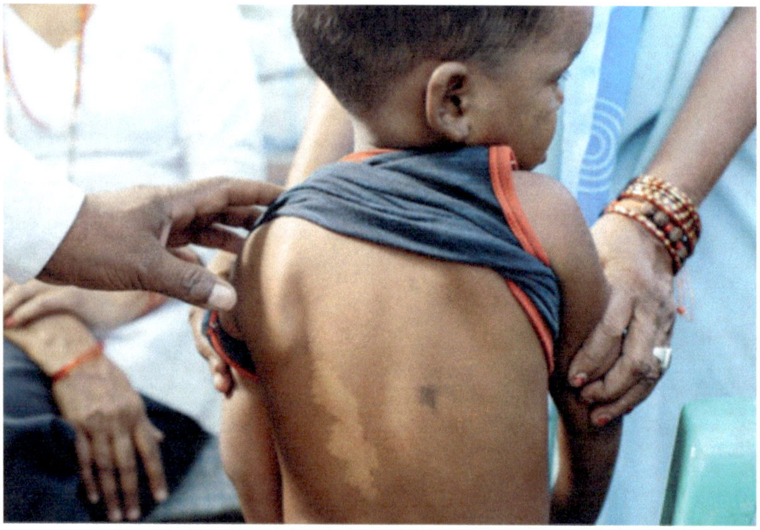

Figure 11.1. Pediatric leprosy.

Source: World Health Organization. (n.d.). *Child with Leprosy.*

11.1. Pathophysiology of Leprosy

Leprosy in kids is a complex affair for the immune system. When *Mycobacterium leprae* slips in, the body immediately sets off a jumble of responses—it's not just one neat attack but a combination of natural and more learned defenses. Early on, macrophages try to wrap things up by trapping the microbe, but how well that works depends on each child's own immune strength. Since many youngsters have defenses that are still getting their act together, they often end up more prone to the multibacillary type. You could say that the tug-of-war between T-helper cell signals—whether leaning toward a Th1 stance that brings about a tuberculoid picture, or a Th2 shift that leaves the immune reaction wanting—ends up drawing the disease's overall outline. And sometimes, inflammation even creeps beyond what you'd expect, affecting areas like the kidneys in ways that oddly resemble damage seen in other neglected tropical illnesses (da Lino et al., 2018). When it comes to the nerves, things get even more complex. The microbe isn't content with just the skin—it finds its way into peripheral nerves, sneaking into Schwann cells and causing myelin to fall apart, which then leads to nerve fibers breaking down. Kids often show up with numbness, weakness, and even visible deformities. Ironically, even though the immune response is critical for fending off the infection, its very attack—through inflammatory chemicals and clumped cell formations—can sometimes end up harming the nerves it intends to protect. Even after most of the bacteria are cleared, the damage may stubbornly persist, contributing to long-term difficulties. Generally speaking, unpicking the molecular triggers behind this nerve loss opens doors to treatments aimed at calming the inflammation and encouraging nerve repair—an especially key goal when you're dealing with growing bodies (da Lino et al., 2018). But leprosy's havoc isn't limited to skin and nerves alone. Underneath the surface, a constant low-level inflammation can stir up damage all over the body. This persistent immune buzz often leads to bouts known as lepra reactions, which make tissue damage even worse and complicate treatment efforts. It's interesting—this overall inflammatory state shares a lot of similarities with what we see in other chronic conditions, where things like macrophage slip-ups can throw off both metabolism and immune balance. The ongoing clash between persisting bacteria and the body's defenses shows that fighting leprosy means tackling both the infection and the overzealous immune response. For kids, catching the disease early and tailoring the treatment are absolutely crucial if we want to ease the burden of systemic inflammation on their organs and overall well-being.

11.1.1. Causative Agent: Mycobacterium leprae

Understanding the microbe behind childhood leprosy isn't just an academic exercise—it's key to grasping how the disease acts in real life. *Mycobacterium leprae*, the microbe we're up against, has its own set of characteristics that make it complex to pin down. It lives inside cells and reproduces at a snail's pace, which helps explain its long incubation period and the persistent nature of the illness. This microbe stubbornly refuses to grow on regular lab media, so researchers often have to rely on armadillo or mouse footpad models instead (Cogneau & Rigouts, 2021). Its acid-fast cell wall not only lets it dodge our immune defenses but also provides a handy marker during biopsies, a point especially important when kids show early or subtle symptoms. The way *Mycobacterium leprae* works is complex up with how a child's immune system responds—a kind of complicated interaction between parasite and host. It turns out that our genes have a say in this too. Variations in immune-related genes, particularly the ones that build toll-like receptors (TLRs), seem to meddle with how well our body recognizes and fights the microbe. Typically, TLRs are the first to spot damage by detecting parts of the bacterium, initiating the immune response. But when there are differences in these receptors, the alarm system might not work as it should, making it easier for the microbe to settle in and eventually cause nerve damage—a classic sign of leprosy. As a result, the disease can show up in very different ways in kids, ranging from mild, localized issues to full-blown, widespread infections (Hart &Tapping, 2012). When it comes to practical treatment, knowing these details about *Mycobacterium leprae* directly shapes both diagnosis and therapy in kids. Because the microbe grows slowly and hides inside cells, doctors tend to lean on what they can observe clinically, supported by histopathology and molecular techniques to find bacterial DNA. This approach is particularly vital for children who might show only slight or even unusual symptoms that can easily be overlooked. Further, understanding the microbe's behavior helps in crafting multidrug regimens that aim to weed out resistance while targeting the bacterium effectively. With kids facing the risks of nerve damage and other complications due to their developing immune systems, treatment plans have to be carefully adjusted. In short, combining insights from microbiology, immunology, and clinical practice is essential for improving care for these young patients (Hart & Tapping, 2012; Cogneau & Rigouts, 2021) (Figure 11.2).

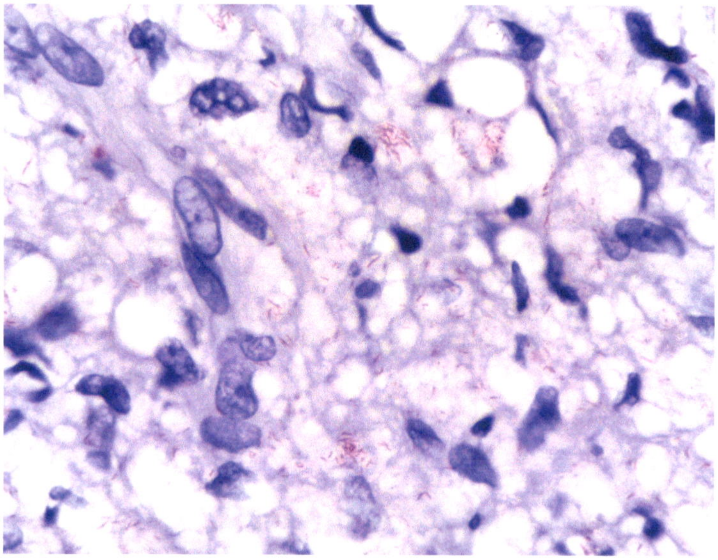

Figure 11.2. *Mycobacterium leprae*: The lazy cousin of tuberculosis.

Source: By Department of Pathology, Calicut Medical College - Calicut Medical College, CC BY-SA 4.0, https://commons.wikimedia.org/w/index.php?curid=36650707

11.1.2. Transmission Methods Among Children

Kids' exposure to leprosy is a complex matter that needs our attention. Grasping how the disease sneaks into their lives is crucial for coming up with ways to stop it. In many instances, leprosy spreads through long, close encounters with someone who hasn't been treated yet, especially when kids, who depend so much on their caregivers and hang out in crowded places like schools, are involved. It isn't only about sharing the same roof, either; sometimes just living near someone affected increases the risk, which tells us that the community plays its own part. The fact that the illness takes its time to show up only adds to the confusion, often causing diagnoses to come too late and letting the infection slip by unnoticed. Clearly, tracking down contacts both in families and in the wider neighborhood is key (Jaganath et al., 2019). Then there's the matter of where and how these kids live. Overcrowded spaces, poor sanitation, and limited access to good healthcare all push up the chances of meeting *Mycobacterium leprae*. Weather conditions, rainy seasons—seem to have a say in how our immune systems hold up against bacteria, though we still can't pin down exactly how the patterns for leprosy work. Looking at tuberculosis, researchers have noticed that heavy rains sometimes go hand-in-hand with more diagnoses in children, likely because respiratory issues and weakened defenses come up together during those damp spells. In many endemic areas, this mix of environmental pressures makes the situation even more challenging, leaving kids even more exposed (Jaganath et al., 2019). Keeping an active watch with spot-on detection methods helps reveal these murky transmission routes and can slow or even stop outbreaks. When teams go door-to-door and track down contacts in regions where leprosy is common, they tend to uncover quite a few cases among kids, which points back to the significance of close-contact spread. Contact tracing, and sometimes it works significantly better than other approaches—picks up more cases by checking both households and nearby contacts that could be hiding infections. Not to mention, the little marks left by BCG shots in children seem to offer some shield, hinting at how immunity factors into the picture. And the ongoing spread isn't just among severe cases; even children coming into contact with less obvious forms of the disease are at risk, showing that leprosy's pathways are as complex as they are complex (Mahato et al., 2023) (Figure 11.3).

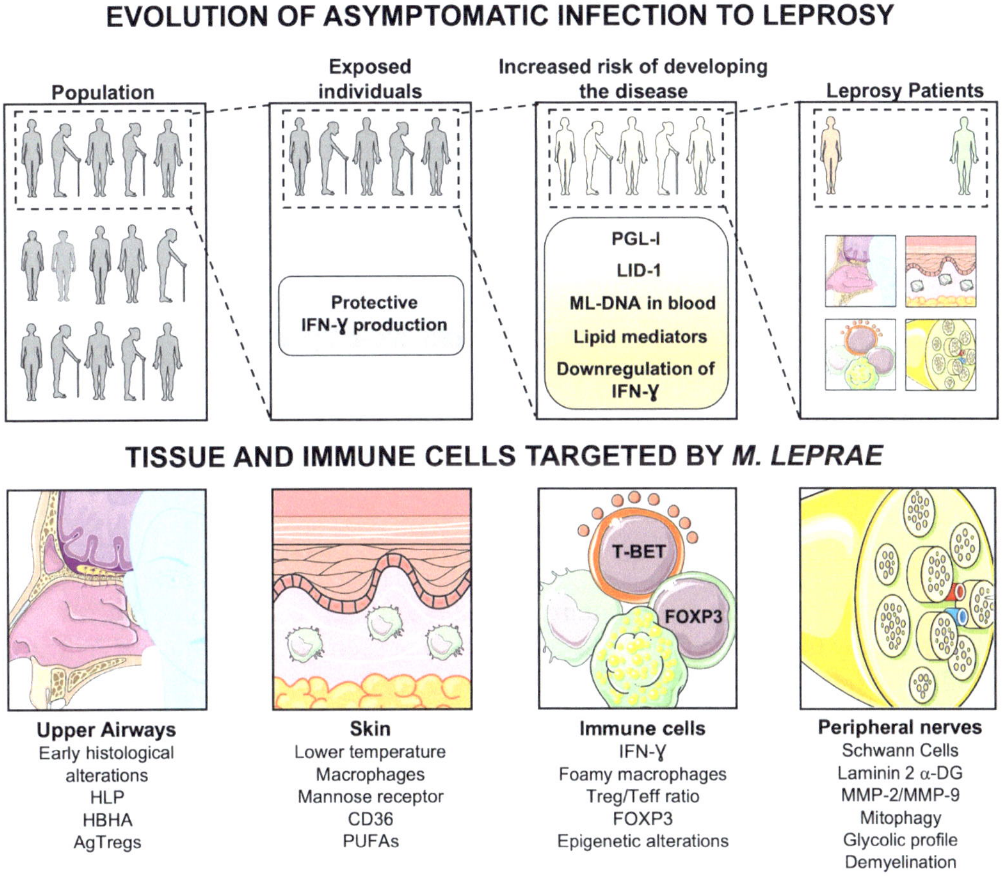

Figure 11.3. Overview of leprosy transmission routes, infection, and symptoms. *Mycobacterium leprae* is the causative agent of leprosy.

Source: Cabral N, de Figueiredo V, Gandini M, de Souza CF, Medeiros RA, Lery LMS, Lara FA, de Macedo CS, Pessolani MCV and Pereira GMB (2022) Modulation of the Response to Mycobacterium leprae and Pathogenesis of Leprosy. Front. Microbiol. 13:918009. doi: 10.3389/fmicb.2022.918009***11.1.3. Immune Response in Pediatric Patients***

Leprosy in kids doesn't quite follow the same route it does in adults. Their bodies seem to deal with the bacteria in unique ways, often showing up as forms with fewer bacteria, a sign that a cell-driven immune response is already at work. Even though their immune systems are still growing, it appears that children are generally less prone to the heavy, more severe forms of the disease. The time from infection to symptoms can stretch on for years, meaning the body might be quietly keeping the bacteria in check without obvious signs. All of this paints a picture of an immune system in progress when facing *Mycobacterium leprae*, with boys and girls equally at risk, and close, long-lasting contact (especially in families) remaining the main way the microbe spreads (Kattan et al., 2006). Shifting focus, the way kids handle leprosy points to a curious mix of innate and adaptive defenses. In most cases, they experience less nerve damage and fewer hypersensitivity reactions, suggesting a kind of immune tolerance or modulation different from what adults show. Cytokine-driven pathways help control inflammation and curb bacterial growth, which is important since the disease's long-running inflammation can hit peripheral or trigeminal nerves and lead to sensory issues. Historical reports even note that traditional remedies—rich in compounds that boost nitric oxide production, seem to step in by enhancing skin cell antimicrobial activity. This combination of the body's own defenses and environmental factors adds another layer of complexity to how children manage the infection (Kattan et al., 2006). New studies are now looking at less obvious parts of the immune story, like mucosal defenses and other potential markers. Take saliva—it isn't just a watery substance; it carries anti-inflammatory cytokines along with a host of microbes, giving us a non-invasive glimpse into a child's overall immune status. Using saliva as a marker might reduce the need for more invasive blood tests or nerve biopsies that can be hard on young patients. In many cases, this fresh approach dovetails with traditional methods, and it might even help us catch and monitor the infection earlier. Advances in how we profile the immune system could eventually lead to treatments that better respect the delicate nature of a child's developing defenses.

11.2. Clinical Manifestations

Pediatric leprosy often shows up with a jumble of skin and nerve signs that can complicate early detection. Kids typically have lighter or reddish patches that seem to lose some feeling when touched, in terms of pain or temperature changes. Often, these minor differences are brushed off or mistaken for common childhood skin issues, which then delays pinpointing the disease. In some cases, the nerves swell and become tender, leading to muscle weakness or even fingers that curl into a claw-like shape, which clearly hints at nerve involvement. Interestingly, rather than the pattern seen in adults, young patients more often develop a multibacillary form, likely because their immune systems have not fully matured yet. Recognizing these hints early is crucial, as untreated leprosy generally leads to irreversible damage. In most instances, careful skin checks and nerve examinations in regions where the disease is common can make a difference in timely treatment. It isn't just the skin and nerves at play. Some children might also experience more general symptoms—think low-grade fevers, a general feeling of malaise, or even swollen lymph nodes, especially during brief reaction episodes that tend to cause sudden inflammation against *Mycobacterium leprae* parts. These flare-ups sometimes worsen the existing skin patches and spike nerve pain or swelling, potentially mimicking other infections or inflammatory conditions. While the skin issues often steal the spotlight initially, clinicians mustn't overlook these systemic signs, since prompt anti-inflammatory treatment can be key to preventing lasting nerve harm. Given that a child's immune response is still evolving, their reaction may be more intense, adding another layer of complexity to the clinical picture. So, understanding the delicate balance between the infection and the body's immune reaction is essential for handling how leprosy varies in young patients. Skin manifestations in pediatric leprosy don't always follow a clear-cut pattern, which makes it complex to separate them from other common skin changes in newborns and young children. For example, those harmless marks that you might see in neonates, like Mongolian spots or sebaceous gland bumps—need careful differentiation from the more worrisome lesions linked with leprosy. Misreading these signs can induce unnecessary worry or even delay the right treatment altogether; experts should consider both what they see on the skin and the child's potential exposure risk.

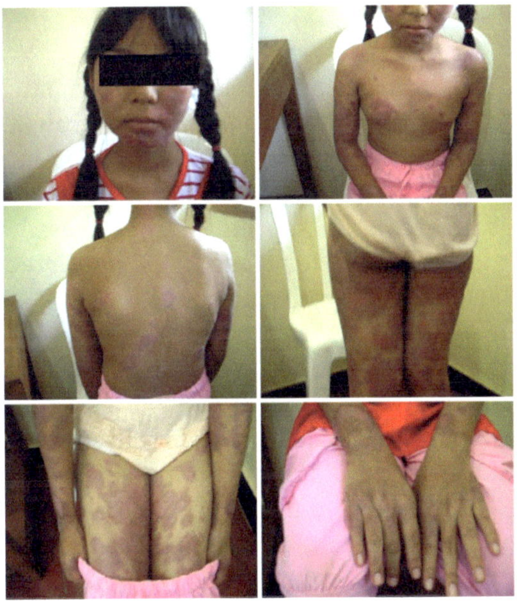

Figure 11.4. Clinical manifestations.

Source: Springer Nature. (n.d.). *Clinical Manifestations of Leprosy.*

Unlike the temporary, physiological skin changes usually seen in newborns, leprosy lesions tend to persist, are often numb, and come with thickened nerves. A comprehensive check of the skin alongside a detailed nerve assessment can boost diagnostic accuracy. Further, spreading awareness about these subtle early signs might improve detection in endemic areas and help lessen the disease's long-term impact. By combining everyday clinical observations with an understanding of typical neonatal skin features, doctors get a valuable framework for diagnosing and treating pediatric leprosy (Pujitha et al., 2023; Zhao et al., 2024) (Figure 11.4).

11.2.1. Early Signs and Symptoms in Children

Kids with infections can be complex to diagnose because early warnings are subtle and shift around a lot. With leprosy in little ones, the first hints might just look like minor skin issues and get mixed up with other skin problems. Sometimes you see patches that seem less sensitive or even totally numb—even though they're painless, and without a careful check, these signs are easy to miss. Occasionally, you might find that the nerves get a bit thicker too, which can be an important clue, yet the absence of real pain or discomfort often means doctors don't suspect leprosy right away. It shows how important it is for clinicians to dig deep with patient history and perform thorough sensory exams; using checklists can help make sure that nothing, like numbness or nerve swelling—is overlooked (Ahmad et al., 2024). Recognizing these early, often sleepy, indicators is key to jumping in with treatment before the disease gets a chance to worsen. Often, tiny neurological hints come up before any major breakdown is noticeable in pediatric leprosy. You might see signs like numbness, weak muscles, or problems with the body's automatic functions, yet these details can slip past both parents and sometimes even doctors. Oddly enough, these nerve issues can appear at the same time as skin lesions or even before obvious skin changes happen, which only complicates the issue further. Kids sometimes struggle to explain what they feel, and factors like limited access to healthcare or other socioeconomic issues can cause delays in getting help. In many cases, just as with other children's diseases, for example, tuberculous meningitis, where early symptoms are super vague (Ahmad et al., 2024), being extra watchful is necessary in high-risk zones. A slight change in sensation, a tingle, or a bit of weakness might be all it takes to remind a doctor that time is of the essence. Combining everyday tools with a structured way of checking can boost the early detection of leprosy in kids. In those busy clinical settings, where distractions and the overload of information sometimes get in the way, important signs may accidentally be missed. Custom checklists that focus on kids' skin and nerve assessments can help curb these oversights. These lists prompt health professionals to ask about things like numbness or notice if nerves seem thicker, and they also help in jotting down essential details like immunization records and related factors (Eshraghi et al., 2021). Generally speaking, this approach has shown promise in not only sharpening diagnostic accuracy but also in cutting down on avoidable mistakes across different areas of care. To summarize, systematically taking in early symptoms and keeping clinicians on alert paves the way for a quicker diagnosis and treatment, ultimately stopping the disease from stepping into more serious territory.

11.2.2. Differences in Presentation Compared to Adults

Leprosy in kids doesn't always show up the same way as it does in adults. Often, subtle skin patches appear that are fewer in number and not as clearly defined as the lesions seen in grownups, which can easily throw off early detection. Their immune systems are still coming into their own, so generally speaking, they're more prone to a widespread (multibacillary) form rather than the leaner (paucibacillary) version more common in adults. This mix-up means the disease can sneakily progress—affecting nerves extensively and setting the stage for disability if not detected in time. Other factors, like malnutrition or concurrent infections, may obscure or alter these signs further, so doctors have to keep an extra careful watch. All these age-related twists highlight the pressing need for diagnostic rules and treatment plans aimed squarely at children, which stand apart from those used for adults (Grønningen et al., 2024). Not only do the visible signs differ, but the way leprosy spreads and reacts to treatment in children is also uniquely different. Kids often end up with a more disseminated infection thanks to their developing immune defenses, and this can induce episodes of leprosy reactions—think of flare-ups resembling erythema nodosum leprosum or sudden reversal events—that might worsen nerve damage and complicate treatment plans. In most cases, children's bodies process medication differently from adults,' meaning that the standard mix of drugs might need a alter here and there to work properly while keeping toxicity in check. On top of that, the social side of things weighs in heavily, as kids are more exposed to stigma and disruptions in their growth and development, which calls for combining both medical and social support in their care.

Recognizing these nuances is crucial for crafting comprehensive pediatric care plans that address health and overall development (Grønningen et al., 2024). Figuring out a correct diagnosis in pediatric leprosy can be quite the puzzle. The symptoms often overlap with those of other local infections and even nutritional deficiencies, leading to potential misdiagnoses or delays compared to adult cases. For instance, when children show signs outside the lungs—something that sometimes mirrors tuberculosis in resource-scarce settings—the process becomes even complex, since our conventional diagnostic tools were mostly validated based on adult presentations (Grønningen et al., 2024). Adding to the challenge, there aren't reliable rapid tests designed specifically for kids, and relying on invasive procedures isn't always practical. Furthermore, treatment adherence can suffer because youngsters depend on caregivers and tend to have a heightened sensitivity to drug-related side effects. To summarize, understanding these presentation differences is essential for adjusting diagnostic protocols and enhancing pediatric leprosy control programs, especially in communities that already face other medical and socioeconomic hurdles (Figure 11.5).

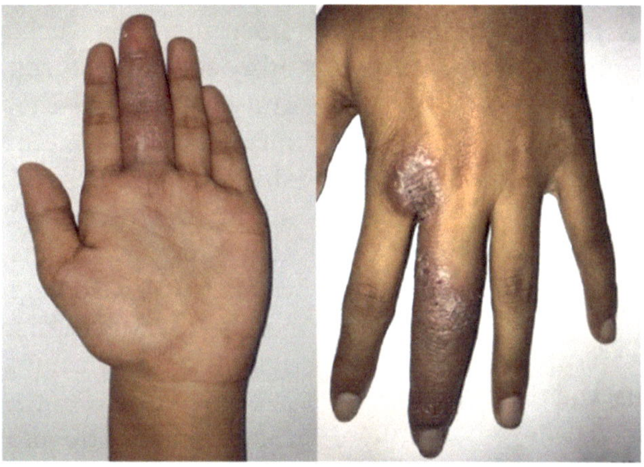

Figure 11.5. Differences in presentation compared to adults.

Source: Leprosy Review. (2022). *Differences in Leprosy Presentation.*

11.2.3. Complications Arising from Untreated Leprosy

Untreated infections in kids can trigger a whole cascade of problems that interfere with both their bodies and how they feel about themselves. With leprosy, missing that window for intervention might lead to nerve damage—kids end up losing some sensation and their muscles just can't keep up. This can leave them open to extra bumps and even deformities that get worse as care slips away. Further, when diagnosis and treatment get pushed back, there's a much higher chance of disabilities that stick around and slow down growth and development. Studies generally show that factors like poverty and not knowing enough about the disease tend to fuel these delays, making the physical symptoms even harsher. To summarize, catching the signs early is key if we're going to cut down on the complications connected to pediatric leprosy. Leaving leprosy untreated doesn't just wreck the body; it also sets up a space for deep psychological stress and social isolation. Visible changes bring on stigma that circles back to fuel anxiety and push kids into social exclusion, a cycle that can last a long time. It's not only about mental health, either; nerve damage can hide pain, so small injuries might be missed until they cause bigger tissue damage down the road. Research, in most cases, shows that these children are more likely to face anxiety disorders, which clearly points to the need for good psychological backup along with physical care. Methods like cognitive-behavioral therapy and even audiovisual aids have, at times, shown promise in easing preoperative jitters in pediatric cases and might be altered to help those wrestling with the mental weight of leprosy (Achule et al., 2025). In short, combining physical treatment with a bit of mental health support becomes important in light of all these challenges. If you stop to think about it, the social and economic side of untreated leprosy in kids plays a huge part in how these complications shape up. Research generally reveals that lower social standing, and even some gender differences—can slow down diagnosis and push kids toward disability. For example, boys tend to end up with advanced disabilities, possibly because of differences in how they seek help or access care. Money issues often get in the way of prompt treatment, letting the disease run unchecked until it turns into Grade 2 complications with clear deformities and serious functional problems. Clearly, this underlines how essential community-based healthcare and programs that target those at risk are (Sinha et al., 2024). Ultimately, a well-rounded, community-focused approach seems not only beneficial but absolutely necessary to break this cycle of neglect.

11.3. Diagnosis of Pediatric Leprosy

Pediatric leprosy is tough to spot early. Kids often show very subtle signs, and the infection—*Mycobacterium leprae*—can take anywhere from 2–6 years to fully burst onto the scene, so those early hints easily get brushed off as routine skin issues. Unlike in adults, where obvious skin spots or nerve pain quickly set off alarm bells, children's symptoms tend to fly under the radar. Often, families delay seeking care partly because social stigma creeps in, which only makes matters worse. In most cases, combining thorough clinical checkups with new diagnostic gadgets is key to catching the disease sooner rather than later (Rodriguez-Marin et al., 2025). Recently, people in the field have been combining methods that look at clinical signs together with bacteriological and immune tests, generally speaking, to get a more complete picture. Traditional slit-skin smears still play a role in picking up acid-fast bacilli, yet their sensitivity can be quite limited, especially in those forms of the disease with very few bacteria—a situation frequently seen in children. Some immunological tests now try to gauge how hosts react to the leprosy antigens, and these offer promising backup for finding infections that don't shout out their presence. Interestingly, machine learning approaches like logistic regression are starting to make a mark: these models sift through a combination of biometric and demographic details to flag changes that could hint at early disease, offering a sort of clarity that aids in tough clinical calls (Bhavika, 2024; Rodriguez-Marin et al., 2025). Given the serious risks of delaying treatment in young patients, a combined, multidisciplinary approach becomes almost inevitable. Merging emerging tools, such as logistic regression and other machine learning algorithms, with tried-and-true clinical checks seems to be the way forward; these methods help highlight subtle shifts in growth or immune response that might otherwise slip by. Training programs and awareness campaigns aimed at frontline health workers can also help in detecting telltale signs early—even if the disease hides behind modest symptoms, and combat stigma that discourages prompt care. Continued, careful altering of these diagnostic models, and widening the data combination—will be vital if we hope to better diagnose pediatric leprosy and, in turn, reduce disease spread and long-term damage (Bhavika, 2024; Rodriguez-Marin et al., 2025) (Figure 11.6).

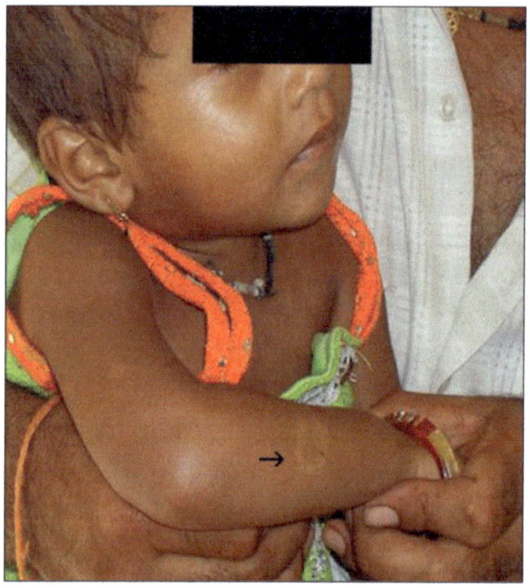

Figure 11.6. Diagnosis of pediatric leprosy.

Source: Indian Journal of Dermatology, Venereology and Leprology. (2013). *Pediatric Leprosy Diagnosis.*

11.3.1. Clinical Evaluation Techniques

When evaluating leprosy in kids, it's important

to realize the disease sometimes shows up in a subtler way than in adults. Kids often display fewer or milder signs, so a careful checkup is a must, looking closely at skin spots and even subtle changes in nerves. Often, young patients might carry the infection longer than expected and lean towards a form with fewer bacteria. Doctors then need to inspect every detail, like how many lesions there are and whether any nerves seem thicker than usual, to steer clear of mistakes. A good physical exam alone isn't enough; digging into the child's health history, especially any contact with sick family members—is key, given that intrafamilial spread happens a lot. This whole-picture approach can catch things sooner, which is crucial because delays (sometimes stretching over a year) might worsen nerve damage and add to problems during critical growth years (Kattan et al., 2006). New imaging methods have, generally speaking, carved out a useful role in checking for pediatric leprosy, especially where resources are tight. Point-of-care ultrasound—or POCUS, as many call it—has popped up as a promising add-on to the standard exam, letting clinicians see real-time details about peripheral nerves and even pinpoint internal organ involvement when the infection goes beyond just the skin. In many tropical infectious diseases, for example, this gadget has proven quite handy, and its ability to reveal even slight nerve swelling or early inflammation in kids is a refreshing bonus. Handheld ultrasound devices, being portable, affordable and rather simple to use, seem to fit the bill for endemic regions, boosting diagnostic accuracy and helping ensure prompt actions to ward off permanent nerve damage (Bélard et al., 2016). Even with these cool new techniques, standardizing how examinations are done and giving proper training remains super important in pediatric leprosy. In areas where the disease is common, healthcare workers often struggle because special expertise is scarce and kids can show a wide range of symptoms. Protocols that push for systematic neurological checks and the thoughtful use of tests like slit-skin smears, histopathology, and ultrasound can tip the scales toward accuracy. It's also vital to coach frontline providers on catching early signs and even odd presentations, like subtle nerve function loss or unexpected hypersensitivity reactions. Altogether, this kind of integrated strategy not only speeds up diagnosis and treatment but also helps dodge long-term complications while improving the everyday lives of young patients (Kattan et al., 2006; Bélard et al., 2016).

11.3.2. Laboratory Tests and Imaging Studies

Diagnosing leprosy in children isn't a one-step process. Doctors start by checking for uneven skin patches—sometimes lighter, sometimes reddish—that seem to have lost feeling. They then back up these observations with lab tests. For example, a classic method involves taking a skin smear and staining it with the Ziehl-Neelsen technique to hunt for the acid-fast bacilli that signal *Mycobacterium leprae*. Even though this method is more common in adult cases, it's often used for kids when there's a heavy bacterial load. There's also been a rise in using serological assays to look for phenolic glycolipid-I antibodies, which offer a non-invasive way to lend support to the clinical picture. Still, these tests usually serve as supplements since, in most cases, their sensitivity and specificity in kids aren't consistent, so a careful clinical evaluation, and histopathology when possible—remains crucial. Sometimes, imaging steps in to add another layer of insight into nerve issues and other complications that come with pediatric leprosy. An ultrasound, for instance, can unexpectedly reveal nerve swelling and inflammation in areas like the ulnar or posterior tibial nerves, offering an early glimpse of neuropathy without any invasive procedure. When more detail is needed, an MRI can show nerve thickening, edema, or even small abscesses developing in advanced situations. Radiographs, on the other hand, help pick up on bone deformities, resorption, or secondary infections that result from nerve damage and repetitive trauma. These scans, combined loosely with lab findings, not only boost diagnostic accuracy but also guide treatment choices in cases where the symptoms aren't completely straightforward. This combination of imaging and lab data lets clinicians track disease progression and see how well kids are responding to multidrug therapy—a key step in avoiding permanent disabilities. Blood tests, too, play a major role in the overall clinical picture. During episodes of inflammation, such as Type 1 (reversal) and Type 2 (erythema nodosum leprosum) reactions, markers like C-reactive protein and the erythrocyte sedimentation rate tend to go up, often flagging the need for corticosteroid treatment. Even though direct studies on children remain a bit scarce, evidence from similar infectious diseases generally supports the idea that these markers can reflect pediatric immune responses (Ben-Ozer et al., 2011). In addition, routine hematological profiles help differentiate coinfections or nutritional deficiencies that might complicate the situation. To summarize, this combination of lab tests and imaging isn't just academic; it's a practical necessity for catching the disease early, managing it comprehensively, and ultimately improving the daily lives of young patients (Fink et al., 2021) (Figure 11.7).

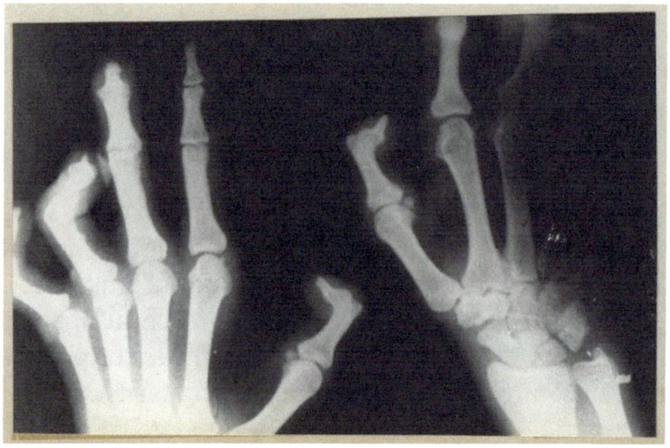

Figure 11.7. Leprosy found in California child: How doctors diagnosed it.

Source: Live Science. (n.d.). *Childhood Leprosy Diagnosis.*

11.3.3. Challenges in Diagnosing Leprosy in Children

Identifying leprosy early in kids is no easy task. The signs are so subtle that they often slip under the radar, children typically show milder symptoms than adults. Light-colored skin spots and slight nerve thickening might not be obvious without some specialized know-how. Further, there's the long incubation period of *Mycobacterium leprae*; in most cases, symptoms don't emerge until years later, especially because younger patients seem to respond differently. All these factors can delay diagnosis and treatment, which in turn raises the risk of permanent nerve damage and disability. Kids might also have damage explaining changes in sensation or pain, which only adds to the diagnostic puzzle. Overall, the mix of unexpected symptoms and communication gaps means extra care and better diagnostic tools are needed, particularly in places where resources are tight (Bett et al., 2012). Another hurdle is the scarcity of diagnostic technologies that work well for children, especially in tropical areas where the disease is more common. Traditional tests like skin smears and biopsies need special equipment and expertise that local clinics just don't always have. For example, point-of-care ultrasound (POCUS) has generally been a game changer in handling other tropical infections by delivering quick, non-invasive results, even in low-resource setups. Yet, using ultrasound to detect leprosy in kids is still not getting the attention it deserves. Integrating targeted ultrasound methods for pediatric leprosy might boost early detection of nerve issues and related problems, though this approach is still pretty much in its infancy. The current mix of clinical, lab, and imaging tools isn't enough, highlighting a clear need for new technology and better training in these high-need regions (Bélard et al., 2016). Social and cultural issues add another layer of complexity when it comes to detecting leprosy in children. The stigma that comes with the disease often pushes families to hide symptoms or wait too long before seeking help. In many communities, outdated ideas about leprosy still persist, which means that people are reluctant to go to clinics—resulting in cases being identified only when the condition has worsened. This delay is especially serious for kids, who depend on caregivers to notice early signs and act quickly. It's also true that many healthcare workers might not be trained enough to tell leprosy apart from other common skin or nerve ailments in children, leading to misdiagnosis or even overlooking the disease. Resolving these issues calls for not only better medical tools but also community education and outreach programs that clear up misconceptions and help reduce stigma, so kids can get treatment before long-term damage becomes a real problem (Bett et al., 2012).

11.4. Treatment Options

Treating leprosy in children isn't just about slapping on antibiotics—it's a balancing act that mixes drug therapy with the often-unexpected characteristics kids bring along. Generally speaking, the go-to plan is multidrug therapy (MDT), where drugs such as dapsone, rifampicin, and clofazimine team up against *Mycobacterium leprae*; the idea here is to slow down spread and curb drug resistance. Still, kids sometimes wrestle with taking medications—they may struggle with tolerance or simply forget to take them—so dosages need altering and close watching. You can kind of see a parallel with other childhood infections: local resistance patterns often steer choices, much like studies in pediatric appendicitis point out the benefits of using gentamicin and metronidazole for their safety and system (Adhehani et al., 2025). In many cases, knowing the local bacterial scene isn't just extra information—it's key to preventing complications down the road. But the fight against this disease goes well beyond just antibiotics. Leprosy can jump-start an immune reaction that, if left unchecked, might end up damaging nerves and causing permanent issues. In most cases, a short burst of corticosteroids helps manage both type 1 and type 2 lepra reactions—pretty similar to what's seen in other inflammatory conditions in youngsters. Yet, as we notice in conditions like Behçet's, these steroids aren't without their limits, so they're usually kept to the short term and paired with other treatments (Giani et al., 2023). Sometimes, when inflammation won't settle down, immunomodulators like thalidomide or newer biologic drugs step in. Given that children typically have a longer battle with the disease and can be more vulnerable to medication side effects, a carefully tuned, team-based approach is critical; early aggressive action often makes all the difference in avoiding lifelong problems. On top of fighting the infection and keeping inflammation under control, supportive care turns the tide in a child's recovery. Rehabilitation, physical therapy, and effective wound care all work together to mend physical issues that come with nerve damage—even if sometimes it feels like a patchwork solution. Managing any secondary infections or disabilities means the family and care providers have to be hands-on, and that collective effort can't be understated. Further, a little psychological support goes a long way for kids wrestling with social stigma and the weight of a chronic condition. Recent advances in drug research, like emerging immunomodulators—offer hope for better long-term outcomes, although many of these options still aren't officially approved for children (mirroring hurdles seen in other pediatric inflammatory diseases [Giani et al., 2023]). To summarize, truly winning against pediatric leprosy means tackling the microbe, tuning the treatments to a child's needs, and weaving in social and emotional care as part of the overall plan (Figure 11.8).

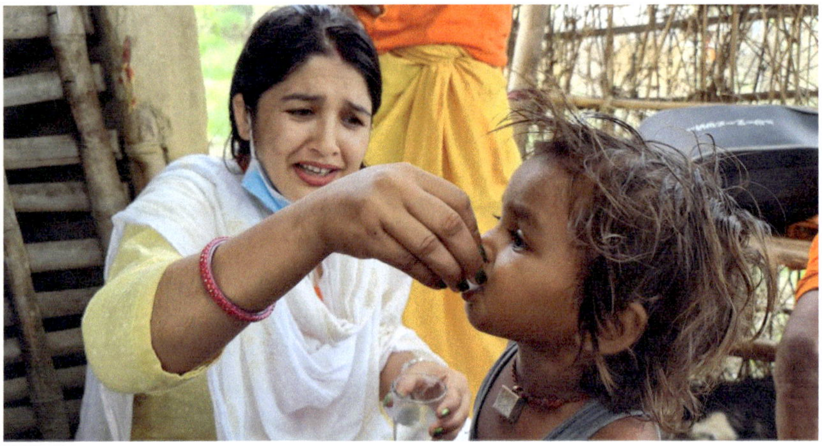

Figure 11.8. Leprosy treatment in children.

Source: NLR International. (2023). *SDR-PEP in Nepal.*

11.4.1. Multidrug Therapy (MDT) Protocols

Treating leprosy in kids is no small feat—it calls for a drug plan that works well while keeping these vulnerable ones safe. MDT, or multidrug therapy, sits at the heart of this approach by combining different antibiotics aimed squarely at the microbe *Mycobacterium leprae*, all while trying to keep drug resistance from creeping in. Generally speaking, the World Health Organization suggests different routines for light versus heavy cases (paucibacillary and multibacillary), meaning children often receive a combination of dapsone, rifampicin, and clofazimine over long stretches; doctors also alter doses and keep a close watch because kids metabolize drugs differently. It's a balance between efficacy and safety, ensuring youngsters stick with the regimen and avoid nasty side effects. To summarize, this standard MDT method has been a real game changer in cutting down leprosy cases across the globe, underlining why following these protocols in pediatric cases is so crucial for stopping spread and reducing long-term problems from delayed treatment (Rodriguez-Morales, 2019, 2022). Staying on track with the full MDT course can be complex for young patients, completing a long, drawn-out drug schedule often means caregivers and healthcare providers need to be fully in the mix. Missing doses or going off schedule not only weakens the treatment but can also pave the way for drug resistance, which is a major issue for public health. The design of these regimens is all about balancing how well the treatment works with how tolerable it is—sometimes even using strategies like directly observed therapy to help maintain proper compliance. At the same time, keeping an eye out for side effects, for example, hemolysis from dapsone or skin pigmentation shifts from clofazimine—is essential so that any complications can be managed quickly without having to scrap the whole treatment plan. Overall, this well-rounded approach highlights the critical role of MDT protocols in both fighting the infection and protecting the wellbeing of pediatric patients during their treatment (Rodriguez-Morales, 2019). Looking past just the medications, it's clear that these MDT plans need to be part of a bigger picture in children's healthcare, especially in places where leprosy is common and social factors weigh heavily on disease spread. This means mixcombining in community education to lessen stigma, catching cases early, and giving healthcare workers the know-how to navigate the finer points of pediatric dosing and side-effect management. In most cases, the success of MDT in young patients goes hand-in-hand with wider national and regional efforts to boost health infrastructure and ensure fair access to care—an aim that jives with global sustainable development goals for curbing infectious diseases. When all these elements work together, multidrug therapy isn't just a treatment plan; it becomes a key part of a broad-based response to cut transmission and improve children's health outcomes in endemic settings (Rodriguez-Morales, 2019, Singh, 2022) (Figure 11.9).

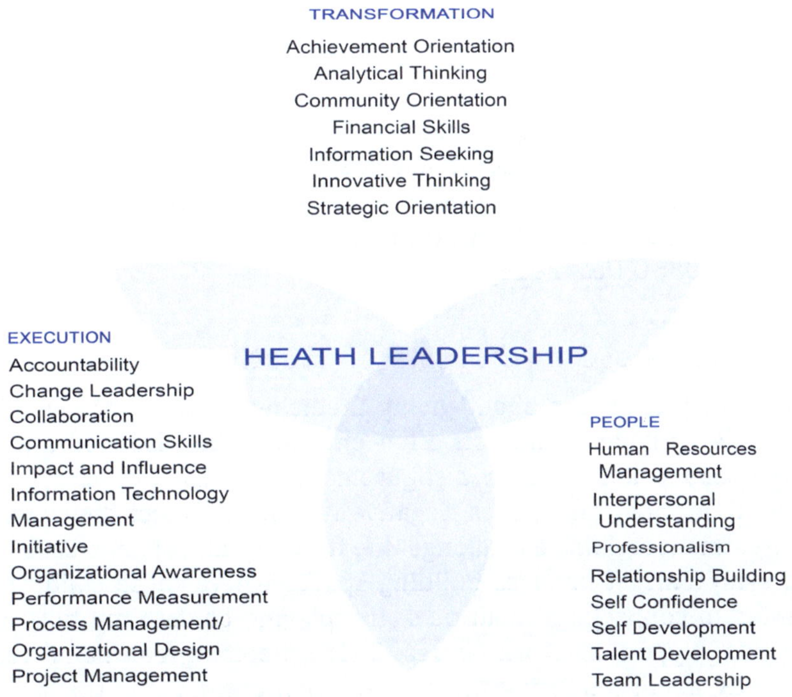

Figure 11.9. Addressing leprosy.

Source: Awofeso N. Leprosy: International Public Health Policies and Public Health Eras. *Administrative Sciences*. 2011; 1(1):32-44. https://doi.org/10.3390/admsci1010032

11.4.2. Role of Supportive Care and Rehabilitation

Kids dealing with leprosy face challenges that go far beyond just getting medicine, they have to cope with a lot of emotional and social hurdles too. Often, they struggle with physical limitations, harsh social judgments, and that deep-down stress that can interfere with their growth and daily lives. It helps, in many cases, to combine regular treatments with real support for their feelings and social needs. Building good self-esteem and inner strength turns out to be key when kids are trying to handle the stigma that comes with their condition. Adding a combination of social and mental support into their treatment can give them the tools to deal with isolation, bullying, and other tough scenarios caused by the disease (O'Dea, 2018). Rehabilitation also jumps in as a big help for these kids. Getting started early with things like physiotherapy, occupational therapy , and sometimes even surgery - can lessen the impact of any physical deformities and make it easier for them to move around. This kind of rehab isn't only about healing; it's about helping the kids find their independence again so they can join in on daily life and community activities. When health services are carefully checked and resources are directed where they're most needed, especially in places hit hard by pediatric leprosy—a lot of these issues can be managed better. Regular reviews of how care is delivered play a crucial role in keeping treatment effective and making sure kids see improvements eventually (Ministry of Health and Welfare, 2008). Beyond clinical care, getting communities and families involved makes a big difference. Public education that busts myths about leprosy, especially those based on looks or mistaken ideas about contagion, helps make kids feel more accepted. When everyone, from family members to local leaders and health workers—gets on board with the rehab process, it creates a safety net that boosts a child's confidence and resilience. Training sessions that pinpoint the unique needs of young patients add another layer of support, fostering an environment where social acceptance goes hand in hand with medical care. All these efforts, when combined, show that beating leprosy isn't just about medicine; it's about weaving together care, rehabilitation, and community strength to help children get back on track (Ministry of Health and Welfare, 2008; O'Dea, 2018).

11.4.3. Addressing Psychosocial Aspects of Treatment

Managing pediatric leprosy isn't just about giving medicine—it goes deeper into the everyday struggles kids face. Kids with this condition often end up feeling isolated and labeled because their skin shows signs like lesions or even disfigurement, and that can lead to bullying at home or in the neighborhood. In most cases, such negative reactions impact their self-worth and even make sticking with treatment feel like a challenge due to worry and shame. Care isn't simply about curing the physical symptoms; it involves building spaces where these children feel secure and understood. Combining in counseling, small peer groups, and community talks that clear up old myths helps create this support network (O'Dea, 2018). Boosting emotional resilience in these young patients is mostly about nurturing their self-esteem and making them a part of choosing their own care. When kids get a say in how they're treated, it not only validates what they're going through but also makes the tough journey feel a bit more theirs. Practical steps like talk-therapy, sessions with family, and learning programs all contribute to lightening the mental load. Often, a pinch of faith or a touch of spirituality serves as an extra pillar of strength for both the children and their families in trying times. This mindful focus on their emotional health tends to lead to better treatment follow-through and overall well-being (O'Dea, 2018). It's also key to remember that leprosy might affect more than just the skin—sometimes, it even involves organs like the kidneys, adding extra layers of concern. For example, kidney damage in neglected tropical illnesses such as leprosy can stir up a combination of medical challenges and emotional stress, ramping up anxiety for both kids and their caregivers. Generally speaking, catching these complications early on helps ease the uncertainty that families face. By combining insights from nephrology, mental health care, and social support networks, a more complete and holistic care model comes together. This combined approach not only highlights the need for ongoing research into new diagnostic tests and biomarkers but also aims to trim down the overall psychosocial burdens on these youngsters (O'Dea, 2018) (Figure 11.10).

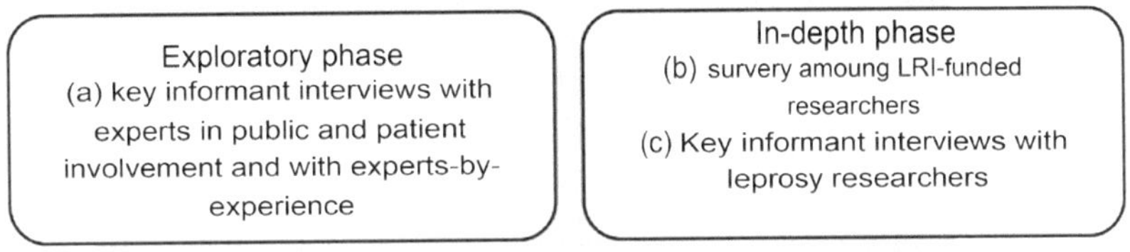

Figure 11.10. Addressing psychosocial aspects of treatment.

Source: de Groot L, van 't Noordende AT, Duck M, Oraga J, Rai SS, Peters RMH, Veldhuijzen N. Meaningful Engagement of Persons Affected by Leprosy in Research: An Exploration of Its Interpretation, Barriers, and Opportunities. *Tropical Medicine and Infectious Disease.* 2023; 8(1):52. https://doi.org/10.3390/tropicalmed8010052

A CLOSER LOOK

DIFFERENTIAL DIAGNOSIS OF LEPROSY IN CHILDREN

The clinical suspicion of leprosy is facilitated in children with a familial case, more reasonably if multibacillary.

Diagnosis of leprosy in children should be based on the cardinal signs of leprosy (clinic, bacteriology, histopathology).

Other skin diseases resulting in similar hypopigmented lesions such as pityriasis alba, early vitiligo, birthmarks, and pityriasis versicolor should be considered in differential diagnosis of leprosy.

With regard to nerve involvement, inherited peripheral nerve disorders, for example, hereditary sensory and sensory-motor neuropathies of various types, neurofibromatosis, neuropathies associated with developmental defects, and acquired neurological conditions, including traumatic neuropathies, should also be taken into consideration in differential diagnosis (Figure 11.11).

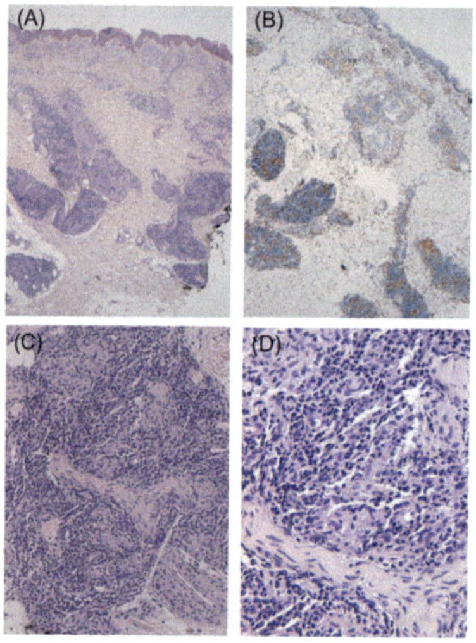

Figure 11.11. The differential diagnosis of leprosy in children.

Source: Beltrame, Anna, Maria Concetta Fargnoli, Charlotte Avanzi, Laura Sollima, Elena Pomari, Antonio Mori, Silvia Stefania Longoni, Lucia Moro, Pierantonio Orza, Mary Jackson, and et al. 2023. "Leprosy in an Adopted Woman Diagnosed by Molecular Tools: A Case Report from a Non-Endemic Area" Pathogens 12, no. 2: 165. https://doi.org/10.3390/pathogens12020165

SUMMARY

Pediatric leprosy throws up a combination of challenges that demand a flexible, sometimes unpredictable, approach. Early detection – which, quite frankly, is crucial for avoiding permanent nerve damage and cutting down disability – isn't as simple as it might sound. Kids often show a range of symptoms, meaning diagnoses can be delayed, and the disease can sneak its way through communities. There's a real need for care that isn't just about medicine; it has to include social and emotional support too. Stigma and isolation only add extra strain on these young patients, and, generally speaking, understanding the characteristics of kids' immune responses means that we have to keep exploring treatments that strike a balance between being effective and keeping them safe. Looking toward the future, the fight against pediatric leprosy hinges on strong, multidisciplinary research that goes beyond just clinical outcomes. Research in this area often runs into ethical puzzles—issues like informed consent and the delicate nature of vulnerability, for example—so adaptive and sensitive protocols become essential. When you consider children dealing with disabling conditions, long-term effects on neurodevelopment and social well-being naturally come into play (Alkattan et al., 2024; Yankulovska et al., 2024). While personalized medicine shows a lot of promise, it must be paired with careful ethical oversight to ensure fair access and true protection of patient rights, ultimately working to reduce disparities and boost care quality. In short, handling pediatric leprosy demands a broad, collaborative strategy that covers early detection, smart treatment, and ethically grounded research practices. The disease isn't just a medical challenge—it also wraps in social issues and potential impacts on brain development. That's why clinicians, researchers, and policymakers need to join forces. Generally, evidence-based approaches that consider both medical and ethical imperatives should be front and center—ensuring treatments are safe, accessible, and in tune with cultural contexts. Continuous, sometimes imperfect, review of treatment protocols alongside ethical guidance will help lessen the burden on these vulnerable youngsters and, eventually, reduce the worldwide impact of pediatric leprosy.

Pediatric leprosy throws up a lot of hidden challenges—its early signs can be so subtle and tucked away behind a long incubation period that catching it in time feels like searching for a needle in a haystack. Kids skip out on help partly because of the usual social stigma and discrimination, which only makes the situation worse, in most cases. Early detection matters, and a combination of medical care, mental support and even a dash of community help is key to keeping both physical and emotional wellbeing on track. It all comes down to having solid clinical evidence backing up treatments and public health drives that spread the word about these age-specific symptoms and responses, even if it means occasionally rethinking the approach. Nowadays, MDT is the main strategy to drop those bacterial levels and stop resistance in its tracks, but it's not as simple as mimicking adult doses—kids process medication differently. Dosing needs careful altering to match their unique metabolism and less mature immune systems, plus adverse reactions and sticking with treatment are pretty big hurdles here; caregiver support often makes or breaks this effort. Monitoring nerve damage and any deformities calls for keen eyes and speedy action to avoid long-term disability. Recent boosts in immunological insights and easier, more accessible diagnostic tools have induced hope: catching the disease early means starting treatment promptly, which in most cases paves the way for a better outcome. Then there's the broader socio-legal jumble that affects treatment availability—policies can shape what kids end up getting. Inconsistencies in regulatory rules, especially around drug efficacy checks, sometimes hold up the rollout of medications meant for children. Sure, a few laws insist on tight efficacy certification for initial treatments, but off-label prescribing can slip by with much looser controls, raising questions about safety and overall effectiveness. Conversations with healthcare pros tend to lean toward keeping stringent, uniform standards for both first-time and off-label drug uses, all in the name of protecting our most vulnerable. All of this highlights the pressing need for clear, consistent policies that balance innovative treatment options with patient safety within pediatric leprosy care (Morgan et al., 1980; Klein &Tabarrok, 2003).

KEY TERMS FROM THIS CHAPTER

- Anti-inflammatory cytokines
- Cognitive-behavioral therapy
- Cytokine-driven pathways
- Immune balance
- Logistic regression
- Metabolism
- Mucosal defenses
- Untreated infections
- Audiovisual aids
- Curb bacterial growth
- Histopathology
- Kidneys
- Machine learning algorithms
- Molecular techniques
- Pediatric leprosy

References

1. Bélard, S., Tamarozzi, F., Bustinduy, A. L., Wallrauch, C., Grobusch, M. P., Kuhn, W., Brunetti, E., Joekes, E., & Heller, T. (2016). Point-of-Care Ultrasound Assessment of Tropical Infectious Diseases--A Review of Applications and Perspectives. *The American journal of tropical medicine and hygiene*, *94*(1), 8–21. https://doi.org/10.4269/ajtmh.15-0421 (accessed on 10th May 2025).
2. Achule, A., Gedeno, K., & Aweke, Z. (2025). Management of preoperative anxiety with non-pharmacological methods in pediatric patients in resource-limited settings: a literature review. *Annals of medicine and surgery (2012)*, *87*(2), 780–790. https://doi.org/10.1097/MS9.0000000000002912 (accessed on 10th May 2025).
3. Adhehani, E., Assi, Z., Shmueli, M., Streltsov, R., & Ben-Shimol, S. (2025). Microbiologic and Clinical Characteristics of Pediatric Appendicitis: A Retrospective Cohort Study on Antibiotic Resistance and Treatment Options. *The Pediatric infectious disease journal*, 10.1097/INF.0000000000004800. Advance online publication. https://doi.org/10.1097/INF.0000000000004800(accessed on 10th May 2025).
4. **Khurshid Ahmad, Vypashi, and Iftikhar Ali (2024);** CHILDHOOD TUBERCULAR MENINGITIS: INSIGHTS INTO CLINICAL PRESENTATION, RADIOLOGICAL FINDINGS, AND OUTCOME DETERMINANTS *Int. J. of Adv. Res.* (Jul). 1569-1573] (ISSN 2320-5407(accessed on 10th May 2025).
5. Alkattan, W., Sabbah, B., Alghafees, M., Sabbah, A., Alsaleem, A., Alqahtani, M., Almadani, A., et al. (2024). Pediatric anesthesia exposure: Decoding its neurodevelopmental implications and navigating the nuances. *Cureus, 16*. https://www.semanticscholar.org/paper/e3352ce8bc26066ef35dd49220bca5e22d6935fe (accessed on 10th May 2025).
6. Alves, A. R., Cabral, P. B. E., Cabral, T. C. B. E., Camara, C. C., et al. (2013). Anti-PGL1 salivary IgA/IgM, serum IgG/IgM, and nasal *Mycobacterium leprae* DNA in individuals with household contact with leprosy. *Int. J. Infect. Dis., 17*(11), e1005–1010. https://core.ac.uk/download/37740204.pdf (accessed on 10th May 2025).
7. Fink, T. T., Marques, H. H. S., Gualano, B., Lindoso, L., Bain, V., Astley, C., Martins, F., Matheus, D., Matsuo, O. M., Suguita, P., Trindade, V., Paula, C. S. Y., Farhat, S. C. L., Palmeira, P., Leal, G. N., Suzuki, L., Odone Filho, V., Carneiro-Sampaio, M., Duarte, A. J. S., Antonangelo, L., ... Zheng, Y. (2021). Persistent symptoms and decreased health-related quality of life after symptomatic pediatric COVID-19: A prospective study in a Latin American tertiary hospital. *Clinics (Sao Paulo, Brazil)*, *76*, e3511. https://doi.org/10.6061/clinics/2021/e3511 (accessed on 10th May 2025).
8. Assadi, G. (2016). *Identification and Functional Characterization of Gastrointestinal Disease Genes*. https://core.ac.uk/download/70344112.pdf (accessed on 10th May 2025).
9. Mahato, R. K., Ghimire, U., Lamsal, M., Bajracharya, B., Poudel, M., Napit, P., Lama, K., Dahal, G., Hayman, D. T. S., Karna, A. K., Pandey, B. D., Das, C. L., & Paudel, K. P. (2023). Evaluating active leprosy case identification methods in six districts of Nepal. *Infectious diseases of poverty*, *12*(1), 111. https://doi.org/10.1186/s40249-023-01153-5 (accessed on 10th May 2025).
10. Ben-Ozer, E. Y., & Spiegelberg, T. A. (2011). *Poster 101: Pediatric Mononeuritis Multiplex*

Secondary to a Nonsystemic Vasculitis: A Case Report. http://deepblue.lib.umich.edu/bitstream/2027.42/147008/1/pmr2s203a.pdf (accessed on 10th May 2025).

11. Bett, J. B., Carter, E. J., Kiptoo, I. N., Maswai, P., et al. (2012). Successes and challenges in an integrated tuberculosis/HIV clinic in a rural, resource-limited setting: Experiences from Kericho, Kenya. *AIDS Res. Treat, 2012*, 238012. https://core.ac.uk/download/pdf/8686823.pdf (accessed on 10th May 2025).
12. Hotez PJ, Biritwum N-K, Fenwick A, Molyneux DH, Sachs JD (2019) Ghana: Accelerating neglected tropical disease control in a setting of economic development. PLoS Negl Trop Dis 13(1): e0007005. https://doi.org/10.1371/journal.pntd.0007005 (accessed on 10th May 2025).
13. Jaganath, D., Wobudeya, E., Sekadde, M. P., Nsangi, B., Haq, H., & Cattamanchi, A. (2019). Seasonality of childhood tuberculosis cases in Kampala, Uganda, 2010-2015. *PloS one*, *14*(4), e0214555. https://doi.org/10.1371/journal.pone.0214555(accessed on 10th May 2025).
14. Cogneau, S., & Rigouts, L. (2021). *Chapter 33: The Genus Mycobacterium*. Book: Practical Handbook of Microbiology. URI
15. https://library.oapen.org/handle/20.500.12657/51539(accessed on 10th May 2025).
16. Bezerra da Silva Junior G, Amélia Reis Jereissati A, Karoline Medina Neri A, Oliveira da Costa Lino D, Gomes Ramalho de Oliveira J, De Francesco Daher E. Neglected Tropical Diseases with an Impact on Kidney Function [Internet]. Current Topics in Tropical Emerging Diseases and Travel Medicine. IntechOpen; 2018. Available from: http://dx.doi.org/10.5772/intechopen.78981(accessed on 10th May 2025).
17. Eshraghi, B., Shaygan, P., Lajevardi, N., & Fazel, M. (2021). Nicolau syndrome, a rare though important complication of hyaluronic acid injection. *International journal of dermatology*, *60*(7), e285–e286. https://doi.org/10.1111/ijd.15487(accessed on 10th May 2025).
18. Giani, T., Luppino, A., & Ferrara, G. (2023). Treatment options in pediatric Behçet's disease. *Pediatric Drugs*, *25*, 165–191. https://www.semanticscholar.org/paper/e0e04204f2ae61b7ad01bad3ffe68614a3589307 (accessed on 10th May 2025).
19. Grønningen, E. (2024). *Extrapulmonary Tuberculosis in the HIV Endemic Setting in Tanzania: Challenges with Diagnosis, Comorbidities, and Association with Mortality*. https://core.ac.uk/download/644959073.pdf (accessed on 10th May 2025).
20. Hart, B. E., & Tapping, R. I. (2012). Genetic Diversity of Toll-Like Receptors and Immunity to M. leprae Infection. *Journal of tropical medicine*, *2012*, 415057. https://doi.org/10.1155/2012/415057 (accessed on 10th May 2025).
21. Jaiswal B, Rajpurohit P, Munot Y, et al. International journal of therapeutic innovation. Medic Scientific. 2024; 2 (4) : 192-202. (accessed on 10th May 2025).
22. Kattan, Jessica Anne, "The Epidemiology and Clinical Presentation of Leprosy in the Pediatric Population of Paraguay" (2006). Yale Medicine Thesis Digital Library. 251. http://elischolar.library.yale.edu/ymtdl/251(accessed on 10th May 2025).
23. Klein, Daniel B. and Tabarrok, Alexander T., Do Off-Label Drug Practices Argue Against Fda Efficacy Requirements? Testing an Argument by Structured Conversations with Experts (March 18, 2003). Available at SSRN: https://ssrn.com/abstract=425791 or http://dx.doi.org/10.2139/ssrn.425791 (accessed on 10th May 2025).

24. Annamreddi Leelavathi, Binu Mathew. Pediatric Obesity: Nursing Strategies for Prevention. Asian Journal of Nursing Education and Research. 2024; 14(2):129-2. doi: 10.52711/2349-2996.2024.00025 (accessed on 10th May 2025).
25. Mehariya, K. R. (2016). *Distinct Blue Print to Restrain Neglected Tropical Diseases*. Mehariya K R. Epidemiology International. 2016; 1 (3) : 14-20. https://core.ac.uk/download/354383009.pdf (accessed on 10th May 2025).
26. Ministry of Health and Social Welfare (MoHSW). (2008). *Health Sector Performance Profile Report: Mainland Tanzania July 2006 – June 2007*. https://core.ac.uk/download/pdf/11307141.pdf (accessed on 10th May 2025).
27. Morgan, R. W. (1980). *Basic Health Needs in Africa*. https://open.bu.edu/bitstream/2144/40428/1/WP_29_Morgan_1980.pdf (accessed on 10th May 2025).
28. J. Rodriguez-Morales, A. (Ed.). (2019). Current Topics in Neglected Tropical Diseases. IntechOpen. doi: 10.5772/intechopen.73918 (accessed on 10th May 2025).
29. Poonam Khetrapal Singh. (2022). *Elimination of Infectious Diseases from the South-East Asia Region*. SpringerBriefs in Public Health; DOI
30. https://doi.org/10.1007/978-981-16-5566-1(accessed on 10th May 2025).
31. O'Dea, Z. (2018). The Ayes have it!. *The Qualitative Report, 23*(10), 2313-2336. https://doi.org/10.46743/2160-3715/2018.2897 (accessed on 10th May 2025).
32. Oz, H. S. (2019). *Dirt, Saliva and Leprosy: Anti-Inflammatory and Anti-Infectious Effects*. https://core.ac.uk/download/232599684.pdf (accessed on 10th May 2025).
33. Pujitha, B., Joweriya, R., & Ramadevi, B. (2023). Spectrum of cutaneous manifestations in neonates at a tertiary care center. *Our Dermatology Online*. https://www.semanticscholar.org/paper/65198b1cd66538771ef9da74313bc28b9b501cd3 (accessed on 10th May 2025).
34. Rodriguez-Marin, M., & Orozco-Alatorre, L. G. (2025). Advancing pediatric growth assessment with machine learning: Overcoming challenges in early diagnosis and monitoring. *Children, 12*. https://www.semanticscholar.org/paper/267bae1a08ee664d5cd5d9bda7a5af5dd781a053 (accessed on 10th May 2025).
35. Russo, R. (2023). *Outpatient Medicine: A Comparison Between Low and High Resource System Settings*. https://core.ac.uk/download/579954902.pdf (accessed on 10th May 2025).
36. Safarabadi, M., Motallebirad, T., Azadi, D., & Jadidi, A. (2024). Healthcare-associated infections in Iranian pediatric and adult intensive care units: A comprehensive review of risk factors, etiology, molecular epidemiology, antimicrobial sensitivity, and prevention strategies during the COVID-19 pandemic. *Journal of intensive care medicine*, 8850666241249162. Advance online publication. https://doi.org/10.1177/08850666241249162(accessed on 10th May 2025).
37. Schmitt, K., & Leisinger, K. (2012). *Corporate Responsibility and Corporate Philanthropy*. https://core.ac.uk/download/75781320.pdf (accessed on 10th May 2025).
38. Sinha, S., Haq, M. A., Ahmad, R., Banik, S., Kumar, S., & Haque, M. (2024). Unmasking the Hidden Burden: A Delayed Diagnosis of Leprosy Patients With Grade 2 Disability and Its Effects on the Healthcare System in Bangladesh. *Cureus, 16*(4), e58708. https://doi.org/10.7759/cureus.58708(accessed on 10th May 2025).
39. Valencia, A., Schijman, A. G., De Andrade, A. L., Luquetti, A. O., Fernandes, C. D., Segura, E., Guhl, F., et al. (2009). Feasibility, drug safety, and effectiveness of etiological treatment

programs for Chagas disease in Honduras, Guatemala, and Bolivia: 10-year experience of Médecins Sans Frontières. *PLoS Negl. Trop. Dis., 3*(7), e488. https://core.ac.uk/download/pdf/9417445.pdf (accessed on 10th May 2025).

40. Yankulovska, S., Stolte, F., Thiemicke, P., Orzechowski, M., & Steger, F. (2024). Research ethics implications in the development of personalised therapy for pediatric SIRS patients. *The European Journal of Public Health, 34*(Suppl 3), ckae144.083. https://doi.org/10.1093/eurpub/ckae144.083(accessed on 10th May 2025).

41. Zhao D, Xiong Q, Lv Y, et al. Pediatric pulmonary embolism: unveiling clinical manifestations, diagnostic challenges, and outcomes in Southwest China. *Pediatr Discov.* 2025; 3(1):e83. **https://doi.org/10.1002/pdi3.83**(accessed on 10th May 2025).

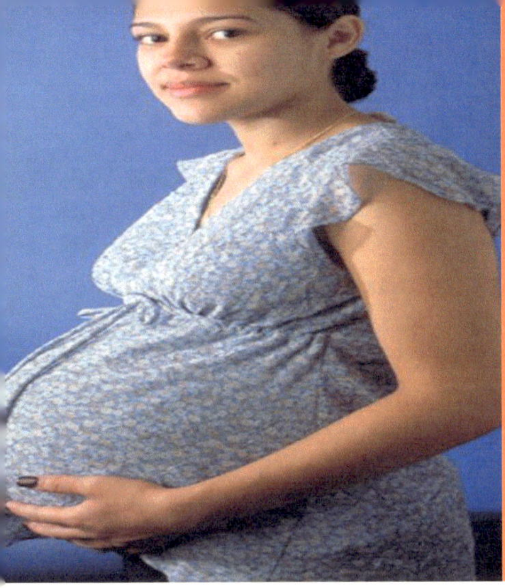

Chapter 12

LEPROSY IN PREGNANCY

Contents

Introduction

In many parts of the world where poverty is deep-rooted and healthcare is hard to come by, infectious diseases mixed with challenges in maternal care complicate global health. Pregnant women in these low-resource settings often face infections that not only hurt them but also endanger their unborn babies. Leprosy, caused by *Mycobacterium leprae*, even with improved treatments, still remains on the radar. Its quiet progression and the all-too-common delays in diagnosis often lead to complications that become especially worrisome during pregnancy. High maternal mortality, widespread poverty, and a shortage of skilled birth attendants only add to the mix, making the overlap of leprosy and pregnancy something that generally needs closer, more nuanced examination to cut down on risks and boost care delivery (Lorenz et al., 2005). This disease's hidden, insidious behavior allows it to keep spreading, and the stigma that surrounds it in many communities further complicates the issue for effective medical intervention during pregnancy. The immune changes a woman goes through can sometimes alter the disease's course or even interfere with treatment effectiveness. On top of that, social factors, like gender inequality, early marriages, and limited access to quality health services—tend to worsen the outcome. In most cases, understanding these intertwined biological and social factors is essential for shaping targeted health policies and clinical strategies that aim to safeguard both mother and baby (Lorenz et al., 2005). Given leprosy's persistent presence and its potential to cause irreversible damage, examining its impact on pregnant women is key to pushing forward better care for both mothers and their little ones. Early detection, prompt treatment, and well-rounded prenatal care tailored to this fragile group can go a long way in reducing complications and curbing transmission risks. Recent epidemiological work points to the importance of actively hunting for cases and combining leprosy management more tightly into maternal health services, especially in regions juggling multiple health crises like rising non-communicable diseases and infectious outbreaks. To summarize, delving into the challenges of leprosy during pregnancy not only tackles clinical issues head-on but also brings to light broader concerns related to health equity and the need for stronger healthcare systems in resource-limited areas (Lorenz et al., 2005) (Figure 12.1).

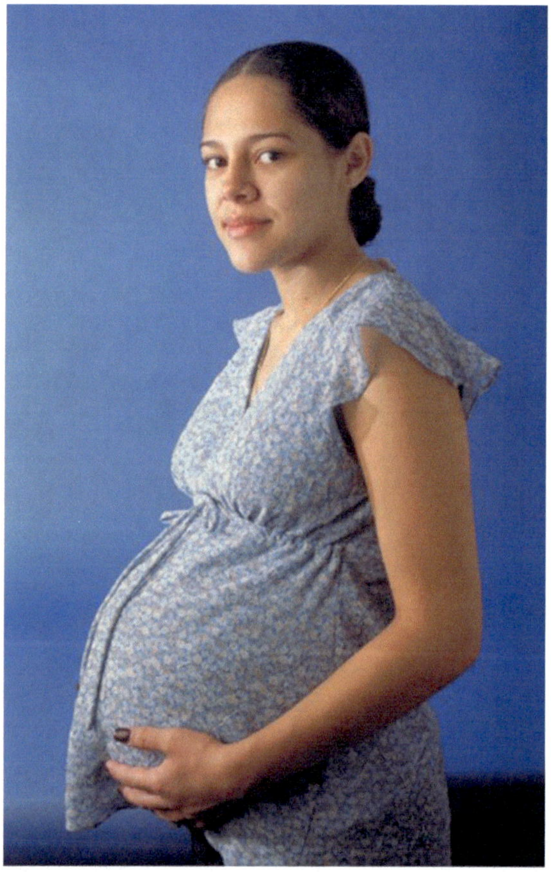

Figure 12.1. Leprosy in pregnancy.

Source: https://en.wikipedia.org/wiki/File:PregnantWoman.jpg

12.1. Pathophysiology of Leprosy

Leprosy's inner workings can be pretty complex, and they shape how the disease shows up and takes hold over time, especially for pregnant women. *Mycobacterium leprae* tends to settle in cooler parts of the body, like the skin and nerves, and it cleverly hides in Schwann cells to slip past immune defenses. You end up seeing nerve damage that brings on numbness and muscle weakness. People don't react the same way, either; some mount a solid cell-based response that keeps things mostly localized, while others develop a more diffuse lepromatous form with rampant bacteria. With pregnancy naturally shifting the immune system to protect the baby, these variations get even complex to sort out (Wojcik et al., 2019). Pregnancy itself stirs up major changes in immunity—generally speaking, a state of tolerance meant to safeguard the developing fetus, but this can backfire when it comes to infections like leprosy. The softening of cell-mediated immunity leaves a door open for *Mycobacterium leprae* to multiply or even push the disease into a more severe form. Hormonal swings and changes in cytokine levels during pregnancy can also alter the inflammatory reactions that end up damaging nerves. All these factors not only blur the clinical picture but also might throw a wrench into treatment plans, raising the stakes for both mother and baby (Wojcik et al., 2019). It's not just the microbes at play either; the link between nerves and immunity in leprosy gets even more complicated under the weight of stress and mood shifts during pregnancy. Anxiety and depression, which can emerge quite naturally, fiddle with immune responses through hormone and cytokine pathways. This mix of mental state and biological reaction isn't trivial—it can stimulate the disease along a different course. On top of that, having support and managing emotions well can make a difference in how a woman copes with a chronic condition like leprosy. In short, looking at leprosy during pregnancy means putting biological factors side by side with social and emotional ones to get a handle on care (Wojcik et al., 2019).

12.1.1. Causative Agent: Mycobacterium leprae

Mycobacterium leprae is the hidden culprit behind leprosy, invading not only skin cells but also peripheral nerves in ways that often catch us off guard. This bacterium replicates so slowly that its effects might only show up months—or even years—later, which becomes especially complex during pregnancy when the body's many changes can mask early signs. The organism lives inside cells, so the immune system has to work overtime to keep it in check; yet, since pregnancy naturally shifts immune defenses to welcome a fetus, those very changes can inadvertently give the bacterium a free pass. In most cases, these overlapping factors mean that careful, close monitoring is essential for women at risk (Jamieson et al., 2006). Pregnancy, by softening the cell-mediated response recharged to prevent fetal rejection, can set the stage for a more aggressive attack by *M. leprae*. Generally speaking, when the body draws back its usual immune firepower, the bacterial load can build up and speed along the disease's progression—leading to more severe skin lesions or nerve issues than one might typically expect. A nuanced look at these immune adjustments is, in most cases, indispensable for managing the infection properly, since unchecked leprosy might end up affecting both mother and baby, including potential issues during delivery and even transmission (Jamieson et al., 2006). Looking at the broader public health picture, leprosy in expecting mothers has plenty in common with other mycobacterial diseases like tuberculosis. Factors such as HIV co-infection, substance abuse, and challenging socioeconomic conditions all complicate the situation further; naturally, pregnant women in medically underserved communities can find themselves especially vulnerable. Health providers, therefore, need to be extra attentive when it comes to detecting and treating *M. leprae* during pregnancy. Approaches borrowed from TB control—think targeted screening and integrated maternal care—are, in most cases, crucial steps for reducing the overall health burden in these at-risk populations (Figure 12.2).

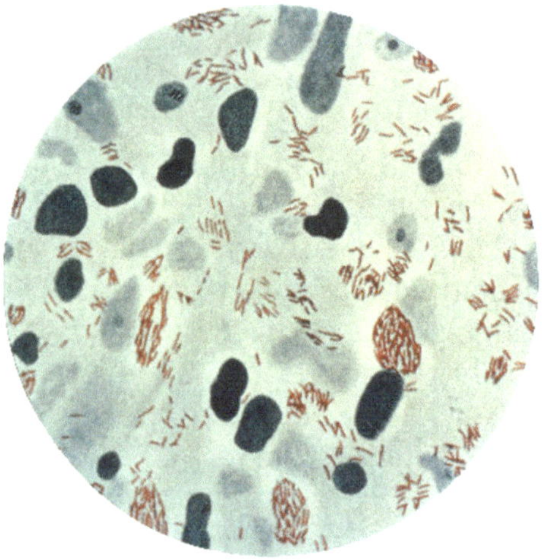

Figure 12.2. The causative agent: *Mycobacterium leprae.*

Source: Wikipedia. (n.d.). *Mycobacterium leprae.*

12.1.2. Mechanism of Infection and Transmission

Leprosy spreads in a complicated, drawn-out way – you get exposed to *Mycobacterium leprae*, the microbe behind it, over a long period. When someone untreated coughs or sneezes, tiny droplets carrying the bacteria float around; being near that person for too long increases your risk. The microbe grows slowly, sometimes taking months and in many cases more than five years to show its work, which complicates early detection. Once inside, *M. leprae* heads straight for the skin and peripheral nerves, favoring cooler spots on the body to settle in. Its tendency for invading Schwann cells eventually damages nerves—a signature sign of the disease, and figuring out these steps is key to stopping both vertical and horizontal spread, especially among individuals like pregnant women whose immune responses might be off-kilter (Kelbessa, 2017). Understanding these routes is crucial if we want to lighten the disease's heavy toll. Being pregnant seems to change up the immune system quite a bit, generally leaving way for the microbe to take hold or even worsen an already creeping infection. This relative drop in immune reaction might not allow the body to defend itself as well, which ups both the chances of spreading and the severity of the illness. Add to that the fact that in many cases people live in tight quarters, often in economically challenged areas where tropical diseases are common—the risk only grows. Leprosy isn't just about physical issues; it brings along lasting disabilities and social stigma, meaning infections during pregnancy can affect both moms and their babies. Tackling this spread head on is a must if we're to break the cycle of sickness and poverty that hits these regions hard (Asian Development Bank, 2014). Some studies point out that while the main way leprosy jumps from one person to another is through direct contact, other factors might alter how easily someone gets infected. Researchers have poked around ideas like environmental spots—soil or water—as possible hideouts for the microbe, though their roles still aren't crystal clear. Living in the same household with an infected person adds a whole new layer to the risk, given the constant close contact. Even though passing the infection from a mom to her child during pregnancy or while nursing seems to be very rare, the immune lull that comes with pregnancy might trigger a dormant infection to flare up. Grappling with these complex factors is key for mapping out strategies to break the spread, especially in places where poverty and crowded living make people even more vulnerable (Asian Development Bank, 2014; Kelbessa, 2017).

12.1.3. Immune Response to Leprosy

Pregnancy throws up a tough challenge when it comes to how our bodies handle infections – especially in conditions like leprosy. The body switches gears during pregnancy, usually creating an environment that shields the fetus while still keeping an eye out for harmful microbes. Looking at leprosy, for example, you see that different immune responses lead to its different flavors, from the localized tuberculoid type to the widespread lepromatous kind. Studies on microbes like Chlamydia abortus even show that the tug-of-war between T helper cells and regulatory T cells at the maternal-fetal boundary can tip the scale toward outcomes like preterm labor or even, at times, fetal loss (Caspe et al., 2023). In most cases, these findings hint that the way a mother's immune system adapts in leprosy might change not just the course of the illness but also the baby's health – a reminder that looking deeply into immune shifts is important. When you consider leprosy's complex immunopathology, it all comes down to how the body reacts to *Mycobacterium leprae*. Generally speaking, a strong cell-based response tends to keep the disease in check, leading to the tuberculoid form. However, if the Th1 response isn't quite up to snuff and the Th2 pattern takes over, the disease can spread out as lepromatous leprosy.

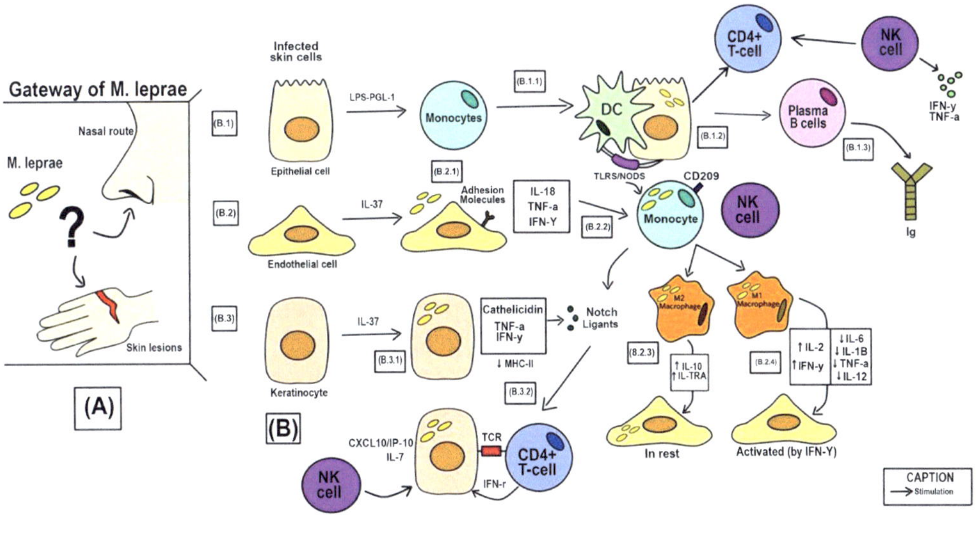

Figure 12.3. Phases of the generation of the human immune response against *M. leprae* since bacterial entry into the initial site of infection.

Source: ilva MJA, Silva CS, Brasil TP, Alves AK, dos Santos EC, Frota CC, Lima KVB and Lima LNGC (2024) An update on leprosy immunopathogenesis: systematic review. Front. Immunol. 15:1416177. doi: 10.3389/fimmu.2024.1416177

Pregnancy itself stimulates the immune system to be a bit more tolerant (to avoid rejecting the fetus), which might further alter these responses. Look at emerging research on infections like SARS-CoV-2 – even though vertical transmission seems rare, the mother's immune kick-starts changes in the fetus via cytokines and different lymphocyte subsets crossing the placenta (González-Mesa et al., 2022). So, this back-and-forth between maternal and fetal immune responses might mean that leprosy in the mom could subtly influence the newborn's immune setup, altering susceptibility in regions where the disease is common. It isn't just about the mom's health – understanding these immune dynamics in pregnant women with leprosy matters for the baby too. Immune mix-ups in leprosy can make complications like miscarriage, preterm birth, or low birth weight more likely. If you compare this to other infections during pregnancy, then it becomes clear that striking the right balance between fighting off pathogens and not overreacting is key. In most cases, therapeutic strategies need to be tailored carefully to lower excessive inflammation while still keeping enough firepower to fight *Mycobacterium leprae*. Additional research into immune cell types, the nuances of cytokine expression, and how exactly the maternal and fetal systems chat with each other is bound to shine a light on better clinical moves – all aiming for improved outcomes for both mom and baby (Caspe et al., 2023; González-Mesa et al., 2022) (Figure 12.3).

12.2. Effects of Leprosy on Pregnancy

Pregnancy brings about many bodily changes that complicate leprosy management in ways one wouldn't always expect – both mom and baby can feel the impact. Immune shifts during this time tend to wake up or worsen old leprosy spots, making it complex to keep the disease in check. In most cases, women carrying the condition run a higher risk of sudden inflammatory flare-ups (lepra reactions) that push nerve damage and skin issues even further; these episodes, if not handled quickly, can end up causing lasting harm. The usual cocktail of drugs, although key for clearing the bacteria, needs a careful balancing act because of its potential risks to the growing fetus. Also, the natural dampening of cellular defenses in pregnancy might tip the scales between the microbe and the body, opening the door for extra infections and influencing outcomes in subtle ways (IJCP Group, 2023). It calls for extra watchfulness during prenatal checkups and flexible treatment plans that match the shifting needs. Looking beyond the immediate health of the mother, leprosy tends to throw a wrench into the works of the baby's development and the birth process itself. Studies generally point out that pregnancies affected by leprosy often end up with issues like low birth weight, babies arriving too soon, or even restricted growth inside the womb – partly thanks to the body's own inflammatory response and placental upset caused by *Mycobacterium leprae*. In fact, an ongoing maternal infection may impact the placenta's ability to deliver vital oxygen and nutrients; this is critical for a healthy baby. Adding to the mix, social stigma and the resulting delays in seeking care can lead to less-than-ideal prenatal attention, which in turn bumps up risks for both mother and child. Even if passing the infection directly is pretty rare, the knock-on effects on fetal growth mean that a more integrated approach to caring for both mother and baby is needed (IJCP Group, 2023). It's a complex web of immune shifts, infection, and the everyday challenges of pregnancy. Now, mix in some metabolic concerns, and the outlook for pregnant women with leprosy gets even murkier. Recent research has started to shine a light on how things like blood sugar control and overall nutrition can influence the journey when an infection is already in play. For instance, with rising issues like obesity and high blood sugar in women of childbearing age, these metabolic glitches might make the inflammatory backdrop of leprosy even worse, eventually shaping the course of the pregnancy in unpredictable ways. There's also some chatter about the longer-term effects that could pass on to the child, prompting calls for more detailed studies tracking these outcomes over time. Bringing regular metabolic screening into the picture alongside infection management could, in most cases, refine prenatal care by addressing these dual challenges and, ultimately, help ensure that both mother and baby have a better shot at staying healthy.

12.2.1. Maternal Health Complications

Pregnancy with leprosy is full of extra challenges. The disease mixes with the natural body changes during pregnancy, usually making maternal health issues even complex. Women dealing with leprosy sometimes end up facing painfully long labors, infections that just persist, and bleeding that can quickly become dangerous if not kept under control. This problem tends to get worse in many rural areas—places where home births are common and help typically comes from untrained individuals—because skilled, on-call care just isn't always available. Factors like long distances to hospitals, limited transportation, and money worries delay needed help, which in turn ups the risk for both mom and baby. Lower education and tough job conditions further link up with lower rates of professional support, worsening outcomes overall (Dhakal et al., 2011). It's also true that missing out on proper postnatal care adds fuel to the fire of maternal health complications connected to leprosy. After childbirth, especially for women fighting off infections, timely care becomes super important so that any arising issues can be detected early. In many resource-poor settings, though, postnatal services are oddly underused, often because people just aren't aware of their importance or cultural norms get in the way. Women with leprosy might also feel even more isolated due to persisting stigma, making them hesitate to seek help promptly. In most cases, the complex mix of social standing, ethnicity, and access to healthcare shows just how much we need targeted interventions, and it means improving the quality of post-delivery services so they meet these women's diverse needs (Bolam et al., 2007). Tackling the health problems in pregnant women with leprosy calls for a broad, multifaceted approach.

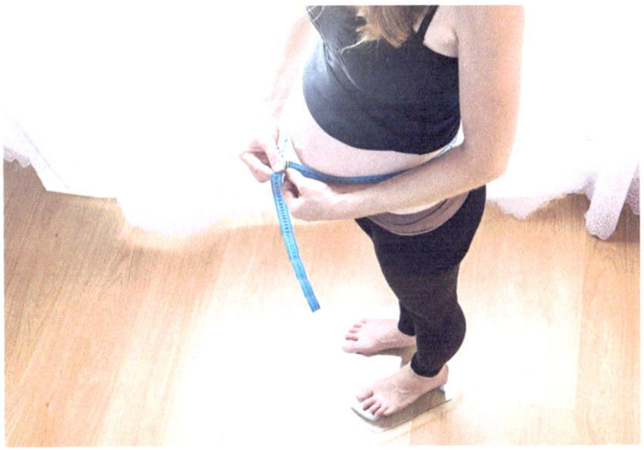

Figure 12.4. Maternal health complications.

Source: By Urvi Goratela - Own work, CC BY-SA 4.0, https://commons.wikimedia.org/w/index.php?curid=131964870

It isn't only about one aspect but involves boosting education, making care easier to access, and lifting the overall quality of services. Increasing awareness about the benefits of delivering in a health facility and the importance of follow-up care, especially in rural spots where home births dominate, can help tip the scales in favor of better outcomes. Empowering women—through better education and improved financial conditions—might encourage more of them to seek out skilled care, thereby reducing the risks that accompany leprosy. Meanwhile, healthcare systems need to be ready with trained professionals who can handle not only emergent obstetric issues but also the special challenges leprosy brings along. Finally, collaboration between public health agencies and community programs stands as a vital piece in lowering maternal mortality and improving results for both mothers and their little ones (Bolam et al., 2007; Dhakal et al., 2011) (Figure 12.4).

12.2.2. Fetal Health Risks Associated with Leprosy

Leprosy mostly messes with the skin and nerves, but when it shows up during pregnancy, things quickly get more complex - not only is the mom at risk, but the baby might suffer too. It's concerning that the microbe, *Mycobacterium leprae*, might pass from mother to child—even if that's pretty rare, and then the usual immune shifts in pregnancy can stir up more damage, inducing inflammation that isn't great for anyone involved. This complex mix of the mother's infection and the baby's fragile state calls for careful, all-around prenatal check-ups. There have been instances of premature births, low birth weights, and even higher newborn mortality; so, it's not just the microbe itself, but broader health issues like malnutrition and systemic inflammation that come into play (Arlen et al., 2015). Treating leprosy when someone is pregnant adds another layer of complication. Some of the drugs used, like thalidomide—famously linked in the 1960s with severe birth defects—still remain key for dealing with conditions like erythema nodosum leprosum, even though they carry serious risks. In regions where leprosy is common, keeping thalidomide on hand means accepting the possibility of problems like limb defects or other birth issues that fall under the so-called thalidomide embryopathy phenotype. Because of that, doctors need to keep a close eye on drug dosages and timing, balancing the mom's need for treatment with the baby's safety (Castilla et al., 2019). It's a tough juggling act that, generally speaking, demands treatment plans that are as flexible as they are cautious. Socioeconomic challenges in regions hit hard by leprosy only add fuel to the fire. Limited healthcare access, spotty prenatal check-ups, and poor nutrition can all interfere with fetal health, even aside from the infection itself. When a mother's immune defenses are already down and the disease persists, the placenta might not deliver enough nutrients to the growing baby, upping the risk for intrauterine growth issues. These overlapping factors aren't just a call for more medicine—they shout out for broader community support, better access to care, and more education on prenatal health. In short, handling the many complications associated with leprosy in pregnancy calls for an approach that tackles both the mother's condition and the baby's well-being, side by side (Arlen et al., 2015; Castilla et al., 2019).

12.2.3. Impact on Labor and Delivery Outcomes

Pregnancy isn't just a matter of the usual birth challenges—when a chronic infection like leprosy steps into the picture, things get complicated. Women dealing with leprosy often face a rougher ride during labor, where nerve damage and persistent skin sores can sap their ability to move easily and fight through pain. This condition also tends to weaken the immune system, leaving them more open to infections that complicate not only labor but also recovery afterward. In many places, such as Niger where poverty and high birth rates mix, these issues are compounded by scarce healthcare and the weight of social stigma (Heller, 2015). Thus, both the direct effects of leprosy and the harsh realities of socio-economic hurdles end up putting a double whammy on delivery outcomes. Labor patterns themselves can go off-kilter for women with leprosy; labor might drag on or get obstructed, paving the way for complications like fetal distress or even forcing a move towards surgical delivery. Often, the nerve damage typical of leprosy dulls pain sensations just enough that a woman may not realize the seriousness of her labor until it's nearly too late, sometimes delaying hospital visits until labor is very advanced. This lag, in turn, sometimes results in a spike in cesarian rates and other maternal problems, as well as more severe issues like obstetric fistula, which is a dire consequence of prolonged blocked labor (Heller, 2015). To summarize, the clash between an infectious disease and not-so-great obstetric care makes it clear that we need better-integrated prenatal and perinatal strategies for these vulnerable women. It isn't only the medical side of things that complicates the issue; the social and political scene plays its part as well. Topics like pregnancy and breastfeeding under the shadow of infectious diseases barely get a mention in public debates or political discussions—East Java, Indonesia for example, sometimes shows only the faintest media coverage. Generally speaking, that lack of attention means policies often overlook the specific needs of mothers affected by leprosy, limiting both the availability and quality of care they receive. Without focused interventions addressing both medical challenges and broader social factors, these women face steep odds during labor and delivery. Boosting awareness, advocating for change, and sharpening healthcare provider training could all help ease the heavy load that leprosy can place on maternal health (Figure 12.5).

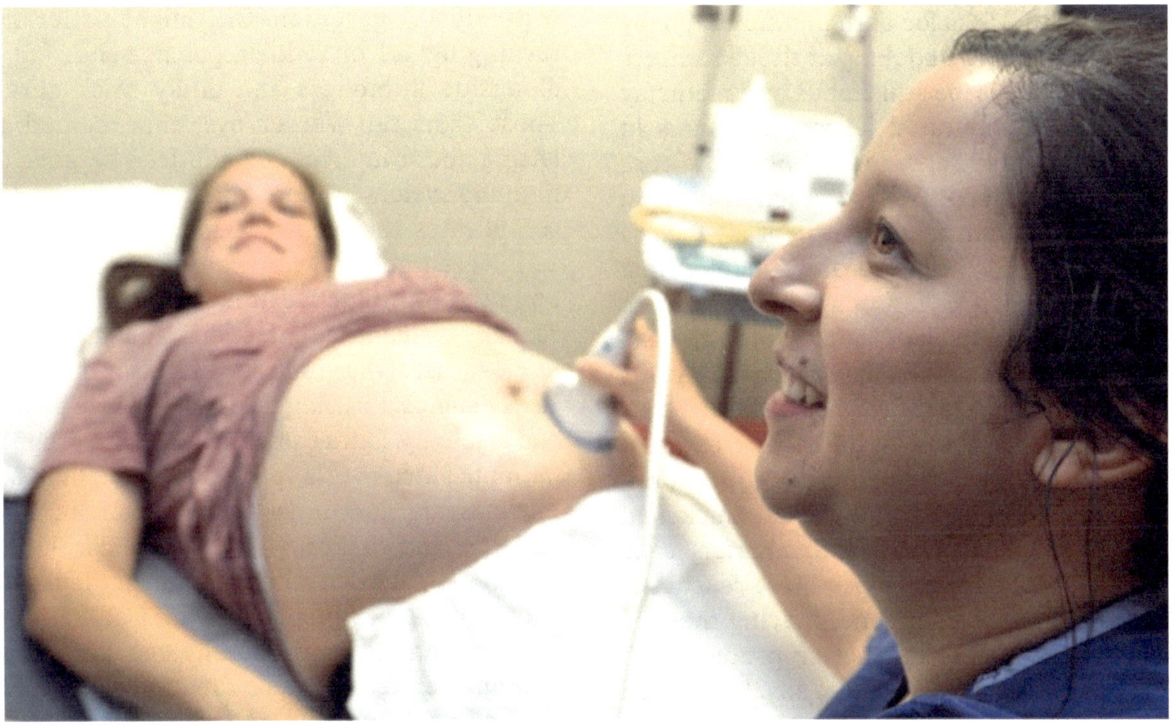

Figure 12.5. The impact on labor and delivery outcomes.

Source: By Jacob Sippel - https://health.mil/News/Gallery/Photos/2017/04/27/During-Pregnancy, CC BY-SA 4.0, https://commons.wikimedia.org/w/index.php?curid=74814735

12.3. Diagnosis of Leprosy in Pregnant Women

Diagnosing leprosy in pregnant women is complex because the body's shifting immune state and physical changes during pregnancy often hide or alter the usual signs of the disease. Pregnancy lowers immune defenses in a way that can flare up dormant *Mycobacterium leprae* infections or even bring on unusual symptoms—ones that aren't easy to pinpoint. Some leprosy signs look a lot like normal skin changes seen during pregnancy, so clinicians have to take a closer look. Usually, a hands-on exam is backed up with lab work, tissue studies and culture tests, to boost diagnostic accuracy. Yet, in many resource-poor areas, missing or outdated diagnostic tools slow down early detection. The lack of solid data on both tuberculosis and leprosy in expecting mothers only adds to the need for better lab services. Quick, sensitive tests are key to getting treatment started sooner, which helps lower the risks for both mother and baby (Kapata et al., 2011). Looking at tissue samples under the microscope still stands as a mainstay for catching complicated leprosy reactions in pregnant patients. Take, for example, the rare Lucio phenomenon, a severe reaction seen in untreated diffuse lepromatous leprosy, where a microscopic exam can reveal a subepidermal grenz zone, foamy macrophages stuffed with acid-fast bacilli, and even spots of blood vessel damage in the deeper skin layers. These signals do more than just confirm the disease; they guide doctors in choosing the right treatment for moms at extra risk. In several reports, detailed histopathologic findings like thickened vessel walls and clusters of inflammatory cells have led clinicians to diagnose these reactional states with greater confidence, paving the way for treatment plans that better protect both mother and child (Fiqnasyani et al., 2023). Even with clinical evaluations and tissue studies available, diagnosing leprosy during pregnancy remains hampered by broader, systemic issues, especially in low-income regions. Limited access to advanced labs that can run tests such as bacillary and morphological index assessments makes a full diagnosis and careful monitoring a challenge. And when conditions like HIV and tuberculosis emerge, which is common in many endemic areas, teasing out the right diagnosis gets even more complicated; an integrated approach becomes necessary. In most cases, boosting diagnostic protocols with rapid, sensitive, field-ready tools is essential to address this public health concern. Improved collaboration between TB and leprosy programs could help doctors better diagnose and treat pregnant women, ultimately leading to improved outcomes for both mothers and their newborns (Kapata et al., 2011).

12.3.1. Clinical Signs and Symptoms

Leprosy in pregnancy is a complex mix of changes. The disease hits in ways that overlap with the body's own immune and hormonal shifts during gestation. One might notice skin turning lighter or reddish patches showing up alongside numbness and oddly thick nerves. These signs can worsen over time, sometimes letting minor injuries go unnoticed because the immune system is acting differently, which only complicates the picture. Genital signals—such as lowered gonadal function or lesions higher up in the reproductive area—can look a lot like sexually transmitted infections (Richens, 2004). In most cases, these subtle hints early on delay a clear diagnosis, raising the risk for nerve damage and disability. Extra care is needed with pregnant patients since overlapping symptoms may blur the lines and slow down proper treatment. Some patients even go through bumps like flare-ups or reactions—think erythema nodosum leprosum and type 1 lepra responses—that add another layer of complexity. Generally speaking, these immune-related episodes can induce extra skin inflammation, nerve pain (neuritis), and other systemic issues that might result in fetal distress or even preterm labor if left unchecked. Visible skin issues and disfigurement often lead to a real toll on mental well-being, compounded by social stigma and isolation (Van Haaren et al., 2016). These psychosocial factors, quite naturally, affect how symptoms are reported, and sometimes even access to care gets more complicated. Further, because leprosy can stick around in different ways even after biomedical treatment, its signs may ebb and flow over time, making a case for a treatment plan that looks after both body and mind. The nervous system gets deeply involved, which is one of leprosy's hallmark challenges, especially during pregnancy. Sensory loss, muscle weakness, and increasingly thick nerves can creep in slowly as pregnancy progresses, boosting the chance of disability if nothing changes. The body's shifting immune responses during pregnancy might either hide or exaggerate these issues, sometimes leading to an underestimation or an overinterpretation of how serious the nerve problems are. At times, genital issues like hydrocele or other lesions overlap with tropical infections common in certain regions, so a careful, deep look is important (Richens, 2004). In many cases, tackling these overlapping problems calls for teamwork, a combination of obstetric, dermatological, and neurological know-how, to try to get the best outcomes for both mom and baby (Figure 12.6).

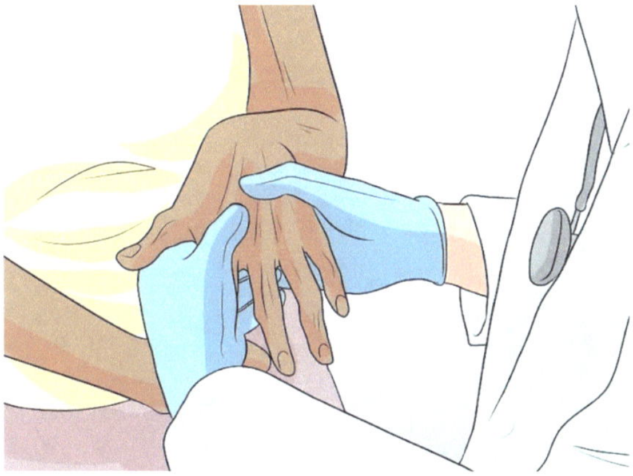

Figure 12.6. A doctor determines the form of leprosy.

Source: WikiHow. (n.d.). *Determining Leprosy Type.*

12.3.2. Diagnostic Tests and Procedures

Leprosy in pregnancy is a real headache because its signs easily mix with other skin issues and body-wide problems common to expecting moms. Getting this diagnosis right early on matters a lot, it sets off treatment fast and helps keep both the mother and the baby on safe ground. Usually, doctors lean on clinical exams and skin biopsies to spot those acid-fast bacilli, but these tests can be quite invasive and sometimes don't give a clear answer at all. Lately, however, people have been trying out safer, more sensitive methods. Some new non-invasive skin tests and immune-based assays—ones that check for delayed-type hypersensitivity or certain antibody responses—look promising. They can pick up an active infection much sooner, so treatment plans can be altered on the fly, which is critical when worrying about drug side effects on the fetus. More recently, fresh developments in leprosy testing have brought in specific skin antigens derived from *Mycobacterium leprae*. Two formulations, MLSA-LAM and MLCwA, have already gone through phases I and II clinical trials and seem to do well on safety and specificity—a big deal when you want to avoid exposing pregnant patients to risky substances. These skin tests depend on delayed-type hypersensitivity (DTH) responses, tapping into immune reactions to flag an infection even before typical signs emerge. On top of that, throwing in interferon gamma release assays seems to boost accuracy for the tuberculoid form; this nicely backs up the antibody tests that work better for the lepromatous kind. To summarize, this immune-based method not only refines disease classification but also helps adjust maternal treatment protocols, keeping the little one safe and reducing the chance of spreading the infection (Rivoire et al., 2012). When you compare this with other mycobacterial issues like Buruli ulcer, there's been a push toward strict antimicrobial trial. These studies stress that getting the diagnosis right and choosing treatments that the patient can handle are important. Fully oral antibiotic courses have shown themselves to be just as effective, and often are even better tolerated—than the injectable versions, hinting at a general switch to less invasive, more secure therapies. Even if these results focus on Buruli ulcer, they underscore ideas that apply to leprosy during pregnancy too. Better diagnostic tests that give clear, measurable outcomes, like confirming that a lesion is healing or checking immune response markers—might cut down on needless surgeries and make it easier to track how well the treatment is working, paving the way for safer management of leprosy in expectant mothers (Phillips et al., 2020) (Figure 12.7).

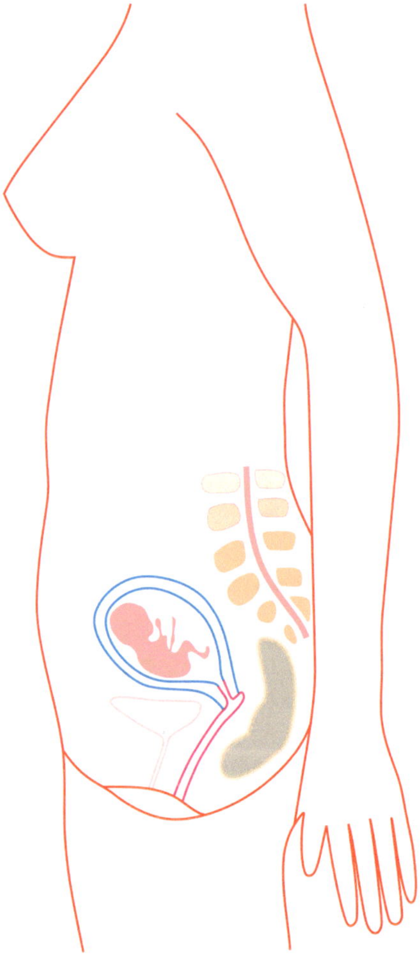

Figure 12.7. The diagnostic tests and procedures.

Source: By Miraceti - Own work, CC BY-SA 3.0, https://commons.wikimedia.org/w/index.php?curid=904212

12.3.3. Challenges in Diagnosing Leprosy During Pregnancy

Pregnancy shakes up the body in unexpected ways, and it's not always easy to tell what's going on when diseases show up. Take leprosy, for example, shifts in hormones and changes in the immune system, along with skin adjustments, can blur the picture. The body, in most cases, calms its defenses to protect the growing baby, which can unintentionally quiet down the cell-based responses needed to fight off *Mycobacterium leprae*. This mix of natural immune softening and altered skin behavior means that what looks like a common pregnancy blemish or nerve tingle might be hiding leprosy signs. Sometimes, a skin lesion or numbness that you'd normally flag as danger gets brushed off as just another pregnancy characteristic. In general, such uncertainties call for doctors to keep a closer, more skeptical eye and use screening methods that with a bit of extra caution, help spot problems early. Standard tests that work well under normal circumstances often hit a snag when used with pregnant patients. For instance, skin smears and tissue biopsies—usually seen as top-notch methods—can end up with mixed, unpredictable results because pregnancy changes blood flow and inflames tissues, interfering with sample quality. Serological tests that aim to pick up anti-phenolic glycolipid antibodies tend to fall short too, struggling to tell an active infection apart from a quiet, latent one in a body that's already set to a different immune tone. Even imaging approaches, like those that check nerve involvement, get used sparingly (or even skipped altogether) to avoid any risks to the baby, leaving clinicians to often depend on their judgment rather than a clear-cut test result (Luong et al., 2025). It's a situation where careful interpretation of lab data and hands-on clinical sense become all the more important. On top of these challenges, there are bigger, systemic problems. In many of the regions where leprosy still shows up often, pregnant women might not have quick access to specialists who can offer a proper skin or nerve examination. Further, social stigma—an ever-present worry with leprosy—can make women hesitant to report symptoms, so the chance for early treatment slips away. Balancing the need to keep the fetus safe with the need to treat effectively can force doctors into delaying treatment until the picture is crystal-clear. This balancing act is similar to what happens in other pregnancy-related issues, like diabetic retinopathy, where the body's shifting state complicates the issue even more (Rosu et al., 2024). Altogether, these layers of difficulty underscore why more awareness, better teamwork among specialists, and refined approaches to diagnosis are so crucial in managing leprosy during pregnancy.

12.4. Treatment Options for Pregnant Women

When leprosy shows up in a pregnant woman, keeping both her health and the baby's safety in check can get pretty complex. Not treating the condition can spell damage for them both. The usual game plan is multidrug therapy—commonly known as MDT—but when a woman is expecting, you have to alter things because pregnancy can change how drugs work, and there's a worry about possible harm to the fetus. Drugs like dapsone, rifampicin, and clofazimine are standard fare, yet their use during pregnancy calls for extra caution, smart dose alters, and constant checking. Generally speaking, stopping the treatment isn't a good idea since the disease might flare up or spread, although sometimes adjusting the dose while offering extra support can ease unwanted effects. A combination of skin experts, pregnancy doctors, and infection specialists usually huddle together to keep both mom and baby as safe as possible. It isn't all about taking pills, though. Teaching pregnant women about leprosy can make a difference in how well they stick to their treatment. Think about how, in cases like opioid use disorder, simple brochures that explain the options, benefits, and risks helped patients feel more in control (Jeminiwa et al., 2024). If similar, clear-cut material is made just for expecting women with leprosy, it could help them feel more confident about staying on track, even when there are pregnancy risks involved. Such resources can fill in the gaps, clear up persisting myths, and stimulate patients toward better adherence, which in turn helps both the mother and her baby get through the treatment smoothly. Extra supportive care can also play a big part when things get complicated. For example, in pregnancies affected by conditions like rhesus immunization, combining in additional therapies and even specialized blood transfusions has shown better perinatal outcomes by looking out for the baby while handling the mom's condition (Vetrov et al., 2023). Though the underlying issues differ from leprosy, the idea remains the same: pairing the main drug treatment with extra supportive measures can lower fetal risks. In most cases, this kind of multipronged approach, tackling not just the infection but its broader effects, is key to ensuring that both mother and baby receive the best possible care during such challenging times (Figure 12.8).

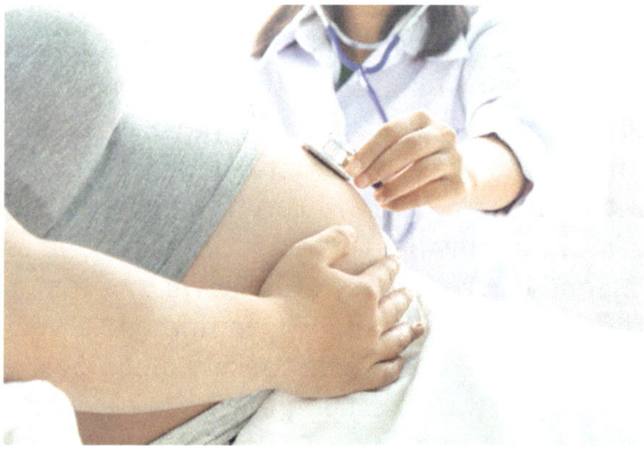

Figure 12.8. Treatment for pregnant women.

Source: iStock. (n.d.). *Pregnant women and doctors check the symptoms. https://media.istockphoto.com/id/1054612538/photo/pregnant-women-and-doctors-check-the-symptoms.jpg?s=170667a&w=0&k=20&c=8XdAbSxoj83jHhmdIulQ9Ag9U7a9Cw5oq_l_pN8xHqU=.*

12.4.1. Recommended Medications and Their Safety

Leprosy treatment during pregnancy is a complex area. Doctors have to juggle the benefits of drugs with the potential risks if the disease is left untreated. The usual approach is a combination of drugs—dapsone, rifampicin, and clofazimine, which work well to keep the infection in check and stop it from spreading, yet each drug carries its own set of concerns. Dapsone, for instance, is mostly safe but can sometimes lead to hemolytic anemia in the mother or cause issues for the newborn. Rifampicin, which can slip past the placental barrier, hasn't shown clear harmful effects in humans, even though careful monitoring is usually advised. On the other hand, there isn't much data on clofazimine during pregnancy, so its use remains a bit of a gamble. In most cases, this means treatment plans are tailored to each individual, steering clear of drugs known for embryo toxicity or those that need extra-precise oversight. Ultimately, this balanced strategy is key for keeping both the mother and the developing baby safe. When it comes to leprosy medications, safety isn't only about how the drug works inside the body—it's also about wider public health issues, especially in places where drug rules might not be very strict. For example, thalidomide sometimes shows up as a treatment for leprosy complications, even though it's infamous for its severe risks to unborn children. Its documented ability to cause congenital defects makes its use during pregnancy completely off the table. Even with regulations meant to keep it in check, occasional lapses in monitoring have unfortunately led to fresh cases of thalidomide embryopathy (Leal & Mota, 2021). Generally speaking, this serves as a stark reminder of the necessity of vigilance, ensuring pregnant women with leprosy avoid these dangerous drugs, while also stressing the importance of proper education and routine checks to prevent accidental exposure. Everyday realities also play a big role in how safe medications are used. In indigenous populations, for example, especially in remote Aboriginal communities, treatment isn't just about handing out pills – it's about building care that feels personal and respects cultural traditions. Issues like longstanding mistrust, language or communication gaps, and even other competing health concerns can sometimes get in the way of proper medication use (Oliver, 2022). As a result, keeping treatment on track means healthcare providers might need to alter their approach to align with local cultural values and ensure patients truly understand and follow the therapy plan. To summarize, medication safety isn't seen purely through the lens of drug properties; it's deeply connected to culturally sensitive, responsive care that helps both mothers and babies in the challenging fight against leprosy (Figure 12.9).

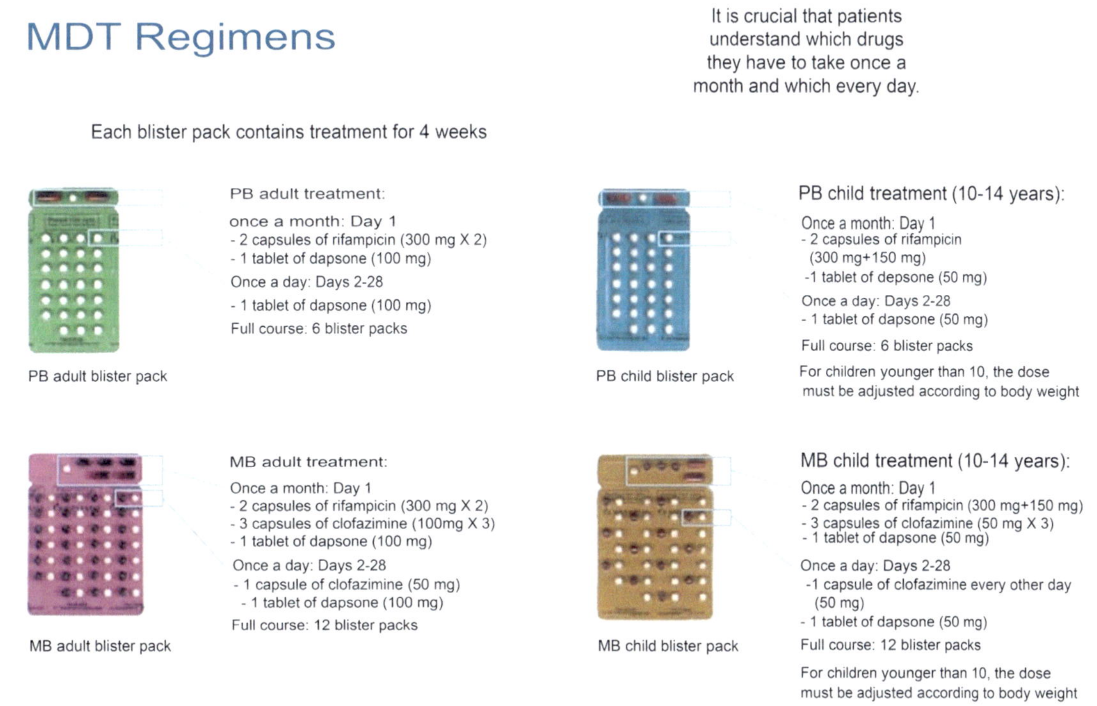

Figure 12.9. Treatment of leprosy.

Source: Public Domain, https://commons.wikimedia.org/w/index.php?curid=1840307

12.4.2. Management of Leprosy Symptoms During Pregnancy

Managing leprosy symptoms in a pregnant woman means walking a fine line, keeping the disease in check while protecting both mom and her baby. Pregnancy sets the immune system into a different gear, which can sometimes make leprosy reactions even worse, so keeping a close, almost casual watch is essential. Generally speaking, multidrug therapy (MDT) is seen as safe and helps stop the condition from getting further out of hand; stopping it can let the disease persist. It also doesn't hurt to keep an eye on signs in the genital area because leprosy might show up as unexpected sores or lumps that could complicate delivery and overall comfort (Richens, 2004). Dealing with these genital signs not only eases discomfort but may even cut down the risk of extra infections affecting both mom and baby. A team effort among dermatologists, obstetricians, and infectious disease experts often ends up being the best way to manage both symptoms and pregnancy outcomes. Taking care of the emotional and social side is just as important as treating the physical aspects. The stigma linked with leprosy can feel even heavier during pregnancy, and that extra weight sometimes makes it tougher for a woman to stick to her treatment. Research, in many cases, shows that patients end up seeing their condition as something lifelong and isolating, which, in turn, stirs up additional anxiety and a sense of shame (Van Haaren et al., 2016). In most cases, healthcare providers are encouraged to offer not just medications but also real talk through counseling and constant supportive care. These conversations help improve treatment follow-through and ease some of the mental stress, while community education efforts—aimed at loosening the old stigmas about leprosy—can create a kinder social environment for pregnant women, making the whole process a bit less overwhelming. Sometimes, particular care is needed when it comes to the body's immune responses during pregnancy, especially with the type 1 and type 2 lepra reactions. Hormonal shifts and changes in immunity can induce up nerve pain, swelling, or even a temporary loss of function if these reactions aren't detected early. In many instances, timely use of corticosteroids or similar immunosuppressive agents becomes a crucial step to rein things in while trying to avoid any side effects on the baby. Nutritional support and regular prenatal checkups also play supporting roles in keeping both mom's diet and fetal growth on track, despite the challenges thrown up by the disease. To summarize, a plan that's tailored to the individual—one that combines medical treatment with psychological and social support—is key to handling both the physical and emotional layers of leprosy during pregnancy (Richens, 2004; Van Haaren et al., 2016).

12.4.3. Considerations for Postpartum Care

After childbirth, new mothers dealing with leprosy—whether the condition first emerged during pregnancy or was managed then, often run into a combination of challenges that sometimes catch everyone off guard. Right after delivery, as the immune system begins to bounce back, leftover *Mycobacterium leprae* can stir up damage, making it easier for the infection to flare or for unexpected reaction states to develop. In many cases the body's own rebound triggers a surge of inflammation, and if that isn't kept in check, nerve pain and worsening skin sores can follow. Newborn care and the sheer exhaustion of early motherhood may even throw off the regularity of taking a full multidrug cocktail, which, honestly, could tip the balance of treatment success. Doctors generally stress sticking to medication plans and popping in for check-ups, while a team that might include dermatologists, obstetricians, and infection experts strives to help both the leprosy symptoms and overall mom's recovery in a way that feels less clinical and more, well, human. Nutrition and how wounds are handled take on extra weight during the postpartum stretch for women with leprosy. When pregnancy and the illness itself drag down nutritional status, it not only hinders the immune system but also slows the healing of ulcers or nerve injuries. Breastfeeding mothers, in particular, face extra head-scratchers because some antileprosy drugs pose risks to the baby—so, weighing the perks of ongoing treatment against potential side effects becomes a must. Providers need to guide these moms through informed choices while juggling the advice on basic hygiene and preventing extra infections, especially since leprous plaques can leave the skin looking and feeling more vulnerable. And, let's be honest, a little emotional and social support goes a long way at a time when sticking to treatment feels like an uphill battle. After delivery, the immune landscape tends to shift unpredictably, sometimes opening the door to intracellular pathogens like *Mycobacterium leprae*. The calm-over-pregnancy immune state changes, often inducing sharper inflammatory responses that can trigger flare-ups or even a relapse of leprosy. Keeping a close watch for signs of immune reconstitution inflammatory syndrome is crucial, this is especially true when another infection, like tuberculosis, persists nearby with overlapping risks (Abdel-Rahman et al., 2015; Jamieson et al., 2006). In most cases, this means tailoring follow-up routines to mix infection vigilance with ongoing postpartum care. Some doctors even suggest that joining clinical studies, geared towards new moms, might shed more light on the best ways to treat these conditions, since current research is sometimes murky due to pregnant and postpartum women being left out of trials (Abdel-Rahman et al., 2015). In the end, a focus on evidence-based, personalized postpartum care can help lower health risks and smooth the long road ahead for mothers dealing with leprosy (Figure 12.10).

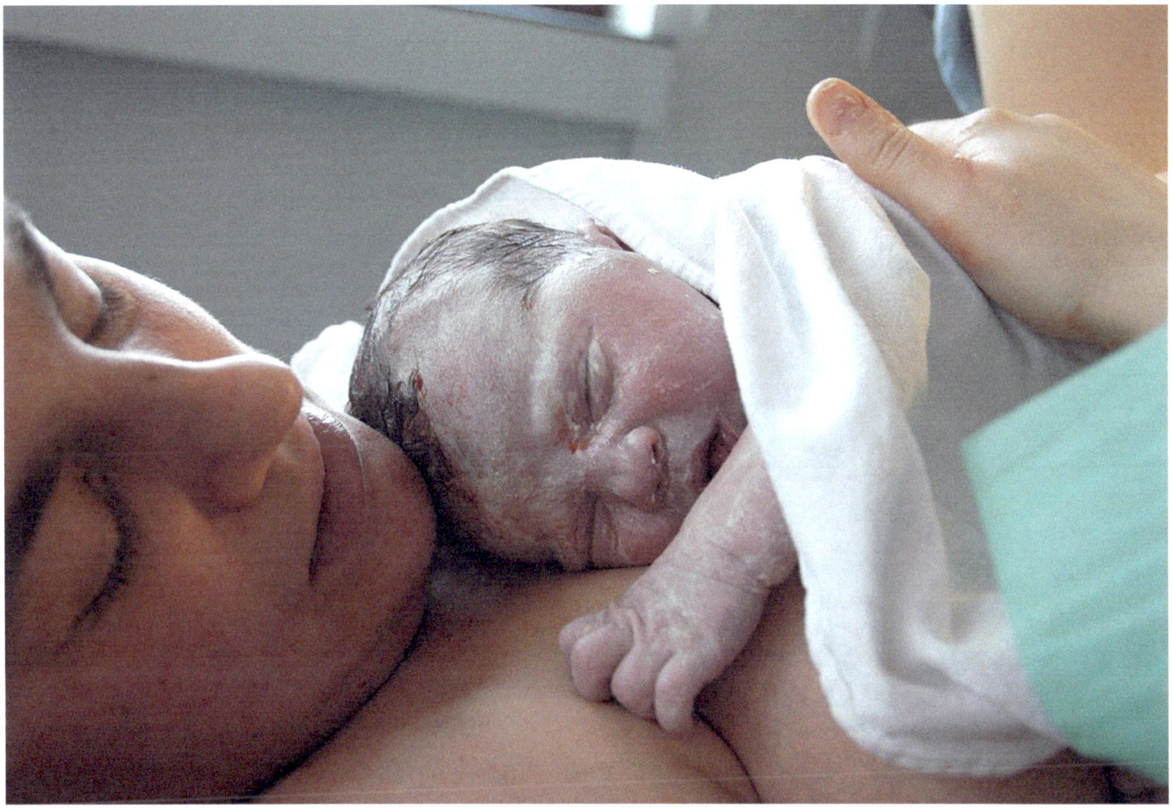

Figure 12.10. Recently delivered mother attending leprosy clinic.

Source: By Tom Adriaenssen - https://www.flickr.com/photos/inferis/110652572/, CC BY-SA 2.0, https://commons.wikimedia.org/w/index.php?curid=639667

A CLOSER LOOK

BIOLOGICAL IMMUNOSUPPRESSION IN WOMEN

All women of reproductive age are immunosuppressed for six months every year and for 10 months during pregnancy and lactation, the immunosuppression "coming off" abruptly, literally overnight, about 40 days after the birth of the baby. Women with leprosy therefore need to be understood and treated differently from men.

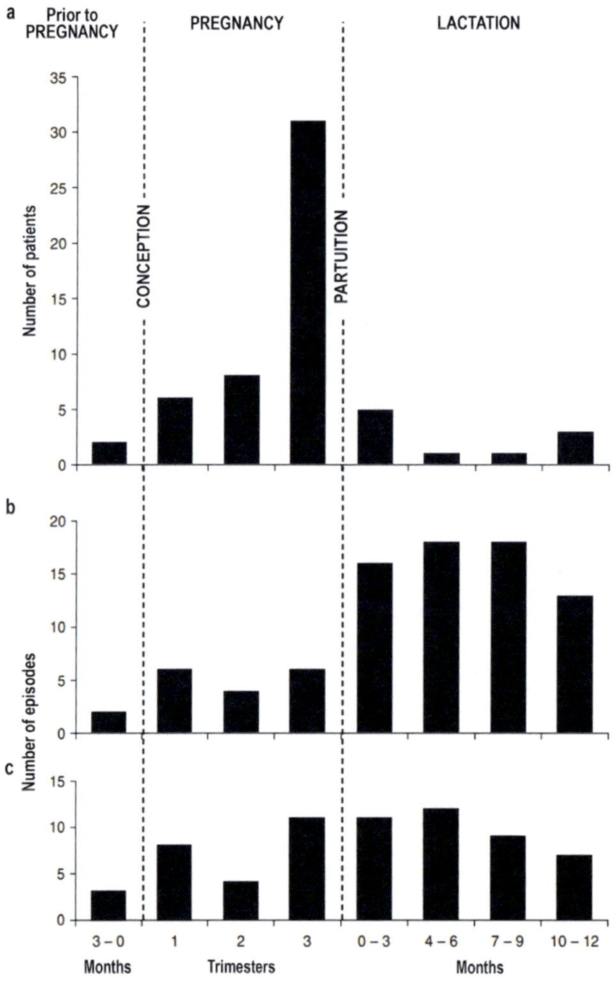

Figure 12.11. (a) Relapse, reactivation, and appearance of new cases of leprosy; (b) reversal reaction; and (c) erythema nodosum leprosum (ENL) are for first episode only.

Source: Springer Nature. (n.d.). Leprosy Relapse and Reaction Types.

Women have cyclic immunosuppression during the menstrual cycle. Immunosuppression starts with ovulation and comes off at the onset of menstruation. Eight women of reproductive age associated with the Armauer Hansen Research Institute in Addis Ababa had lymphocyte transformation tests with phytohemagglutinin thrice weekly for two months. All showed a biphasic pattern with immunosuppression starting abruptly with ovulation and continuing through the second half of the menstrual cycle, coming off at the onset of menstruation with one exception; she had continuing immunosuppression and pregnancy confirmed one month later [Reitan and Duncan, unpublished data].

Immunosuppression during pregnancy is physiological, so that the fertilized ovum, later to become the fetus, is not rejected because its genetic makeup (50% from each parent) is incompatible with the mother. Without our own mothers being immunosuppressed, not one of us would be here today.

Many of the damaging complications of leprosy are caused by an unstable host– parasite relationship related to changes in the host's immune response potential Immunosuppression results in new cases of leprosy becoming overt and apparently cured women showing relapse and reactivation. Others may have the emergence of drug-resistant leprosy as drug-resistant *Mycobacterium leprae* multiply freely during the 10 months of immunosuppression during pregnancy and the puerperium. Type 2 leprosy reaction (T-2-R) or erythema nodosum leprosum (ENL), frequently with nerve function impairment (NFI), occurs during pregnancy, initially in the first trimester when it may be the first indicator of pregnancy, and especially during the third trimester, and continues postpartum. With the recovery of cell-mediated immunity six weeks postpartum, type 1 leprosy reaction (T-1-R) or reversal reaction in skin and nerve with NFI is a major problem, with persistent NFI for up to two years postpartum (Figure 12.11). In severe cases, this can result in crippling paralysis and extensive foot and hand ulceration.

The recommendations made in this chapter are based on observations made on women of reproductive age followed for almost 30 years and amounting to 3000 "reproductive life years." The "A9" study was a collaborative study with the Medical Research Council (MRC) Leprosy Project, the Armauer Hansen Research Institute, and the Addis Ababa Leprosy Hospital (ALERT). For review of leprosy in women.

For the majority of people with leprosy, it is a disease of poverty. With no state security, pension, or sickness benefit, mothers with leprosy need enough living healthy children to care for them in sickness and old age as carers and breadwinners. These women run the risk of further pregnancies, although they know and have stated that the maximum number of pregnancies that they should risk is two. For women with leprosy who have to undergo several pregnancies to achieve the desired family size, repeated immunosuppression can result in a progressive shift across the Ridley–Jopling scale from borderline tuberculoid (BT) to borderline (BB), to borderline lepromatous (BL), and even to subpolar lepromatous (LLs) in successive pregnancies.

With urbanization and the rising cost of food, traditional nourishing diets of pulses and vegetables are unaffordable, and a cheaper Western diet of pasta now supplies calories without nutritional factors essential for cell-mediated immunity. Immunosuppression is further aggravated by ethnic unrest and war, food and drought, crop failure and famine, and poverty, all causing massive displacement of people. HIV/AIDS and tuberculosis also compound the problem. Intestinal parasitosis such as amebiasis and giardiasis, especially the latter, is per se immunosuppressive.

SUMMARY

Managing leprosy in pregnancy is a complex challenge , one that brings together clinical puzzles and social hurdles, all of which push us to think broadly about both medical and public health approaches. Pregnancy itself shifts the immune system in ways that can sometimes worsen leprosy symptoms or even change the course of the disease, so generally speaking, women need careful check-ups and treatment plans made just for them. It's a complex balance, trying to look after the mother's health while also guarding against problems in the newborn, which calls for a combination of different specialists and a strong focus on patient care. And, of course, the stigma around leprosy often slows down diagnosis and makes it hard to stick with treatments – a complication that adds yet another layer of difficulty. All of this suggests that weaving prenatal care into wider leprosy programs is key, ensuring that affected women get both the medical help and emotional support they need. Taking these factors together, even with some overlaps, can lower the risk of bad outcomes and boost the overall well-being of both mom and baby, underscoring why broad healthcare policies are so important for vulnerable communities. Looking into current treatments shows that while multidrug therapy has truly revolutionized how we treat leprosy, its use in pregnant women should be approached with extra caution. In most cases, some antileprosy drugs carry teratogenic risks – a reminder that each treatment plan must be picked and managed with the fetus in mind, without leaving the mother unprotected. Adverse reactions to drugs and the natural immune shifts during pregnancy can stir up complications, meaning that close clinical oversight is absolutely needed. To add to that, there's not enough data on the long-term effects of these medications when used during pregnancy, which, frankly, calls for more research and stronger pharmacovigilance. It all comes down to ensuring that healthcare providers stay updated with the safest treatment protocols; this kind of evidence-based mindset not only refines clinical decisions but also helps shape guidelines that meet pregnant women's unique needs. When all's said and done, the mix of leprosy and pregnancy highlights a public health issue that's as complex as it is pressing. Reactive neurological complications in other infections have been well documented (Tolera, 2023), yet the pregnancy-specific problems related to leprosy and how best to manage them are still not fully mapped out. Sometimes, drawing on lessons from similar infectious diseases can offer some useful insights into managing these challenges. And it doesn't end there – looking at social factors like stigma and limited access to healthcare uncovers deep-rooted obstacles that persist even after major biomedical breakthroughs. Future research should, in most cases, prioritize long-term studies to better understand outcomes for both mother and child, work to optimize treatment safety and support the creation of outreach programs that are culturally sensitive. Ultimately, a combined effort in clinical practice, policy updates, and community involvement is necessary to lift healthcare outcomes for pregnant women facing leprosy, thereby pushing us a step closer to real equity and health justice (Oligbu et al., 2018; Tolera, 2023).

Leprosy mixed with pregnancy isn't a simple matter—it comes with its own set of challenges that studies, both clinical and epidemiological, have pointed out over time. Pregnant women dealing with leprosy often face extra risks like miscarriages, early births, or babies with low birth weight. In many cases, the immune shifts that happen during pregnancy can not only worsen leprosy symptoms but also induce reactional episodes. Additionally, the hormonal and physical changes of pregnancy might even alter the bacteria load, which sometimes ends up interfering with treatment. All this stresses why early diagnosis and a careful, sometimes bespoke, approach to treatment (using multidrug therapy where needed) become so important in keeping both the mother and her baby safe. There's also a significant social and mental side to all this. The stigma connected to leprosy frequently forces affected women into isolation, which in turn messes with their mental health and often discourages them from seeking care promptly. This isolation tends to make it harder for them to stick with their treatment plans and get timely access to health services. In most cases, community-based initiatives that involve health education and counseling have proven essential in reducing the stigma and boosting treatment adherence. Moreover, frontline health workers play a crucial role, often acting as the bridge between these women and the broader healthcare system – a fact that's been underscored in wider public health strategies (Bajpai et al., 2011). Such social factors knit together with medical needs to form a more complete picture of care during pregnancy when leprosy is involved. When you put all these findings together, it becomes clear that handling leprosy in pregnancy calls for a combination of strategies. Medical care alone isn't enough; it needs to be accompanied by strong social support and targeted public health policies to lessen the disease's burden on vulnerable groups. Generally speaking, training and empowering healthcare providers, especially at the community level, is key—they must grasp how leprosy can affect pregnancy so they can guide treatments properly. Evidence from resource-limited settings shows that localized health programs have managed to yield real improvements in both maternal and child outcomes (Morgan et al., 1980). To summarize, combining these approaches is vital for reducing risks for mothers and improving newborn health, thereby supporting broader goals of effective disease control and health issues.

KEY TERMS FROM THIS CHAPTER

- Buruli ulcer
- Depression
- Gender inequality
- Maternal health
- Obstetric fistula
- Prolonged blocked labor
- Sensory loss
- Stress
- Coughs
- Fetal distress
- High blood sugar
- Obesity
- Pregnancy
- Schwann cells
- Sneezes
- Substance abuse

References

1. Phillips, R. O., Robert, J., Abass, K. M., Thompson, W., Sarfo, F. S., Wilson, T., Sarpong, G., Gateau, T., Chauty, A., Omollo, R., Ochieng Otieno, M., Egondi, T. W., Ampadu, E. O., Agossadou, D., Marion, E., Ganlonon, L., Wansbrough-Jones, M., Grosset, J., Macdonald, J. M., Treadwell, T., ... study team (2020). Rifampicin and clarithromycin (extended release) versus rifampicin and streptomycin for limited Buruli ulcer lesions: a randomised, open-label, non-inferiority phase 3 trial. *Lancet (London, England)*, *395*(10232), 1259–1267. https://doi.org/10.1016/S0140-6736(20)30047-7(accessed on 10th May 2025).

2. Abdel-Rahman, S. M., Albano, J. D., Botgros, R., Brown, D., et al. (2015). Toward earlier inclusion of pregnant and postpartum women in tuberculosis drug trials: Consensus statements from an international expert panel. *Clin. Infect. Dis.*, *62*(6), 761–769. https://core.ac.uk/download/304662919.pdf (accessed on 10th May 2025).

3. Abubakar, I., Dalglish, S. L., Angell, B., Sanuade, O. A., Abímbọ́lá, Ṣ., Adamu, A. L., Adetifa, I., et al. (2022). The Lancet Nigeria Commission: Investing in health and the future of the nation. *The Lancet, 399*, 1155–1200. https://doi.org/10.1016/s0140-6736(21)02488-0 (accessed on 10th May 2025).

4. Kapata, N., Chanda-Kapata, P., O'Grady, J., Schwank, S., Bates, M., Mukonka, V., Zumla, A. and Mwaba, P. (2011), Trends of Zambia's tuberculosis burden over the past two decades. Tropical Medicine & International Health, 16: 1404-1409. https://doi.org/10.1111/j.1365-3156.2011.02849.x (accessed on 10th May 2025).

5. Aksoy S (2015) Strong Local Scientific Communities Are Essential to Reach the Millennium Development Goals. PLoS Negl Trop Dis 9(10): e0004136. https://doi.org/10.1371/journal.pntd.0004136(accessed on 10th May 2025).

6. Gaither, K., & Apuzzio, J. J. (1996). Tuberculosis in pregnancy. *Infectious diseases in obstetrics and gynecology*, *4*(2), 92–96. https://doi.org/10.1155/S1064744996000208 (accessed on 10th May 2025).

7. Arlen, R. R., Hamanishi, C., Jonsson, N. A., Lenz, W., Livingstone, G., McBride, W., et al. (2015). *Thalidomide-Induced Teratogenesis: History and Mechanisms.* https://core.ac.uk/download/30435704.pdf (accessed on 10th May 2025).

8. Asian Development Bank. (2014). *Addressing Diseases of Poverty: An Initiative to Reduce the Unacceptable Burden of Neglected Tropical Diseases in the Asia Pacific Region.* https://core.ac.uk/download/20125985.pdf (accessed on 10th May 2025).

9. Babu, G. R., Murthy, G., Deepa, R., Yamuna, Prafulla, Kumar, H. K., Karthik, M., Deshpande, K., Benjamin Neelon, S. E., Prabhakaran, D., Kurpad, A., & Kinra, S. (2016). Maternal antecedents of adiposity and studying the transgenerational role of hyperglycemia and insulin (MAASTHI): a prospective cohort study : Protocol of birth cohort at Bangalore, India. *BMC pregnancy and childbirth*, *16*(1), 311. https://doi.org/10.1186/s12884-016-1088-4 (accessed on 10th May 2025).

10. Bajpai, N., & Dholakia, R. H. (2011). *Improving the Performance of Accredited Social Health Activists in INDIA.* https://core.ac.uk/download/161441854.pdf (accessed on 10th May 2025).

11. Bolam, A., Shariff, A., Raja, A. E., Sharma, B., Simkhada, B., Nwakoby, B. N., Vlassoff, C., et

al. (2007). *Utilization of Postnatal Care Among Rural Women in Nepal.* https://core.ac.uk/download/75502.pdf (accessed on 10th May 2025).

12. WÓJCIK, Magdalena, BOREŃSKI, Grzegorz, SZABAT, Przemysław, POLESZAK, Julita, SZABAT, Marta and MILANOWSKA, Joanna. Depression during pregnancy. *Journal of Education, Health and Sport.* Online. 5 April 2019. Vol. 9, no. 3, pp. 465-473. (accessed on 10th May 2025).
13. Caspe, S. G., Ewing, D. A., Livingstone, M., Underwood, C., Milne, E., Sargison, N. D., Wattegedera, S. R., & Longbottom, D. (2023). The Immune Response in the Uteri and Placentae of *Chlamydia abortus*-Infected Ewes and Its Association with Pregnancy Outcomes. *Pathogens (Basel, Switzerland), 12*(6), 846. https://doi.org/10.3390/pathogens12060846(accessed on 10th May 2025).
14. Castilla, E. E., Dutra, M. G., Leite, J. C. L., López, C. J. S., et al. (2019). *Epidemiological Surveillance of Birth Defects Compatible with Thalidomide Embryopathy in Brazil.* https://core.ac.uk/download/pdf/296423486.pdf (accessed on 10th May 2025).
15. Dhakal, S., van Teijlingen, E., Raja, E. A., & Dhakal, K. B. (2011). Skilled care at birth among rural women in Nepal: practice and challenges. *Journal of health, population, and nutrition*, *29*(4), 371–378. https://doi.org/10.3329/jhpn.v29i4.8453(accessed on 10th May 2025).
16. Ediati, A., Hadisaputro, S., Pramono, N., Wahyuni, S., et al. (2024). *Factors Associated with Pregnancy-Related Anxiety: A Health Facility-Based Study*. https://core.ac.uk/download/618287433.pdf (accessed on 10th May 2025).
17. Fiqnasyani, S. E., Mudigdo, A., Novriana, D. E., Oktavriana, R., et al. (2023). *Lucio Phenomenon in Pregnancy: A Histopathology Review.* https://core.ac.uk/download/639385429.pdf (accessed on 10th May 2025).
18. González-Mesa, E., García-Fuentes, E., Carvia-Pontiasec, R., Lavado-Fernández, A. I., Cuenca-Marín, C., Suárez-Arana, M., Blasco-Alonso, M., Benítez-Lara, B., Mozas-Benítez, L., González-Cazorla, A., Egeberg-Neverdal, H., & Jiménez-López, J. S. (2022). Transmitted Fetal Immune Response in Cases of SARS-CoV-2 Infections during Pregnancy. *Diagnostics (Basel, Switzerland), 12*(2), 245. https://doi.org/10.3390/diagnostics12020245(accessed on 10th May 2025).
19. Hambridge, T. (2024). *Shortening leprosy case detection delay: Narrowing the window of transmission and disease progression*. [Doctoral Thesis, Erasmus University Rotterdam]. (accessed on 10th May 2025).
20. Heller, A. (2015). *Interrogating the Superlative Sufferer: Experiencing Obstetric Fistula and Treatment Seeking in Niger*. https://core.ac.uk/download/233212176.pdf (accessed on 10th May 2025).
21. IJCP Group. (2023). *News and Views.* https://core.ac.uk/download/572373426.pdf (accessed on 10th May 2025).
22. Jamieson, D. J., Theiler, R. N., & Rasmussen, S. A. (2006). Emerging infections and pregnancy. *Emerging infectious diseases, 12*(11), 1638–1643. https://doi.org/10.3201/eid1211.060152 (accessed on 10th May 2025).
23. Jeminiwa, R., Park, S., Popielaski, C., Gannon, M., Myers, R., & Abatemarco, D. J. (2024). Development of an educational brochure about treatment options for pregnant women with opioid use disorders. *Pharmacy, 12*. https://www.semanticscholar.org/paper/8dd613dd57d8943c66a60db5a4cc04768d844954 (accessed on 10th May 2025).

24. van Haaren MA, Reyme M, Lawrence M, Menke J, Kaptein AA. Illness perceptions of leprosy-cured individuals in Surinam with residual disfigurements – "I am cured, but still I am ill". *Chronic Illness*. 2016;13(2):117-127. doi:10.1177/1742395316657398
25. (accessed on 10th May 2025).
26. Kelbessa, T., & ALERT/AHRY Staff, A. S. (2017). Bibliography on Leprosy in Ethiopia: Preliminary compilation. *The Ethiopian Journal of Health Development*, *1*(2). Retrieved from https://ejhd.org/index.php/ejhd/article/view/1380 (accessed on 10th May 2025).
27. Leal, L. F., & Mota, D. M. (2021). Thalidomide surveillance and pharmacovigilance in Brazil – an overview. (2021). *Vigilância Sanitária Em Debate* , *9*(2), 14-20. https://doi.org/10.22239/2317-269x.01557(accessed on 10th May 2025).
28. Lorenz, N., & Mpemba, C. (2005). *Review of the State of Health in Tanzania 2004*. https://core.ac.uk/download/pdf/11307056.pdf (accessed on 10th May 2025).
29. Luong, T. V., Le, L. D., Nguyen, N. V. D., & Dang, H. N. N. (2025). Persistent challenges in the diagnosis of acute pancreatitis due to primary hyperparathyroidism during pregnancy. *World journal of gastroenterology*, *31*(7), 100973. https://doi.org/10.3748/wjg.v31.i7.100973(accessed on 10th May 2025).
30. Morgan, R. W. (1980). *Basic Health Needs in Africa*. https://open.bu.edu/bitstream/2144/40428/1/WP_29_Morgan_1980.pdf (accessed on 10th May 2025).
31. Oligbu, G., Fallaha, M., Pay, L., Ahmed, L., Children, I. N., Oligbu, O., & Saroey, P. (2018). G329(P) Risk of seizure following Zika virus infection in children. *Archives of Disease in Childhood, 103*, A133–A133. https://www.semanticscholar.org/paper/d2d0bf87842c3109ef44ab39278e4683c5b51efa (accessed on 10th May 2025).
32. Oliver, S. J. (2022). From Isolation to Inclusion: Embracing Local Perspectives in Examining the Treatment Model of Care for Aboriginal Persons Affected by Tuberculosis or Leprosy in the Kimberley Region, North Western Australia [Doctor of Philosophy (College of Medicine)]. The University of Notre Dame Australia. https://researchonline.nd.edu.au/theses/386(accessed on 10th May 2025).
33. Richens J. (2004). Genital manifestations of tropical diseases. *Sexually transmitted infections*, *80*(1), 12–17. https://doi.org/10.1136/sti.2003.004093 (accessed on 10th May 2025).
34. Ridlo, I.A. (2023), "Frequency and specificity of health issues in local political campaigns", International Journal of Health Governance, Vol. 28 No. 4, pp. 368-382. https://doi.org/10.1108/IJHG-03-2023-0034 (accessed on 10th May 2025).
35. Rivoire, B. L. (2012). *Development and Evaluation of New Leprosy Skin Test Antigens as Diagnostic Tools*. https://core.ac.uk/download/354378292.pdf (accessed on 10th May 2025).
36. Rosu, L. M., Prodan-Bărbulescu, C., Maghiari, A. L., Bernad, E. S., Bernad, R. L., Iacob, R., Stoicescu, E. R., Borozan, F., & Ghenciu, L. A. (2024). Current Trends in Diagnosis and Treatment Approach of Diabetic Retinopathy during Pregnancy: A Narrative Review. *Diagnostics (Basel, Switzerland)*, *14*(4), 369. https://doi.org/10.3390/diagnostics14040369(accessed on 10th May 2025).
37. Harpur, A., Goodfellow, A., Garbe, F., & Wilson, S. (2023). Complex social factors in pregnancy - a Scottish health needs assessment. *The European Journal of Public Health*, *33*(Suppl 2),

ckad160.140. https://doi.org/10.1093/eurpub/ckad160.140(accessed on 10th May 2025).

38. Thangaswamy, G. C., Arulappan, J., Anumanthan, S., & Jayapal, S. K. (2021). Trends and determinants of mental health during COVID-19 pandemic. *International Journal of Nutrition Pharmacology Neurological Diseases, 11*, 1–6. https://doi.org/10.4103/ijnpnd.ijnpnd_86_20 (accessed on 10th May 2025).

39. Tolera, M. (2023). The "smart city" between urban narrative and empty signifier: Shaggar in focus. *World Journal of Education and Humanities*. Scho Link Vol 5 (4) DOI: https://doi.org/10.22158/wjeh.v5n4p1(accessed on 10th May 2025).

40. Vetrov V.V., Ivanov D.O., Reznik V.A., Romanova L.A., Kurdynko L.V., Nikolaev A.V., Sadykova G.K., Menshikova S.V., Ovsyannikov P.A., Vyugov M.A., Avrutskaya V.V., Vladimirova N.Y., Chermnykh S.V., Zheleznaya A.A., Koroteev A.L., Barinov V.A. Gestation outcomes in various options of help for pregnant women with Rh-immunization // Pediatrician (St. Petersburg). - 2023. - Vol. 14. - N. 2. - P. 5-16. doi: 10.17816/PED1425-16(accessed on 10th May 2025).

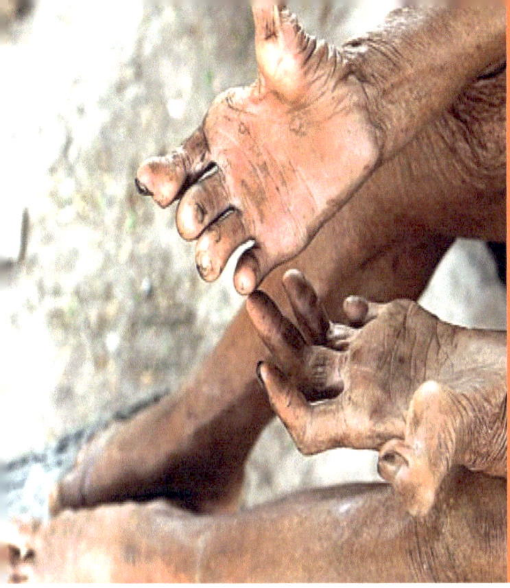

Chapter 13

LEPROSY-RELATED DISABILITIES AND REHABILITATION

Contents

Introduction

Leprosy still showing up as a public health issue makes it clear that handling all its aftermath, especially the disabilities people end up with, is no simple task. Modern antimicrobial treatments have cut down on the spread quite a bit, yet many still wrestle with long-lasting physical setbacks. Nerve damage, for example, can lead to lost feeling, weakened muscles, and even noticeable deformities, all of which take a toll on everyday life. Generally speaking, getting a grip on the many faces of these impairments is crucial if we're to build rehab plans that work; these plans must go well beyond just medical fixes to also cover physical, psychological, and social support, partly to combat the stigma and isolation so often encountered. When it comes to helping individuals with leprosy-related disabilities, a broad and flexible game plan is needed, one that emphasizes getting back function and easing the journey back into society. The complex nature of these challenges calls for treatments tailored to each person's needs, from physical exercises and focused work therapy to providing helpful assistive tools. In many cases, these efforts aren't solely about boosting physical strength but about fostering independence and opening up job prospects too. One can't ignore that the wider living environment, with its prevailing attitudes and real-life access issues, also plays a big role in creating a more inclusive setting. Looking at similar conditions, say spinal cord injuries, generally points to the need for standardized education and evidence-based moves to get better outcomes while keeping side effects in check (Zupo et al., 2024). Success in rehabilitation also leans heavily on teamwork across different disciplines and a willingness to mix in new technologies with tried-and-true methods. Just like occupational therapists and driver rehab experts have jumped on board with fresh assistive and even automated vehicle tech to support people with disabilities, comparable modern alters could help those dealing with leprosy's fallout as well (Classen et al., 2024). This sort of collaborative approach keeps the focus on the individual, stimulating them toward greater independence while narrowing gaps in disability care. Further, steady research and smart policymaking remain essential to guide best practices and distribute resources efficiently. In short, giving serious thought to the hurdles posed by leprosy-related disabilities and the rehab needed lays the groundwork for broader strategies aimed at cutting down disability, boosting overall quality of life, and promoting real social inclusion (Figure 13.1).

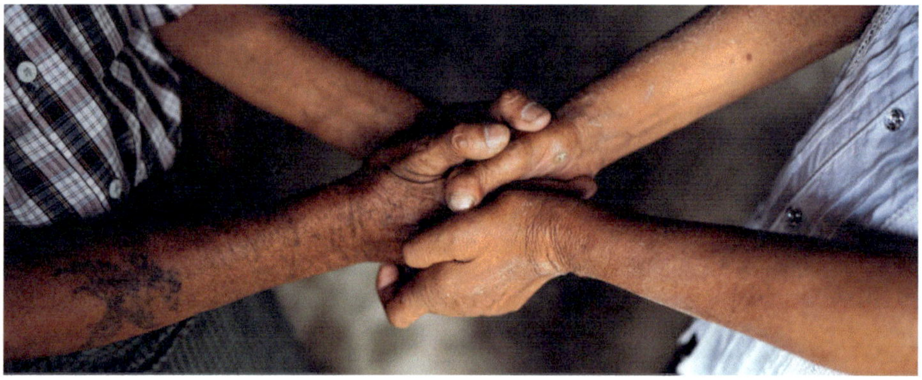

Figure 13.1. Leprosy-related disabilities.

Source: The Leprosy Mission Myanmar. (2023). *Leprosy-Related Disabilities.*

13.1. Physical Disabilities Associated with Leprosy

Leprosy hits people in a surprisingly stealthy way—it starts off by attacking the skin and nerves, and if it's not detected early, the damage to nerves can take a toll. Nerves begin to fail, leading to a loss of feeling, muscle weakness, and even paralysis in places like the hands, feet, and face. This lack of sensation makes everyday bumps, burns, and other injuries way more likely, which only piles on more problems over time. Often the situation gets worse because the disease isn't diagnosed fast enough or managed properly from the start. Treatment isn't just about fixing the physical problems; it also has to help improve overall quality of life. In most cases, research shows that once patients leave the hospital, a mixed approach with good post-discharge care helps keep further decline at bay and eases social reintegration (Pinheiro et al., 2019). Beyond the initial nerve issues, individuals can end up with deformities such as a claw-like hand, foot drop or noticeable changes in the face. These aren't just cosmetic problems—they make moving around more difficult and can bring about social stigma that leaves people feeling isolated. A combination of care is needed: physical therapy, occasional reconstructive surgery, and supports like braces can all play a role in trying to restore some function. Education is key here too; when the public understands the importance of early detection, it helps cut down on the irreversible damage. And then there are laws and policies that, by creating job opportunities and other supports, help improve outcomes, as has been seen in different areas around the world (InFocus Program on Skills, 2003). It turns out that combining smart clinical care with a supportive social network can make a big difference. When it comes to getting someone back on track after leprosy-related disabilities, the journey doesn't stop at treatment—it continues with ongoing support. Rehabilitation has to cover everything from prevention to consistent treatment and social care, ensuring that affected individuals feel included and valued. Generally speaking, combining policies that welcome people with disabilities and focused rehabilitation services helps boost functional recovery and community participation. Research suggests that understanding local healthcare systems, policy environments, and even cultural factors is crucial for effective care after discharge (Pinheiro et al., 2019). Further, providing easy access to jobs and fair, inclusive legislation can counter the economic setbacks that disabled individuals often face (InFocus Program on Skills, 2003). All these efforts, taken together, work to uplift both the quality of life and the dignity of those living with leprosy-related challenges (Figure 13.2).

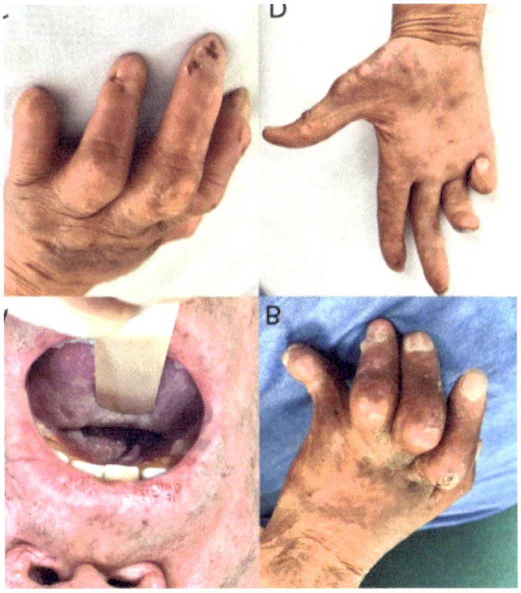

Figure 13.2. Patients with lepromatous leprosy and grade 2 disability. First patient: absence of the uvula and nasal infiltration (a); finger and nail dystrophy secondary to bone resorption (b). Second patient: claw hand, bone resorption, and traumatic erosions (c). Third patient: benediction sign (d).

Source: ResearchGate. (n.d.). *Patients with Lepromatous Leprosy and Grade 2 Disability.*

13.1.1. Common Physical Impairments Caused by Leprosy

Leprosy can lead to many physical setbacks, often hitting the skin, peripheral nerves, and even the mucous layers. In most cases, untreated infections tend to cause serious disabilities. One key sign is that nerves get damaged—this damage usually shows up as numbness, weakened muscles, or even paralysis, which in turn ups the risk of injuries and secondary infections. Early on, a person might notice numbness or a drop in muscle power, mainly in the hands, feet, or face, caused by nerve inflammation. When these nerves falter, the natural ability to sense pain or temperature may vanish, so minor wounds can worsen without anyone noticing. All this gradually speeds up the onset of deformities and functional impairments, a fact that is central when planning interventions meant to restore ability and ward off further harm. The range of impairments due to leprosy is broad—many people end up with visible deformities that disrupt everyday life and social contacts. Some only experience subtle losses in feeling, while others develop more severe changes like claw hand, foot drop, or even facial palsy.

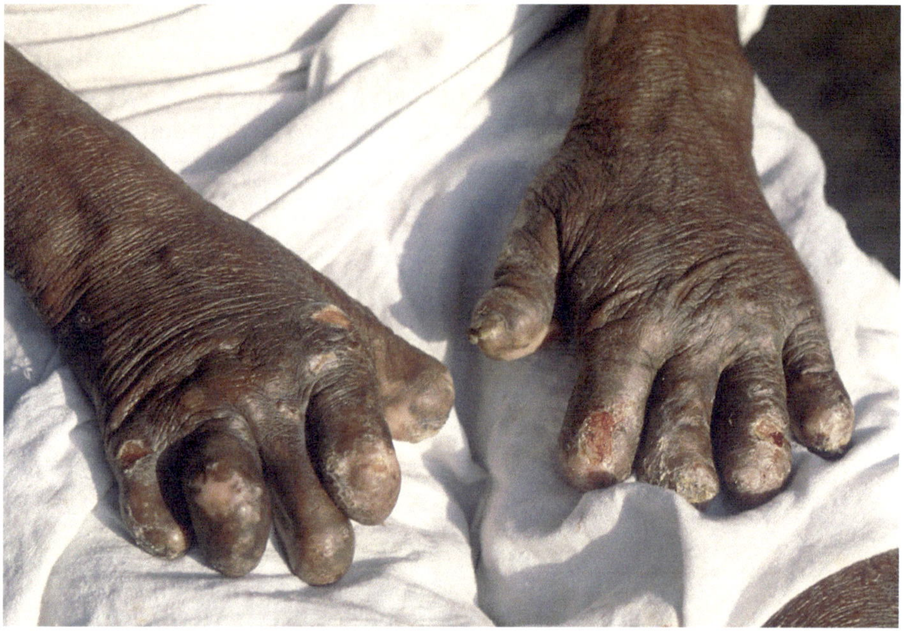

Figure 13.3. Typical deformity in a patient with leprosy.

Source: By B.jehle - Own work, CC BY-SA 3.0, https://commons.wikimedia.org/w/index.php?curid=27098744

These changes not only restrict movement and fine motor skills but often lead to stigma and social exclusion, which only makes recovery tougher. In many endemic areas, statistical reports show a high occurrence of grade I and grade II disabilities, and generally speaking, the multibacillary forms of the disease tend to cause more intense nerve damage (Sy Savané et al., 2024). Often, individuals end up seeking help late—when the nerve damage is already advanced—highlighting the importance of early detection and regular medical, as well as rehabilitative, care to keep long-term impairments at bay. When it comes to rehabilitation, a combination of approaches is needed to handle both the physical challenges and the social fallout. Vocational rehabilitation, for example, plays a critical role in helping people adapt and find their way back to work, even when faced with significant physical issues. Research generally indicates that custom-fit rehab methods—using assistive devices and targeted exercises—can boost function, although there remain noticeable gaps in both access and quality of care among different groups (Ahonle et al., 2025). It seems essential to pay attention not only to the severity of the physical impairments but also to the surrounding social factors, including gender and education, which can heavily impact recovery and job prospects. In most cases, merging well-rounded rehabilitation strategies with solid medical treatment is key to lessening the disability burden and empowering those affected by leprosy to live a fuller, better life (Figure 13.3).

13.1.2. Impact on Mobility and Daily Activities

Leprosy can hit hard physically, it often damages nerves so that people lose feeling and their muscles just aren't as strong, which damages everyday movement and simple tasks. Over time, these issues can snowball into deformed limbs, painful ulcers, and other infections that further limit what someone can do. Treatment doesn't always mark the end of the problems; in many cases, things keep getting worse after medical care, suggesting that these disabilities tend to be long-lasting. A person might find that even basic actions like moving around, picking up objects, or handling daily activities such as dressing, cooking, or personal hygiene become a struggle. This gradual loss of independence not only degrades one's quality of life but also means leaning more on caregivers or special tools, showing that continuous support is often needed even after a cure. Besides these physical setbacks, there's also a whole layer of social and psychological hurdles. Stigma and discrimination, real issues that most affected individuals face, can lead to social withdrawal, lower self-esteem, and less involvement in community life. This isolation, in turn, often fuels a vicious cycle where reduced activity leads to further muscle loss and falling mobility. The result? Not only is it harder to get a job or education, but one's mental health also takes a hit, which matters a lot for staying motivated in rehabilitation. In most cases, the best approach to address mobility issues is a combination of physical therapy, initiatives that ease stigma, and programs that boost social inclusion (InFocus Program on Skills, 2003). Good rehabilitation, then, needs to cover both the medical side and the social or legal support systems to truly help people regain function and rejoin society. National policies and disability laws are key here; they open doors to vocational training, adaptations at work, and a range of social services tailored to those dealing with leprosy's aftereffects. Initiatives that push for better employment opportunities and guard against discrimination can empower someone by turning mobility challenges into manageable hurdles that can be overcome with meaningful work. The proper setup and follow-up of these programs are crucial for boosting recovery and long-term independence. Essentially, rehabilitation isn't just about one thing—it calls for a combination of clinical care, social rehabilitation, and legal backing to lessen the heavy toll leprosy takes on everyday movement and living (InFocus Program on Skills, 2003).

13.1.3. Long-Term Consequences of Untreated Leprosy

Neglecting early treatment can quickly morph what might be a manageable infection into a lifelong ordeal. With leprosy, for instance, leaving the infection untreated paves the way for nerve damage that's creeping in as a gradual loss of feeling and muscle power. This weakening sensation often makes individuals vulnerable to repeated injuries that can end up distorting limbs into forms like clawed hands or even causing a foot to drop. Over time, this chain reaction not only hampers motor skills but also ruins daily activities and slashes social participation. The lack of proper sensory feedback tends to open the door for unnoticed injuries, infections, and even ulcers – all of which throw extra curveballs into the rehabilitation process. In many cases, such a prolonged condition ends up burdening not just the individual, but also their family and community, underscoring why a timely diagnosis matters. Living with the persisting aftermath of untreated leprosy isn't just about the physical struggle. People often end up wrestling with heavy social and emotional challenges too. Disabilities that spring from leprosy can saddle someone with stigma and social isolation, making it tougher to bounce back and feel part of society again. These social juggernauts tend to cut off access to the kind of support that's critical for recovery. There's also a tangible emotional toll – a drop in self-esteem and a heightened risk for mental health issues further complicate the issue of rehabilitation. Generally speaking, research, including studies on trauma and chronic illness recovery (Borysova et al., 2024; Wróbel et al., 2024), shows that combining approaches to care for both the body and the mind is key to improving function and overall quality of life. Rehabilitation for those hit by the lasting effects of leprosy isn't a one-step fix—it demands a combination of ongoing strategies. It's not just about patching up physical impairments; the emotional and behavioral hurdles deserve attention too. Techniques like customized physical therapy, focused sensory retraining, and even some surgical fixes can help curb the decline. Behavior change approaches and solid social support also play standout roles in getting people to stick with their rehab routines, as noted in studies around stroke recovery (Wróbel et al., 2024). When family and community step up, they serve as a vital buffer against the isolating effects of disability, creating spaces where recovery and social reintegration can take hold. Ultimately, combining medical care with psychological support and a push for social inclusion is what tackles the complex, enduring challenges that arise from unattended leprosy (Figure 13.4).

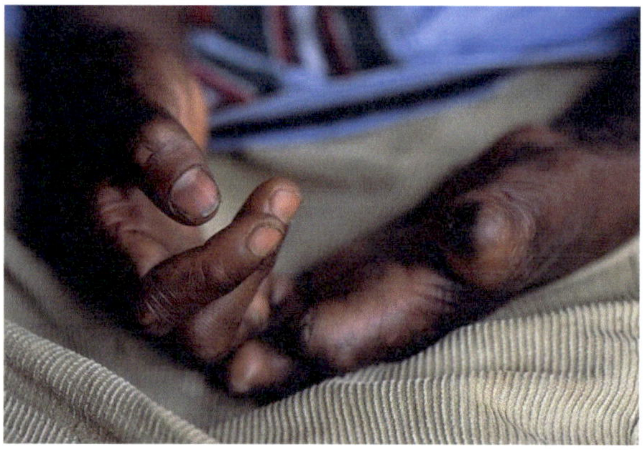

Figure 13.4. If leprosy is not treated, it can cause deformity, especially in the hands, feet, and face.

Source: Healthdirect Australia. (n.d.). *If Leprosy is not Treated, it Can Cause Deformity, Especially in the Hands, Feet and Face.*

13.2. Psychological Impact of Leprosy

Living with leprosy isn't simply about the physical symptoms; its effects seep into one's inner world in unexpected ways. Many people, after going through their medical rehabilitation, describe a combination of ups and downs. They might feel happier and more confident because their physical look and abilities have improved, yet there remains a persisting sense of sadness, shame, or uncertainty, often connected to the visible changes like loss of limbs. Society doesn't always make things easier either, as judgments, stigma, or even subtle social exclusion can push some individuals to withdraw or choose to live in specialized communities. In most cases, this combination of regained physical strength and ongoing social bias creates a complex impact on mental health (Nasution et al., 2012). Even once the body has healed, the label "leprosy" can stick, casting a long shadow over self-esteem and identity. Often, external prejudice deepens the internal feelings of inferiority and vulnerability, making everyday routines and jobs even harder to resume normally. Sometimes, the ongoing weight of discrimination can disrupt one's ability to settle back into work or adjust life's rhythms, hindering economic independence. Generally speaking, the degree of acceptance in the social environment plays a crucial role in either softening or sharpening these mental health challenges, suggesting that recovery must attend equally to the psychological as it does to the physical (Nasution et al., 2012).

Looking past individual healing, broader, system-wide strategies prove necessary to tackle the psychological fallout of leprosy-related disabilities. Opportunities employment, proper legal protections, and active support for disabled persons can help carve out spaces in which mental and emotional well-being start to recover. For instance, measured initiatives, like disability-inclusive labor policies seen in parts of East Africa and Asia—aim to boost both economic standing and personal dignity, indirectly fostering better mental health. Still, such frameworks need rigorous enforcement and a genuine change in public attitudes to truly lower societal bias. To summarize, rehabilitation programs that combine medical care with social and legal support seem to promise a more rounded path to recovery, even if the journey remains complex.

13.2.1. Stigmatization and Social Isolation

People's lives with leprosy aren't defined only by the medical facts, they're also deeply influenced by how society tends to see them. Many individuals dealing with leprosy face a kind of stigma that isn't limited to physical challenges; often, the emotional and psychological impacts can be just as heavy. Studies from specialized leprosy centers, in most cases, show that patients and their families feel this layered judgment even long after a clinical cure, which seems to stick around. This kind of stigma can dampen self-confidence and make social interactions awkward, and factors such as gender, marital status, and religious background may further skew just how intense that feeling gets (Adedeji et al., 2023). In a way, getting a grasp on these social dynamics is key when one is putting together recovery plans that attend to both the body and the mind. Beyond that sense of being judged, many leprosy patients also end up feeling isolated. The overlap between physical limitations and society's tendency to push people aside frequently ends up causing bouts of depression, anxiety, and sometimes plain old stress—that impact everyday quality of life. Research, generally speaking, indicates that a good number of individuals experience moderate to severe psychological distress, which often goes hand in hand with reduced social participation and even withdrawal from community activities. In many instances, this mental strain not only hurts personal well-being but also stops individuals from engaging fully with rehabilitation programs, further compounding their challenges (Barakat & Zaki, 2019). As a result, weaving mental health support into leprosy care is seen as essential even if, at times, its benefits might come across in unpredictable ways. Tackling both the stigma and isolation means that solutions can't rely solely on medical treatment. Instead, a combination of wider, psychosocial strategies is needed. Educational programs that fight ignorance and prejudice are crucial for slowly shifting those negative public attitudes, while tailored counseling and support services can bolster self-esteem and counter the internalized stigma that sometimes makes people retreat socially. The interplay between feeling shamed, enduring psychological stress, and becoming isolated creates a complex cycle to break, one that clearly needs every part addressed at once. In most cases, targeted interventions that factor in cultural backgrounds and demographic nuances better support successful reintegration, ultimately helping restore dignity and empowerment for individuals with leprosy-related disabilities (Barakat & Zaki, 2019; Adedeji et al., 2023). Overall, this broad and sometimes imperfect approach is critical to achieving lasting rehabilitation and a more inclusive society (Figure 13.5).

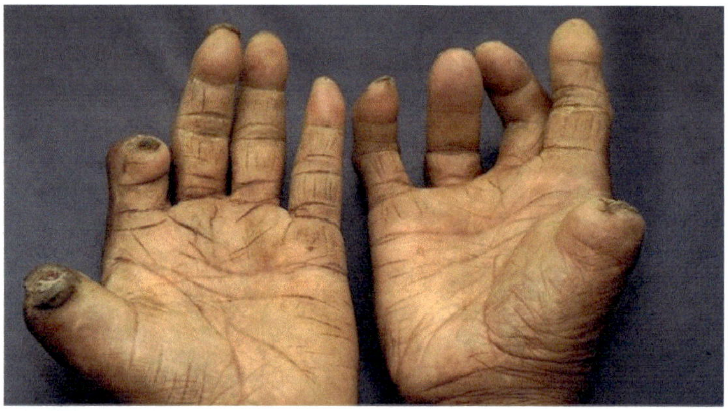

Figure 13.5. Ending social stigma against leprosy patients.

Source: India Tomorrow. (2021). *Ending Social Stigma Against Leprosy Patients.*

13.2.2. Mental Health Issues Related to Leprosy

Leprosy carries a heavy social tag that only makes the mental struggles for those affected even tougher. People living with the condition, often misunderstood and even feared—find themselves battered by isolation and subtle discrimination, which can spiral into feelings of shame, anxiety, and depression. There's this awkward mix when a visible physical challenge meets the harsh glare of society's rejection; it piles on the emotional load and often limits efforts to fully recover. Sometimes community support is just missing, and old stereotypes still hold decide, deepening the sense of exclusion and mental strain. To summarize, these interconnected issues point to the need for care that isn't just about treating the body but also mending the mind, so healthcare providers can roll out interventions that help rebuild social ties and uplift the overall quality of life. Those who care for people with leprosy-related disabilities face their own heavy burden of emotional strain that ripples into their mental well-being. Much like what's seen with caregivers supporting individuals with intellectual disabilities (Wormald et al., 2023), those on the front lines dealing with leprosy often end up wrestling with extra bouts of loneliness, isolation, and even exhaustion, especially when the available health or social resources just aren't enough. In many cases, the stress these caregivers experience directly colors the rehabilitation journey of the patients they support. It seems natural then that giving caregivers a breather through proper emotional support or respite services isn't just a nice extra; it's a crucial piece of a comprehensive strategy to help leprosy-affected families get back on their feet. Schooling and social life for children and adults with leprosy aren't any easier, as exclusion in educational settings and broader society deepens the mental health challenges they face. Think about how other marginalized groups are treated, for example, children with disabilities often end up facing higher rates of suspension (Cleary et al., 2024), and you'll see that people affected by leprosy bump head-on with systemic barriers that shut down many chances for genuine social or educational participation. This kind of exclusion not only elevates psychological distress but can also hold back the growth of essential coping skills and social confidence. Recognizing this link between isolation and mental strain is key if we want policies that build emotional resilience and encourage community ties. Combining mental health care into the mix of educational and rehabilitation frameworks is, generally speaking, essential to soften the harsh effects of leprosy-related challenges.

13.2.3. Coping Mechanisms and Support Systems

Leprosy-related disabilities can be tough to manage. People dealing with these challenges not only struggle with physical issues but also wrestle with the harsh weight of social stigma. It's not uncommon for individuals to feel isolated or lose a sense of self-worth when family dynamics shift because of outdated attitudes. In most cases, individuals try to push through by leaning on personal resilience—connecting with others and rethinking their experiences in ways that ease the psychological burden. Families, when they're supportive and informed about leprosy, often make a palpable difference, helping break down the internalized stigma.

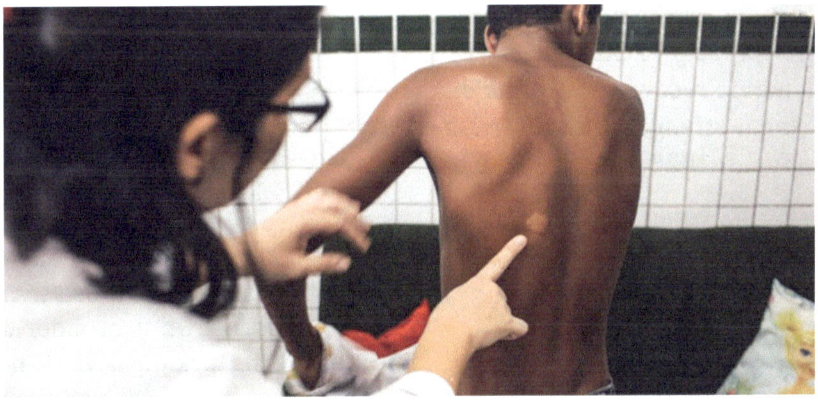

Figure 13.6. Preventing leprosy-related disabilities.

Source: Pan American Health Organization. (n.d.). *Preventing Leprosy-Related Disabilities.*

Yet, if family members adopt stigmatizing views, that support network turns into a barrier, underlining the need for community education and timely intervention (Cornell University, World Health Organization, and World Bank, 2011). Beyond personal and family efforts, formal support systems are equally crucial. Employment and being part of the economy help build up self-esteem and independence, yet many people with disabilities—including those with leprosy-related issues—face systemic roadblocks like discrimination and scarce job opportunities. Generally speaking, international policies like the United Nations Convention on the Rights of Persons with Disabilities push for job markets that are more inclusive and freer from unfair bias. Vocational rehab, which offers job training and counseling, plays a key role in equipping people with the kind of skills that lead to real work opportunities. Further, workplace adjustments and anti-discrimination laws impact structural barriers, not only restoring livelihoods but also gradually shifting societal attitudes in a positive direction (Cornell University, World Health Organization, and World Bank, 2011). Outside the individual and formal spheres, the broader community and health services form a critical piece of the puzzle. Local attitudes and how accessible healthcare is can either widen the gap of stigma or help mend it—sometimes community judgment hurts even more than the physical challenges themselves. When healthcare providers adopt a non-judgmental approach and take the time to educate both patients and their neighbors, they become vital in reducing stigma and easing access to care. This kind of multi-pronged support—touching on individuals, families, and entire communities, often builds resilience and slowly erodes the negative impacts of bias. In a way, it shows that sustainable recovery depends on mixcombining personal strength with effective systemic backing (Yusuf, 2025) (Figure 13.6).

13.3. Rehabilitation Strategies

Rehabilitation for people with leprosy-related challenges isn't just about treating the symptoms—it's about looking at the full picture, including how a person's physical signs mix with their everyday social and environmental hurdles. Often, patients end up with more advanced issues by the time they're diagnosed, largely because treatment got delayed and there wasn't enough public awareness; you can see this in the high number of cases showing grade I or II disabilities at specialized centers (Sy Savané et al., 2024). This situation generally points to how essential early intervention is, paired with active physical rehab to keep further damage at bay. In many programs, medical management, like using corticosteroids to ease nerve inflammation—is combined with exercises designed to keep joints moving and reduce the risk of contractures. Also, patient education and self-care skills are repeated themes since they help in slowing down additional complications. When rehab plans are adjusted to meet both physical and emotional needs, patients tend to see improvements in how well they function daily and in their overall quality of life. Traditional rehab isn't standing still either; there's a big shift happening thanks to new technologies. Digital tools—think telemedicine, wearable trackers, and even immersive virtual reality—are opening up fresh and sometimes unexpected ways to offer personalized rehabilitation that pushes past common barriers like distance or cost (Willingham et al., 2024). In many cases, these devices allow for ongoing monitoring, remote therapy sessions, and exercise setups that adapt to a person's individual progress. This tech-driven approach is particularly key in areas where specialized services are hard to come by, and it also tends to boost patient engagement, which is critical for long-term success. Generally speaking, giving emerging technologies a more central role in rehab strategies not only cuts down health disparities but also makes care more accessible for those living with leprosy-related issues. On a broader scale, addressing rehab means tackling a whole host of obstacles—physical, psychosocial, and financial—that make it tough for individuals with leprosy-related disabilities to take part in regular activities. Often, these layered challenges block steady access to rehab services, reinforcing cycles of disability and social exclusion (Willingham et al., 2024). To break this cycle, many experts are turning to community-based rehab methods. These approaches don't focus solely on clinical treatment; they also work on social integration, offer vocational training, and use peer support to empower patients. Building networks that deliver psychological support and work to ease stigma is also seen as crucial since even small boosts in social confidence can help with reintegration and improved mental health. In most cases, health systems that expand both classic and innovative rehabilitation services create fairer opportunities for those affected to reclaim independence and a better quality of life (Figure 13.7).

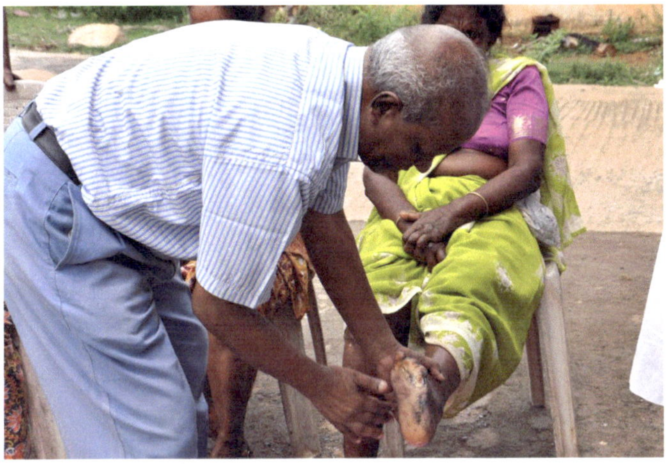

Figure 13.7. Leprosy rehabilitation.

Source: Christian Missions India. (2015). *Leprosy Rehabilitation.*

13.3.1. Medical Interventions and Treatments

Managing disabilities linked to leprosy isn't just about a quick medical fix, it calls for a combination of early detection, ongoing treatment, and long-term rehab. It starts when doctors catch the infection early and put patients on multidrug therapy (MDT), which usually stops *Mycobacterium leprae* cold and helps avoid nerve damage. Still, in many low- and middle-income places, shaky health infrastructure and a lack of well-trained staff make it hard to roll out care the way it's needed. Often, a team made up of doctors, nurses, therapists, and community health workers ends up shouldering the responsibility, not only helping with the clinical side of things but also acting as a front line against further disability. Simple steps, regular nerve checks, proper wound care, and mobility tests, can, in most cases, greatly cut down the severity of disability. When effective post-treatment rehab is woven into everyday practice, long-term issues tend to drop while quality of life shoots up, especially when mixed with a dash of psychosocial support and patient as well as caregiver education (Rahman, 2025). Rehabilitation doesn't stop at medical treatment; it jumps in to restore function and ward off extra problems connected to leprosy. Think physical therapy, using splints to steer clear of deformities, or even reconstructive surgery when the situation calls for it—all aiming to salvage as much function as possible. Yet, in many under-resourced regions, the healthcare system struggles to deliver ongoing, well-rounded rehab. Socioeconomic challenges play their part, too; patients working informal jobs or subsistence farming often miss regular follow-ups and suffer treatment gaps. Add in issues like stigma and poverty, and the whole picture becomes even murkier. That's why tailored approaches, ones that factor in economic limitations, local community education, and capacity building, are so essential. Further, when families and caregivers get some structured training, care can spill over from clinics into everyday life, making a real difference in outcomes (Yévèdo Tossou et al., 2025). Looking at the bigger picture, giving solid, all-around care for leprosy-related disabilities means systems need to back up healthcare delivery and social integration wholeheartedly. Medical interventions on their own can't cover all the challenges people with disabilities face—what's needed is a combination of prevention, rapid treatment, steady rehab, and ongoing social support. Strengthening the healthcare backbone through extra funding, better training, and more accessible services goes a long way in bridging the gaps. At the same time, public health programs that raise awareness, help lessen stigma, and promote economic inclusion also play their part in easing the burden of leprosy. It's a collaborative effort: government bodies, NGOs, and community groups all need to work together to create intervention models that are both sustainable and fit the local culture. Generally speaking, mounting evidence shows that when rehab is given equal weight alongside clinical treatment, the overall disability impact drops and quality of life improves for those living with the condition (Rahman, 2025; Yévèdo Tossou et al., 2025) (Figure 13.8).

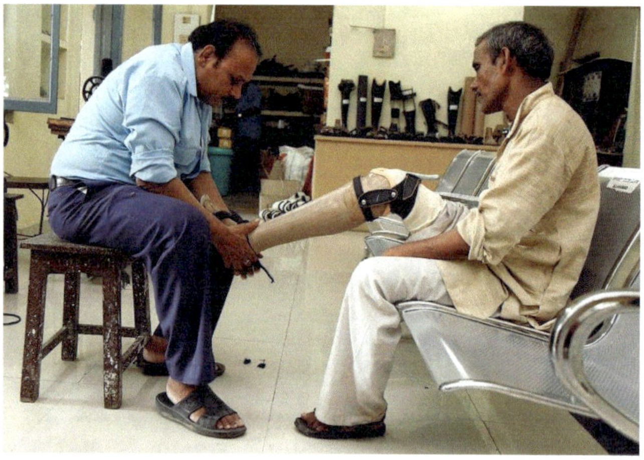

Figure 13.8. The importance of physical rehabilitation of leprosy patients cannot be emphasized enough.

Source: Leprosy Awareness Campaign. (2021). *The Importance of Physical Rehabilitation of Leprosy Patients Cannot be Emphasized Enough*. Facebook.

13.3.2. Physical Therapy and Occupational Therapy

Rebuilding everyday independence is the heart of life after leprosy. Many people try to regain control over their daily routines with rehabilitation techniques that combining physical and occupational therapies. Physical therapy, for example, works on restoring muscle strength and mobility with targeted exercises, gait training, and sometimes splinting to manage nerve damage and paralysis. At the same time, occupational therapy helps people tackle everyday tasks, promoting self-care and even skills for work life. In some communities where survivors are welcomed back into everyday life, these combined methods have been linked to a better quality of life and increased social connection (Chinguo et al., 2011). Accessing proper rehabilitation remains a huge challenge, especially in low-income regions. There's often a real shortage of trained professionals and facilities needed to deliver effective physical and occupational therapy. Lately, a number of government initiatives have started dedicating resources to expanding rehabilitation services, generally speaking, these plans focus not only on boosting available care but also on putting evidence-based practices into use to help people cope with disabling conditions like leprosy. By developing sustainable training and service models, countries can better meet the complex needs of this affected group; such measures significantly support both physical recovery and social reintegration (Dhakal et al., 2019). Moreover, having multidisciplinary teams on board is crucial so that both bodily functions and the emotional aspects of disability are addressed. Physical and occupational therapy work best when they complement each other, each bringing its own set of strategies to assist recovery. While physical therapy typically concentrates on maintaining joint movement, reducing contractures, and improving circulation through daily exercises, occupational therapy takes a more adaptive approach—adjusting environments and teaching alternative techniques that let patients continue enjoying meaningful activities despite persisting impairments. Together, these therapies tend to cut down on the need for extra surgeries and help lessen the visible signs of disability, which in turn can reduce social stigma. When rehabilitation programs are designed with keeping in mind the cultural sensitivities, they not only uplift physical improvement but also enhance overall life quality (Chinguo et al., 2011; Dhakal et al., 2019) (Figure 13.9).

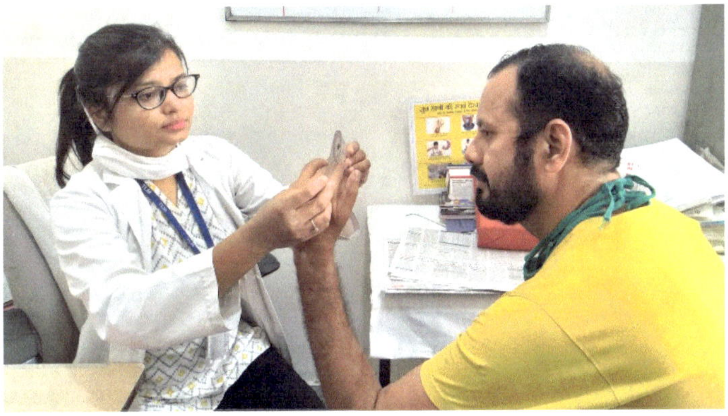

Figure 13.9. Occupational therapy.

Source: The Leprosy Mission Shahdara. (2021). *Occupational Therapy.*

13.3.3. Role of Assistive Devices in Rehabilitation

Recovery after tough conditions depends on combining in new tech that fits individual needs. When leprosy throws in damage with movement and feeling, these handy devices, from basic splints to high-tech robotic exoskeletons—step in not just as add-ons but as core parts of rehab. It all comes down to whether the tool can shift to match someone's own body characteristics and mental state. Research generally points out that matching what device you use along with altering training to suit someone's cognitive and emotional vibes can boost how comfortable individuals feel with them. Something as simple as letting people get used to the equipment beforehand can ease nerves and lift performance, showing that a people-first approach is key in rehab (Bertuccelli et al., 2025). To summarize, these assistive tools can work together with other therapies to help manage challenges linked to leprosy. Another important bit in rehab is how these devices support everyday tasks. For people dealing with leprosy—where issues in both upper and lower limbs can make it hard not just to move but also to handle everyday stuff like driving or using common tools—gadgets designed to cover for lost function step up as true lifesavers. In many cases, when the technology is made to cope with reduced limb use or lost senses, it helps make daily tasks both safer and more practical. For example, specialized alters in vehicles or gadgets that help with driving have shown clear improvements in performance, safety, and overall quality of life (Lee, 2024). These kinds of adjustments let individuals hold onto their autonomy and keep in touch with social circles. Using similar ideas for those touched by leprosy might just bridge gaps in independence and help people reconnect with their communities, proving the irreplaceable role of these assistive devices. Combining assistive devices into rehab calls for a broad, teamwork-based approach—one that values not just physical fixes but also how people think and feel. It matters how usable these devices seem and how naturally they slip into everyday routines. Studies, in most cases, have noted that things like mental reserve and anxiety levels can significantly affect how someone gets used to and benefits from such gadgets. When it comes to leprosy-related disabilities, minding these emotional and mental factors during device choice and training can boost both engagement and overall gains. Often, when a person feels a personal tie to the tool and finds it not too burdensome to use, the gear works even better, underlining why personalized, human-tailored strategies can be so important. In the end, linking thoughtful design, users' cognitive profiles, and good supportive therapy tends to bring about better rehab results and helps people maintain that hard-won independence—even while dealing with leprosy (Bertuccelli et al., 2025) (Figure 13.10).

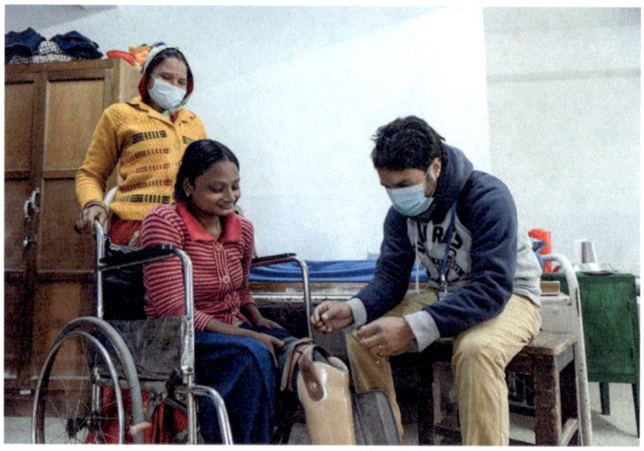

Figure 13.10. The role of assistive devices in rehabilitation.

Source: The Leprosy Mission International. (n.d.). *The Role of Assistive Devices in Rehabilitation.*

13.4. Community-Based Rehabilitation Programs

Leprosy rehabilitation goes well beyond just medical treatment, it is about helping individuals rebuild their lives socially and economically. Community rehab programs, often known as CBR, emerge as a keyway of getting people back on their feet in their own neighborhoods. These local initiatives usually mix basic health care, classes, job training, and a bit of social support to tackle the many hurdles that come with leprosy-related disabilities. They lean on local resources and community efforts, which generally helps break down stigma and pave the way for inclusion—even though the social isolation can be stubborn. Since the setup is decentralized, these programs tend to be more accessible, especially in rural or underserved spots where healthcare may be thin on the ground. To summarize, CBR seems to offer a sustainable mix that not only boosts physical recovery but also lifts overall quality of life. Often, putting a community-based rehab program together means that local healthcare providers, NGOs, and government agencies need to work hand-in-hand. This kind of teamwork usually optimizes resource use and fine-tunes service delivery, making sure things like prosthetic and orthotic care are both thorough and tuned to local needs. In most cases, various reports on disability services in different areas stress just how important this coordination is. For instance, the success seen in Cambodia with USAID-supported rehabilitation initiatives (Fund et al., 2001) suggests that a multi-stakeholder approach can make a difference for people with disabilities, including those stemming from leprosy. In various regions, these initiatives have shown notable results by leaning on community engagement and even setting up self-supporting units, which help keep care going and allow for intervention plans that truly have a local touch. That said, not everything is smooth sailing. Challenges still persist when it comes to fine-tuning community-based rehabilitation for leprosy-related disabilities. Studies looking at prosthetic and orthotic services in low-resource settings such as Uganda, for example, reveal ongoing gaps in both quality and accessibility, issues that run parallel to challenges seen in other leprosy rehabilitation efforts (Fund et al., 1998). Addressing these shortcomings generally calls for more investment in training, better resource distribution, and more reliable monitoring within the CBR framework. Moreover, upping rehabilitation quality means being culturally sensitive and adaptable to local social dynamics—a must when trying to combat deep-seated stigma. Balancing standardized methods with room for local alters can improve outcomes. Ultimately, building stronger community rehab programs is about merging the medical, social, and economic aspects in a way that lets people with leprosy-related disabilities regain not just physical function, but also their place in society (Figure 13.11).

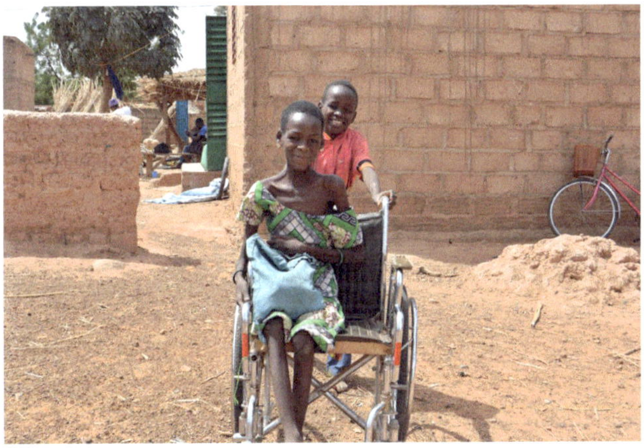

Figure 13.11. Community based rehabilitation (CBR).

Source: Afri-Can. (2017). *CBR.*

13.4.1. Importance of Community Involvement

Community involvement makes a difference in rehab programs for leprosy-related disabilities. Health workers, who often know the local scene inside and out, generally say that when people pitch in, it cuts through those long-held stigmas and the unfair social setup that can block proper care. They sometimes point out issues like gender imbalances, scarce resources, and not enough community participation, which all seem to interfere with the longevity of these programs. In most cases, dialing up open talks and trust within the community lets locals get more involved as partners in preventing and fixing these issues. This kind of shared effort helps tailor solutions to local needs and builds culturally aware interventions, ultimately boosting both health outcomes and social inclusion for those affected by leprosy (Martos-Casado et al., 2022). It isn't just about health services either—the social side matters a lot, too. Beyond the quick health fixes, getting communities involvement often helps in dealing with the people with leprosy-related disabilities. Often, grassroots actions and the unique insights of community members challenge common stereotypes and push for fair treatment. In spots like India, where formal support can be spotty at times, local acts of solidarity sometimes lay the groundwork for vital support networks and even new opportunities for making a living. Further, when communities gather accurate data and work on research themselves, it helps shine a light on groups that might otherwise be overlooked, paving the way for more focused education and job training programs. This repeated effort to break the cycle of exclusion opens doors for training and work opportunities, giving those affected a shot at greater independence and self-respect (Rungta et al., 2004). Combining community participation into leprosy rehabilitation stretches care well beyond just the medical angle. When locals get involved, they not only encourage health pros to be more compassionate but also push for approaches that keep gender issues in mind, addressing specific vulnerabilities. The model here is kind of a shared-responsibility deal—health workers, families, and affected individuals all collobaroate, which tends to heal not just the body but also the social and emotional sides. Typically, the ongoing success of these programs depends on this kind of widespread bond, ensuring that services remain accessible yet genuinely respected. In the end, a strong community role often induces broader moves toward universal health care and rights-based systems, aligning health efforts more closely with wider quests for social justice (Martos-Casado et al., 2022).

13.4.2. Successful Case Studies from Various Regions

Leprosy-related disabilities present a tough challenge, and several regions are trying out rehab ideas that seem to work in unexpected ways. In parts of Asia, community programs mix health support with job training, helping individuals find independence and a place in society again. They lean on local know-how and cultural flavors to create steady work opportunities, which in most cases eases both stigma and the economic setbacks that often come with the condition. Tailoring skill-building to what each person can do has turned out to be key for boosting work chances and self-reliance. These grassroots efforts, by opening up spaces for people with disabilities to contribute at work, do fit—albeit in their own informal way, with international guidelines calling for accessible, inclusive job options (Cornell University, World Health Organization, and World Bank, 2011). To summarize, such success stories underline that a combination of physical care and social support truly makes a difference. Outside Asia, many Latin American countries have also made noticeable headway in rehabilitating leprosy disabilities. In several urban centers, integrated teams are putting together streams of medical care, psychological counseling, and community inclusion – a combination that has noticeably improved lives in many ways. Often, these collaborative approaches help cut down discrimination by getting local governments, NGOs, and other community figures involved directly. They don't just provide treatment; they also pave the way for people to return to schools or jobs, reflecting a commitment to human rights and equal access that international conventions usually highlight. In most cases, the experiences there show how important a coordinated system and culturally aware methods are to untangle the complex mix of disease, disability, and social isolation (Cornell University, World Health Organization, and World Bank, 2011). Across the globe, digital platforms and networks now play a big part in sharing promising rehab practices. Experts and stakeholders link up through international gatherings and online archives—places where case studies get exchanged and evidence-based ideas are quietly refined as our grasp of disability rights deepens. This open flow of information stimulates many to try innovative models that have been proven effective in various settings, expanding the reach and impact of these programs. Encouraging simple, user-friendly communication forms part of a broader plan to break down the stigma and misinformation that often surrounds leprosy. By connecting successful stories from different regions, these digital hubs help push forward practices that support not just physical recovery but also dignity, independence, and lasting livelihoods.

13.4.3. Challenges Faced by Rehabilitation Programs

Leprosy rehabilitation isn't just about medical treatment—it's a tough journey marred by deep-seated prejudice and scant resources. Many individuals dealing with leprosy ends up isolated by widespread stigma that cuts them off from support and decent job opportunities. Often, community participation is the lifeblood of these programs, so when people are shunned, efforts to reintegrate them fizzle out. Health centers, already strapped for specialized care and skilled staff, add another layer of difficulty in addressing patient needs fully.

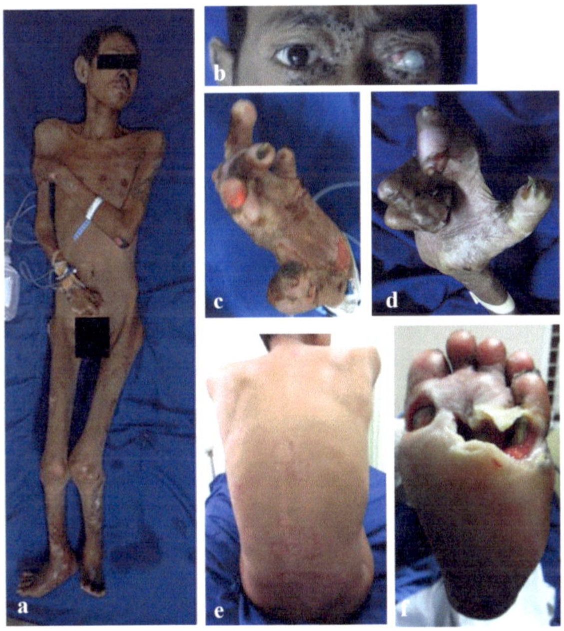

Figure 13.12. The challenges faced by rehabilitation programs.

*Source*Gunawan, H., Johan, R., Achdiat, P.A. *et al.* Challenging diagnosis of leprosy in a psychotic homeless patient with atypical clinical manifestations: an interesting case report. *BMC Infect Dis* **21**, 540 (2021). https://doi.org/10.1186/s12879-021-06242-0

In most cases, it seems that the complex interplay of societal bias and faltering institutional support ends up making recovery and inclusion a patchwork process (Cornell University, World Health Organization, and World Bank, 2011). Another big hurdle shows up when it comes to reintroducing people affected by leprosy into the workforce. Although many are more than capable of contributing productively, discrimination alongside structural barriers generally makes the labor market feel like a closed door. Prevailing prejudices in hiring practices often leave them with higher unemployment rates, even when their skills are undeniable. Sometimes, even disability benefits inadvertently create an economic trap that discourages getting back to work. Vocational training and job services remain essential; yet, due to inconsistent funding and weak policy oversight, their overall impact tends to fall short highlighting the clear need for more inclusive legal structures and proactive workplace adjustments (Cornell University, World Health Organization, and World Bank, 2011). Sustainability of these programs also suffers from a lack of community involvement and noticeable gender gaps. Health professionals frequently report that engaging local communities isn't as straightforward as hoped, a factor which dulls the intended impact of self-care, disability prevention and the push for social inclusion. Women, in particular, find themselves detected in a double bind, as uneven gender treatment restricts their access to essential services and curtails empowerment in rehabilitation activities. Without more sensitive, context-aware approaches that take local and social nuances into account, achieving broad health coverage and long-lasting success becomes even more elusive. In essence, a balanced focus on reducing stigma, shoring up resources, boosting community engagement, and addressing gender disparities seems necessary to truly overcome these systemic challenges (Martos-Casado et al., 2022) (Figure 13.12).

A CLOSER LOOK

SURGICAL REHABILITATION

This section will limit itself to the more common paralytic conditions that result from leprosy neuropathy. Neurolysis as a surgical procedure to restore or prevent nerve function impairment (NFI) will not be discussed. This remains a controversial issue in leprosy surgery, whose possible benefits have not been established.

Some important principles related to reconstructive limb surgery are listed below:

1. Reconstructive surgery should only be performed by surgeons with sufficient training in leprosy reconstructive surgery. The surgeon should ideally have spent time with an experienced leprosy reconstructive surgeon.
2. Surgeons and therapists should be confident that patients understand that movements will be restored, not sensation. Patients should have shown good understanding and practice of living with a limb, or limbs, with loss of protective sensation.
3. No tendon transfer surgery should be done without the assurance that patients will be followed with postoperative therapy.
4. Assess corrected hands and feet after 6–12 months to determine occurrence of possible secondary impairments (wounds, contractures) and to assess functional social benefits (Figure 13.13).

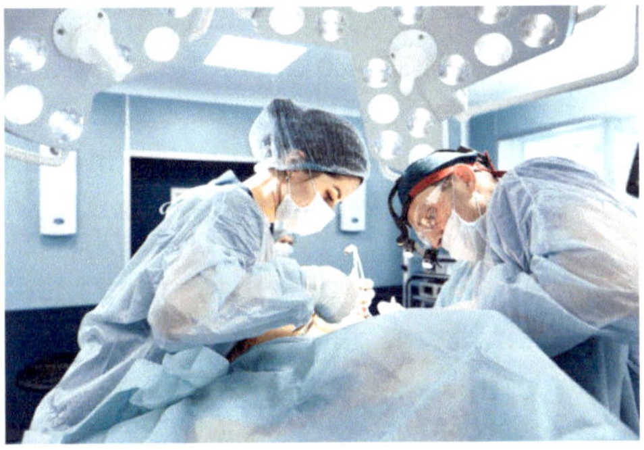

Figure 13.13. Surgical rehabilitation.

Source: AIFO India. (2023). Surgical Rehabilitation.

SUMMARY

People struggling with leprosy keep facing serious challenges, which means we need a combination of strategies to prevent disabilities and help with rehabilitation. Studies show that stepping in early , using vaccines like BCG or MIP , might lower both how severe and how common these disabilities become in kids. There's even a noticeable trend: kids without obvious BCG scars often end up with a tougher version of the disease, more multibacillary cases, notable reactions, and even grade 2 disabilities. In most cases, this curious link hints that more research could clear up how protective these shots are. If we dig a bit deeper, we might fine-tune vaccine practices and shape public policies to stave off long-term issues. Boosting vaccine coverage along with early detection could ease both the physical and social toll that leprosy brings on children (Narang et al., 2025). Looking closer, healthcare setups and support that put patients first show up as key to effective rehabilitation. It turns out that people recovering from reconstructive surgery often do better when they have solid family backing and even see small psychologic gains from it, which goes right along with the surgery's functional benefits. Yet, persisting stigma and deep-seated fears keep many from seeking treatment promptly, and that only makes disabilities worse over time. In most cases, addressing these issues means improving our healthcare delivery by upgrading facilities, ensuring enough funding, and backing programs such as the National Leprosy Eradication Program. Clearly, combining sound medical care with some psychological and social support paves the way for earlier treatment and better post-surgical recovery (Shrivastava et al., 2024). To wrap this up, the complex nature of leprosy disabilities shows that there isn't a one-size-fits-all fix. Generally speaking, a smart combination of prevention, timely treatment, and broad rehabilitation is critical. Continued focus on vaccine research, along with real efforts to impact stigma and expand access to reconstructive procedures, creates a powerful combo that can curb disabilities and boost everyday function. Policymakers and caregivers alike need to invest more and help raise community awareness so that medical advances turn into gains for patients. To summarize, a genuine, multidimensional commitment seems to be our best shot to ease leprosy's lifelong impacts and build more inclusive rehabilitation paths (Shrivastava et al., 2024; Narang et al., 2025).

Leprosy-related disabilities hit people hard, not just on the medical side but also by interfering with everyday life. Many end up feeling cut off from society and drained of quality of life. It seems that when physical difficulties mix with social hurdles, rehab can't be a one-track fix; it has to address both issues simultaneously. Jobs play a huge part here. Even when individuals have proven skills, they're often sidelined in the job market because of discrimination, patchy policies, and other systemic blips. Generally speaking, these disparities come down to a combination of workplace bias, market imperfections, and lacking enforcement of rules. For instance, international guidelines like the United Nations Convention on the Rights of Persons with Disabilities call for equal access to work by supporting vocational rehab, self-employment initiatives, and reasonable adjustments at work (Cornell University, World Health Organization, and World Bank, 2011). All of these social factors need to be tackled for rehab and long-term disability management to work well. In remote or low-resource areas, the picture gets even murkier since rehab services are few and far between—adding to the exclusion many already experience. To bridge this gap, specialized manuals and communication tools tailored for low- and middle-income countries have started to show promise. A broad mix of individuals, from healthcare professionals and community aides to volunteers and families, get a boost from these tools, even when infrastructure is minimal. The development of these manuals is an ongoing experiment—feedback and early tests shape them in ways that lean on smart, available technology in tough settings. This iterative strategy not only helps achieve more consistent rehab results but also bolsters equitable access for marginalized groups (Theint et al., 2022). Clearly, crafting such targeted resources is a key piece in scaling rehab efforts where they're needed most. When you look at all this together, it's apparent that handling leprosy-related disabilities means combining medical, social, and even technological angles. It starts with fighting workplace discrimination through better laws and adaptive work conditions, plus offering vocational training and counseling to strengthen labor market inclusion. At the same time, widening access to rehab information and tools that work in resource-poor environments builds a much-needed support network for real recovery and community integration. All these measures—coordinated in sometimes complex, human ways, show just how multifaceted rehabilitation is. They empower individuals, impact stigma, and nurture environments where everyone can thrive. Continuously fine-tuning and applying these varied strategies promises not only improved personal well-being but also a stronger sense of inclusion at the community level (Cornell University, World Health Organization, and World Bank, 2011; Theint et al., 2022).

KEY TERMS FROM THIS CHAPTER

- Burns
- Facial palsy
- Personal dignity
- Physical therapy
- Smart clinical care
- Social exclusion
- Social network
- Stereotypes
- Education
- Intellectual disabilities
- Physical impairments
- Quality of life
- Social dynamics
- Social fallout
- Solid medical treatment
- Vocational rehabilitation

References

1. Adedeji P, Olabisi I, Aladegbami O, Adedeji O. Perceived stigmatization, psychosocial well-being and self-esteem among individuals living in leprosy center in south-west, Nigeria . J Ideas Health [Internet]. 2023 Sep. 7 [cited 2025 May 31];6(3):908-19. Available from: https://www.jidhealth.com/index.php/jidhealth/article/view/296(accessed on 10th May 2025).
2. Ahonle ZJ, Wei T, Rumrill PD, Dillahunt-Aspillaga C. Comparing competitive integrated employment outcomes in the state-federal vocational rehabilitation program among individuals with cognitive, physical, and sensory functional impairments. *Journal of Vocational Rehabilitation*. 2025;62(2):168-177. doi:10.1177/10522263241310068 (accessed on 10th May 2025).
3. Barakat, M., & Zaki, H. (2019). *Relationship Between Psychological Problems and Quality of Life Among Leprosy Patients*. https://core.ac.uk/download/524771812.pdf (accessed on 10th May 2025).
4. van Brakel, W. H., Sihombing, B., Djarir, H., Beise, K., Kusumawardhani, L., Yulihane, R., Kurniasari, I., Kasim, M., Kesumaningsih, K. I., & Wilder-Smith, A. (2012). Disability in people affected by leprosy: the role of impairment, activity, social participation, stigma and discrimination. *Global health action, 5*, 10.3402/gha.v5i0.18394. https://doi.org/10.3402/gha.v5i0.18394 (accessed on 10th May 2025).
5. Bertuccelli M, Tortora S, Trombin E, Negri L, Bisiacchi P, Menegatti E, Del Felice A. Human–Robot Interactions: A Pilot Study of Psychoaffective and Cognitive Factors to Boost the Acceptance and Usability of Assistive Wearable Devices. *Multimodal Technologies and Interaction*. 2025; 9(1):5. https://doi.org/10.3390/mti9010005(accessed on 10th May 2025).
6. DOROTHY CHINGU*, MADELEINE DUNCAN** & SEYI AMOSUN (2011). *A Comparison of the Quality of Life Between Survivors of Leprosy Living in a Leprosarium and Those Re-Integrated in their Communities in the Southern Region of Malawi*. Lepr Rev (2013) 84, 292–301 https://core.ac.uk/download/185398263.pdf (accessed on 10th May 2025).
7. Classen, S., Gélinas, I., Barco, P., Gibson, B., Haffner, E., Jeghers, M., Wandenkolk, I. C., et al. (2024). Automated vehicles: Future initiatives for occupational therapy practitioners and driver rehabilitation specialists. *OTJR: Occupation, Participation and Health*. https://www.semanticscholar.org/paper/e05266fd6334c0841421a0c181586ef734ca2137 (accessed on 10th May 2025).
8. Cleary, M., West, S., Johnston-Devin, C., Kornhaber, R., McLean, L., & Hungerford, C. (2024). Collateral Damage: The Impacts of School Exclusion on the Mental Health of Parents Caring for Autistic Children. Issues in Mental Health Nursing, 45(1), 3–8. https://doi.org/10.1080/01612840.2023.2280718(accessed on 10th May 2025).
9. Cornell University, World Health Organization, & World Bank. (2011). *World Report on Disability, Chapter 8: Work and Employment*. https://core.ac.uk/download/5131044.pdf (accessed on 10th May 2025).
10. Dhakal, R., & Groves, C. C. (2019). *Rehabilitation in Nepal*. https://core.ac.uk/download/333957093.pdf (accessed on 10th May 2025).
11. Donovan, H. (2023). A novel national family caregiver advocacy training program: Lessons

learned. *Innovation in Aging, 7*, 251–251. https://www.semanticscholar.org/paper/31b871d1da51f2bd44149ee6a04150a386bce9c7 (accessed on 10th May 2025).

12. Martos-Casado, G., Vives-Cases, C., & Gil-González, D. (2022). Community intervention programmes with people affected by leprosy: Listening to the voice of professionals. *PLoS neglected tropical diseases*, *16*(3), e0010335. https://doi.org/10.1371/journal.pntd.0010335 (accessed on 10th May 2025).
13. Pinheiro, M. G. C., Lins, S. L. D. F., Gomes, B. R. D. S., Simpson, C. A., Mendes, F. R. P., & Miranda, F. A. N. (2019). Contextual analysis of health care at discharge in leprosy: an integrative review. Análise contextual da atenção à saúde na alta em hanseníase: uma revisão integrativa. *Revista gaucha de enfermagem*, *40*, e20180258. https://doi.org/10.1590/1983-1447.2019.20180258(accessed on 10th May 2025).
14. Holubenko, T., Ivzhenko, I., & Kuznetsova, O. (2024). Social policy regarding veterans, people with disabilities and other vulnerable population groups. *Social Work and Education*. https://www.semanticscholar.org/paper/66718ad7c4486a66dae710c07e56af7233373950 (accessed on 10th May 2025).
15. Zin Mar Theint, Zin Lynn Htun, Khin Mar Swe, Kathy Kuipers, Pim Kuipers;
16. Remote disability and leprosy services via basic communications technology ; Leprosy Review; 2022; 93; 2; 166-171; DOI: 10.47276/lr.93.2.166 (accessed on 10th May 2025).
17. InFocus Program on Skills, Knowledge and Employability, International Labor Office. (2003). *India Country Profile*. https://core.ac.uk/download/5129441.pdf (accessed on 10th May 2025).
18. InFocus Program on Skills, Knowledge and Employability, International Labor Office. (2003). *Ethiopia Country Profile*. https://core.ac.uk/download/5129442.pdf (accessed on 10th May 2025).
19. Lee, M. Y. (2024). A systematic review of assistive devices and vehicle modifications for safe driving. *Society of Occupational Therapy for the Aged and Dementia*. https://www.semanticscholar.org/paper/5c2f1d7387bac7eeffce40613526563c8c618eb1 (accessed on 10th May 2025).
20. Bhattacharya, S. (Ed.) (2003). Public health in Calcutta. *Wellcome History*, *22*, 1-24. http://www.wellcome.ac.uk/stellent/groups/corporatesite/@msh_publishing_group/documents/web_document/wtd006093.pdf (accessed on 10th May 2025).
21. Narang, T., Sharma, A., Kaushal, I., Chatterjee, D., & Dogra, S. (2025). Protective effects of BCG vaccination against multibacillary disease, reactions, and disabilities in childhood leprosy: Insights from a retrospective observational study from a tertiary care center in India. *International journal of dermatology*, *64*(6), 1086–1091. https://doi.org/10.1111/ijd.17636 (accessed on 10th May 2025).
22. Nasution, S., Ngatimin, M. R., & Syafar, M. (2012). *Dampak Rehabilitasi Medis Pada Penyandang Disabilitas Kusta*. https://media.neliti.com/media/publications/39476-ID-dampak-rehabilitasi-medis-pada-penyandang-disabilitas-kusta.pdf (accessed on 10th May 2025).
23. Rahman, M. S. (2025). Rehabilitation of stroke survivors with disabilities in low- and middle-income countries: Barriers and opportunities. *Journal of Enam Medical College*. J Enam Med Col 2022; 12(3): 148–154https://www.semanticscholar.org/paper/023d8f8d1594ef081a1f64c50497906ec5ff2c19 (accessed on 10th May 2025).

24. Raj, S. P., & Joseph, J. (2025). Empowering Persons with Disabilities through Grassroots Organisations: A Case Study of Disabled People's Organisations in Kerala. Manatri: Journal of Multi-Disciplinary Research, 1(1), 44–51. https://doi.org/10.4038/manatri.v1i1.5 (accessed on 10th May 2025).

25. Rungta, S. K. (2004). *Training and Employment of People with Disabilities: India 2002*. https://core.ac.uk/download/5119037.pdf (accessed on 10th May 2025).

26. Shrivastava, K., Ray, S., Rathod, H., Wahegaonkar, A. L., Jadhav, S. L., Mahajan, A., S, J., Verma, P., Palal, D., & Sengupta, S. (2024). Transforming Lives: A Qualitative Study Seeking Insights Into Reconstructive Surgery for Leprosy Patients in Western Maharashtra. *Cureus, 16*(9), e68416. https://doi.org/10.7759/cureus.68416(accessed on 10th May 2025).

27. Sy Savané, I. S., Sidibe, S., Kolié, D., Camara, M., Sakho, F., Sidibé, S., Chérif, M. S., Doumbouya, S., Nabé, A. K., & Delamou, A. (2024). Frequency and Factors Associated with Disabilities among Leprosy Patients Admitted to the Kindia Disability Prevention and Physical Rehabilitation Centre (Pirp) in Guinea from 2017 to 2021. *Tropical medicine and infectious disease, 9*(10), 237. https://doi.org/10.3390/tropicalmed9100237(accessed on 10th May 2025).

28. Tossou YB, Gbaguidi FNC, Agbo SIE, Zanvo SDE, Codjo-Seignon KLM, Biaka PH, Guedou FA, Kouadio KJ, Anagonou SGE, Mignanwande FZ, Djossou P, Yemadje BV, Houndjrebo FS, Arrawo JdNL, Faihoun Y, Johnson H, Sopoh GE, Houezo JG, Kaloga M, Dizoe AS, Nichter M, Juan Jimenez C, Gine-March A and Johnson RC (2025) Factors associated with the management of people affected by disabilities in communities endemic to skin-related neglected tropical diseases in Benin and Côte d'Ivoire. Front. Trop. Dis. 6:1522660. doi: 10.3389/fitd.2025.1522660(accessed on 10th May 2025).

29. United Nations Economic and Social Commission for Asia and the Pacific (UN.ESCAP). (1987). *Handbook on Funding and Training Resources for Disability-Related Services in Asia and the Pacific*. https://core.ac.uk/download/641691033.pdf (accessed on 10th May 2025).

30. USAID Leahy War Victims Fund. (1998). *Uganda Prosthetic/Orthotic Needs Assessment – Leahy War Victims Fund Report*. https://core.ac.uk/download/346453607.pdf (accessed on 10th May 2025).

31. USAID Leahy War Victims Fund. (2001). *Veterans International Technical and Medical Rehabilitation Support Services in Cambodia*. https://core.ac.uk/download/346453606.pdf (accessed on 10th May 2025).

32. Wang, Q., & Yang, T. (2025). A Study on the Optimization Path of Medical Rehabilitation Policy for People with Disabilities in Hong Kong. *Highlights in Business, Economics and Management, 47*, 327-335. https://doi.org/10.54097/48rvz617(accessed on 10th May 2025).

33. Willingham, T. B., Stowell, J., Collier, G., & Backus, D. (2024). Leveraging Emerging Technologies to Expand Accessibility and Improve Precision in Rehabilitation and Exercise for People with Disabilities. *International journal of environmental research and public health, 21*(1), 79. https://doi.org/10.3390/ijerph21010079(accessed on 10th May 2025).

34. Wormald, A., McGlinchey, E., D'Eath, M., Leroi, I., Lawlor, B., McCallion, P., McCarron, M., O'Sullivan, R., & Chen, Y. (2023). Impact of COVID-19 Pandemic on Caregivers of People with an Intellectual Disability, in Comparison to Carers of Those with Other Disabilities and with Mental Health Issues: A Multicountry Study. *International journal of environmental research*

and public health, *20*(4), 3256. https://doi.org/10.3390/ijerph20043256(accessed on 10th May 2025).

35. Wróbel, A. E., Cash, P., Maier, A., & Paulin Hansen, J. (2025). Determining the Prioritization of Behavior Change Techniques for Long-Term Stroke Rehabilitation: Delphi Survey Study. *Interactive journal of medical research*, *14*, e59172. https://doi.org/10.2196/59172(accessed on 10th May 2025).

36. Yusuf, A. (2025). *The Effect of Individual, Family and Environmental Factors on Family Stigma with Leprosy*. Conference: Advances in Social Science, Education and Humanities Research (ASSEHR), volume 98 1st International Conference Postgraduate School Universitas Airlangga: Implementation of Climate Change Agreement to Meet Sustainable Development Goals (ICPSUAS 2017). https://core.ac.uk/download/296887582.pdf (accessed on 10th May 2025).

37. Zupo, R., Poggi, B., Caggiano, N., Varrone, G., Castellana, F., Natoli, S., Sardone, R., Nardone, A., & Pavese, C. (2025). Methods of diagnosis and rehabilitation of dysphagia in patients with spinal cord injury: a systematic review. *European journal of physical and rehabilitation medicine*, *61*(1), 41–51. https://doi.org/10.23736/S1973-9087.24.08614-3(accessed on 10th May 2025).

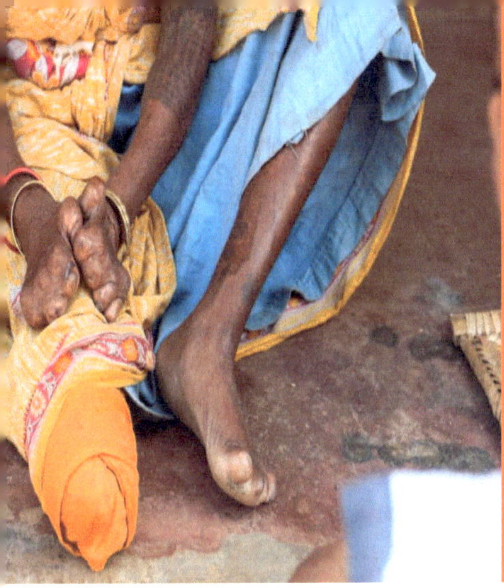

Chapter 14

PSYCHOSOCIAL ASPECTS AND QUALITY OF LIFE

Contents

Introduction

Leprosy has long been seen as a crippling, stigmatized disease, and even today it poses challenges that stretch well beyond just the physical symptoms. Its chronic nature tends to spiral into long-term problems that mix body, mind, and society , hitting people from all different walks of life around the globe. Even with effective multidrug treatments on hand, social stigma and discrimination still block patients from accessing proper health care and being truly included in society. This vicious loop not only worsens physical disabilities but also deepens emotional distress and isolation, ultimately denting one's quality of life quite a bit (Rahman et al., 2022). When you step back and consider the complex interplay of medical and social issues, it becomes clear that grasping leprosy's full impact means looking at both the body and the burden on the heart. Looking at the bigger picture with neglected tropical diseases like leprosy, socio-political and economic conditions generally play a huge part in letting these illnesses persist. In many cases, vulnerable communities in areas with scant resources face compounded hardships due to weak healthcare systems, poverty, and deep-seated cultural misconceptions. Poor sanitation, lack of health education, and longstanding cultural norms often delay diagnosis and treatment, which in turn makes coping with the disease even tougher (Elizabeth et al., 2021). All of these factors tend to hamper disease control and add layers to the psychosocial strain experienced by affected individuals; so, addressing these issues means taking a multi-layered look at the underlying economic and social roots that keep people trapped in cycles of illness and deprivation. Understanding how leprosy affects quality of life comes down to appreciating the diverse ways people experience and manage their illness. The way someone feels about having leprosy—shaped by personal experiences, family dynamics, and community reactions—invariably influences whether they stick to treatment plans or struggle with mental and emotional pressures. Social exclusion, economic hardships, and emotional stress often arrive alongside physical impairments, weaving together a tangle of difficulties. Studies tend to bring these aspects into themes that span the physical, social, economic, and emotional realms, all of which impact overall well-being. Therefore, effective interventions need to go beyond just medical treatment and also offer tailored psychosocial support that acknowledges the everyday realities of those involved, thereby fostering resilience and, ultimately, a better quality of life (Rahman et al., 2022) (Figure 14.1).

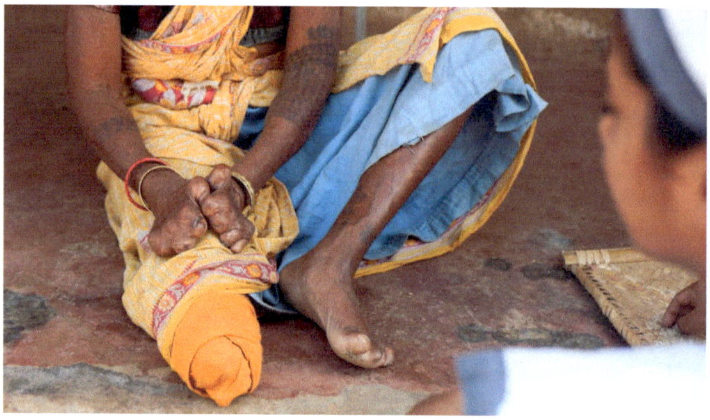

Figure 14.1. Leprosy mental health.

Source: Gospel for Asia. (2023, November). *Physical Effects of Leprosy.*

14.1. Medical Aspects of Leprosy

Leprosy comes from the bacterium *Mycobacterium leprae* and runs a long course as an infection. It tends to hit the skin, nerves, and even moist tissues, showing up in all kinds of ways. Generally speaking, the nerve damage that follows can lead to numbness, weak muscles, and even odd shifts in automatic body functions. These issues aren't just numbers on a chart—they often evolve into lasting physical changes and disabilities that many people recognize as classic signs of the disorder. What's more, once those nerves are affected, it isn't just a medical problem; it spills over into everyday life, stirring up serious social and emotional struggles. Patients might deal with pain that doesn't slot efficiently into standard definitions, sometimes it's a jumble of sensations that mix together, making treatment efforts all the more complicated (Freynhagen et al., 2018). Getting a full grasp on these layered health issues is pretty key to tackling the wider social and quality-of-life challenges too. The long haul of living with leprosy almost always drags along a stigma that goes far beyond any visible symptoms. Irreversible nerve damage can leave lasting marks on the body, and those changes often push people into social isolation and emotional distress. Much like other tough, long-term conditions, the stigma here is multidimensional, it twists not only how others see someone but also how a person might start seeing themselves. In most cases, this negative label can worsen mental stress, disrupt adherence to treatment routines, and limit social encounters, which all impact overall well-being. Detecting nerve damage early, handling pain with care, and working to prevent further disabilities are all vital steps that seem to help ease that weight of shame and isolation, as some studies on similar chronic issues suggest (Keefer & Taft, 2016). In the end, pairing practical medical care with support that addresses those deeper social wounds seems to matter. On top of it, treating leprosy goes beyond just a straightforward antibiotic fix—it means juggling a combination of drugs aimed at squashing the infection while also stepping in to guard against or repair nerve damage. Even when the diagnosis comes early and treatment starts on time, challenges like ongoing neuropathic pain and lost sensations might still persist, hampering everyday activities. Clinicians, in most cases, need to keep a close watch for symptoms that blur the lines of typical pain categories; this mixed picture often calls for a tailored treatment plan (Freynhagen et al., 2018). When these stubborn symptoms hang around, they can pile on extra burdens such as anxiety, bouts of depression, and issues with social interaction, all of which drag down a person's daily life. That's why a broad approach—one that weaves medical strategies with extra psychological support—is so important, aiming not only to lift clinical numbers but also to boost overall life satisfaction.

14.1.1. Symptoms and Progression of the Disease

Leprosy sometimes sneaks up in ways that are easy to miss, making early diagnosis a real challenge and paving the way for complications that hit both the body and the spirit. Early on, you might notice pale or slightly reddish skin patches that lose feeling gradually—if these signs go unchecked, they can worsen. Nerve involvement may start to show up as numbness or even muscle weakness, and before you know it, disabilities and deformities appear that carry a heavy social stigma. In many cases, the slow shift from a quiet infection to clear, distressing symptoms leaves patients feeling anxious and isolated—a situation made even worse by society's reactions (Lira et al., 2014). As the condition progresses, everyday life can become unexpectedly difficult. Patients begin to experience declining motor skills and a loss of sensation, which puts a strain on even simple tasks. Neuropathic effects might lead to muscle shrinkage, a hand that curls into a claw-like shape, or even a foot that tends to drop—all of which can cause lasting disabilities if treatment is delayed. These visible changes not only disrupt daily routines but also often result in social exclusion and deep emotional distress. Over time, the chronic nature of the ailment can induce anxiety and bouts of depression, feeding a cycle that steadily erodes self-esteem. Clearly, the complex progression of these symptoms calls for a mixed approach that combines clinical care with steady psychosocial support (Bonkass et al., 2024). Even with the advances in multidrug therapy that have lowered the infectious and physical toll of the disease, challenges remain—mainly because the nerve-related and inflammatory reactions can be unpredictable. For instance, reactions like Type 1 (reversal) and Type 2 (erythema nodosum leprosum) may trigger sudden bouts of inflammation that end up damaging nerves in unexpected ways. Such flare-ups often worsen neurological deficits and lead to fluctuating levels of disability, which can unsettle patients' emotional stability and strain social interactions. Given this erratic trajectory, the visible signs tend to reinforce stigma and can leave people feeling hopeless. It becomes essential, then, to tackle these shifts with targeted psychosocial measures that not only help improve coping mechanisms but also promote resilience and enhance overall quality of life (Bonkass et al., 2024; Lira et al., 2014) (Figure 14.2).

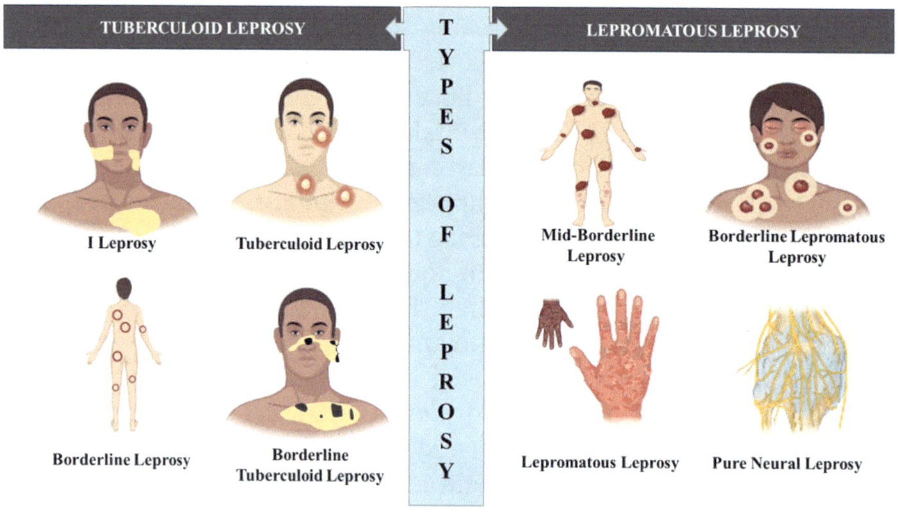

Figure 14.2. Signs and symptoms of Hansen's disease.

Source: Kimta N, Majdalawieh AF, Nasrallah GK, Puri S, Nepovimova E, Jomova K and Kuča K (2024) Leprosy: Comprehensive insights into pathology, immunology, and cutting-edge treatment strategies, integrating nanoparticles and ethnomedicinal plants. Front. Pharmacol. 15:1361641. doi: 10.3389/fphar.2024.1361641

14.1.2. Treatment Options and Their Effectiveness

Leprosy isn't just about visible skin changes, it leaves a mark that runs deep, touching every corner of a person's life. The main treatment, a multidrug regimen (MDT), works well to slow the disease and cut down its spread but doesn't fix the emotional fallout. In most cases, simply treating the body won't mend the isolation, stigma, or disability that patients often contend with. Pairing MDT with some real-world support, like counseling and community rehab, for instance, tends to ease feelings of loneliness and help rebuild self-esteem. Research generally shows that when you mix the physical treatment with a bit of mental and social care, patients stick with their therapy better and feel more capable of rejoining society (Nergiz, 2023). Clearly, tending to both body and mind is a must for real progress against leprosy. For many facing leprosy, the mental strain is as heavy as its physical toll. Simple approaches like talking it out, joining support groups, or even trying cognitive-behavioral sessions seem to help ease anxiety and bouts of depression. These methods work by chipping away at the inner stigma and encouraging a sense of empowerment, which is key to feeling better overall. Often a family-centric care style—where relatives get involved in learning about the disease and share in the emotional ups and downs—can quietly break down long-held misconceptions and build a warmer home atmosphere. This kind of catch-all care, much like approaches used in other lasting illnesses, truly boosts both recovery and social well-being (Alkhaywani et al., 2023). In many cases, combining mental health services with the standard leprosy treatments fills in the gaps that a one-track approach leaves behind. Even with major strides in treatment, staying connected with full, ongoing care remains tough, especially when unexpected crises like pandemics emerge. Restrictions on in-person visits—reminds me of what happened in some prisons during COVID-19—drove home how isolation can hurt mental health (Nergiz, 2023). Lately, telemedicine and remote counseling have started stepping in, letting patients get the support they need even when they can't meet face-to-face. Alongside these, job-training and rehab programs, which are crucial for regaining economic independence and social ties, also need to be rethought to overcome current obstacles. In most cases, recognizing and tackling these systemic hurdles is the only way to boost how effective treatment is, ensuring that both the body and the spirit get the care they deserve.

14.1.3. Stigma Associated with Medical Diagnosis

Getting a medical diagnosis can flip your world in unexpected ways—it's not just about the clinical facts but the mix of emotions and social responses that come along with it. Take leprosy, for example: finding out you have it is more than a health update. The disease carries a heavy social weight, one that isn't only connected to visible symptoms but also comes from long-standing cultural fears and misunderstandings. People might end up feeling shunned or even start to believe the negative ideas tossed their way, which can then delay reaching out for help. In most cases, this extra burden can trap someone in a cycle of distress, making treatment and support even harder to get. Understanding how these layers of stigma work is key if we're going to help individuals get back on track both medically and socially. Stigma seems to hit even harder when there isn't enough community awareness or proper education about the disease. In leprosy, research generally speaking shows that even patients who are just beginning their treatment journey face a deep social stigma, often because their diagnosis drags on and gets confused with other skin conditions. Sometimes, people hide their symptoms, fearing that opening up will lead to being ostracized, and this delay only deepens the problem. Basic health education and local outreach can make a real difference here.

Studies using tools like the Dermatology life quality index (DLQI) have pointed out that patients, regardless of gender or job, experience major interruptions in their everyday lives. Further, the emotional toll of stigma even messes with educational and employment chances, highlighting the need to combine psychosocial support with medical care (Widasmara & Menaldi, 2019). Dealing with the stigma connected to medical diagnoses isn't something one field can handle alone—it calls for a real team effort that mixes medical treatment, mental health support, and community involvement. We see a similar approach working with other conditions, like Disorders of Sex Development, where groups of psychiatrists, endocrinologists, and social workers come together to handle both the physical and emotional parts of the condition. In many cases, personalized counseling and a broader care strategy can empower patients and help ease that feeling of isolation and shame. Letting patients have a say in their treatment, even if it makes the process a bit complex at times, often ends up making them stick with their care plans and feel more accepted. This kind of approach could work well for leprosy too, tackling stigma on multiple fronts and paving the way for better social reintegration. In most cases, new models in healthcare will have to put stigma reduction at the forefront if we want lasting improvements in quality of life (Saktini et al., 2024) (Figure 14.3).

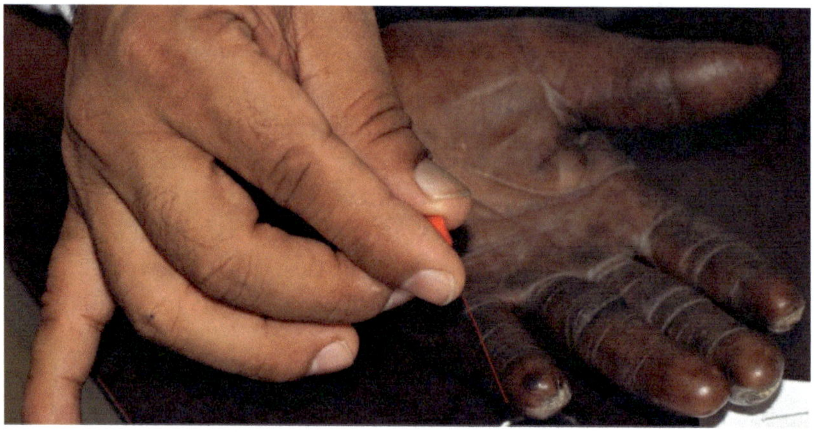

Figure 14.3. Stigma and discrimination prevent early diagnosis and treatment of Leprosy in the Americas.

Source: Pan American Health Organization. (2019). *Leprosy Treatment.*

14.2. Psychological Impact of Leprosy

Living with a visible skin condition isn't just about the physical marks—it can interfere with how someone feels inside. Conditions like leprosy, for example, bring skin lesions that change a person's appearance in ways that unsettle their sense of self. These changes mix up social interactions, leaving many with a heavy dose of shame and isolation. Generally speaking, common misunderstandings, like the idea that leprosy means moral failings or that it's contagious—only make things worse, pushing stigma and discrimination even further. This stigma can knock self-esteem down and leave a persisting sense of being cut off from others. Even when the disease isn't raging, these mental and social pressures disrupt daily life and erode overall quality of life. The gap between visible medical improvement and the need for emotional healing suggests that we need focused help to deal with the ongoing social and emotional challenges (Mehta & Gupta, 2022). It is not just about the individual either. Skin conditions such as leprosy can ripple out to affect community health statistics and strain local healthcare services. Those obvious skin signs often lead to social shunning, which feeds into mental health issues and highlights just how complex the link is between disease stigma and everyday well-being. Some epidemiological studies remind us that it's not only about counting deaths; we also have to reckon with disability-adjusted life years (DALYs) to see how long people live with the burden of the condition. In most cases, leprosy's long-lasting complications pile on substantial DALYs, showing just how heavy the toll is. This mix of economic and emotional costs doesn't stop at the individual, spilling over to families and communities, and making a strong case for care strategies that combine psychological support with conventional medical treatment (Flohr & Hay, 2021). Tackling leprosy's psychological side means recognizing the many layers of stigma that drain mental health. Beyond the visible signs, there's an unseen weight—feelings of anxiety, bouts of depression, and a shrinking sense of self-worth—that many suffer while also facing society's rejection. Research on similar skin issues even suggests that these mental health problems don't always match up efficiently with how severe the physical symptoms are. This discrepancy calls for targeted support: counseling, community efforts to clear up myths, and creative ways of boosting social inclusion. By aiming at lifting overall life quality through better mental health care, providers can support a more complete recovery, help build resilience and slowly impact the long-term social and emotional fallout that leprosy leaves behind (Flohr & Hay, 2021; Mehta & Gupta, 2022) (Figure 14.4).

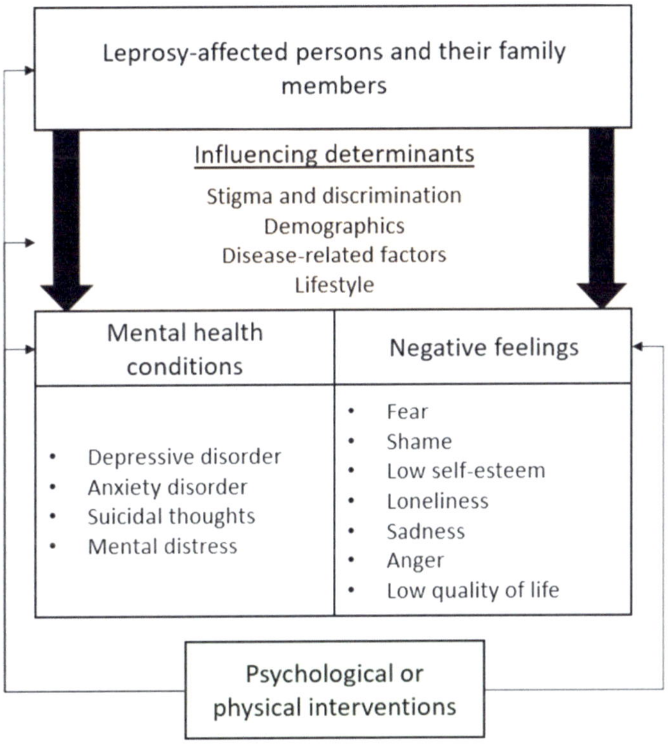

Figure 14.4. Model of the impact of leprosy on the mental health.

Source: Cambridge University Press. (2020). *Impact of Leprosy on Mental Health.*

14.2.1. Mental Health Challenges Faced by Individuals

Chronic diseases hit more than just the body—they dig into the mind too. Take leprosy, for example: in many cases, the weight of social stigma piles on top of the physical issues, triggering anxiety and chipping away at self-esteem. Research shows that people with leprosy, and even their families, often feel persistently marked by rejection, a feeling that's closely linked to their overall sense of worth. When social isolation and internalized shame mix, they form a vicious cycle that makes bouncing back mentally a real struggle. It turns out the mental hardships aren't just side effects of the illness but are also driven by a broader, often unforgiving, social environment (Adedeji et al., 2023). In short, true care means addressing both the clinical and social wounds. People dealing with leprosy quickly find that their social world and personal identity don't stay the same. The link between disease-related stigma and being pushed aside can leave someone feeling isolated, depressed, and lacking in confidence. Studies have pointed out that, even after a person's physical recovery—the mental scars can persist, changing how they see themselves and making community life hard to reclaim. Factors like age, gender, marital status, and even religious background tend to shape how this stigma is experienced, meaning that support needs to be as unique as each individual. In most cases, tailoring mental health assistance to one's personal and cultural landscape makes all the difference (Adedeji et al., 2023). This nuanced view is key if long-term recovery and social healing are to ever become a reality. When you compare leprosy to other neglected tropical illnesses, you see that the mental strain they impose isn't an isolated phenomenon. For instance, studies on cutaneous leishmaniasis show that fears, issues with body image, and social rejection can all crank up anxiety and emotional distress. And sometimes, the treatment itself, often long, painful, and disruptive, adds yet another layer of hardship, trapping patients in a cycle of worry and helplessness. All of this suggests that a people-centered healthcare approach, one that combines solid medical treatment with sensitive mental health support, could make a difference. Integrating psychosocial care seems to help not only with sticking to treatment plans but also with building resilience and improving everyday life. Recognizing this complex interplay of issues is essential when shaping policies and programs aimed at leprosy and similar conditions (Figure 14.5).

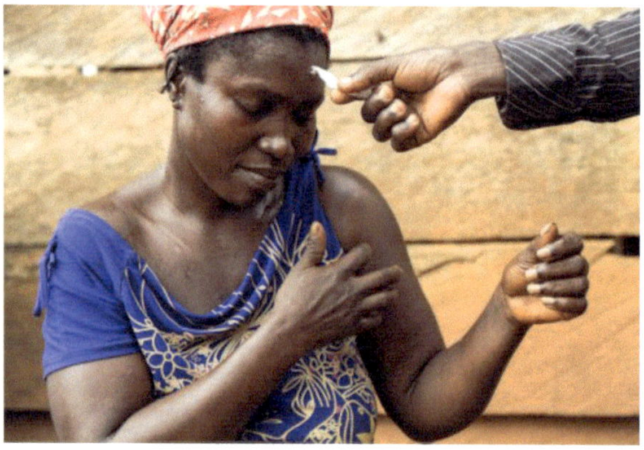

Figure 14.5. The mental health challenges faced by individuals.

Source: Royal Society of Tropical Medicine and Hygiene. (2023). *Mental Health Challenges and Leprosy.*

14.2.2. Coping Mechanisms and Resilience

Living with leprosy isn't just about physical symptoms, it often brings along an undercurrent of mental strain that wears on a person over time. Some people, though, seem to muster a kind of natural grit; they adjust and cope in ways that might surprise you. There's a lot of variability here, and frankly, it shows we need to pay attention to what helps or hinders this inner strength. In most cases, staying mentally steady under constant stress involves a combination of clear-headed thinking, supportive interactions, and healthy ways to deal with problems, even though falling back on negative habits or facing repeated trauma threatens that balance. And when you add in the extra weight of stigma and discrimination that comes with leprosy, understanding these factors (and even repeating them, if you think about it) becomes even more crucial. Recognizing and boosting things like faith, community backing, and close personal ties can help caregivers shield patients from the broader psychosocial blow of the disease (Johnson et al., 2024). The way personal support systems and everyday coping behaviors mesh plays a huge role in how someone manages long-term health challenges. For leprosy patients, keeping on track with complex treatment plans often depends a great deal on how well they can handle everyday stress and stay positive about their health. Generally speaking, solid community networks and flexible mental habits are key to sticking with treatment and feeling better overall. On the contrary, high stress levels and unhelpful health beliefs can disrupt this balance and lead to worse outcomes. That's why looking at both mental outlooks and stress management strategies is so, so important. Incorporating a bit of psychosocial support into routine medical care not only makes keeping up with treatments easier but also gives patients a boost of confidence and optimism to face their challenges head-on (Pokhodenko et al., 2024). When it comes to building resilience in those affected by leprosy, relying only on medications just doesn't cut it. A broader, more mixed approach is needed—one that also taps into social, emotional, and community resources. Detecting early signs of damage by checking in on someone's social life, coping style, and overall mental health can make all the difference; sometimes, a simple conversation or a community meeting helps shift the tide. Interventions that encourage fresh ways of thinking, rally community support, and even directly challenge stigma have shown promise in beefing up a person's inner strength. These efforts, even if they might sometimes feel redundant or overlapping, help maintain wellbeing in spite of leprosy's heavy physical and social toll. Ultimately, if care models weave together both treatment and these softer, yet vital, psychosocial supports, they do more than treat a disease, they truly work to improve quality of life by embracing all the complex, human parts of the experience (Johnson et al., 2024; Pokhodenko et al., 2024) (Figure 14.6).

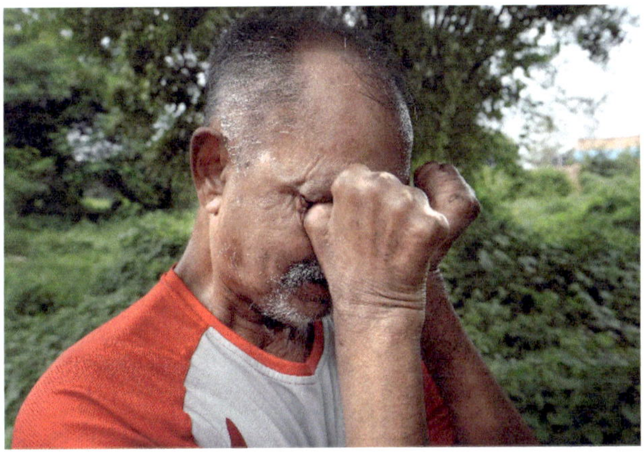

Figure 14.6. Resilience and survival: Documenting the lives of people diagnosed with leprosy.

Source: Pulitzer Center. (2023). *Resilience and Survival in Leprosy.*

14.2.3. Role of Support Systems in Mental Well-Being

People dealing with leprosy face more than just physical struggles—it's a whole mix of emotional and social challenges. Often, the way someone feels mentally hinges on having a few good people around. Research seems to show that you can build resilience by involving not only the individual but also their family. For example, one ten-week, family-oriented program in Odisha, India, managed to boost both resilience and overall quality of life among the participants, hinting that sticking together can ease the stigma and discrimination (Van't Noordende et al., 2021). Family support, after all, creates a sort of safe space where emotions get validated and strength is shared, which is important for feeling mentally well. Apart from the family itself, the role of the community can't be overlooked. Studies in Mozambique reveal that many people with leprosy wrestle with deep mental distress, stiff stigma in their daily lives, and even restrictions on social participation, all of which hurt their psychological health. Interestingly, joining self-care or peer support groups seems to help ease these pressures. When individuals come together, share their experiences, and encourage one another, the sense of isolation tends to dwindle a bit, making it easier for them to get involved in their neighborhoods. This sort of communal backing not only steadies mental well-being but also bumps up life quality by promoting inclusion and a shared resilience against stigma (Van Wijk et al., 2024). Community engagement, in many cases, works hand in hand with family support in tackling the overall challenges of leprosy. Integrating deep, supportive networks into leprosy care isn't a quick fix—it's the result of consistent, thoughtful effort. Generally speaking, scaling up these family and community-based programs so they're accessible and culturally in tune is essential for long-term mental benefits. And, even after initial interventions wind down, keeping these support systems active is key to locking in gains in resilience and avoiding slips back into isolation or poor mental health. Tackling broader issues, like deep-rooted stigma in society, calls for a multi-layered strategy where these networks, combined with both family and community bonds—also serve as platforms for advocacy and education. In the end, a combine of support from family, peers, and the wider social circle remains vital for sustaining mental well-being and truly enhancing the everyday lives of people affected by leprosy (Van't Noordende et al., 2021; Van Wijk et al., 2024).

14.3. Social Stigma and Discrimination

Leprosy's effects run deeper than just the physical signs. It seeps into how people connect with one another, often leaving them feeling isolated. Individuals with leprosy regularly face exclusion, bias, and harsh labels that only strengthen feelings of being cast aside. When these negative views start to sink in, they can cause a kind of self-stigma that makes everyday life even tougher by heightening stress and chipping away at overall wellbeing. This isn't just about treating the disease; it also means addressing the negative, ingrained attitudes persisting in society. When healthcare workers and policy individuals understand all these layers, they can craft plans that aim for real inclusion and try to ease the relentless grip of stigma on quality of life (Pereira et al., 2021). Resilience, in most cases, stands out as a key savior against all this social stigma. Research suggests that supportive bonds—whether in families, among friends, or within neighborhoods—help nurture both mental strength and the ability to rejoin society. Sometimes self-help and support groups form naturally, creating pockets of safety where people share their struggles, encourage one another, and learn in ways that click with their cultural background. Sharing clear, correct information about leprosy can also defuse myths and cut down on fear, which too often fuels discrimination. Alongside this, personal beliefs and spirituality lend important emotional backup. When formal mental health approaches back these natural supports, affected individuals can better handle the rough patches of stigma, improving their everyday lives (Pereira et al., 2021). Even though medical treatments have come a long way, social discrimination still stands in the way of a full recovery and genuine community acceptance for those with leprosy-related disabilities. Research has shown that the stigma not only increases psychological stress but also complicates the normal ways people adjust and thrive. Self-stigma, in particular, can become an extra burden, often bringing along anxiety, depression, and a battered sense of self-worth. Still, many people display surprising, very human ways of coping, they jump into problem-solving, try to see their experiences from a fresh, positive angle, and keep busy with activities that give them a sense of purpose.

These coping routes often help them adapt and even strengthen their personal identity. Encouraging such responses is a key step for interventions aiming to lessen discrimination's harmful effects and support the overall mental recovery of those affected by leprosy (Jatimi et al., 2020) (Figure 14.7).

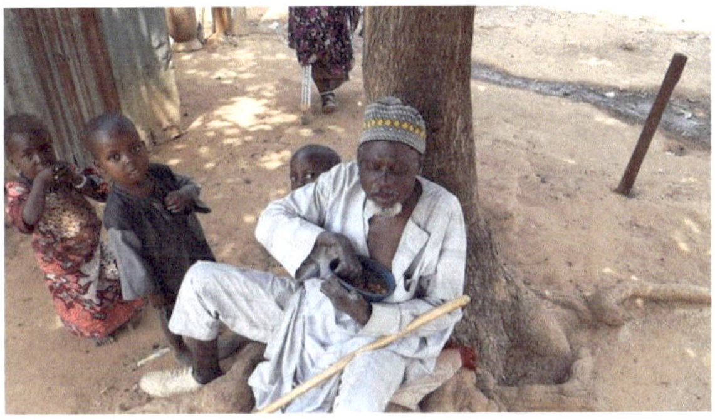

Figure 14.7. End leprosy discrimination.

Source: Qualitative Magazine. (2022). *End Leprosy Discrimination.*

14.3.1. Sources of Stigma in Communities

History and long-held cultural ideas still stir up confusion about leprosy. Many communities cling to old myths and misconceptions that make the risk seem far worse than it truly is. People tend to overreact to the disease's supposed contagion—not because the threat is real, but because outdated stories about transmission and cure have taken hold. This overblown fear isolates those affected, leaving emotional scars that go well beyond any physical signs. When untreated cases show up with visible disabilities or deformities, they become obvious signals that, in turn, fuel negative stereotypes. In many cases, leprosy gets painted as if it were a punishment or a sign of moral failing, and such views end up weighing heavily on an individual's mental state and ability to socially belong (Koschorke et al., 2022; Rahman et al., 2022). Economic struggles only add to the mix. Generally speaking, people from marginalized socioeconomic groups bear the brunt of leprosy, partly because they have less access to the kind of healthcare and education needed to clear up misunderstandings. Job discrimination and pockets of poverty often deepen the stigma, making recovery and reintegration even more of an uphill battle. In most cases, money problems both trigger and worsen the stigma, rreinforcing the idea that leprosy marks someone as socially incapable or unworthy. This double-whammy tends to sap self-esteem and stir up serious distress, further cutting people off from community life. Recognizing just how complex economic hardship and stigma is key to coming up with ways to improve overall wellbeing (Rahman et al., 2022). Social attitudes and policy missteps also play a big role. Many communities still lack solid awareness programs that could bust the myths and show that, after treatment, leprosy isn't contagious. Not having enough support systems leaves affected individuals without the boost they need to regain confidence and resilience. Stigma, then, becomes both something imposed from the outside and something internalized shaping how individuals view themselves, too. Despite vast medical progress, the ongoing exclusion proves that we still need to mix mental health services, real community engagement, and focused stigma reduction efforts to truly raise the quality of life (Koschorke et al., 2022).

14.3.2. Effects of Discrimination on Social Interactions

People struggling with leprosy don't just deal with physical challenges – they also face widespread social bias that messes with how they interact with others. Often, this prejudice winds up turning inward; many end up internalizing those negative views and seeing themselves as burdens or outsiders. This self-imposed stigma can seriously curtail their willingness to join in social activities, leaving them increasingly isolated. Sometimes community members steer clear or outright shun them, further cutting off opportunities for genuine, meaningful connections. In most cases, this ends up looking like a vicious cycle where less social involvement leads to worsening emotional wellbeing, ultimately chipping away at their overall quality of life.

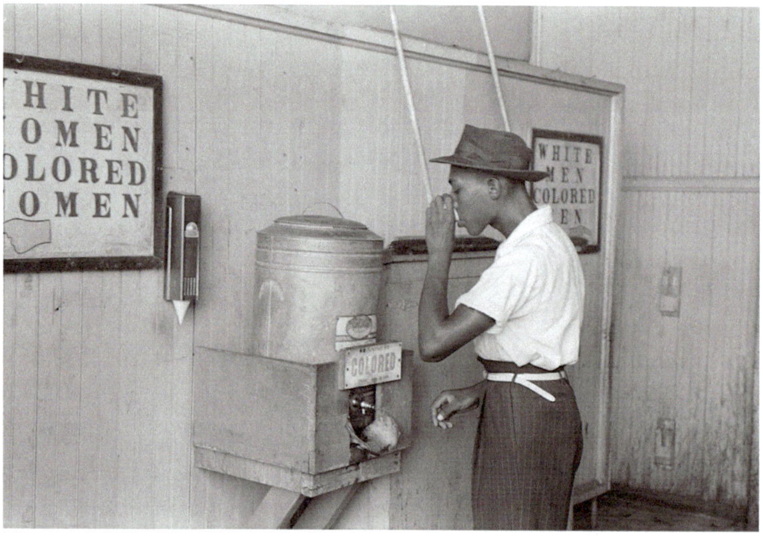

Figure 14.8. The effects of discrimination on social interactions.

Source: By Russell Lee / Adam Cuerden - This image is available from the United States Library of Congress's Prints and Photographs divisionunder the digital ID fsa.8a26761.This tag does not indicate the copyright status of the attached work. A normal copyright tag is still required. See Commons:Licensing., Public Domain, https://commons.wikimedia.org/w/index.php?curid=150747684

Clearly, the challenges people with leprosy face underscore how discrimination can undermine the social bonds that are so key for support and resilience building in marginalized groups (Jatimi et al., 2020). Individuals with visible conditions like leprosy often find themselves edged out of many areas of life – from marriage and employment to even everyday community events. You might see this bias in plain acts like social exclusion, hurtful insults, or even sudden breakups of marital arrangements; such incidents drastically cut off access to important networks and support systems. Generally speaking, these experiences don't just hurt self-esteem, they can also provoke deep feelings of despair—occasionally pushing someone toward thoughts of suicide as a way to escape relentless prejudice. This kind of overt rejection sends a message that affected people are somehow unworthy of being part of a community. Ultimately, discrimination here operates on several levels, attacking one's identity while also limiting the chance to engage fully in everyday social life (Soykan et al., 2014). As the signs of leprosy become more noticeable, the sting of discrimination tends to ramp up, piling on extra emotional stress. When the physical manifestations grow bolder, the likelihood of experiencing open stigma and rejection increases too, and that can intensify feelings of shame and prompt someone to withdraw even further. With fewer chances to lean on family, friends, or local groups, managing day-to-day challenges becomes even complex. Yet, despite these setbacks, many individuals show surprising resilience by adopting active coping strategies that help them confront the stigma head-on and find a way to adapt positively. In most cases, this mix of adversity and inner strength highlights the complex tug-of-war between discrimination's damaging social impact and our innate ability to endure; it also suggests that dedicated efforts to reduce stigma and boost social inclusion are essential for improving overall life quality among leprosy patients (Jatimi et al., 2020) (Figure 14.8).

14.3.3. Strategies to Combat Stigma and Promote Inclusion

Tackling leprosy stigma isn't solved by one simple fix—it needs a combination of approaches that combine hands-on support with broader healthcare ideas. For example, it's not enough to simply treat the physical side; teaching people about how leprosy works (and that, after treatment, it isn't contagious) goes a long way. This kind of effort can slowly break down long-held myths that lead to unfair treatment and exclusion. In most cases, adding a bit of counseling and even cognitive therapy can help those affected manage emotional burdens, boosting their self-worth and easing everyday interactions. New tech tools, for instance, sometimes step in when resources are tight, offering fresh ways to provide mental health support. All these bits, together, seem to improve quality of life and push for more social inclusion, especially when you keep local cultural flavors in mind, say in endemic areas like India (Bonkass et al., 2024). Working together also matters a great deal. Healthcare workers, mental health pros, and local community figures joining forces can change the mood of a whole area—making it feel friendlier and less judgmental. When individuals from all sides get involved, the programs to cut stigma naturally align with what public health policies and local setups already support. It's pretty crucial, generally speaking, to weave mental health into programs for neglected tropical diseases because both patients and their caretakers face deep emotional struggles. Take the Mental Wellbeing and Stigma Task Group, for example—it's one way of ensuring mental health stays a top concern amid broader health challenges (Steinmann et al., 2019). Even if it sounds a bit piecemeal, these coordinated actions show that combining physical care with emotional support can create real, lasting change. Policy changes and advocacy moves play their part too. Shifting national and local health policies so they directly address stigma, by openly including strong, supportive measures, can secure much-needed backing and resources. Raising public awareness in a way that builds empathy can, in most cases, help bring those affected back into the everyday mix of work and social life. It's especially important to tailor these strategies to fit the unique needs of low- and middle-income regions, where systemic hurdles can intensify feelings of isolation. In essence, stitching together these varied methods into a single, holistic care model not only boosts mental health outcomes but also improves the overall quality of life for those living with leprosy (Bonkass et al., 2024).

14.4. Quality of Life Assessments

Quality of life evaluations for people with leprosy go far beyond simply checking physical signs. In most cases the disease not only leaves its physical mark but also deeply alters a person's emotional and social well-being; basic symptoms can easily mask inner struggles. One needs tools to measure not just bodily issues but also to capture distress, social stigma, and practical hurdles in daily life. Generally speaking, these assessments help pinpoint emotional pain and social exclusion, which then guide actions aimed at easing these burdens. Because the links between body, mind, and community are so complex, especially in regions where leprosy is common, evaluations must echo the unique life stories of each patient. By weaving in culturally sensitive checks and taking local realities into account, healthcare professionals can get a clearer view of how the disease shakes up both everyday routines and feelings, setting the stage for a type of care that crosses over physical and hidden psychosocial needs (Bonkass et al., 2024). Reliable quality of life instruments have shown, without a doubt, just how much leprosy disrupts mental balance. Research generally indicates that depression, anxiety, and social withdrawal emerge frequently—much of this stems from the constant shadow of stigma and a persisting fear of exclusion. With a careful look through systematic evaluations, it becomes possible to put numbers on those struggles and then track how well targeted supports work overtime. Recent studies, for example, point to educational programs, personalized counseling, cognitive behavioral therapy, and even tech-based support as making measurable improvements in patient outcomes. In most cases, when these interventions lean on robust quality of life insights, care plans become more tailored, boosting overall satisfaction while easing feelings like shame or isolation (Rodriguez-Morales). Regularly including quality of life assessments in leprosy care is, in many respects, a public health must. Measurements that capture health-related aspects of living not only suggest ways to rethink policy—aiming at reducing stigma and widening mental health access—but also expose gaps that need urgent attention in resource-limited settings, where mental health support sometimes falls short. By adopting a biopsychosocial view (one that also considers environmental, social, and even spiritual aspects), providers are reminded to treat the whole person rather than just the disease. Altogether, this broader understanding supports developing inclusive programs that not only manage leprosy but also help restore dignity and foster better social integration for those living with the disease (Bonkass et al., 2024; Rodriguez-Morales, 2019) (Figure 14.9).

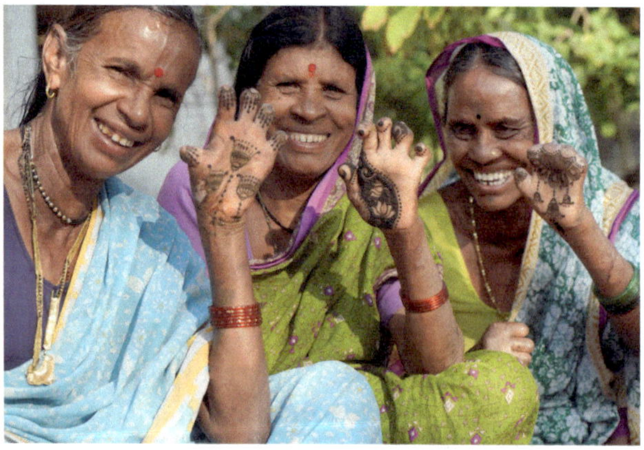

Figure 14.9. Impact of leprosy on the quality of life.

Source: Pulitzer Center. (n.d.). *Leprosy in India.*

14.4.1. Tools and Methods for Measuring Quality of Life

Assessing life quality for people living with leprosy isn't as simple as looking at physical symptoms;

it usually calls for a combination of measures that catch not only the body's condition but also the emotional and social side of things. People often turn to tools like the WHOQOL-BREF, which dives into areas such as bodily health, mood, relationships, and the immediate environment – all in one go. This questionnaire helps clinicians and researchers turn personal feelings into numbers, which is pretty important when you consider the complex, long-lasting effects of stigma and disability on mental well-being. In most cases, adding scales like the Connor-Davidson Resilience Scale (CD-RISC) gives extra insight into how individuals handle discrimination and social sidelining. Sometimes, pairing those quantitative numbers with more open chats, say, semi-structured interviews, fills in the gaps with personal stories about lived experiences and the various contexts that shape daily life (Bonkass et al., 2024). Overall, combining these tools carefully builds a robust way to look at the psychosocial challenges in leprosy care. Beyond the well-known scales, newer psychosocial programs need smart ways to check if they're making a difference. Generally speaking, systematic reviews have shown that educational sessions, counseling, cognitive-behavioral activities, and even tech-supported methods tend to boost both overall well-being and mental health in leprosy patients (Bonkass et al., 2024).

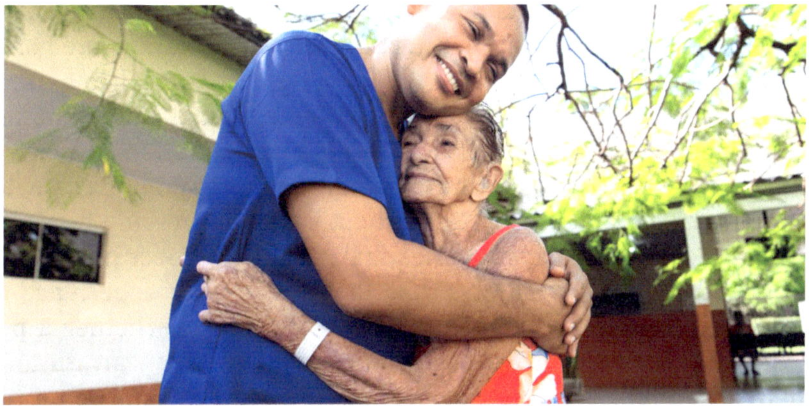

Figure 14.10. The tools and methods for measuring quality of life.

Source: NLR International. (2022, October). *Quality of Life Assessment.*

Researchers often use targeted checks for depression, anxiety, and stress alongside life quality assessments to spot trends before and after interventions. Repeating these measurements helps track changes over time, which in many cases confirms that benefits can last. Combining the rigid numbers with some qualitative feedback, like casual narratives or personal reflections—adds a layer of reliability, paving the way for evidence-based suggestions on growing mental health services in regions hit hardest by the disease, making sure interventions align with individual nuances and cultural contexts (Bonkass et al., 2024). Family-oriented resilience programs are a solid example of how these measurement tools work in real-world settings. A pilot study, for instance, followed a 10-week program that showed clear boosts in both resilience and quality of life among patients and their families, especially in rural spots, as detailed by the CD-RISC and WHOQOL-BREF measurements (Van't Noordende et al., 2021). Scores taken before the start, right after the program, and then again six months later offered a combined picture of short-term gains and lasting impacts. Moreover, qualitative feedback brought out the important role of social support and shared resilience in countering the psychological weight of stigma. To summarize, combining solid quantitative tools with real-life stories gives a deeper understanding to shape focused psychosocial strategies and, ultimately, to improve comprehensive care models for those facing leprosy, thereby enhancing overall quality of life outcomes (Van't Noordende et al., 2021) (Figure 14.10).

14.4.2. Factors Influencing Quality of Life in Leprosy Patients

Leprosy isn't only about physical symptoms—it also messes with people's lives in unexpected ways. Getting on top of the problem early can cut down on lasting disabilities and keep social isolation in check. Local health workers trained through hands-on, social learning methods have shown they can spot cases faster; this, in turn, helps patients get timely treatment, reducing both disability and the heavy burden of stigma. Empowering these health cadres tends to smooth disease management and, indirectly, lifts patients' spirits by setting up a friendly atmosphere that clears away misconceptions about the disease and ushers in early rehabilitation (Hasbi et al., 2024). In a roundabout but very real way, these community-based strategies turn out to be the key drivers that shape a better quality of life for those facing leprosy. Stigma and psychological distress are, frankly, huge roadblocks for these patients. Take, for instance, people with leprosy in incarceration settings, here, the sting of prejudice and social rejection deepens isolation and harms mental health. Studies generally point out that stigma isn't just something that comes from outside pressures; it also festers from within as patients battle feelings of shame, denial, and sometimes even lean on unusual spiritual coping approaches. This mix of external discrimination and internal struggles can sap self-esteem, push people into social withdrawal, and generally interfere with their ability to join rehabilitation programs (Lira et al., 2014). In most cases, addressing these layered emotional challenges is essential for building care strategies that genuinely boost life quality. Social support networks and cultural beliefs play a massive role in the everyday experience of someone with leprosy. Family bonds and ties within the community often decide whether a person can handle the hurdles of stigma and physical limitations. When families offer warmth and understanding, it can soften the blow of prejudice, but a lack of that support may only serve to deepen feelings of abandonment and despair. Many patients end up juggling between relying on divine faith and falling into denial about their condition, choices that shape how they view their illness and whether they take up treatment and push for social integration. These social and cultural variables kind of intertwine to either build resilience or contribute to psychological distress, pointing to the need for care approaches that are sensitive to social, emotional, and even spiritual factors. A nuanced grasp on these influences is, generally speaking, critical for lifting the overall quality of life for people with leprosy (Lira et al., 2014).

14.4.3. Comparative Studies with Other Chronic Illnesses

Individuals with leprosy face deep psychosocial challenges that often mirror those seen in other long-term illnesses. Many people in these conditions find themselves needing more than just physical care—a steady, integrated mental health support. For instance, someone dealing with chronic pain typically ends up with bouts of anxiety and depression that, in turn, worsen their daily struggles. Research from the Federal University of Minas Gerais Pain Center, quite interestingly, shows that as pain intensity rises, so do the mental health issues, leading to isolation and a sense of stigmatization not unlike what is seen in leprosy. All this goes to show, generally speaking, that these intertwined burdens call for interventions that tackle both physical discomfort and mental strain (Costa & Gomez, 2023). Sickle cell disease, too, has emerged as a condition where issues beyond mere physical symptoms are coming to light. Patients and caregivers have benefited from practical educational interventions; even though these efforts tend to lower depression, they don't always shift healthcare patterns or help much with coping. The slight drop in depression echoes what we've noted in leprosy when ongoing mental support is in place – a clear sign that addressing stigma and exclusion is key. Still, the overall modest improvements in quality of life and family dynamics remind us that managing such chronic conditions calls for multifaceted approaches that go well past just boosting disease knowledge (Asnani et al., 2016). When you put leprosy side by side with other chronic illnesses, the physical differences become less important than the shared emotional struggles. Conditions like chronic pain and sickle cell disease show high levels of anxiety and depression, mirroring the psychiatric challenges often found in leprosy cases. What's more, the visible nature of leprosy and the way society views it can make the stigma hit harder, further undermining the quality of life. In most cases, the best results from psychosocial interventions appear when they're finely tuned to the cultural and clinical specifics of each condition. Looking at these varied examples highlights why a well-rounded care model, one that weaves together both mental and physical support—can be so vital for those living with chronic illnesses, leprosy included (Asnani et al., 2016; Costa & Gomez, 2023) (Figure 14.11).

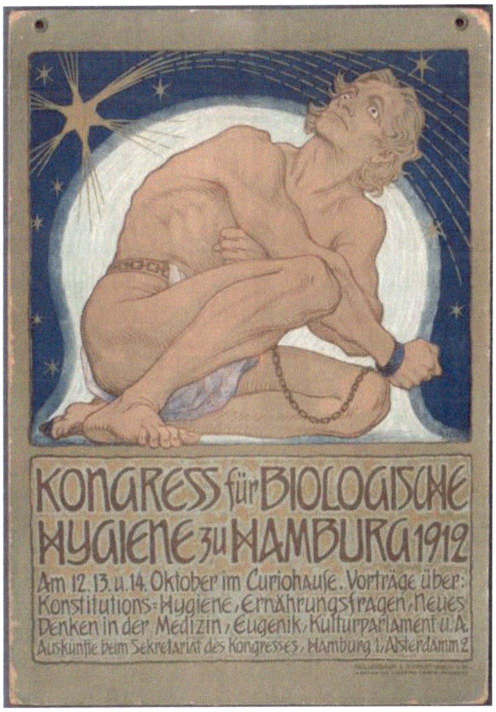

Figure 14.11. Chronic pain.

Source: By Fidus - https://berlinischegalerie.de/en/collection/artists-archives/highlights/hugo-hoeppener Photographer: Kai-Annett Becker, Public Domain, https://commons.wikimedia.org/w/index.php?curid=79689480

A CLOSER LOOK

DAPSONE DRUGS USED TO TREAT LEPROSY

Dapsone (4,4′-diaminodiphenyl sulfone) is a synthetic sulfone similar to the sulfonamides. It is bacteriostatic, acting by blocking folic acid synthesis by targeting dihydropteroate synthase, which is a key bacterial enzyme. Despite early reports of widespread resistance, it remains a very useful drug within MDT regimens. Its role in the PB MDT regimen is to prevent the emergence of rifampicin-resistant organisms. Dapsone in combination with clofazimine, as used in the MB regimen, has bactericidal efficacy, although this is not as powerful as the bactericidal activity of single-dose rifampicin. A daily 100 mg dose of dapsone is incorporated in both MDT regimens for leprosy (Figure 14.12).

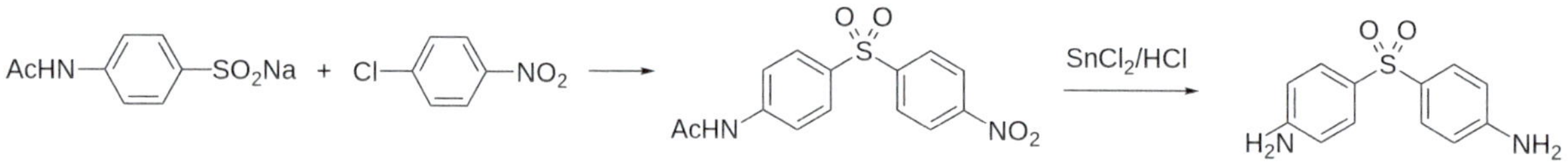

Figure 14.12. Dapsone drugs used to treat leprosy.

Source: By Fidus - https://berlinischegalerie.de/en/collection/artists-archives/highlights/hugo-hoeppener Photographer: Kai-Annett Becker, Public Domain, https://commons.wikimedia.org/w/index.php?curid=79689480

1. Adverse Effects: Dapsone is generally well tolerated. Mild hemolytic anemias are common, and hemolysis is dose-dependent. The doses used in treating leprosy (50–100 mg daily) are usually inconsequential. Severe hemolytic anemias are rare except in those with glucose-6-phosphate deficiency. Dapsone-associated agranulocytosis has also rarely been reported. Dapsone at doses of 100 mg daily may cause methemoglobinemia, but this is usually asymptomatic unless there is hypoxemia secondary to lung disease. Gastrointestinal disturbance with anorexia, nausea, and vomiting may occur. There have been occasional reports of delayed hypersensitivity reactions presenting as "dapsone syndrome" that has skin manifestations similar to Stevens-Johnson syndrome. This typically develops 4–6 weeks after treatment initiation, and patients should be advised to discontinue the drug and seek medical attention because it can be associated with significant morbidity and mortality. Dapsone syndrome is characterized by exfoliative dermatitis, generalized lymphadenopathy, fever, and hepatosplenomegaly. Dapsone is contraindicated in patients known to be sensitive to any of the sulfa drugs.
2. Pharmacology: Dapsone is well absorbed orally. It is distributed throughout body fluids. Its plasma half-life is 28 h, and there is some drug retention up to three weeks. Dapsone becomes acetylated, and 80% is excreted as metabolites in urine. Its dosage must therefore be reduced in renal failure.
3. Drug Interactions: Folic acid antagonists such as pyrimethamine may increase the risk of hematological reactions with dapsone, and therefore patients should be monitored for agranulocytosis during the second and third months of treatment. Concurrent administration of rifampicin may decrease levels of dapsone because of increased renal clearance.

SUMMARY

Leprosy impacts people in ways that go well beyond the usual physical signs. Multi-drug therapy, in most cases, handles the medical side fairly well—even though a lot of psychosocial issues still persist. Studies from around the globe generally show that combining supports like counseling, cognitive behavioral therapy, and even tech-based programs can make a real dent in the mental health load. These kinds of approaches not only lift someone's spirits but also tend to improve the overall quality of life by cutting down on depression, anxiety, and that isolating feeling. In many regions where mental health help isn't plentiful, these points stress the need to incorporate comprehensive care strategies into current health systems (Bonkass et al., 2024). Stigma and self-imposed isolation often come off as the primary triggers for the inner turmoil many with leprosy feel. This sense of internalized stigma can, quite frankly, lead to a maze of negative self-perceptions and social pullbacks that slowly erode resilience and overall well-being. Interestingly, qualitative insights suggest that those who try out active coping methods along with a dose of positive adaptation show a marked bounce-back, often displaying increased productivity and even a measure of altruistic behavior in spite of adversity. It's a reminder, then, of how important it is to back patients with psychosocial support systems that nurture adaptive coping skills and rebuild self-esteem—even if, at times, the journey isn't perfectly linear (Jatimi et al., 2020). To summarize, tackling leprosy means shifting from a narrow biomedical view to one that genuinely considers the psychological, social, and economic hurdles patients face. Generally speaking, a varied mix of psychosocial strategies that are tailored to local cultures and conditions can boost a patient's quality of life. Alongside this, raising awareness and altering policies to lessen stigma are crucial. Ultimately, reducing the overall mental and social burden of this disease demands collaborative efforts from healthcare professionals, policymakers, and local community partners, each playing their part in creating more inclusive environments that support mental health and pave the way for social reintegration (Bonkass et al., 2024).

A look through past research shows that people dealing with leprosy feel the weight—not just in their bodies but also on their minds and in their everyday lives. Studies often point out problems like constant stigma and mental distress, which seem to wear down a person's overall well-being. Researchers have been increasingly zeroing in on these issues, especially those connected to visible conditions like leprosy, but generally speaking, most work has just described the challenges rather than offering hands-on fixes. It turns out that the mental strain isn't only from the physical effects; being socially sidelined and the ever-present shame play huge roles too. This all hints that combining medical treatment with solid psychological support could make the biggest difference (Koschorke et al., 2022). Everyday experiences also remind us that leprosy's impact isn't one-dimensional. Many narratives reveal that the disease often drags individuals into loops of financial hardship, social isolation, and emotional struggles. In many cases, people feel trapped detected in cycles where poverty and exclusion feed one another. How someone understands and follows through with treatment can hinge a lot on their social environment and inner resilience; even repeated mentions of stigma, loss of community roles, and money issues add to the overall burden. Basically, there's a clear call for interventions that aren't only about physical healing but also work to bring people back into society and boost their economic footing (Rahman et al., 2022). On top of that, all the gathered evidence kind of suggests that combining different types of support might work well. Integrated approaches that combine mental health care, steps to reduce stigma, community engagement, and empowerment strategies seem promising. Yet there just aren't enough real-world studies, especially in low- to middle-income settings that test these ideas out properly. In most cases, boosting research in these areas might pave the way for smarter policies and better funding decisions; after all, even slight shifts can have major impacts. Ultimately, taking on the intertwined challenges of physical, emotional, and social struggles with well-rounded, evidence-based approaches may finally help break the cycle of disability, stigma, and mental strain, offering a true glimmer of hope for a better quality of life for those with leprosy (Koschorke et al., 2022; Rahman et al., 2022).

KEY TERMS FROM THIS CHAPTER

- Community involvement
- Cultural norms
- Deep-seated cultural misconceptions
- Emotional stress
- Health education
- Lost sensations
- Mental health support
- Physical impairments
- Community reactions
- Deep-rooted stigma
- Disability-adjusted life years
- Family dynamics
- Heart
- Marital status
- Neuropathic pain

References

1. Abdul, R. N., Rajaratnam, V., Burchell, G. L., Peters, R. M. H., & Zweekhorst, M. (2022). Experiences of living with leprosy: A systematic review and qualitative evidence synthesis. *PLoS Neglected Tropical Diseases, 16*, e0010761–e0010761. https://doi.org/10.1371/journal.pntd.0010761 (accessed on 10th May 2025).
2. Steinmann, P., Dusenbury, C., Addiss, D., Mirza, F., & Smith, W. C. S. (2020). A comprehensive research agenda for zero leprosy. *Infectious diseases of poverty*, *9*(1), 156. https://doi.org/10.1186/s40249-020-00774-4(accessed on 10th May 2025).
3. Adedeji P, Olabisi I, Aladegbami O, Adedeji O. Perceived stigmatization, psychosocial well-being and self-esteem among individuals living in leprosy center in south-west, Nigeria . J Ideas Health [Internet]. 2023 Sep. 7 [cited 2025 May 31];6(3):908-19. Available from: https://www.jidhealth.com/index.php/jidhealth/article/view/296(accessed on 10th May 2025).
4. Nuwangi, H., Dikomitis, L., Weerakoon, K. G., Agampodi, S. B., & Agampodi, T. C. (2024). The psychosocial burden of cutaneous leishmaniasis in rural Sri Lanka: A multi-method qualitative study. *PLoS neglected tropical diseases*, *18*(1), e0011909. https://doi.org/10.1371/journal.pntd.0011909 (accessed on 10th May 2025).
5. Faisal Hussein Alkhaywani et al. Patient's Perspective for their Non-Urgent Presentations to the Emergency Department in Najran City. World Family Medicine. December 2023; 21(11): 50-52. DOI: 10.5742/MEWFM.2023.95256220 (accessed on 10th May 2025).
6. Atika Jatimi, Ah Yusuf, Sestu Retno Dwi Andayani (2020). *Leprosy Resilience with Disabilities Due to Illness: A Qualitative Study*. INJEC Vol 5; No. 2. http://dx.doi.org/10.24990/injec.v5i2.298(accessed on 10th May 2025).
7. Van't Noordende, A. T., Bakirtzief da Silva Pereira, Z., Biswas, P., Ilyas, M., Krishnan, V., Parasa, J., & Kuipers, P. (2021). Strengthening individual and family resilience against leprosy-related discrimination: A pilot intervention study. *PLoS neglected tropical diseases*, *15*(4), e0009329. https://doi.org/10.1371/journal.pntd.0009329 (accessed on 10th May 2025).
8. Bonkass A-K, Fastenau A, Stuetzle S, Boeckmann M, Nadiruzzaman M (2024) Psychosocial interventions for persons affected by Leprosy: A systematic review. PLOS Ment Health 1(3): e0000091. https://doi.org/10.1371/journal.pmen.0000091 (accessed on 10th May 2025).
9. van Wijk, R., Raimundo, L., Nicala, D., Stakteas, Y., Cumbane, A., Muquingue, H., Cliff, J., van Brakel, W., & Muloliwa, A. M. (2024). Leprosy and lymphatic filariasis-related disability and psychosocial burden in northern Mozambique. *PLoS neglected tropical diseases*, *18*(8), e0012342. https://doi.org/10.1371/journal.pntd.0012342 (accessed on 10th May 2025).
10. Costa MD S S, Gomez RS. Quality of life and functionality in patients suffering from chronic pain, anxiety and depression. Archives of Psychiatry and Psychotherapy. 2023;25(1):79-93. doi:10.12740/APP/155142.(accessed on 10th May 2025).
11. Van't Noordende, A. T., Bakirtzief da Silva Pereira, Z., & Kuipers, P. (2021). Key sources of strength and resilience for persons receiving services for Hansen's disease (leprosy) in Porto Velho, Brazil: What can we learn for service development?. *International health*, *13*(6), 527–535. https://doi.org/10.1093/inthealth/ihab001 (accessed on 10th May 2025).
12. Deek, H., & Massouh, A. (2024). Effect of psychosocial aspects on medication adherence

in patients with heart failure amid socioeconomic challenges. *Open heart, 11*(1), e002550. https://doi.org/10.1136/openhrt-2023-002550(accessed on 10th May 2025).

13. Flohr, C., & Hay, R. J. (2021). Putting the burden of skin diseases on the global map. *British Journal of Dermatology, 184*, 189, 190. https://doi.org/10.1111/bjd.19704 (accessed on 10th May 2025).
14. Freynhagen, R., Parada, H. A., Calderón-Ospina, C. A., Chen, J., Emril, D. R., Fernández-Villacorta, F. J., Franco, H. L., et al. (2018). Current understanding of the mixed pain concept: A brief narrative review. *Current Medical Research and Opinion, 35*, 1011–1018. https://doi.org/10.1080/03007995.2018.1552042 (accessed on 10th May 2025).
15. Hasbi, M., & Kurniadi, K. (2024). *The Role of Trained Cadres to Find New Cases of Leprosy with a Social Learning Theory Approach in the City of Bima, Indonesia*. DOI: http://doi.org/10.11591/ijphs.v13i1.23346 (accessed on 10th May 2025).
16. Johnson, S., Tunison, L., Thiruppathi, N., Humphries, N., & Cernak, I. (2024). Demographic, Environmental, and Psychosocial Influences on Resilience Toward Chronic Stress. *Cureus, 16*(8), e67897. https://doi.org/10.7759/cureus.67897(accessed on 10th May 2025).
17. Keefer, L., & Taft, T. (2016). A systematic review of disease-related stigmatization in patients living with inflammatory bowel disease. *Clinical and Experimental Gastroenterology*. https://doi.org/10.2147/ceg.s83533 (accessed on 10th May 2025).
18. Koschorke, M., Al-Haboubi, Y. H., Tseng, P. C., Semrau, M., & Eaton, J. (2022). Mental health, stigma, and neglected tropical diseases: A review and systematic mapping of the evidence. *Frontiers in Tropical Diseases, 3*. https://doi.org/10.3389/fitd.2022.808955 (accessed on 10th May 2025).
19. Lira, M. O. S. C. E., Mistura, C., Sarmento, S. S., Silva, A. L., et al. (2014). *Stigmata and Prejudice: Reality of Carriers of Leprosy in Prisional Units*. https://nbn-resolving.org/urn:nbn:de:0168-ssoar-54505-8. https://core.ac.uk/download/267906344.pdf (accessed on 10th May 2025).
20. Mehta, N., & Gupta, V. (2022). Psychosocial impact of vitiligo in patients with skin of color. *Dermatological Reviews, 3*, 269–275. https://doi.org/10.1002/der2.148 (accessed on 10th May 2025).
21. Menaldi, S. (2019). *The Quality of Life of Leprosy Patients in Dermatovenereology Polyclinic of Dr. Cipto Mangunkusumo Hospital Jakarta: Study on Social Stigma*. https://www.semanticscholar.org/paper/fb34b95424b655971ac4d4c3452eca24f0798f3e (accessed on 10th May 2025).
22. Ochola, E. A., Karanja, D. M. S., & Elliott, S. J. (2021). The impact of neglected tropical diseases (NTDs) on health and wellbeing in sub-Saharan Africa (SSA): A case study of Kenya. *PLoS Neglected Tropical Diseases, 15*, e0009131. https://doi.org/10.1371/journal.pntd.0009131 (accessed on 10th May 2025).
23. Pal, A., Mukhopadhyay, P., & Pal, N. D. (2023). An online mindfulness-based intervention influences the health-related quality of life of Indian children and adolescent during COVID-19 pandemic: a randomized controlled trial. *International Journal of Contemporary Pediatrics, 10*(6), 887–893. https://doi.org/10.18203/2349-3291.ijcp20231495(accessed on 10th May 2025).
24. Pokhodenko, I. V., & Savinykh, E. A. (2024). Study of psychosocial factors affecting patients' adherence to treatment of chronic diseases. *Manager Zdravookhranenia*. DOI: 10.21045/1811-0185-2024-9-130-136(accessed on 10th May 2025).

25. F. Saktini, H. G. Asikin, W. Sarjana A.S, and A. Utari, "Disorders of Sex Development: A Review of Medical and Psychosocial Aspects," Diponegoro International Medical Journal, vol. 5, no. 2, pp. 36-43, Dec. 2024. https://doi.org/10.14710/dimj.v5i2.25084(accessed on 10th May 2025).

26. Tora, A., Franklin, H., Deribe, K., Reda, A. A., & Davey, G. (2014). Extent of podoconiosis-related stigma in Wolaita Zone, Southern Ethiopia: a cross-sectional study. *SpringerPlus*, *3*, 647. https://doi.org/10.1186/2193-1801-3-647(accessed on 10th May 2025).

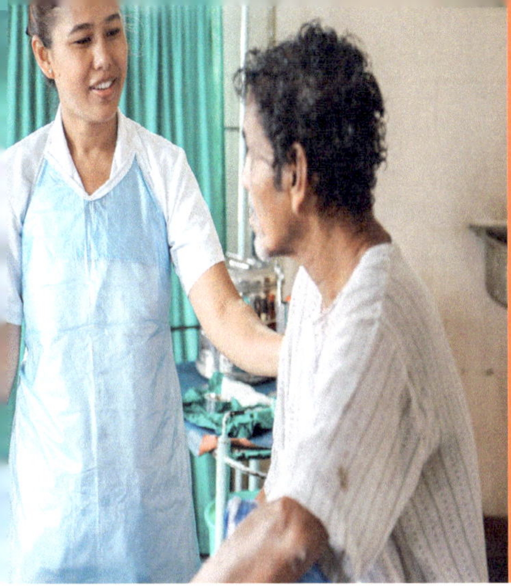

Chapter 15

ETHICAL AND LEGAL CONSIDERATIONS OF LEPROSY CARE

Contents

Introduction

Medical research has come a long way over the decades, reshaping how we treat infectious diseases like leprosy. Yet, even with many treatment advances, complex ethical and legal questions still persist , mostly because leprosy's deep-rooted social stigma and a history of marginalizing those affected make matters anything but simple. In most cases, healthcare providers find themselves scrambling to keep public health safe while still giving patients the freedom to choose, a balancing act that calls for thoughtful legal frameworks and ethical guidelines. Leprosy care gets even murkier when you consider its close ties with social exclusion – a factor that often leads to violations of basic human rights. These problems aren't just medical; they also touch on issues like discrimination, privacy, and a person's right to belong in their community. In many cases, this mix of challenges suggests that a combination of legal safety nets and compassionate care just might be the only way to offer complete support. Advances in fields such as public health genomics and precision medicine open the door to more targeted approaches, but such progress generally must be checked by ethical standards that curb any risk of exploitation or harm (Molster et al., 2018). A steady commitment to justice and equity remains central to shaping successful care policies. On another front, global initiatives tackling neglected diseases show just how essential ethical medical volunteering and aid can be , especially in areas with limited resources where leprosy tends to stick around. Still, some concerns have cropped up about whether medical volunteers are always well-prepared or purely driven by good intentions; a lack of cultural insight or oversight of local needs might inadvertently lead to harm (Bauer, 2017). This only underscores the need for a shift toward care rooted in solidarity, social justice, and equality. Ultimately, legal frameworks should back these values by firmly protecting patient rights, reducing discrimination, and fostering partnerships that empower communities rather than creating new forms of dependency (Figure 15.1).

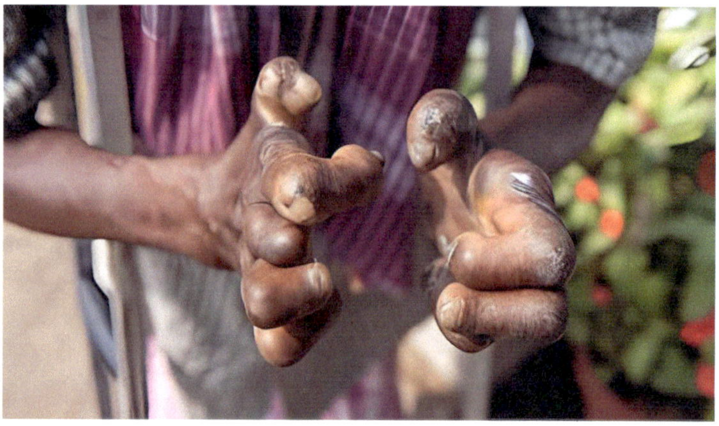

Figure 15.1. The ethical and legal considerations of leprosy care.

Source: OnlyMyHealth. (2023). *Main-leprosy. https://images.onlymyhealth.com/imported/images/2023/December/21_Dec_2023/main--leprosy.jpg.*

15.1. Ethical Principles in Healthcare

Patients battling leprosy don't just deal with physical issues, they face tough social setbacks too. Respect and fairness in care become a must. In most cases, clinicians lean on beneficence, the simple idea of doing good while keeping harm at bay, to shape their treatments. Leprosy's history, steeped in fear and misunderstanding that led to ostracism, makes it even clearer that privacy and sensitivity in clinics are vital; patients need to feel safe reaching out, free from discrimination. Open talk, genuine empathy, and a bit of trust-building let individuals keep control over their own treatment while their caregivers do what they do best. This mix of medical work and the drive for social dignity shows that healing is about caring for both body and spirit. Looking beyond one-on-one care, fairness in the system matters. Generally speaking, everyone deserves the same shot at quality care, no matter their background, wealth, or where they live. Since leprosy tends to impact marginalized groups, often detected in cycles of poverty, these deep-rooted inequities end up shaping health outcomes in harsh ways. Policies, therefore, shouldn't just dish out medication and follow-up checkups; they ought to mix in social support that eases the heavy toll of economic hardship (Schmitt & Leisinger, 2012). Fair treatment isn't merely a logistical puzzle—it's a moral call for governments, local community groups, and even international agencies to work together, tackling structural injustice while promoting inclusion and respect for human rights. Stigma remains a stubborn obstacle in leprosy care. Nonmaleficence—that basic duty to avoid harm—stimulates healthcare providers to be careful not to isolate patients further. Often, fear of being judged or left out stops individuals from getting diagnosed on time, which in most cases, only makes the disease worse (Craig et al., 2018). Reducing such stigma means busting myths through community education and setting up support systems that truly empower patients. This kind of well-rounded approach meets ethical needs by putting patient and community well-being at the forefront, aiming for care that's as compassionate and fair as it is effective (Figure 15.2).

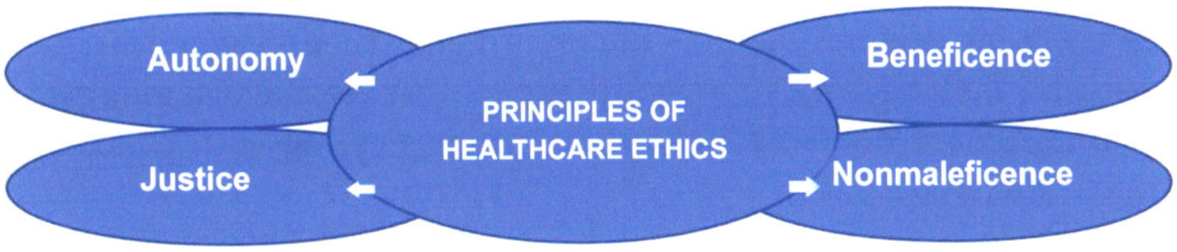

Figure 15.2. Global ethical principles in healthcare.

Source: Mousavi S (April 26, 2024) Global Ethical Principles in Healthcare Networks, Including Debates on Euthanasia and Abortion. Cureus 16(4): e59116. doi:10.7759/cureus.59116

15.1.1. Autonomy and informed Consent in Leprosy Treatment

Leprosy treatment isn't just about clinical care—it's also wrapped up in ethical challenges, especially when it comes to patients' ability to decide for themselves. Many individuals dealing with this disease come from areas where health information is scarce, so, in many cases, they might not fully grasp the available options. Research generally shows that when education is tuned to match the local culture, it boosts understanding and confidence, and that, in turn, helps people make better decisions. For instance, initiatives in schools focusing on Hansen's disease have proven effective at raising basic awareness, which supports informed consent processes by giving people the essential background they need (Pinheiro et al., 2015). In this light, clinicians must work to fill those gaps in knowledge while still fully respecting a patient's right to accept or decline treatment without any undue pressure. informed consent here isn't just a checkbox—it calls for a careful, sometimes nuanced, look at both ethical and legal rules, particularly in places with limited resources. Generally speaking, while international standards push for a one-size-fits-all approach, you need to adjust those expectations to fit local cultural values and historical contexts. It's a sort of balancing act—avoiding a strict, Western-style model that might, inadvertently, lower a patient's autonomy. Many public health studies, in most cases, insist on setting up protocols that are global in integrity yet flexible enough to interaction to the local tune, ensuring consent remains truly informed and voluntary (Pappas & Hyder, 2005). This kind of approach helps guard against exploitation and sets the stage for fairer healthcare interactions. There's also the very real challenge of stigma and discrimination, which can seriously shake a patient's trust and make them hesitant to get fully involved in making care decisions. When someone feels sidelined or judged, it becomes much harder for them to share how they feel or agree to a treatment plan freely. Providers, therefore, need to create a comfortable, supportive space—one where, for instance, tailored counseling meets clear, open communication, and education is delivered in a down-to-earth way. Such efforts, however imperfect at times, help ensure that legal consent isn't just a formality; it's a genuine, well-informed, and voluntary choice that honors both individual rights and the broader community context in leprosy care.

15.1.2. Beneficence and Non-Maleficence in Patient Care

Optimal outcomes in leprosy care depend on a deep commitment to doing good and avoiding harm. Doctors are expected to not only treat the physical symptoms of the disease but also to look after the broader well-being of their patients—mindful that leprosy can upset lives in more than one way. In most cases, this means handling complications before they become a bigger problem and offering support on a personal level, as much as stabilizing the physical signs. At the same time, professionals must be cautious so that the treatments themselves don't worsen a patient's condition or encroach on their dignity. In a way, these ethical ideas work alongside legal measures that ensure patients' rights are respected, especially when dealing with conditions that may lead to lasting disability or social isolation.

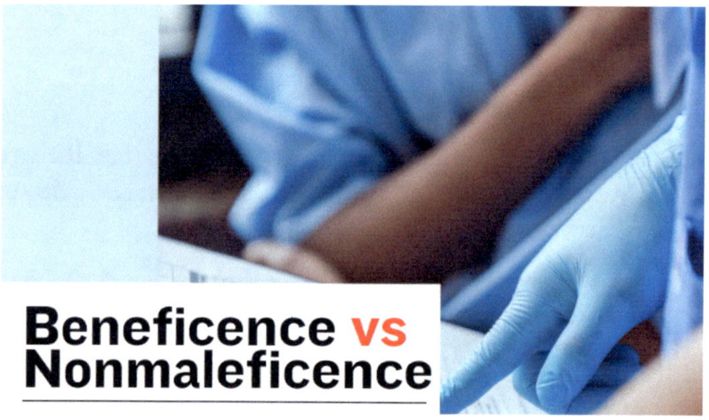

Figure 15.3. Beneficence and non-maleficence in patient care.

Source: Verve College. (2023). *Beneficence and Non-Maleficence in Patient Care.*

When it comes to infectious diseases like leprosy, the balance between public health needs and individual rights becomes even complex. Generally speaking, beneficence pushes healthcare providers to set up strong treatment and educational programs to limit the spread of the disease, aligning personal treatment with community health goals. However, non-maleficence warns against steps that might harm a patient, like imposing isolation without proper cause, which could break down personal freedoms. Legal cases have shown, over time, how difficult it can be to juggle these demands, meaning that clear communication and genuine consent become almost as important as the treatment itself (Ofunne et al., 2017). Sometimes, a slightly irregular punctuation or a minor grammatical slip echoes the real human element in these challenging decisions. Looking back, history teaches us that vigilance in both doing good and avoiding harm is not just theoretical, it's a hard lesson learned from past mistakes. Instances like forced sterilizations remind us that even actions taken in the name of health can spiral into coercion, disproportionately affecting those already on the margins (Welch et al., 2019). In most cases, this painful history pushes modern practitioners to listen more closely to patients' needs and to ask for their informed consent. It's as if the past insists that care must be tailored to each person's cultural, social, and individual background, preventing discrimination and stigma from creeping in. In short, keeping this balance right isn't just about ticking ethical boxes; it's an ongoing effort to protect rights and deliver truly compassionate care (Figure 15.3).

15.1.3. Justice and Equitable Access to Leprosy Care

Leprosy still wears a heavy stigma that blocks fair treatment and justice without much warning. People facing the disease often get shunned, and this social sidelining, with its mix of discrimination and exclusion—keeps many from seeking help when they need it most, which in turn lets the illness spread and deepens both physical and mental distress. In many cases, similar hurdles show up with other feared conditions, where the worry over social backlash stops individuals from getting treated on time. It's not a straightforward fix either; a combination of solid anti-stigma programs, local community talks, and efforts to boost patient voices must join forces. These actions not only lift health outcomes, but also quietly remind everyone that dignity and respect are rights all of us share—even if, sometimes, the system stumbles. When we finally face up to stigma's damaging role, health services can better honor their ethical promise to offer inclusive, non-discriminatory care (Craig et al., 2018).

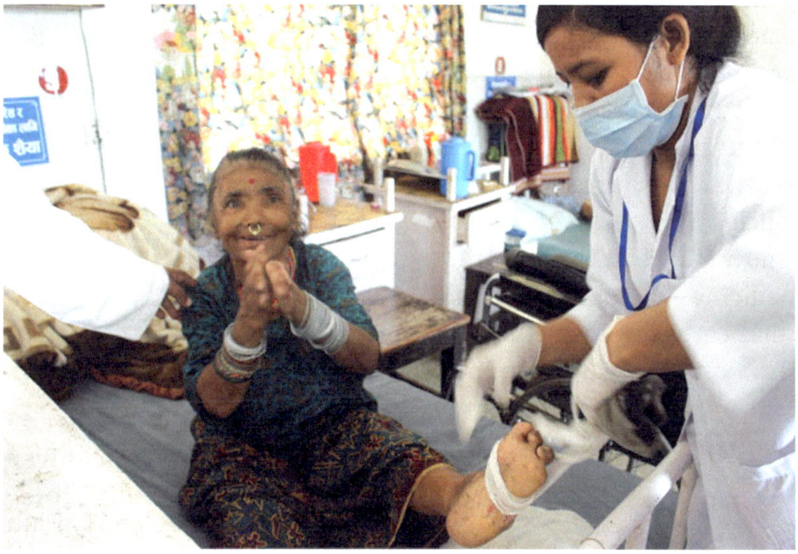

Figure 15.4. The justice and equitable access to leprosy care.

Source: Nepali Times. (2022, November 14). *The Justice and Equitable Access to Leprosy Care.*

Ensuring fair leprosy care isn't only about the details on the ground—it also involves a curious mix of local social vibes with global human rights ideas. Generally speaking, as governments wrestle with mounting challenges in staying true to international rights standards, partnering with local, non-state, and even sub-state players becomes a real game-changer. Here, local know-how and cultural sensitivity play a complex yet essential role in tailoring care to each community's needs. Often, a collaborative push that combines legal, medical, and social outlooks helps unravel deep-seated inequalities. By looking at human rights as evolving tools instead of rigid laws, stakeholders can question outdated stigma-filled norms and push for reforms that lean toward equity and pluralism. In doing so, grounding leprosy care in a broader human rights debate not only builds ethical credibility but also paves the way for steady improvements in access and justice (Chase et al, 2023). Legal rules, too, carry a big responsibility when it comes to fair access to leprosy care—sometimes even more than people might think. In quite a few regions, old-fashioned laws end up criminalizing or pushing aside those with leprosy, which only reinforces negative stereotypes and blocks chances for social and economic inclusion. For the most part, ethical standards insist these outdated policies get a thorough relook and reform, so that patients enjoy nondiscriminatory treatment and secure privacy in healthcare encounters. It is also essential that legal safeguards stretch far enough to guarantee that treatments like multidrug therapy and subsequent rehabilitation services remain both available and affordable, especially in places where resources are tight. When laws and policies start echoing human rights values, it shows a commitment that goes beyond just medicine—it's about stitching together a system that cares for both body and social well-being. This mix of legal and ethical principles is, without a doubt, at the heart of pushing justice in leprosy care (Figure 15.4).

15.2. Legal Framework Surrounding Leprosy Care

Health care for overlooked conditions can get pretty complex. It's not just having solid medical know-how – you also need legal rules that guard patient rights while keeping treatments on track. When it comes to leprosy, the law often steps in to sort out who gets treatment, how privacy is kept, and how discrimination is fought off. Rules have to juggle public health worries with individual freedoms, especially since leprosy's bad name has long made people feel cast out. Setting down clear legal guidelines might ease these rough edges by giving hospitals and doctors a set of standards to follow. At the same time, as technology and data tracking change the game, keeping patient information secure turns even complex. In most cases, tackling these issues means putting strong, flexible measures in place that stick to old laws while letting new ideas in (Mustafa et al., 2024). Ethics and law mix in interesting ways when conflicts emerge between doctors, patients, and even families over leprosy treatment. Sometimes ethical questions arise simply because individuals see things differently, and the old stigma around this disease only makes matters more confusing. Ideally, clear legal rules should help sort out these clashes by encouraging openness and letting everyone have a say. Several practical examples in healthcare show that when doctors talk things through and include patients and their relatives in decisions, things turn out smoother. This kind of approach not only lets patients call some of the shots but can also cut down on the frequent, complex disputes induced by ethical misunderstandings. Further, when resources are scarce and choices get tough, a bit of legal clarity can go a long way in keeping everyone on the same page (Ginting et al., 2024). On another level, making sure leprosy care works right means wrestling with bigger issues—spotty policies and uneven rule enforcement that end up hurting both patient rights and the quality of care. We need laws that push for fair access and ensure that healthcare systems handle both the medical details and the social fallout of leprosy. In plain terms, legal guidelines should set clear accountability for hospitals and clinics and work to shield patients from stigma, whether they're in the clinic or out in the community. It's generally speaking a must that these laws get checked and updated over time, to stay in step with global human rights ideas and the latest advances in treatment and data security. New tech, like blockchain, shows some promise for boosting compliance and keeping data safe, but rolling these out has to be done carefully so that privacy isn't trampled in the rush to modernize. This shows how our legal landscape for leprosy care is always in flux (Mustafa et al., 2024) (Figure 15.5).

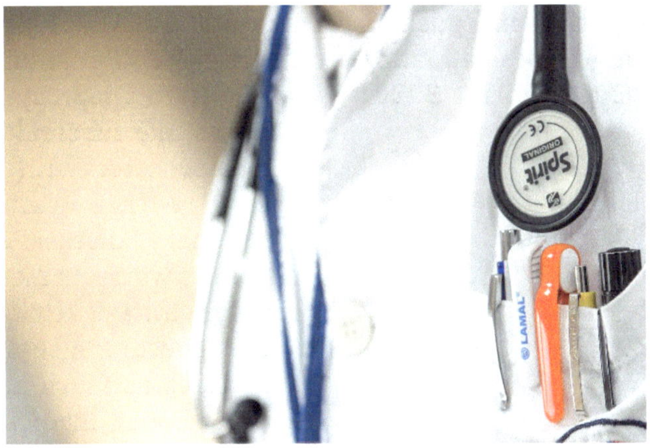

Figure 15.5. Legal framework surrounding leprosy care.

Source: Oxford Human Rights Hub. (2017). *Legal Framework Surrounding Leprosy Care.*

15.2.1. National Laws and Regulations Governing Leprosy Treatment

National laws for leprosy treatment sit right at the crossroads of public health and human rights. In the past, individuals with leprosy were shoved into isolation by outdated rules that stripped away basic dignity and freedom. Today, there's an effort to mix disease control with respect for patients' legal rights—offering chances for proper treatment without coercion or stigma. You'll often see these laws touching on early diagnosis, free multidrug therapy, and steps to stop unfair treatment at work or in daily life. Yet, enforcement can look very different from one country to the next, meaning that what's promised on paper sometimes fails in practice. This gap shows how hard it is to mix health goals with ethical care, pushing us to keep altering policies (Ahmed et al., 2018). Many nations now lean on World Health Organization guidelines when they set up their health systems' protocols for leprosy care. In most cases, the idea is to guarantee free and accessible treatment while insisting on non-discrimination both in healthcare and beyond. Interestingly, some places have even put laws on the books that criminalize discrimination toward people living with leprosy, a sign of a slow but steady move toward inclusiveness and social justice. National laws also tend to get creative by setting up oversight bodies meant to check treatment adherence and look after patient privacy, little details that add up to ethical care. Still, real-world hurdles persist, especially where cultural and legal stigma runs deep; these challenges underline the need for ongoing education and fresh policy efforts to bridge the gap between law and fair treatment (Ullah, 2020). Leprosy care laws often find themselves detected between the need to protect public health and the importance of individual freedom. While the aim is to cut down on disease spread, authorities have to be careful not to trample on patients by enforcing overly harsh or isolating measures. Increasingly, newer models put patients first—basing rules on informed consent, a respect for confidentiality, and community-based treatments that avoid social exclusion. The move away from old laws that once promoted strict isolation shows a broader recognition that leprosy is manageable rather than a reason for fear. Of course, there are still gaps to fill in areas like social support, anti-stigma measures, and even compensation for those who've faced discrimination. To summarize, strong and ethically grounded legal frameworks are key for breaking down barriers to care, helping people grow social ties, and pushing forward toward the global goal of eliminating leprosy (Ahmed et al., 2018; Ullah, 2020) (Figure 15.6).

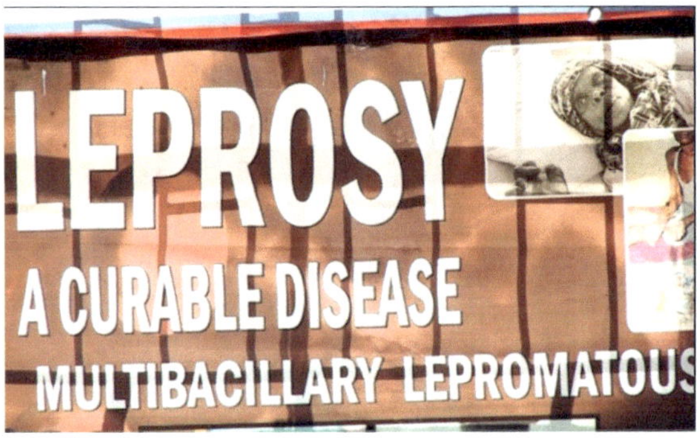

Figure 15.6. Laws against discrimination of leprosy.

Source: iPleaders. (2017, July). *Laws Against Discrimination of Leprosy.*

15.2.2. International Human Rights Standards Applicable to Leprosy Patients

International human rights law has slowly grown to recognize that some groups, like people suffering from leprosy—face obstacles that others don't. For years, those living with leprosy were pushed aside, often sent to institutions or shunned out of fear and a lot of old, mistaken ideas about the disease. Over time, global organizations began introducing guidelines that aim to protect the dignity and basic freedoms of these individuals. These rules go beyond merely offering healthcare; they also try to wipe out bias in schools, jobs, and everyday social life. The UN, for instance, has been a major voice in saying that reintegrating leprosy patients into society and fighting discrimination at all levels is essential. It turns out that making real progress means everyone—governments, health services, community groups—has to work together without leaving anyone behind. A key part of putting these international rights into action is dealing head-on with stigma and bias, factors that still hold back progress in public health. There's a rough similarity between the way society treats leprosy and how it views other diseases like tuberculosis. Generally speaking, our experience with TB shows that stigma doesn't just keep patients from seeking help; it also makes diseases spread faster and health outcomes worse. In most cases, reducing stigma calls for strategies that mix proper medical care with support for mental and social challenges—help that's as much about feeling understood as it is about medicine. Increasingly, global guidelines stimulate us toward approaches that combine community education with the kind of empowerment that helps restore a sense of normalcy and worth to those in need (Craig et al., 2018). All of this points to a simple idea: when people get treated with basic respect, it makes a difference in how they recover. It isn't just about battling stigma, though. The human rights framework also reminds us that people with leprosy deserve enough socioeconomic support to live healthy, dignified lives. Even though treatments have improved, leprosy is still too often complex up with poverty, a condition that only deepens vulnerabilities and curtails access to care. The Millennium Development Goals, for example, pushed for coordinated global efforts—highlighting that real, sustainable change usually needs a team effort across all sectors (Schmitt & Leisinger, 2012). For those battling leprosy, this means laws and policies should guarantee fair access to social safety nets, rehabilitation, education, and job opportunities. Such all-around support not only lessens the harsh social fallout of the disease but also connects closely with the broader ideals of justice and human dignity that underlie international human rights standards. In the end, addressing the economic and social roots of poor health is key to moving forward with truly fair care practices.

15.2.3. Legal Implications of Discrimination and Stigma

Leprosy stigma and discrimination still block fair healthcare in many ways, and the legal impacts run pretty deep. People dealing with leprosy often get shut out of things like jobs, schools, and public services, basically, everyday life. This exclusion isn't just a violation of basic rights; it also tends to break anti-discrimination laws meant to protect vulnerable groups. Often, societal biases mix with legal safeguards in a complicated way that can lead to uneven enforcement: leprosy patients might not get treated equally or could even be overlooked by the law. In most cases, we need strong legal frameworks that go beyond medical treatment and actively guard against discrimination, thus preserving dignity and fairness within our legal system. Without these steps in place, stigma can keep a harmful cycle of legal and social marginalization alive, which hurts public health and individual rights.

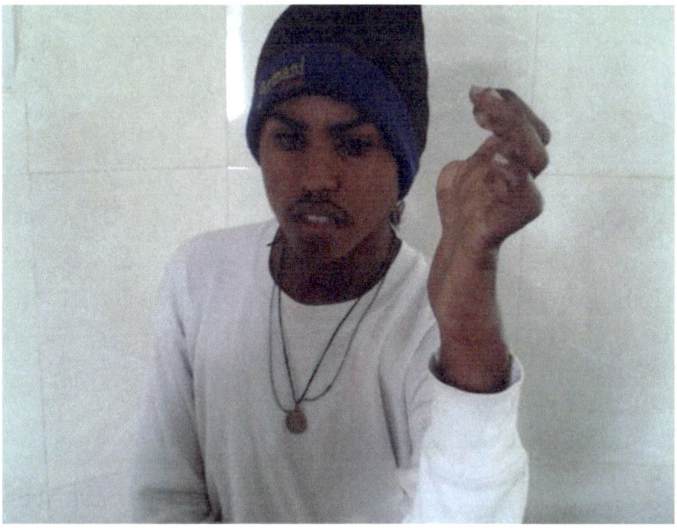

Figure 15.7. Some laws discriminate against people with leprosy.

Source: Hindustan Times. (2015). *Some Laws Discriminate Against People with Leprosy.*

Beyond personal discrimination, legal issues connected to leprosy stigma ripple out to affect broader public health policies and community life. Many individuals, feeling stigmatized, may avoid getting diagnosed or treated out of fear—fear of legal damages or social rejection, for example, which only weakens efforts to control the disease and undermines the right to health. The law plays a critical role here; on one hand, badly framed policies can lock in prejudice, yet on the other hand, thoughtful legal protections can empower people to stand up for themselves and get involved fully in society. Generally speaking, healthcare providers and lawmakers must work together to fix these legal structures that, even unintentionally, let discrimination persist. As seen with other infectious diseases, reducing stigma effectively involves legal steps that try to balance public health goals with respect for personal freedoms and social inclusion (Craig et al., 2018). When it comes to tackling the legal fallout of leprosy-related discrimination, a multi-layered approach is necessary. Legal protections should go hand-in-hand with public awareness efforts aimed at changing outdated, often exaggerated ideas about leprosy, ideas that have long been fueled by misconceptions about contagion and severity (Van Haaren et al., 2016). In addition, health laws and human rights rules need practical enforcement measures to hold institutions accountable for any discriminatory actions, all while protecting patient privacy and preventing unjust isolation. International human rights guidelines can serve as a helpful roadmap for shaping national laws that honor equality and dignity for those affected by leprosy. Ultimately, the legal system can be a stumbling block or a gateway to social change, and its proper operation is key in breaking down the deep-rooted biases that persist and ensuring ethical standards are met in leprosy care (Figure 15.7).

15.3. Patient Rights and Advocacy

Patient rights in leprosy care deserve attention—even if it's easy to overlook how stigma seeps into every layer of the issue. Misguided beliefs still persist and, quite frankly, these old ideas often push people with leprosy into unfair corners, leaving them vulnerable to exclusion and discrimination. Advocacy sets in here, acting much like a shield while also stimulating patients to have more say in their treatment. Trust builds slowly between patients and healthcare providers once we start breaking down these barriers; this, in turn, helps treatment stick better. Overall, standing up for patient rights not only protects an individual's dignity but also connects to larger ethical ideas aimed at safeguarding individuals who have long been marginalized (Craig et al., 2018). Balancing individual rights against the need to keep our communities safe is always a complex puzzle in leprosy care. Generally speaking, keeping everyone healthy shouldn't come at the cost of trampling on personal freedom, even though the two sometimes clash. When individual choices start to conflict with the community's good, a more nuanced ethical framework seems necessary, one that doesn't just see things in black and white. Here, the Mixed Interests Ethics Model (MIEM) comes into play; it weaves together bits from libertarian thought, insights from epidemiology, and ideas around social justice. This model, prioritizing ideas like necessity and proportionality, essentially provides a set of guidelines ensuring every intervention respects both patient rights and the collective well-being (Kamweri et al., 2013).

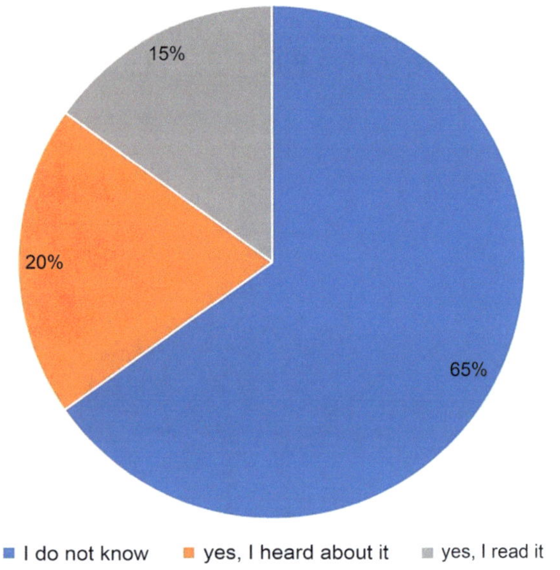

Figure 15.8. Patient rights.

Source: Al-Rebdi M, Rabbani U, Alqahtani S M (November 05, 2021) Are Patients Aware of Their Rights? A Cross-Sectional Study of Visitors to Three Primary Healthcare Centers in Riyadh, Saudi Arabia. Cureus 13(11): e19290. doi:10.7759/cureus.19290

Pushing for patient rights in leprosy care calls for a many-sided approach that tackles both deep-seated stigma and stubborn legal challenges. Solid education, legal protections, and real community involvement help create an environment where patients can stand up for themselves without fear of being sidelined. Sometimes, effective advocacy even means using practical tools to check how much the stigma impacts people and to see if measures designed to cut prejudice are truly working kind of like keeping a progress score, ensuring accountability along the way. By combining down-to-earth human rights principles with strategies backed by evidence, healthcare systems can build a framework that genuinely upholds the dignity of those affected by leprosy. When you step back and look at it, securing these rights isn't just about the individual's well-being; it's also a cornerstone for a broader and ethically sound public health strategy (Craig et al., 2018) (Figure 15.8).

15.3.1. Rights of Leprosy Patients in Healthcare Settings

Access to healthcare is a basic moral duty, especially for people who've been marginalized – like those suffering from leprosy who still face harsh stigma. In the past, biased attitudes have made it difficult for these individuals to get proper treatment and the social support they need. In everyday healthcare settings, every patient should get a prompt, accurate diagnosis and treatment without prejudice, so that their dignity and privacy always come first.

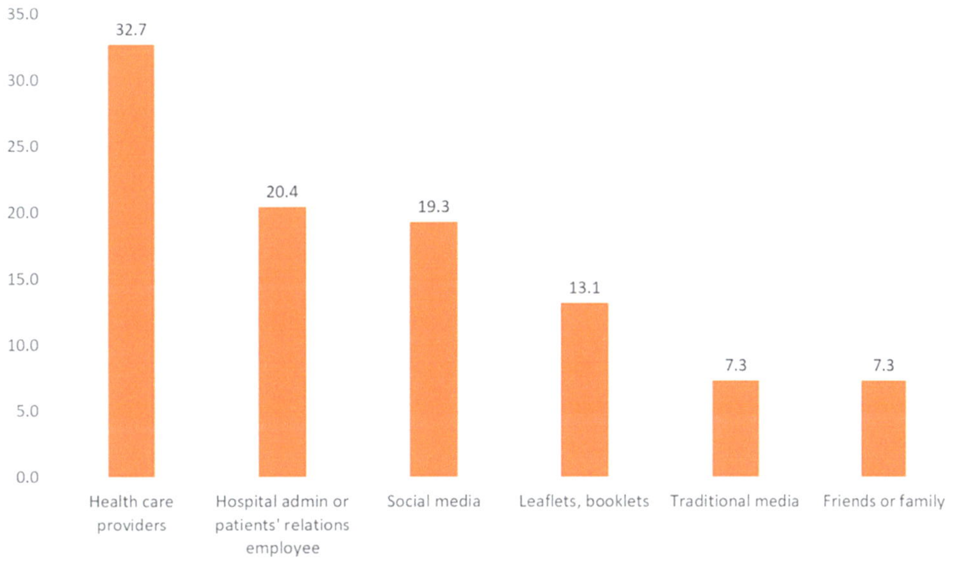

Figure 15.9. Leprosy: The world's oldest human-rights issue.

Source: Al-Rebdi M, Rabbani U, Alqahtani S M (November 05, 2021) Are Patients Aware of Their Rights? A Cross-Sectional Study of Visitors to Three Primary Healthcare Centers in Riyadh, Saudi Arabia. Cureus 13(11): e19290. doi:10.7759/cureus.19290

This basic right, in most cases, means protecting them from being unnecessarily isolated or forced into segregation—a shadow that haunts leprosy care even after significant medical advances. Strong, clear policies that train healthcare workers to act fairly aren't just nice to have; they're essential for breaking down outdated views and building a climate of trust and real compassion. But treatment isn't the whole picture. Leprosy patients also deserve robust protection for their personal health information and a genuine say in their own care. Keeping a patient's condition confidential is vitally important when you consider the stigma connected to the disease. The right to informed consent – ensuring patients actively participate in decisions about their treatment – boosts their independence and helps them stick with care plans. Such legal safeguards must be enforced carefully within health systems to ward off any form of exploitation or abuse, including forced treatment or overly coercive public health moves. At the same time, offering counseling and community reintegration programs touches on the broader needs of patients and reminds us that, generally speaking, health involves much more than just physical well-being. Reviewing healthcare policies and embracing new technologies can further secure the rights of those with leprosy by keeping patient-centered, evidence-based care in clear focus. Using additional data sources and connection tools shows promise in tracking health outcomes and detecting differences in care quality (Ali et al., 2019). In addition, the overlap of leprosy care with factors like migration and environmental pressures calls for global strategies that respect patients' rights in the face of complex social challenges (Johannes et al., 2021). These approaches need to address both ethical values and legal obligations, helping reduce inequalities and bolster human rights in healthcare. Ultimately, sticking to these principles sends a clear message – effective leprosy care goes far beyond simple disease control; it's about honoring the dignity and rights of every patient (Figure 15.9).

15.3.2. Role of Advocacy Groups in Promoting Patient Rights

Many people living with leprosy face struggles that go well beyond just medical treatment. They also wrestle with deep social and emotional hurdles, stigma and discrimination often cast a long shadow over their lives. Advocacy groups step in here, working hard to break down these barriers and champion patient rights. They tackle the stigma head-on, understanding that when people are shamed, they might avoid getting diagnosed or treated promptly. By rallying communities and even local healthcare providers, these groups build environments where respect and decent care come first. In most cases, their work helps cut through the exclusion that can rob patients of autonomy, fitting well within broader public health efforts aimed at fair treatment and better health outcomes (Craig et al., 2018). Balancing an individual's rights with the needs of public health is no simple task in leprosy care. Generally speaking, the MIEM offers one way to manage this complex balance. It tries to mix personal autonomy with population-level goals, and advocacy groups often find themselves putting these ideas into action. Sometimes, they have to negotiate between guarding a patient's confidentiality and meeting public health reporting obligations, an exercise in necessity and reasonableness. These efforts create an ethical approach that respects both the rights of patients and the welfare of the community, keeping in line with international bioethical guidelines (Kamweri et al., 2013). Beyond pushing for policy changes, these organizations work hard to empower patients through education and legal support. They make sure that those affected by leprosy know their rights in systems that can sometimes be biased or even discriminatory. This empowerment is key, especially when dealing with issues like forced isolation or sloppy consent practices that have marred care in the past. By giving patients, a louder voice in decisions about their own health and social lives, advocacy groups encourage both personal autonomy and shared responsibility. In doing so, they nurture a kind of solidarity that helps restore dignity and promote a culture of inclusion. These steps not only strengthen legal protections but also drive a cultural shift toward respect and humane treatment within leprosy care frameworks (Craig et al., 2018; Kamweri et al., 2013).

15.3.3. Case Studies of Successful Advocacy Efforts

Understanding how disease mixes with how we see each other turns out to be pretty important when looking at public health advocacy, especially for conditions like leprosy that often get sidelined. Effective advocacy shows that getting the community involved and running local learning campaigns cuts down on stigma and pushes people to stick with their treatment. Take some efforts that mix cultural understanding with straightforward, evidence-based communication; they seem to foster environments where people affected by leprosy feel a little less jittery about reaching out, without the looming dread of being judged. This kind of approach, which you can also see with other infectious diseases, helps counter the kind of stigma that makes getting proper care and social acceptance nearly impossible. By tackling both the medical needs and the human, everyday side of leprosy, advocates have slowly built-up healthcare setups that respect basic ethical and legal standards—ultimately keeping human dignity and rights in check for vulnerable groups (Craig et al., 2018). Beyond just planting seeds at the grassroots level, working together among different groups has shown itself to be a real game changer in pushing leprosy care efforts forward. Corporate social responsibility programs, for example, illustrate how links between private companies, healthcare groups, and the very communities dealing with these issues can bring in resources and boost awareness in unexpected ways. It's not a neat system by any means, but these partnerships call for a good dose of transparency, accountability, and overall inclusion. Efforts that mix a bit of social entrepreneurship with what they call responsible investment have even led to clever fixes, like skill-building programs for people with leprosy—that impact social exclusion by giving individuals a chance to earn their own keep. This patchwork strategy stresses how a joint push from all sides is needed to break down barriers while keeping ethical treatment and legal rules in balance (Coulson-Thomas, 2015). Look at the way strong advocacy campaigns leave their mark—it's clear from policy alters and better legal protections for leprosy patients. A handful of case studies from countries that have always battled high disease rates show that nonstop, persistent advocacy can eventually make governments rethink and change unfair laws, shifting toward health policies that respect basic rights. Generally speaking, these achievements highlight an urge not only to treat the illness but also to challenge deep-rooted inequalities that block access to care. Regular follow-ups and assessments, even if they aren't perfect, using tools for measuring stigma have been key in tracking progress and flagging spots that still need attention. In most cases, this evidence-driven way of pushing for change makes sure care providers stick to their promises and that legal protections keep up with what people need, reaffirming both ethical duties and human rights standards in leprosy care (Coulson-Thomas, 2015; Craig et al., 2018) (Figure 15.10).

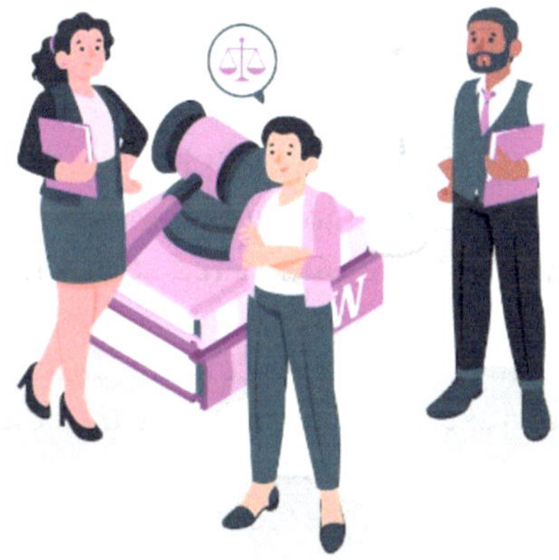

Figure 15.10. Leprosy advocacy.

Source: Freepik. (n.d.). *Leprosy Advocacy.*

15.4. Challenges in Leprosy Care

Worldwide, health systems show so many cracks—this becomes especially obvious when diseases like leprosy are in the picture. It's not just a matter of clinical care; damages also sprout from shaky infrastructure, too few trained hands, and budgets that just don't cut it. This weakness disrupts steady care, particularly in places where leprosy still persists. Generally speaking, it's vital to have systems that can quickly spot issues and keep treatment rolling without a hitch. Building these kinds of systems means putting money in the right places and setting priorities that mix prevention and immediate care. Without such efforts, the promise of fair treatment falls short, and legal rules may not do enough to protect patients' rights (Thiagarajan et al., 2021). In many regions where leprosy is common, getting specialized care is a real struggle mainly because of distance and limited resources. Local providers, who often have not been trained specifically in skin problems, end up finding it hard to offer a diagnosis that fits the situation. Lately, telemedicine, especially in the form of teledermatology—has stepped in as a promising fix. These programs let community health workers touch base with experts remotely, aiming for quicker and more spot-on care. Still, even with its promise, these digital approaches bump up against issues like patchy internet and outmoded tech, challenges that are especially acute in rural or underserved spots. In most cases, overcoming these hurdles is key not just to better clinical outcomes but also to meeting the ethical call to deliver quality care no matter where someone lives or how much they earn (Faye et al., 2018). Stigma and social isolation connected to leprosy add yet another puzzle to the mix, making fair care even harder to achieve. Many patients encounter biases and discrimination that not only scare them away from seeking help but also throw off their long-term treatment routines. While there are legal safeguards intended to protect those affected, these protections often fall by the wayside in real-world practice, leaving people sidelined. And then there are the complex ethical issues when public health goals start to bump up against personal rights and privacy. In many ways, truly effective care for leprosy needs to go beyond just the medical fixes, it should offer solid emotional support and push for legal changes that break down these unfair practices. Overall, such a well-rounded approach helps make sure that care isn't only about battling the disease but also about defending the basic rights that help narrow health gaps (Figure 15.11).

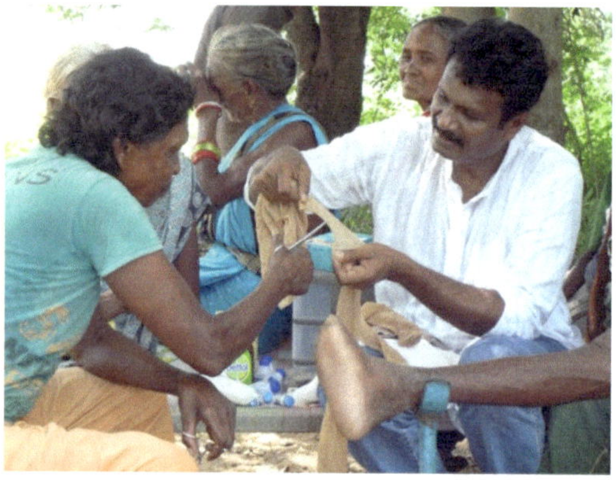

Figure 15.11. Leprosy patient care.

Source: New Hope India. (2013). *Leprosy Patient Care.*

15.4.1. Barriers to Accessing Healthcare for Leprosy Patients

Leprosy patients often run into serious issues getting proper healthcare because it's not just about the disease—it's complex up with problems inside our medical system. Many times, doctors and nurses simply don't know enough about leprosy, so they end up thinking it's more contagious or severe than it is. This kind of mix-up can induce needless fear or even make providers hesitate, which then messes with how quickly or thoughtfully patients get help. When healthcare workers aren't up to speed, stigma and discrimination can quietly creep into clinics, turning what should be routine care into a barrier for people who need help. Early diagnosis suffers too, which is a real problem since catching things early is key to avoiding lasting damage. Generally speaking, better training for medical staff not only improves care but also tackles the ethical issues of fairness and non-discrimination (Kuhns 2012). It points to the importance of ongoing, though sometimes imperfect, learning in healthcare. Stigma around leprosy adds another complex layer to these challenges, and it's not just about medicine—it's also about deep social and legal concerns. A lot of patients hold back on sharing symptoms or looking for treatment because they fear being ostracized or judged harshly, a concern that ends up widening health gaps.

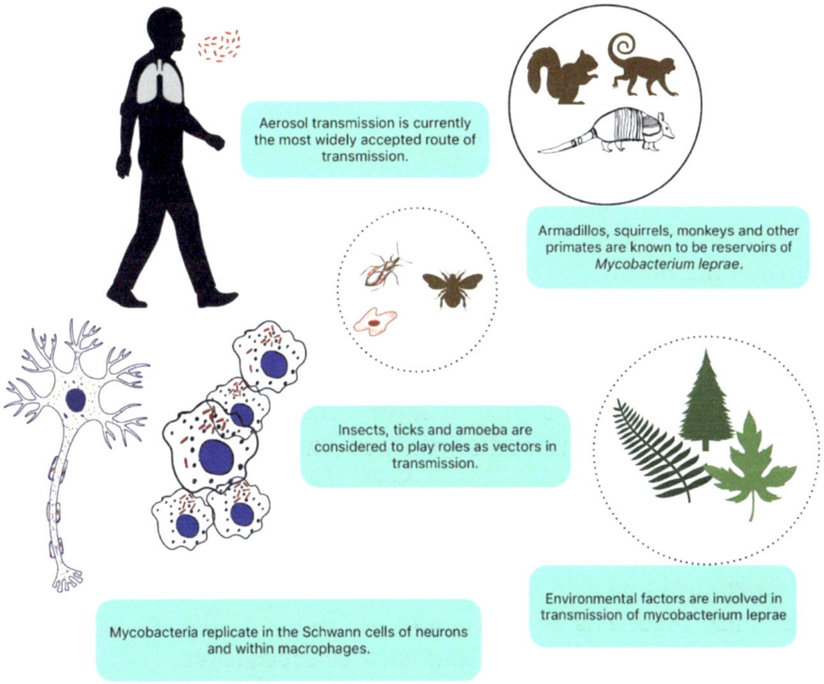

Figure 15.12. Handling leprosy.

Source: Rashidi M, Pitton Rissardo J, Byroju V V, et al. (January 21, 2025) Exploring the Neurological Manifestations of Leprosy: Clinical Insights and Implications. Cureus 17(1): e77799. doi:10.7759/cureus.77799

The dread of social exclusion can delay treatment, letting the disease get worse and even spread in the community. It's kind of ironic that something meant to protect us—patient confidentiality and dignity—ends up being compromised by these very fears. Legal safeguards against discrimination are often too weak or unevenly enforced, leaving the most vulnerable at a disadvantage. Just like how measures have been tried for tuberculosis stigma, a steady yet flexible approach to cutting down on discrimination seems necessary. These efforts not only help shape policy and advocacy to better support leprosy patients, but they also underline our shared commitment to justice and compassion (Craig et al., 2018). There's also the big issue of logistics and money-making access to care even tougher, especially for those already on the margins. In many regions, clinics that focus on leprosy are few and far between, so even when someone recognizes the early signs, getting to a specialist can be a huge challenge. Costs pile up too, from travel expenses to consultation fees and long-term treatments that just don't fit everyone's budget. Here, the debate over fair distribution of healthcare resources becomes very real: everyone deserves proper treatment regardless of income, right? Legally, the promise of a right to health should mean these hurdles are removed, but in practice, things don't always work out that way. When you mix these structural issues with the weight of stigma and occasional biases from providers, you get a complicated situation that keeps many patients away from the help they need. Fixing this isn't purely a matter of medicine or social work—it also requires building stronger ethical and legal systems that truly protect patient rights and encourage accessible, inclusive care (Figure 15.12).

15.4.2. Ethical Dilemmas Faced by Healthcare Providers

Leprosy care isn't a simple fix—it's a jumble of choices where patient freedom tangles with the needs of the whole community. Doctors end up wrestling with the idea that while patients deserve to keep their health details private, the harmful weight of stigma might keep them from getting help at all. Early treatment matters, not only for the sake of that one person, but also to slow down the spread of illness, yet this goal often collides with the duty to keep things confidential. Historically, those living with leprosy have been pushed to the side, so providers have to talk in ways that respect dignity even when urging strict treatment plans. In most cases, clinicians find themselves weighing the downside of both disclosing and holding back information in environments where misinformation and bias still run rampant. Sometimes the challenge isn't just about labs and treatment plans; it's personal, too. The obvious physical signs of leprosy can hit a person's self-image in a big way, which in turn messes with everyday life and feelings of acceptance. Just like other uncommon skin conditions, patients might face discrimination, changes in their social lives, and a heavy psychological load. The emotional strain and the sting of social rejection can make sticking to treatment even tougher, and care that ignores these layers risks failing the patient—not to mention running counter to basic ideas of doing good while avoiding harm. Generally speaking, healthcare experts push for a combination of treatments that weave in mental health and social support alongside the usual medical care (Fournier et al., 2023). Then there's the approach of hunting for cases in communities where leprosy is more common, a move that adds another ethical twist. Targeted screening might help catch more cases and reduce transmission, but if it's done without proper consent or safeguards, patient rights can get trampled. Drawing on lessons from tuberculosis control, some have pointed out that checking the whole community—even when symptoms aren't clear—coupled with prompt treatment, can drop case numbers significantly. Still, when you try to push this strategy in leprosy care, it stokes the debate between individual freedoms and the need for public safety (Coleman et al., 2023). Providers must then craft approaches that are both ethically sound and sensitive to local cultures, aiming for a combination of transparency, patient education, and real engagement with the community—even if that balance sometimes feels awkward or uneven.

15.4.3. Societal Stigma and Its Impact on Treatment Adherence

Infectious diseases hit people in more ways than just physical symptoms—they also stir up some nasty social reactions. Conditions like leprosy, for example, end up carrying heavy social baggage, pushing individuals into isolation, unfair treatment, and mental stress that might make them think twice about getting help. Sometimes the dread of being labeled or shunned even stops them from checking in with a doctor until things get much worse. Once treatment starts, that persisting stigma can still cause problems; patients might ditch their medication if they fear any kind of exposure. This mix of issues naturally forces us to ask tough questions about whether healthcare systems and society at large are doing enough to create welcoming spaces for healing. In most cases, fighting stigma isn't merely a social nicety—it's a core part of controlling diseases, mixcombining ethical care with necessary legal backing. Keeping up with your treatment becomes a real struggle when social judgment creeps in. The weight of stigma can dig deep, making patients feel ashamed or even cut off from others, so they sometimes back off from following through with prescribed routines. We see a similar pattern in other infections too; the negative buzz around an illness often means people are less likely to seek proper, ongoing care, which can even upset efforts to stop further spread. Take tuberculosis for instance, when stigma piles on, patients end up interrupting their treatment, and the health outcomes go downhill (Craig et al., 2018). In the case of leprosy, it's crucial to keep this social angle in mind so that any care strategy respects patient dignity while also supporting proper adherence. Combining a bit of emotional support with traditional medical care might just be the key. A broader, integrated approach to cutting down stigma can help keep treatment on track and offer more lasting results. Looking at what's happened with HIV prevention and care, it turns out that combining behavioral alters, solid medical treatments, and shifts in social structures tends to work better than isolated fixes (van Vermund & Hayes, 2013). With leprosy, this means pairing stigma reduction efforts with legal measures to prevent discrimination, all while running community education initiatives alongside strong medical services. Laws and legal frameworks play a big part in protecting patients' rights and in setting up an environment where going for treatment feels normal rather than intimidating. When neighborhoods chip in through awareness programs, misconceptions gradually fade, letting patients stick with their treatment without that heavy fear of being shunned. In essence, ethics and law need to work together, however imperfectly at times, to break down the barriers of stigma, ensuring fair treatment and better health outcomes for everyone (Figure 15.13).

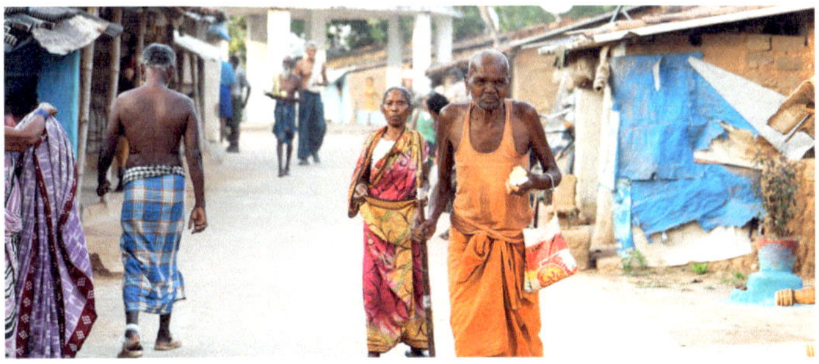

Figure 15.13. Societal stigma and its impact on treatment adherence.

Source: Missions Box. (2019). *Leprosy colony. https://missionsbox.org/wp-content/uploads/2019/01/leprosy-colony.jpg.*

A CLOSE LOOK

ROLE OF PERSONS AFFECTED WITH LEPROSY AND THEIR ORGANIZATIONS

The Human Rights Council of United Nations has recommended that "Persons affected by leprosy and their family members, have the right to be actively involved in decision-making processes regarding policies and programs that directly concern their lives."

WHO has produced guidelines for promoting the participation of affected persons in leprosy control programs. According to these guidelines, people who have personally experienced the disease are important partners in their treatment. Ensuring that persons affected by leprosy are the central focus of the program will have profound implications for the way that services are planned, delivered, and evaluated.

These guidelines identify different areas in which persons affected with leprosy can play an important role. The primary issues are stigma and discrimination; equity, social justice, and human rights; and gender. The central theme of the guidelines is to recognize the expertise of individuals who have had the disease and, through partnership, enable these individuals to support the delivery of leprosy services. For example, persons with personal experience of planter ulcers or loss of sensation can be very effective in reaching out to other affected persons about the importance of a regular routine of prevention of disabilities and selfcare activities (Figure 15.14).

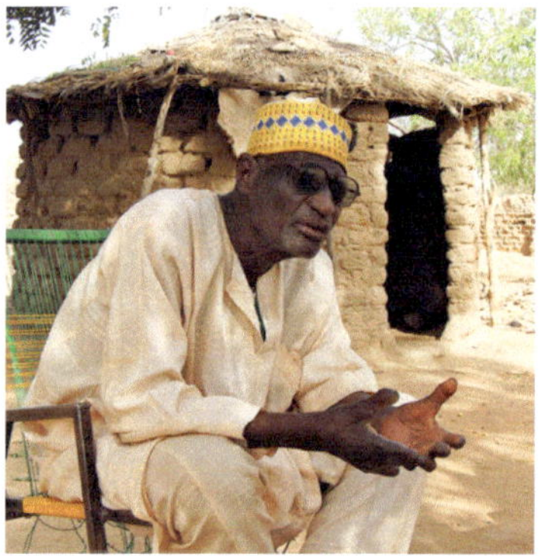

Figure 15.14. Role of persons affected with leprosy and their organizations.

Source: ILEP. (2020, February). Role of Persons Affected with Leprosy and Their Organizations.

At the same time, the guidelines recognize that facilitating the participation of persons affected by leprosy is not simple. It is essential to document the process and results, provide feedback on lessons learned, and disseminate the results to a wider audience to expand the process.

SUMMARY

Leprosy care isn't just about checking off clinical boxes—its ethical and legal twists push us to think far beyond routine treatment. Historical practices and today's challenges alike remind us that handling leprosy means staying aware of social, cultural, and legal characteristics that deeply affect those involved. In most cases, entrenched stigma and persistent discrimination, born from wrong ideas and legal gaps that miss protecting patients' rights, keep fair care out of reach. Research done in postgraduate and professional spheres generally speaking stimulates health workers to reflect on outdated routines and embrace ethical standards that respect human dignity and autonomy (Patel et al., 2007). This kind of thoughtful awareness, even if it seems subtle at first, shifts the whole conversation from treating leprosy as just a medical issue to recognizing it as a matter of social justice—one that calls for real legal backing and care tuned to people's cultural needs. Combining in care methods that are both culturally secure and centered on the individual is another key step, especially in places where Indigenous groups face leprosy. The experience in the Kimberley region, for instance, shows us that typical routines like Directly Observed Therapy and case management often overlook the deep cultural backgrounds and historical traumas that influence Aboriginal communities' trust in health services. It's like we need to recognize, again and again, each community's special needs—encouraging open talks, shared choices, and support those springs from a real cultural connection (Oliver, 2022). Legally speaking, this situation calls on us to mangle away old policies that keep systemic biases going, pushing instead for frameworks that protect patients' rights to culturally competent and effective care. In the end, weaving ethical thinking with legal reform paves the way toward leprosy care that feels a lot more just and balanced. Health interventions must juggle robust medical treatment with respect for a patient's own choices, cultural roots, and community values. The persisting effects of colonial legacies in our health systems clearly point to the need for decolonizing approaches—ones that empower individuals and families through joint care and legal protective measures against discrimination. Drawing on insights from qualitative research, historical snapshots, and a bit of everyday wisdom, future care models can look after not only the body but also the mind and spirit of those affected. This kind of evolution in care doesn't just boost treatment outcomes—it also meets our wider, ethical and legal call to uphold human rights and push for health equity (Patel et al., 2007; Oliver, 2022).

Leprosy care isn't just about fighting an illness—it's a complex mix of ethics and law that aims to protect individual rights while keeping communities healthy. Patient dignity and privacy come first, especially when deep-rooted stigmas still hover around. In most cases, asking for proper consent and letting patients share in decisions builds a kind of trust that matters a lot. This point hits home, particularly in indigenous or socially sidelined communities, where a genuine sense of cultural care is needed. Sometimes, treatment plans that ignore this cultural side can, almost by accident, induce mistrust or even make patients less likely to stick with their treatment. Studies from places like Australia's Kimberley region show that weaving together historical insight with real community feedback helps improve outcomes (Oliver, 2022). To summarize, combining time-tested ethical ideas with practical approaches goes a long way toward solving the everyday dilemmas of leprosy care. On the legal front, the rules around leprosy care strive to keep discrimination out of the picture, safeguard each person's rights, and make it easier for everyone to access proper treatment. National and international guidelines—many of which have been shaped by both affected individuals and experienced health professionals—lay out how to diagnose, treat, and even screen for contacts (External Review Group, 2018). These step-by-step plans provide more than just a clinical checklist; they also act as a protective net against old, isolating practices that only made marginalization worse. Laws, generally speaking, have to juggle public health needs and personal freedom, which means avoiding forced isolation unless the situation is extraordinary and well-supported by evidence. Also, having strong legal protections makes sure that even the most vulnerable groups, like indigenous peoples, aren't pushed to the side by systemic biases or money problems. Bringing together legal standards with care that respects cultural differences seems to build a framework that's both fair and supportive in treating leprosy. When you step back and look at everything, it's clear that truly effective leprosy care means combining cultural respect, trust-building, and patient empowerment right into public health and clinical strategies. History tells us, albeit sometimes painfully, that stigmatizing policies and overly paternalistic methods have hurt people; this forces us to adopt more inclusive, even decolonized approaches where patients and communities play an active role in care (Oliver, 2022). Sticking with guidelines born of global cooperation also makes sure that legal protections remain consistent and shield both personal rights and the welfare of the community (External Review Group et al., 2018). In the end, the best way forward isn't just about medical treatment—it's also about fighting social injustice, setting up solid legal safeguards, and nurturing genuine cultural understanding. This kind of multidimensional approach is key if we truly want to overcome not only the disease itself but also the persisting inequalities and ethical snags that have long plagued leprosy care.

KEY TERMS FROM THIS CHAPTER

- Blockchain
- Equality
- Human rights
- Leprosy care laws
- Medical research
- National laws
- Patient rights
- Social justice
- Discrimination
- Genuine empathy
- International human rights law
- Leprosy stigma
- Mixed Interests Ethics Model
- Nonmaleficence
- Public health genomics

References

1. Craig, G., Meershoek, A., Zwerling, A., Daftary, A., Citro, B., Smyth, C., Lewis, D., Ni Cheallaigh, D., Byrne, E., Mitchell, E. M. H., Leimane, I., Malar, J., Levy, J., van der Land, J., Macintyre, K., Johnston, L. G., Ferris France, N., Engel, N., Mumba, O., ... Nair, T. (2018). *TB STIGMA – MEASUREMENT GUIINTERACTION*. CHALLENGE TB. https://doi.org/10.18745/PB.20489 *Guidance*(accessed on 10th May 2025).
2. Ahmed, A., Bruner, K., Gajewski, A., Kiraly, A., et al. (2018). *Triple Helix, Fall 2018*. University of Texas Libraries. http://hdl.handle.net/2152/72454; https://core.ac.uk/download/211337566.pdf (accessed on 10th May 2025).
3. Ali, M. S., Ichihara, M. Y., Lopes, L. C., Barbosa, G., Pita, R., Carreiro, R., Dos Santos, D. B., et al. (2019). Administrative data linkage in Brazil: Potentials for health technology assessment. *Frontiers in Pharmacology, 10*. https://doi.org/10.3389/fphar.2019.00984 (accessed on 10th May 2025).
4. Bauer, I. (2017). More harm than good? The questionable ethics of medical volunteering and international student placements. *Tropical Diseases, Travel Medicine and Vaccines, 3*. https://doi.org/10.1186/s40794-017-0048-y (accessed on 10th May 2025).
5. Coleman, M., Nguyen, T. A., Luu, B. K., Hill, J., Ragonnet, R., Trauer, J. M., Fox, G. J., et al. (2023). Finding and treating both tuberculosis disease and latent infection during population-wide active case finding for tuberculosis elimination. *Frontiers in Medicine, 10*. https://doi.org/10.3389/fmed.2023.1275140 (accessed on 10th May 2025).
6. Coulson-Thomas, Colin (2015), Responsible Business and Corporate Social Responsibility, in Ahluwalia, J S (Editor), Embedding CSR Mandate into Corporate Strategy, New Delhi, IOD Publishing, February, pp 26-39 ISBN 978-81-930987-9-0 (accessed on 10th May 2025).
7. Dayrit, J. F., Sugiharto, A., Coates, S. J., Lucero-Prisno, D. E., Davis, M. D. D., & Andersen, L. K. (2021). Climate change, human migration, and skin disease: Is there a link? *International Journal of Dermatology, 61*, 127–138. https://doi.org/10.1111/ijd.15543 (accessed on 10th May 2025).
8. External Review Group, Guidelines Development Group, WHO Steering Group. (2018). *Guidelines for the Diagnosis, Treatment and Prevention of Leprosy*. **ISBN:** 978 92 9022 638 3. https://core.ac.uk/download/161992414.pdf (accessed on 10th May 2025).
9. Faye, O., Bagayoko, C. O., Dicko, A., Cissé, L., Berthé, S., Traoré, B., Fofana, Y., et al. (2018). A teledermatology pilot program for the management of skin diseases in primary health care centers: Experiences from a resource-limited country (Mali, West Africa). *Tropical Medicine and Infectious Disease, 3*, 88. https://doi.org/10.3390/tropicalmed3030088 (accessed on 10th May 2025).
10. Fournier, H., Calcagni, N., Morice-Picard, F., & Quintard, B. (2023). Psychosocial implications of rare genetic skin diseases affecting appearance on daily life experiences, emotional state, self-perception and quality of life in adults: A systematic review. *Orphanet Journal of Rare Diseases, 18*. https://doi.org/10.1186/s13023-023-02629-1 (accessed on 10th May 2025).
11. Ginting, G., & Suningrat, N. (2024). Development of a legal framework for the management of ethical and legal conflicts in patient care. *ANAYASA: Journal of Legal Studies*. https://www.

semanticscholar.org/paper/04440ad522b8ea3b1c64f1bc3be1f6b12bed3dc8 (accessed on 10th May 2025).

12. Vermund, S. H., & Hayes, R. J. (2013). Combination prevention: new hope for stopping the epidemic. *Current HIV/AIDS reports*, *10*(2), 169–186. https://doi.org/10.1007/s11904-013-0155-y (accessed on 10th May 2025).

13. Pappas, G., Hyder, A.A. Exploring ethical considerations for the use of biological and physiological markers in population-based surveys in less developed countries. *Global Health* **1**, 16 (2005). https://doi.org/10.1186/1744-8603-1-16 (accessed on 10th May 2025).

14. Kamweri, J. M. M. (2013). *The Ethical Balance Between Individual and Population Health Interests to Effectively Manage Pandemics and Epidemics.* https://core.ac.uk/download/234047812.pdf (accessed on 10th May 2025).

15. van Haaren MA, Reyme M, Lawrence M, Menke J, Kaptein AA. Illness perceptions of leprosy-cured individuals in Surinam with residual disfigurements – "I am cured, but still I am ill". *Chronic Illness.* 2016;13(2):117-127. doi:10.1177/1742395316657398

16. (accessed on 10th May 2025).

17. Kuhns, Kristen E., "What's to Know?: Navigating Knowledge Gaps of Hansen's Disease in the U.S.." Thesis, Georgia State University, 2012. https://scholarworks.gsu.edu/anthro_theses/66 (accessed on 10th May 2025).

18. Pinheiro, M. G. C., Medeiros, I. B. G., Monteiro, A. I., & Simpson, C. A. (2015). The nurse and the theme of leprosy in the school context: case studies. Revista de Pesquisa: Cuidado é Fundamental Online, 7(3), 2774-2780. https:// doi.org/10.9789/2175-5361.2015.v7i3.2774-2780 (accessed on 10th May 2025).

19. Molster, C., Bowman, F. L., Bilkey, G. A., Cho, A. S., Burns, B. L., Nowak, K. L., Dawkins, H. (2018). The evolution of public health genomics: Exploring its past, present, and future. *Frontiers in Public Health, 6.* https://doi.org/10.3389/fpubh.2018.00247 (accessed on 10th May 2025).

20. Mustafa, G., Rafiq, W., Jhamat, N., Arshad, Z., & Rana, F. A. (2024). Blockchain-based governance models in e-government: A comprehensive framework for legal, technical, ethical and security considerations. *International Journal of Law and Management.* https://www.semanticscholar.org/paper/c2ea28685f24d68932a90adeaed8e765007355da (accessed on 10th May 2025).

21. Anthony Tirado Chase (Anthology Editor) , Pardis Mahdavi (Anthology Editor) , Hussein Banai (Anthology Editor) , Sofia Gruskin (Anthology Editor) (2023). *Human Rights at the Intersections.* ISBN 9781350268661; Imprint Bloomsbury Academic; Bloomsbury Publishing(accessed on 10th May 2025).

22. Ofunne, I. (2017). *The Legal and Ethical Implications of Involuntary Detention of Drug-Resistant Tuberculosis (DR-TB) Patients in South Africa.* Master of Law. University of KwaZulu-Natal, Durban, 2017. https://researchspace.ukzn.ac.za/handle/10413/16462 (accessed on 10th May 2025).

23. Oliver, S. J. (2022). From Isolation to Inclusion: Embracing Local Perspectives in Examining the Treatment Model of Care for Aboriginal Persons Affected by Tuberculosis or Leprosy in the Kimberley Region, North Western Australia [Doctor of Philosophy (College of Medicine)]. The University of Notre Dame Australia. https://researchonline.nd.edu.au/theses/386(accessed on 10th May 2025).

24. Patel, D. (2007). *Research and Training Programs.* https://core.ac.uk/download/42630889.pdf (accessed on 10th May 2025).
25. Schmitt, K., & Leisinger, K. (2012). *Corporate Responsibility and Corporate Philanthropy.* https://core.ac.uk/download/75781320.pdf (accessed on 10th May 2025).
26. Thiagarajan, S., Muraleedharan, V. R., & Ranjan, A. (2021). Pandemic resilience and health systems preparedness: Lessons from COVID-19 for the twenty-first century. *Journal of Social and Economic Development, 23*, 290–300. https://doi.org/10.1007/s40847-020-00133-x (accessed on 10th May 2025).
27. Mohammad Ahsan Ullah. (2020). Corporate Social Responsibility in The Sustainable Development Of Bangladesh: An Overview. *Pacific International Journal*, *3*(3), 63–72. https://doi.org/10.55014/pij.v3i3.99 (accessed on 10th May 2025).
28. Welch, B. (2019). *An Ethical Analysis of Reproductive Justice in the Context of the Eugenics Movement in the United States.* A Dissertation Submitted to the McNulty College and Graduate School of Liberal Arts, Duquesne University. In partial fulfillment of the requirements for the degree of Doctor of Philosophy. https://core.ac.uk/download/234050868.pdf (accessed on 10th May 2025).

INDEX